Recent Developments in Anti-Inflammatory Therapy

Recent Developments in Anti-Inflammatory Therapy

Edited by

Parteek Prasher
Department of Chemistry, University of Petroleum & Energy Studies, Dehradun, Uttarakhand, India

Flavia C. Zacconi
Department of Chemistry and Pharmacy, Pontificia Universidad Católica de Chile (PUC), Santiago, Chile

Jeffrey H. Withey
Department of Biochemistry, Microbiology, and Immunology, Wayne State University School of Medicine, Detroit, MI, United States

Michael Rathbone
ULTI Pharmaceuticals, Turangi, New Zealand

Kamal Dua
Discipline of Pharmacy, Graduate School of Health, University of Technology Sydney, Sydney, NSW, Australia

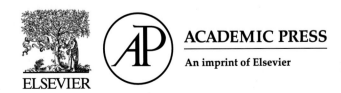

ACADEMIC PRESS
An imprint of Elsevier

ELSEVIER

Academic Press is an imprint of Elsevier
125 London Wall, London EC2Y 5AS, United Kingdom
525 B Street, Suite 1650, San Diego, CA 92101, United States
50 Hampshire Street, 5th Floor, Cambridge, MA 02139, United States
The Boulevard, Langford Lane, Kidlington, Oxford OX5 1GB, United Kingdom

ISBN 978-0-323-99988-5

For information on all Academic Press publications
visit our website at https://www.elsevier.com/books-and-journals

Publisher: Stacy Masucci
Acquisitions Editor: Andre Gerhard Wolff
Editorial Project Manager: Matthew Mapes
Production Project Manager: Paul Prasad Chandramohan
Cover Designer: Victoria Pearson

Typeset by STRAIVE, India

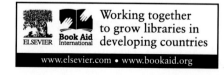

Contents

5. Modulation of intestinal microbiome: Promising therapies in the treatment of inflammatory bowel disease

Koushik Das, Shashi Upadhyay, and
Shalini Oli

6. Advanced therapeutics for renal inflammation

Manish Pal Singh, Rashita Makkar,
Tapan Behl, and Kamla Pathak

7. Advanced therapeutics for targeting inflammatory arthritis

Vikram Jeet Singh, Pooja A. Chawla,
Bhupinder Kumar, and Parteek Prasher

16. Mechanisms of antiinflammatory effects of naturally derived secondary metabolites

Ramakrishna Thilagar Uma Maheswari, Pradeep Kumar, and Mariappan Rajan

17. Antiinflammatory activity of herbal bioactive-based formulations for topical administration

Madhu Sharma, Ritu Rathi, Sukhanpreet Kaur, Inderbir Singh, Erazuliana Abd Kadir, Amir-Modarresi Chahardehi, and Vuanghao Lim

18. Therapeutic potential of plant-derived flavonoids against inflammation

Reyaz Hassan Mir, Roohi Mohi-ud-din, Prince Ahad Mir, Mudasir Maqbool, Nazia Banday, Saeema Farooq, Syed Naeim Raza, and Pooja A. Chawla

19. Heterocycles in managing inflammatory diseases

Bhupender Nehra, Pooja A. Chawla, Parteek Prasher, and Devidas S. Bhagat

20. In vivo models of understanding inflammation (in vivo methods for inflammation)

Poonam Negi, Shweta Agarwal, Prakrati Garg, Aaliya Ali, and Saurabh Kulshrestha

21. Clinical trials and future perspectives of antiinflammatory agents

Kamini, Anoop Kumar, Pooja A. Chawla, and Bhupinder Kapoor

Contributors

Numbers in parentheses indicate the pages on which the authors' contributions begin.

Shweta Agarwal (315), Department of Pharmaceutics, L.R Institute of Pharmacy, Solan, Himachal Pradesh, India

Sattam Khulaif Alenezi (1), Department of Pharmacology and Toxicology, Unaizah College of Pharmacy, Qassim University, Qassim, Saudi Arabia

Khalid Saad Alharbi (1), Department of Pharmacology, College of Pharmacy, Jouf University, Sakakah, Saudi Arabia

Aaliya Ali (315), School of Applied Sciences and Biotechnology; Center for Omics and Biodiversity Research, Shoolini University, Solan, Himachal Pradesh, India

Mohd Nazam Ansari (19,143), Department of Pharmacology & Toxicology, College of Pharmacy, Prince Sattam Bin Abdulaziz University, Al-Kharj, Saudi Arabia

Vimal Arora (183), University Institute of Pharma Sciences, Chandigarh University, Gharuan, India

Nazia Banday (279), Pharmacognosy & Phytochemistry Division, Department of Pharmaceutical Sciences, University of Kashmir, Srinagar, Jammu and Kashmir, India

Tapan Behl (69), School of Health Science and Technology, University of Petroleum and Energy Studies, Bidholi, Uttarakhand, India

Devidas S. Bhagat (295), Department of Forensic Chemistry and Toxicology, Government Institute of Forensic Science, Aurangabad, Maharashtra, India

Nitish Bhatia (11), Department of Pharmacology, Khalsa College of Pharmacy, Amritsar, Punjab, India

Shome Sankar Bhunia (93), School of Pharmacy, The Assam Kaziranga University, Jorhat, Assam, India

Ananya Bishnoi (155), School of Health Sciences and Technology, University of Petroleum and Energy Studies, Energy Acres Bidholi, Dehradun, Uttarakhand, India

Gunjan Vasant Bonde (155), School of Health Sciences and Technology, University of Petroleum and Energy Studies, Energy Acres Bidholi, Dehradun, Uttarakhand, India

Amir-Modarresi Chahardehi (245), Advanced Medical and Dental Institute, Universiti Sains Malaysia, Penang, Malaysia

Yinghan Chan (29,113), School of Pharmacy, International Medical University (IMU), Kuala Lumpur, Malaysia

Silpi Chanda (155), Amity Institute of Pharmacy, Lucknow, Amity University Uttar Pradesh, Noida, UP, India

Pooja A. Chawla (11,81,279,295,331), Department of Pharmaceutical Chemistry and Analysis, ISF College of Pharmacy, Moga, Punjab, India

Viney Chawla (11), University Institute of Pharmaceutical Sciences and Research, Baba Farid University of Health Sciences, Faridkot, Punjab, India

Dinesh Kumar Chellappan (29,113,163), Department of Life Sciences, School of Pharmacy, International Medical University (IMU), Kuala Lumpur, Malaysia

Xiangmei Cui (29), School of Medicine, Faculty of Medicine and Health Sciences, Royal College of Surgeons in Ireland (RCSI), Dublin, Ireland

Koushik Das (57), Department of Allied Health Science, School of Health Science, University of Petroleum and Energy Studies, Dehradun, India

Utsab Debnath (93), School of Health Sciences and Technology, University of Petroleum and Energy Studies, Dehradun, Uttarakhand, India

Hari Prasad Devkota (107), Graduate School of Pharmaceutical Sciences, Kumamoto University, Kumamoto, Japan

Kamal Dua (29,113,163), Discipline of Pharmacy, Graduate School of Health, University of Technology Sydney, Sydney, NSW, Australia

Harish Dureja (183), Faculty of Pharmaceutical Sciences, Maharshi Dayanand University, Rohtak, Haryana, India

Saeema Farooq (279), Pharmacognosy & Phytochemistry Division, Department of Pharmaceutical Sciences, University of Kashmir, Srinagar, Jammu and Kashmir, India

Prakrati Garg (315), School of Applied Sciences and Biotechnology; Center for Omics and Biodiversity Research, Shoolini University, Solan, Himachal Pradesh, India

Ajmer Singh Grewal (183), Guru Gobind Singh College of Pharmacy, Yamunanagar, Haryana, India

Gaurav Gupta (1), Department of Pharmacology, School of Pharmacy, Suresh Gyan Vihar University, Jaipur, India

Mahesh Gupta (163), Department of Biology, University of Saskatchewan, Saskatoon, SK, Canada

Saurav Kumar Jha (107), Department of Biomedicine, Health & Life Convergence Sciences, BK21, Mokpo National University, Muan-gun, Jeonnam, Republic of Korea

Erazuliana Abd Kadir (245), Advanced Medical and Dental Institute, Universiti Sains Malaysia, Penang, Malaysia

Kamini (331), Department of Pharmacology, Delhi Institute of Pharmaceutical Sciences and Research, New Delhi, India

Neha Kanojia (163), Chitkara University School of Pharmacy, Chitkara University, Baddi, Solan, Himachal Pradesh, India

Bhupinder Kapoor (331), School of Pharmaceutical Sciences, Lovely Professional University, Phagwara, Punjab, India

Sukhanpreet Kaur (245), Chitkara College of Pharmacy, Chitkara University, Punjab, India

Saurabh Kulshrestha (315), School of Applied Sciences and Biotechnology; Center for Omics and Biodiversity Research, Shoolini University, Solan, Himachal Pradesh, India

Abhitinder Kumar (11), University Institute of Pharmaceutical Sciences and Research, Baba Farid University of Health Sciences, Faridkot, Punjab, India

Anoop Kumar (331), Department of Pharmacology, Delhi Institute of Pharmaceutical Sciences and Research; School of Pharmaceutical Sciences, Delhi Pharmaceutical Sciences and Research University, New Delhi, India

Bhupinder Kumar (81), Department of Pharmaceutical Chemistry and Analysis, ISF College of Pharmacy, Moga, Punjab, India

Pradeep Kumar (233), Wits Advanced Drug Delivery Platform Research Unit, Department of Pharmacy and Pharmacology, School of Therapeutic Sciences, Faculty of Health Sciences, University of the Witwatersrand, Johannesburg, South Africa

Hui Shan Liew (113), School of Postgraduate Studies; Center for Cancer and Stem Cell Research, Institute for Research, Development and Innovation (IRDI), International Medical University (IMU), Kuala Lumpur, Malaysia

Jun Sing Lim (29), School of Medicine, Faculty of Medicine and Health Sciences, Royal College of Surgeons in Ireland (RCSI), Dublin, Ireland

Vuanghao Lim (245), Advanced Medical and Dental Institute, Universiti Sains Malaysia, Penang, Malaysia

Xin Wei Lim (29), School of Health Sciences, Faculty of Biology, Medicine and Health, University of Manchester, Manchester, United Kingdom

Ramakrishna Thilagar Uma Maheswari (233), Department of Natural Products Chemistry, School of Chemistry, Madurai Kamaraj University, Madurai, Tamil Nadu, India

Neeraj Mahindroo (19), School of Pharmacy, MIT World Peace University, Pune, Maharashtra, India

Rashita Makkar (69), Chitkara College of Pharmacy, Chitkara University, Rajpura, Punjab, India

Mudasir Maqbool (279), Pharmacy Practice Division, Department of Pharmaceutical Sciences, University of Kashmir, Srinagar, Jammu and Kashmir, India

Prince Ahad Mir (279), Amritsar Pharmacy College, Amritsar, Punjab, India

Reyaz Hassan Mir (279), Pharmaceutical Chemistry Division, Chandigarh College of Pharmacy, Landran, Punjab; Pharmaceutical Chemistry Division, Department of Pharmaceutical Sciences, University of Kashmir, Srinagar, Jammu and Kashmir, India

Roohi Mohi-ud-din (279), Sher-I-Kashmir Institute of Medical Sciences, Srinagar, Jammu and Kashmir, India

Poonam Negi (315), School of Pharmaceutical Sciences, Shoolini University, Solan, Himachal Pradesh, India

Bhupender Nehra (295), Department of Pharmaceutical Sciences, Guru Jambheshwar University of Science & Technology, Hisar, Haryana, India

Sin Wi Ng (29,113), School of Pharmacy, International Medical University (IMU), Kuala Lumpur, Malaysia

Shalini Oli (57), Department of Allied Health Science, School of Health Science, University of Petroleum and Energy Studies, Dehradun, India

Nisha Panth (107), College of Pharmacy and Natural Medicine Research Institute, Mokpo National University, Muan-gun, Jeonnam, Republic of Korea

Kamla Pathak (69), Faculty of Pharmacy, Uttar Pradesh University of Medical Sciences, Etawah, Uttar Pradesh, India

Jeevan Patra (19), School of Health Sciences and Technology, University of Petroleum and Energy Studies, Dehradun, Uttarakhand, India

Keshav Raj Paudel (107), Department of Oriental Medicine Resources, Mokpo National University, Muan-gun, Jeonnam, Republic of Korea

Parteek Prasher (81,295), Department of Chemistry, University of Petroleum & Energy Studies, Dehradun, Uttarakhand, India

Lesley Jia Wei Pua (113), School of Postgraduate Studies; Center for Cancer and Stem Cell Research, Institute for Research, Development and Innovation (IRDI), International Medical University (IMU), Kuala Lumpur, Malaysia

Vivek Puri (163), Chitkara University School of Pharmacy, Chitkara University, Baddi, Solan, Himachal Pradesh, India

Alan Raj (171), Department of Pharmaceutics, College of Pharmaceutical Sciences, Government Medical College Kannur, Pariyaram, Kerala; Department of Pharamceutical Biotechnology, Manipal College of Pharmaceutical Sciences, Manipal Academy of Higher Education, Manipal, Karnataka, India

Mariappan Rajan (233), Department of Natural Products Chemistry, School of Chemistry, Madurai Kamaraj University, Madurai, Tamil Nadu, India

Lata Rani (163,183), Chitkara University School of Pharmacy, Chitkara University, Baddi, Solan, Himachal Pradesh, India

Ritu Rathi (245), Chitkara College of Pharmacy, Chitkara University, Punjab, India

Syed Naeim Raza (279), Pharmaceutics Division, Department of Pharmaceutical Sciences, University of Kashmir, Srinagar, Jammu and Kashmir, India

Abdul Samad (143), Faculty of Pharmacy, Tishk International University, Erbil, Kurdistan Region, Iraq

C. Sarath Chandran (171), Department of Pharmaceutics, College of Pharmaceutical Sciences, Government Medical College Kannur, Pariyaram, Kerala, India

Ameya Sharma (163), Chitkara University School of Pharmacy, Chitkara University, Baddi, Solan, Himachal Pradesh, India

Kushal Sharma (107), College of Pharmacy and Natural Medicine Research Institute, Mokpo National University, Muan-gun, Jeonnam, Republic of Korea

Madhu Sharma (245), Amravati Enclave, Panchkula, Haryana, India

Gurpreet Singh (11), Department of Pharmaceutical Sciences, Guru Nanak Dev University, Amritsar, Punjab, India

Inderbir Singh (245), Chitkara College of Pharmacy, Chitkara University, Punjab, India

Manish Pal Singh (11,69), Department of Pharmacology, Agra Public Pharmacy College; Anand College of Pharmacy (SGI), Agra, Uttar Pradesh, India

Vikram Jeet Singh (81), Department of Pharmaceutical Chemistry and Analysis, ISF College of Pharmacy, Moga, Punjab, India

Laura Soon (113), School of Pharmacy, International Medical University (IMU), Kuala Lumpur, Malaysia

K. Sourav (171), Department of Pharmaceutics, College of Pharmaceutical Sciences, Government Medical College Kannur, Pariyaram, Kerala, India

Manvi Suri (19,143), School of Health Sciences and Technology, University of Petroleum and Energy Studies, Dehradun, Uttarakhand, India

K.K. Swathy (171), Department of Pharmaceutics, College of Pharmaceutical Sciences, Government Medical College Kannur, Pariyaram, Kerala, India

Joycelin Zhu Xin Tan (113), School of Pharmacy, International Medical University (IMU), Kuala Lumpur, Malaysia

Komal Thapa (163), Chitkara University School of Pharmacy, Chitkara University, Baddi, Solan, Himachal Pradesh, India

Nidhi Tiwari (19,143), Institute of Nuclear Medicine and Allied Sciences, Defence Research and Development Organization, New Delhi, Delhi, India

Raj Kumar Tiwari (155), School of Health Sciences and Technology, University of Petroleum and Energy Studies, Energy Acres Bidholi, Dehradun, Uttarakhand, India

Jyoti Upadhyay (19,143), School of Health Sciences and Technology, University of Petroleum and Energy Studies, Dehradun, Uttarakhand, India

Shashi Upadhyay (57), Department of Allied Health Science, School of Health Science, University of Petroleum and Energy Studies, Dehradun, India

Nitin Verma (163), Chitkara University School of Pharmacy, Chitkara University, Baddi, Solan, Himachal Pradesh, India

Chapter 1

Pathophysiology and pathogenesis of inflammation

Khalid Saad Alharbi[a], Sattam Khulaif Alenezi[b], and Gaurav Gupta[c]

[a]*Department of Pharmacology, College of Pharmacy, Jouf University, Sakakah, Saudi Arabia,* [b]*Department of Pharmacology and Toxicology, Unaizah College of Pharmacy, Qassim University, Qassim, Saudi Arabia,* [c]*Department of Pharmacology, School of Pharmacy, Suresh Gyan Vihar University, Jaipur, India*

1 Introduction

Inflammation is a complicated cellular event that primarily involves vasculature and leukocyte responses. Plasma proteins and circulating leukocytes, along with tissue phagocytic cells produced by circulating cells, are the body's main defenses toward external pathogens. Proteins and white blood cells in the bloodstream have the potential to migrate to any location in which they are demanded. While intruders such as bacteria and necrotic cells are usually found in tissues outside of the circulatory system, circulating cells and proteins are quickly attracted to these extravascular regions. Vasculature and intracellular responses of the inflammation are initiated by dissolved substances released by the different proteins present in plasma or diverse cells, which will be formed, stimulated, and released in response to strong stimuli [1,2]. Microorganisms, dead cells, or even oxygen deprivation can cause the production of inflammatory mediators, resulting in inflammation. Based on the kind of the stimulus and the efficiency of the first response in removing the stimuli or injured tissues, inflammation can be acute or chronic. Acute inflammation is characterized by quick onset (usually minutes) and short duration (hours or days); its key types include efflux of fluids and proteins present in plasma and migration of WBC, primarily neutrophils. Whenever short-term inflammation is effective in removing intruders, the cellular response decreases; however, when responses fail to eliminate intruders, the response might develop to further later stage known as chronic stage. When acute inflammation is left untreated it will develop into chronic inflammation or appear gradually [3–5].

Whenever the harmful substance is removed, the inflammation stops. Since the mediators are degraded and dispersed, and because leukocytes have limited lives in tissues, the response occurs quickly. Antiinflammatory systems are also triggered, which help to moderate the response and keep it from inflicting too much harm to the organism. The inflammatory response is intricately linked to the healing process. Simultaneously the inflammation dissolves, diminishes, and seals off the harmful substances, it also puts in motion a chain of actions that attempt to repair the injured tissue. Healing tends to occur during inflammation but is generally completed after the harmful impact has been removed [6,7]. When the wound is healed, the wound's native parenchymal cells regenerate, and new fibrous tissue fills the defect or a mix of all different mechanisms occur in the healing process.

2 Pathophysiology and pathogenesis of inflammation

2.1 Acute inflammation

Acute inflammation is a fast-acting systemic action that transports leukocytes and plasma proteins such as immunoglobulin to the location of infectious and damaged tissue. Acute inflammation entails three key factors: (a) changes in vascular circumference that enhance blood supply, (b) anatomical modifications in the vascular endothelium which allow protein present in plasma and white blood cells to exit the circulatory system, and (c) leukocyte outflow from the vasculature, aggregation in the injured area, and stimulation to eradicate the accusing substance [8].

2.2 Stimuli for acute inflammation

Reaction developed by acute inflammation can be stimulated through various factors or stimuli:

- Inflammation is not just a sign of illness; it is caused by a number of microbial pathogens and infections. A variety of mechanisms exist in mammals to detect microorganisms. TLRs are perhaps the most significant

Recent Developments in Anti-Inflammatory Therapy. https://doi.org/10.1016/B978-0-323-99988-5.00006-1

microbial product receptors, and they are called after Drosophila Toll, a cytosol withal molecule, which can identify bacteria, viruses, and fungi. Signaling pathways are activated as a result of these receptors getting engaged, which causes the synthesis of numerous mediators.

- Cell death due to tissue ischemia, trauma, or chemical injury. Some chemicals that are produced from dead cells, such as uric acid, ATP, and HMGB-1, are believed to promote inflammation. In addition to inciting the inflammatory response, hypoxia is also a common factor in cell damage.

- When the ordinarily defensive immune system harms the body's own cell, the reaction is known as hypersensitivity reaction. Autoimmune disorders or anaphylactic shock could be the result of harmful immune responses targeting self-antigens. The main reason of tissue damage in these disorders is inflammation. In many cases, autoimmune reactions do not terminate when the triggering stimulus is withdrawn. As a result, most of these reactions are difficult to eradicate and difficult to get rid of. They are also closely associated with chronic inflammation, which is a common and serious health problem. T lymphocytes and various other inflammatory mediators can produce cytokines that cause inflammation. When speaking of this particular set of illnesses, it is more common to refer to immune-mediated inflammatory illness [9,10].

2.3 Blood vessels reactions in acute inflammation

The redness, swelling, and warmth that you see with inflammation is the result of certain changes in the blood arteries that increase the migration of proteins present in blood plasma and cells present in circulation to the location of damage or wounded site. Exudation is a process by which fluid, proteins, and blood cells enter the interstitial tissue and surrounding tissues leaving the vascular system. A cytoplasmic fluid that is extravascular, highly protein-rich, and consists of waste organic materials after cell dies has an excessive relative density called exudate. This occurrence indicates that the body's typical tiny blood vessel permeability has increased in the damage site or location, and so, there is an inflammatory reaction. A transudate is a solution that has tiny or no cellular material, low protein contents, and little or no specific gravity. An imbalance in two different pressures, hydrostatic pressure and colloid osmotic pressure in the artery wall, will cause the leakage of plasma by increasing the vascular or capillary permeability known as microvascular ultrafiltrate. Pus, a purulent exudate, is an inflammatory discharge containing a large amount of white blood cell granulocytes, i.e., neutrophils, as well as a significant amount of leukocytes (Fig. 1) [11–13].

3 Changes in vascular flow

Early postinjury that alters vascular flow and ability comprises the following:

- The earliest sign of inflammation is vasodilation, which occurs within a few seconds of a brief constriction of the arteries. First, the arterioles are vasodilated, and then new capillary beds open in the area. Inflammation is a consequence of a higher movement of blood to the area, causing redness (erythema) and heat. Although histamine and nitric oxide (NO) causes the dilation of blood vessels by acting on smooth muscle of blood vessels, various other mediators contribute as well.

- Vasodilation is rapidly followed by increases in microvasculature permeability resulting in extravascular fluid ooze that includes protein-rich fluids.

- Reduced blood flow, elevated red cell volume in tiny vessels, and high viscosity of the blood are all associated with fluid loss. Due to these alterations, the vessels containing a large number of gradually moveable red cells are expanded, a characteristic of stasis, which causes redness in the affected tissue.

- The more stasis that is developed, the more blood neutrophils (a type of white blood cell) gather along the vascular endothelium. Simultaneously, mediators released at the infection regions and tissue injury boost the number of endothelial cells, resulting in enhanced adhesion molecule expression. Once leukocytes stick to the endothelium, they move into the tissue that surrounds the vessel (interstitial tissue) [14–16].

3.1 Increased vascular permeability or vascular leakage

An important characteristic of acute inflammation is the development of vascular permeability, which allows extravascular fluid to enter the tissue, resulting in edema. The enhancement in vascular permeability is attributable to several factors.

- Chemical mediators such as histamine, leukotrienes, bradykinin, substance P, and many more can cause an increase in intervascular spaces by contracting endothelial cells, a condition known as vascular leakage. After exposure to and contact with the mediator an immediate reaction will occur, this type of response is known as transient response and typically lasts for 15–30 min. Leakage of red blood cells begins 2–12 h after a mild injury such as burn, irradiation, or exposure to bacterial toxins. There may be prolonged blood leakage because of the constriction of endothelial cells or mild endothelial injury.

- In burn wound, bacterial infection of endothelial cells, major injury or damage to endothelium cells lead to cell

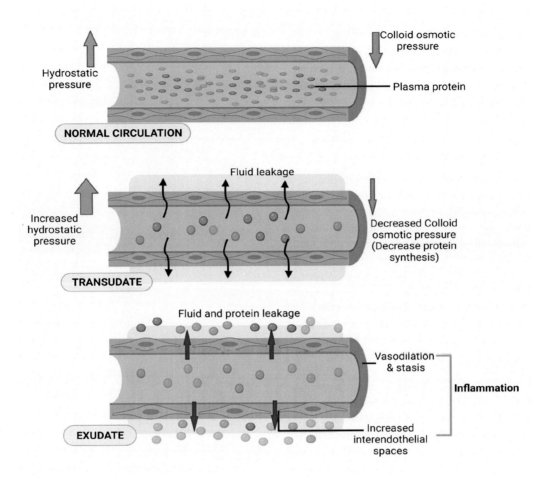

FIG. 1 Formation of transudates and exudates.

death and endothelial cell necrosis due to the detachment of endothelial cells. During inflammation some neutrophils may remain attached to endothelium layer, and this may contribute to endothelial cell injury and hence the responsiveness to inflammation. Injuries caused by a leak typically begin shortly after the injury occurs and are sustained for several hours until thrombosis or repair occurs.

- Transcytosis is the enhancement in the movement of fluids and proteins within the endothelial cell. Some intercellular connections are associated with vesiculovacuolar organelle, a network of interconnected, uncoated vesicles and vacuoles. In addition to their ability to be recruited into new blood vessels, certain substances, such as VEGF, appear to increase vascular leakage by increasing the number and possibly the mass of these channels [17–19].

4 Chronic inflammation

The word chronic, which means "continuing or existing for a long time," describes long-term inflammation. Acute

inflammation may follow; however, more commonly, chronic inflammation starts as a low-grade, smouldering response that lacks any obvious acute signs. Persistent and continuous inflammation of tissues can cause several prevalent and severe diseases such as autoimmune disease, rheumatoid arthritis, atherosclerosis, tuberculosis, and pulmonary fibrosis. Alzheimer disease and several cancers, which were previously assumed to be solely degenerative, are also believed to be associated with inflammation [20,21].

4.1 Causes of chronic inflammation

Chronic inflammation arises in the following settings:

- Recurring infections caused by mycobacteria, viruses, fungi, and parasites are hard to treat. These organisms generally induce a delayed-type hypersensitivity immunological reaction.
- It is well established that chronic inflammation is a major player in certain disorders in which immune system activation is extreme and inappropriate. Auto-antigens

in disorders such as rheumatoid arthritis and multiple sclerosis stimulate an autoimmune response that causes chronic tissue damage and inflammation. In some circumstances, uncontrolled immune responses are provoked by microorganisms, resulting in persistent inflammation such as in inflammatory bowel disease. Allergic illnesses, such as bronchial asthma, are caused by immune responses to common environmental agent [22–24].

4.2 Mediators of inflammation

Thus far, we have studied the sequence of events that occur in the process of inflammation, so it is now time to focus on the chemical mediators that are involved. It has been established that numerous mediators exist, and their roles in a coordinated manner have yet to be fully understood. Mediators are usually formed from proteins found in blood plasma or from tissue cells. Some mediators are stored in cell membranes and are then released when cells are stimulated. One well-known example is histamine in mast cell granules, which is secreted swiftly when a stimulus is applied. Others are made anew in response to a stimulus, such as prostaglandins or cytokines, and are also called cell-derived mediators. Most, but not all, of the primary cell types that are involved in mediating acute inflammation include platelets, neutrophils, monocytes/macrophages, and mast cells. The major source of plasma-derived mediators is the liver, and they are nonactive progenitor cells that should be stimulated or activated to gain their biological qualities, for example, complement protein and kinins.

Various stimuli stimulate the production of active mediators. Microbial products, necrotic cell products, and complement proteins, which are themselves triggered by microorganisms and injured tissues, are included among these stimuli. In this way, the cytokine TNF stimulates endothelial cells to produce more cytokines and chemokines. In contrast to the initial mediators, secondary mediators exhibit same behaviors but may have additional, contradictory actions. The types of mediators can vary depending on their spectrum of target cells. Their target cells can be one or several, diversified, or they may have varying impacts on different cell types. Most of these mediators, once activated and discharged from the cell, will have shorter lives (Table 1) [25–28].

4.3 Cell-derived mediators

Histamine and serotonin are the two primary vasoactive amines that have an important effect on blood vessels. When inflammation starts, the first mediators to be released into the system are retained inside cells. Histamine is most abundant in the connective tissue associated with blood

TABLE 1 Principal mediators of inflammation and their actions.

Mediator	Principal sources	Actions
Cell-derived		
Histamine	Mast cells, basophils, platelets	Vasodilation, increased vascular permeability, endothelial activation
Serotonin	Platelets	Vasodilation, increased vascular permeability
Prostaglandins	Mast cells, leukocytes	Vasodilation, pain, fever
Leukotrienes	Mast cells, leukocytes	Increased vascular permeability, chemotaxis, leukocyte adhesion and activation
Platelet-activating factor	Leukocytes, mast cells	Vasodilation, increased vascular permeability, leukocyte adhesion, chemotaxis, degranulation, oxidative burst
Reactive oxygen species	Leukocytes	Killing of microbes, tissue damage
Nitric oxide	Endothelium, macrophages	Vascular smooth muscle relaxation, killing of microbes
Cytokines (TNF, IL-1)	Macrophages, endothelial cells, mast cells	Local endothelial activation (expression of adhesion molecules), fever/pain/anorexia/hypotension, decreased vascular resistance (shock)
Chemokines	Leukocytes, activated macrophages	Chemotaxis, leukocyte activation
Plasma protein derived		
Complement products (C5a, C3a, C4a)	Plasma (produced in liver)	Leukocyte chemotaxis and activation, vasodilation (mast cell stimulation)
Kinins	Plasma (produced in liver)	Increased vascular permeability, smooth muscle contraction, vasodilation, pain
Proteases activated during coagulation	Plasma (produced in liver)	Endothelial activation, leukocyte recruitment

vessels, which contains mast cells. A study also revealed that it is present in blood basophils and platelets. Histamine is found in the granules of mast cell and is produced by the degranulation of mast cell upon exposure to many stimuli, including trauma, cold, or heat; the binding of antibodies to mast cells, which leads to allergic reactions; anaphylatoxins derived from fragments of complement; and histamine-releasing proteins synthesized by leukocytes, cytokines (IL-1, IL-8), and neuropeptides (e.g., substance P) [29,30].

Histamine: Histamine enhances the permeability of venules and expands the arterioles. It is commonly accepted as the direct mediator of enhanced vascular permeability in the transitory phase, causing interendothelial gaps in venules. The vasoactive effects of histamine are activated by H1 receptors on microvascular endothelial cells.

Serotonin: Histamine and serotonin are both preformed vasoactive mediators, and their effects are somewhat similar. Whenever platelets interact with collagen, thrombin, ADP, and antigen antibody complexes, serotonin and histamine are released from the platelets. Thus, coagulation, a fundamental step in blood clotting, enhances vascular permeability. Inflammation and coagulation are interconnected, as shown in Fig. 2 [31–33].

5   Arachidonic acid (AA) metabolites: Prostaglandins and leukotrienes

Prostaglandins and leukotrienes are both produced when AA is activated in cells by various stimuli such as

microbiological substances and different inflammatory mediators. In addition to acting as an intracellular or extracellular signal, these physiologically active lipid mediators act on numerous physiological processes, including inflammation and hemostasis. Essential fatty acid linoleic acid can be used to synthesize AA. AA is a polyunsaturated fatty acid of 20 carbon atoms that is acquired from diet. The compound is esterified in phospholipids in the cell membrane. Phospholipid of cell membrane will synthesize AA with the help of enzyme phospholipase A2 by stimulating several stimuli. A surge in cytosolic Ca^{2+} and stimulation of many kinases in response to an external stimulus activate phospholipase A2. COX (which generate prostaglandins) and LOX (which produce leukotrienes and lipoxins) both produce AA-derived mediators known as eicosanoids [34,35].

Mastocyte, macrophages, endothelial cells, and several different cells make prostaglandins (PGs), which are crucial in vascular and systemic effects of inflammation. Cyclooxygenases (COX-1 and COX-2) are the catalysts responsible for the production of prostaglandins. Prostaglandins (PGE2, PGD2, PGF2α), prostacyclins, and thromboxanes are the three most prominent mediators of inflammation, each originating from an enzyme acting on an intermediary in the path. TxA2, a strong platelet-aggregating agent and vasoconstrictor, converts to its inactive form TxB2. Prostacyclin (PGI2) and end product of prostacyclin PGF1α are synthesized by endothelial cells lacking thromboxane synthase but possesses prostacyclin synthetase. Prostacyclin is a

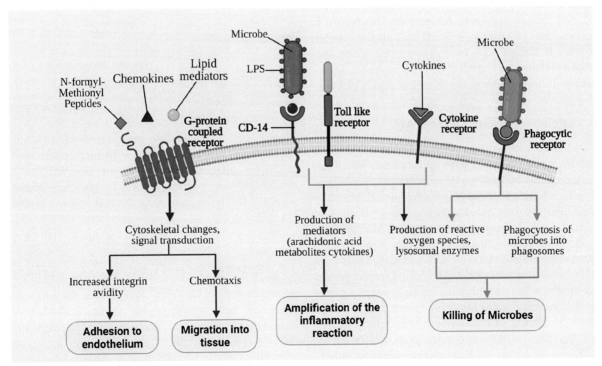

FIG. 2 Leukocyte receptors and responses.

vasodilator, and its influence on platelet aggregation is also significant which produces inhibitory action. Mast cells synthesize PGD2, the most important prostaglandin involved in the initiation of the process of fluid accumulation in the body; alongside PGE2, PGD2 promotes dilation in blood vessels and enhances the permeability of postcapillary small blood circulation, thus increasing the risk of edema development. PGF2α regulates uterine and bronchial smooth muscle contraction, as well as arterioles and venules, while PGD2 acts as a chemokine for neutrophils. The prostaglandins, besides acting locally, are important in the development of pathogenesis of pain and heat in inflammation. PGE2 is a painful substance which makes the skin hypersensitive to histamine and bradykinin because PGE2 is a proinflammatory agent, it has the undesirable effect of making the skin more sensitive to pain [36–38].

Leukotrienes are formed via lipoxygenase enzymes, which are released predominantly by leukocytes, attract leukocytes, and affect the blood vessels. While there are three distinct lipoxygenases, the most prevalent lipoxygenase is 5-lipoxygenase, which is found in neutrophils. This enzyme that is active in this system transforms arachidonic acid to 5-hydroxyeicosatetraenoic acid, which would be chemotactic for neutrophils, and this is a progenitor or starting point for the leukotrienes. The LTB4 acts as a chemotactic agent and a neutrophil activator, resulting in increased cell aggregation and adherence to venular endothelium, increased ROS production, and discharge of lysosomal enzymes. LTC4-, LTD4-, and LTE4-containing cysteinyl leukotrienes produce vasoconstriction, bronchospasm, and increased vascular permeability. In contrast to histamine, vascular leakage is found only in the venules. Even while histamine is far more potent at increasing vascular permeability and producing bronchospasm, leukotrienes are 10 times more powerful in this regard [39,40].

5.1 Platelet-activating factor (PAF)

PAF has been identified as another mediator which is derived from phospholipids. Although shown to play a role in the aggregation of platelets, this compound has now been discovered to have inflammatory effects as well. PAF can be secreted into the bloodstream by various cells such as platelets, basophils, mastocyte, neutrophils, macrophages, and endothelial cells. Although PAF causes platelet aggregation, it also constricts blood vessels and narrows airways, as well as causes vasodilation and increased venular permeability at very small concentration having a potency over a hundred to thousand times larger than histamine. PAF also enhances the binding of leukocytes to endothelium, as well as their migration, activation, degranulation, and the release of oxidative chemicals. PAF can trigger the most inflammatory responses of the vascular and cellular systems.

TABLE 2 Role of mediators in different reactions of inflammation.

Response in inflammation	Mediators
Vasodilation	Prostaglandins
	Nitric oxide
	Histamine
Increased vascular permeability	Histamine and serotonin
	C3a and C5a (by liberating vasoactive amines from mast cells, other cells)
	Bradykinin
	Leukotrienes C_4, D_4, E_4
	PAF
	Substance P
Chemotaxis, leukocyte recruitment and activation	TNF, IL-1
	Chemokines
	C3a, C5a
	Leukotriene B_4
	(Bacterial products, e.g., N-formyl methyl peptides)
Fever	IL-1, TNF
	Prostaglandins
Pain	Prostaglandins
	Bradykinin
Tissue damage	Lysosomal enzymes of leukocytes
	Reactive oxygen species
	Nitric oxide

Eicosanoids, which include prostaglandins, are also produced via the PAF pathway. The evidence supports the existence for platelet-activating factor in vivo, as some synthesized antagonist of PAF receptor are shown to decrease the inflammation in several research (Table 2) [41–43].

5.2 Reactive oxygen species

After a leukocyte has been exposed to pathogens, chemokines, and immune complexes, or after it has been challenged by a phagocytic encounter, oxygen-derived free radicals may be produced extracellularly. Initiation and stimulation of the NADPH oxidase system is required for their synthesis. The primary by-products of cellular activity are superoxide anion, H_2O_2, and hydroxyl radical •OH, with O being able to interact with NO to form reactive nitrogen species. While ROS are produced in leukocytes to assist in removing microorganisms that have been phagocytosed, too much of these substances might be detrimental to the host [44,45].

5.3 Nitric oxide (NO)

Endothelial cells secrete NO, a soluble gas, although macrophages and certain neurons in the brain create it as well. It triggers a chain of actions within target cells, such as the relaxation of vascular smooth muscle cells, by acting as a paracrine agent and increasing cyclic guanosine monophosphate. In vivo, the half-life of NO is merely seconds, and the gas has only a short range. When one compares the chemical activity of NO in the tissues with its dual physiological effect in the relaxing vascular smooth muscle, it is seen that the first component likewise works to promote vasodilation while blocking the cellular response to inflammation. NO is a modulator of host defense against infection because it is a microbicidal agent. In reaction to microorganisms, the high quantities of iNOS-induced NO are produced by leukocytes, especially neutrophils and macrophages [46,47].

5.4 Cytokines and chemokines

The cytokines regulates the activity of several neighboring cells. One of these has been shown to play a role in cellular immune responses, but new findings have shown that it has additional impacts on acute and chronic inflammation [48,49].

5.5 Tumor necrosis factor and interleukin-1

The primary cytokines that influence inflammation are TNF and IL-1. Activated macrophages are responsible for producing the majority of these compounds. Endotoxin, immunological complexes, physical damage, and a range of inflammatory stimuli can promote the release of TNF and IL-1. Inflammation is mainly marked by an increase in endothelial cells, leukocytes, and fibroblasts, and the development of acute-phase reactions in the whole body. When they are present in the endothelium, they can cause a wide range of physiological changes, including endothelial activation. The compound most likely to be involved in mediating endothelial adhesion molecule expression is. As a result, production of other cytokines such as chemokines, growth factors, eicosanoids, and NO; enzyme production; and changes in endothelial thrombogenicity are all most likely to occur. TNF (tumor necrosis factor) increases the number of neutrophils that respond to endotoxin, which is bacterial origin. There is a multiprotein cellular complex

called the "inflammasome" that responds to bacteria and dead cells, and it is known to govern the synthesis of IL-1. This combination stimulates proteases in the caspase family, which cleave the freshly generated IL-1 parent into the functional cytokine [50–52].

6 Summary

In order to end on a high note, let's now recap the elements, mediators, and pathological symptoms associated with acute inflammatory responses. As soon as a pathogen or dead cells (like cancer cells) are encountered, phagocytes in all tissues actively attempt to destroy these harmful substances. Other host cells in addition to phagocytes release cytokines, lipid messengers, and other inflammatory mediators in response to the presence of an outside or aberrant substance. In a small area around the location of the source of the problem, these mediators induce the release of plasma and accumulation of circulating leukocytes to the area. A stimulated leukocyte recruits other leukocytes to eliminate the damaging agent through phagocytosis. The health of the host improves as the damaging factor is removed and anti-inflammatory mechanisms begin to function. Chronic inflammation may ensue if the damaging agent cannot be immediately removed.

A number of reactions are responsible for both the clinical and pathologic aspects of the inflammatory response. An acute inflammatory vascular inflammation is defined by a rise in blood flow to the wounded area; this rise is mostly due to an increase in arteriolar dilatation and opening of capillary beds that are accompanied by the presence of mediators such as histamine. The production of exudate due to the aggregation of fluid from protein-rich capillaries produces an increase in vascular permeability. In almost all cases, plasma proteins exit the vessel by spreading out through the interendothelial cell connections of the small vessels. Elevation in blood flow and edema are characteristic of acute inflammation and its manifestations such as redness (rubor), warmth (calor), and swelling (tumor) induced by the blood flow. Toxic metabolites and proteases can be released from active leukocytes and endogenous mediators, damaging tissue. Another localized sign is pain (dolor) in response to the lesion and in part due to the release of prostaglandins, neuropeptides, and cytokines.

References

[1] T. Adage, V. Konya, C. Weber, E. Strutzmann, T. Fuchs, C. Zankl, et al., Targeting glycosaminoglycans in the lung by an engineered CXCL8 as a novel therapeutic approach to lung inflammation, Eur. J. Pharmacol. 748 (2015) 83–92.

[2] N.R. Aggarwal, L.S. King, F.R. D'Alessio, Diverse macrophage populations mediate acute lung inflammation and resolution, Am. J. Physiol. Lung Cell. Mol. Physiol. 306 (8) (2014) L709–L725.

[3] I.C. Allen, Bacteria-mediated acute lung inflammation, Methods Mol. Biol. (Clifton, N.J.) 1031 (2013) 163–175.

[4] G.K. Aulakh, J.A. Brocos Duda, C.M. Guerrero Soler, E. Snead, J. Singh, Characterization of low-dose ozone-induced murine acute lung injury, Phys. Rep. 8 (11) (2020), e14463.

[5] G.K. Aulakh, M. Kaur, V. Brown, S. Ekanayake, B. Khan, H. Fonge, Quantification of regional murine ozone-induced lung inflammation using [(18)F]F-FDG microPET/CT imaging, Sci. Rep. 10 (1) (2020) 15699.

[6] M.B. Beasley, T.J. Franks, J.R. Galvin, B. Gochuico, W.D. Travis, Acute fibrinous and organizing pneumonia: a histological pattern of lung injury and possible variant of diffuse alveolar damage, Arch. Pathol. Lab. Med. 126 (9) (2002) 1064–1070.

[7] J. Becker, C. Delayre-Orthez, N. Frossard, F. Pons, Regulation of inflammation by PPARs: a future approach to treat lung inflammatory diseases? Fundam. Clin. Pharmacol. 20 (5) (2006) 429–447.

[8] C. Beisswenger, R. Bals, Antimicrobial peptides in lung inflammation, Chem. Immunol. Allergy 86 (2005) 55–71.

[9] D.K. Bhalla, Ozone-induced lung inflammation and mucosal barrier disruption: toxicology, mechanisms, and implications, J. Toxicol. Environ. Health B Crit. Rev. 2 (1) (1999) 31–86.

[10] R. Bhargava, W. Janssen, C. Altmann, A. Andrés-Hernando, K. Okamura, R.W. Vandivier, et al., Intratracheal IL-6 protects against lung inflammation in direct, but not indirect, causes of acute lung injury in mice, PLoS One 8 (5) (2013), e61405.

[11] J. Bhattacharya, K. Westphalen, Macrophage-epithelial interactions in pulmonary alveoli, Semin. Immunopathol. 38 (4) (2016) 461–469.

[12] J.B. Borges, E.L. Costa, M. Bergquist, L. Lucchetta, C. Widström, E. Maripuu, et al., Lung inflammation persists after 27 hours of protective acute respiratory distress syndrome network strategy and is concentrated in the nondependent lung, Crit. Care Med. 43 (5) (2015) e123–e132.

[13] J. Boskabadi, A. Mokhtari-Zaer, A. Abareshi, M.R. Khazdair, B. Emami, N. Mohammadian Roshan, et al., The effect of captopril on lipopolysaccharide-induced lung inflammation, Exp. Lung Res. 44 (4-5) (2018) 191–200.

[14] H.M. Braakhuis, M.V. Park, I. Gosens, W.H. De Jong, F.R. Cassee, Physicochemical characteristics of nanomaterials that affect pulmonary inflammation, Part. Fibre Toxicol. 11 (2014) 18.

[15] J. Britto, R.H. Demling, Aspiration lung injury, New Horiz. (Baltimore, Md.) 1 (3) (1993) 435–439.

[16] J. Cai, C. Zhao, Y. Du, Y. Huang, Q. Zhao, Amentoflavone ameliorates cold stress-induced inflammation in lung by suppression of C3/BCR/NF-κB pathways, BMC Immunol. 20 (1) (2019) 49.

[17] A.M. Cantin, D. Hartl, M.W. Konstan, J.F. Chmiel, Inflammation in cystic fibrosis lung disease: pathogenesis and therapy, J. Cyst. Fibros. 14 (4) (2015) 419–430.

[18] A. Caretti, V. Peli, M. Colombo, A. Zulueta, Lights and shadows in the use of mesenchymal stem cells in lung inflammation, a poorly investigated topic in cystic fibrosis, Cell 9 (1) (2019).

[19] I. Cattani-Cavalieri, V.H. da Maia, J.A. Moraes, L. Brito-Gitirana, B. Romana-Souza, M. Schmidt, et al., Dimethyl fumarate attenuates lung inflammation and oxidative stress induced by chronic exposure to diesel exhaust particles in mice, Int. J. Mol. Sci. 21 (24) (2020).

[20] W.C. Chou, M.C. Kao, C.T. Yue, P.S. Tsai, C.J. Huang, Caffeine mitigates lung inflammation induced by ischemia-reperfusion of lower limbs in rats, Mediat. Inflamm. 2015 (2015), 361638.

[21] P.L. Davies, N.C. Maxwell, S. Kotecha, The role of inflammation and infection in the development of chronic lung disease of prematurity, Adv. Exp. Med. Biol. 582 (2006) 101–110.

[22] B. Dhooghe, S. Noël, F. Huaux, T. Leal, Lung inflammation in cystic fibrosis: pathogenesis and novel therapies, Clin. Biochem. 47 (7-8) (2014) 539–546.

[23] J. Dong, Signaling pathways implicated in carbon nanotube-induced lung inflammation, Front. Immunol. 11 (2020), 552613.

[24] M. Duan, M.L. Hibbs, W. Chen, The contributions of lung macrophage and monocyte heterogeneity to influenza pathogenesis, Immunol. Cell Biol. 95 (3) (2017) 225–235.

[25] M.G. Duvall, T.R. Bruggemann, B.D. Levy, Bronchoprotective mechanisms for specialized pro-resolving mediators in the resolution of lung inflammation, Mol. Asp. Med. 58 (2017) 44–56.

[26] E.A. Engels, Inflammation in the development of lung cancer: epidemiological evidence, Expert. Rev. Anticancer. Ther. 8 (4) (2008) 605–615.

[27] J.M. Felton, R. Duffin, C.T. Robb, S. Crittenden, S.M. Anderton, S.E.M. Howie, et al., Facilitation of IL-22 production from innate lymphoid cells by prostaglandin E(2) prevents experimental lung neutrophilic inflammation, Thorax 73 (11) (2018) 1081–1084.

[28] S. Fröhlich, J. Boylan, P. McLoughlin, Hypoxia-induced inflammation in the lung: a potential therapeutic target in acute lung injury? Am. J. Respir. Cell Mol. Biol. 48 (3) (2013) 271–279.

[29] N. Fuentes, M. Nicoleau, N. Cabello, D. Montes, N. Zomorodi, Z.C. Chroneos, et al., 17β-Estradiol affects lung function and inflammation following ozone exposure in a sex-specific manner, Am. J. Physiol. Lung Cell. Mol. Physiol. 317 (5) (2019) L702–116.

[30] M. Gomes, A.L. Teixeira, A. Coelho, A. Araújo, R. Medeiros, The role of inflammation in lung cancer, Adv. Exp. Med. Biol. 816 (2014) 1–23.

[31] M. Guilliams, F.R. Svedberg, Does tissue imprinting restrict macrophage plasticity? Nat. Immunol. 22 (2) (2021) 118–127.

[32] K. Hellbach, F.G. Meinel, T.M. Conlon, K. Willer, A. Yaroshenko, A. Velroyen, et al., X-ray dark-field imaging to depict acute lung inflammation in mice, Sci. Rep. 8 (1) (2018) 2096.

[33] R.S. Hoehn, P.L. Jernigan, L. Japtok, A.L. Chang, E.F. Midura, C.C. Caldwell, et al., Acid sphingomyelinase inhibition in stored erythrocytes reduces transfusion-associated lung inflammation, Ann. Surg. 265 (1) (2017) 218–226.

[34] G. Hu, J.W. Christman, Editorial: Alveolar macrophages in lung inflammation and resolution, Front. Immunol. 10 (2019) 2275.

[35] M. Ilves, P.A.S. Kinaret, J. Ndika, P. Karisola, V. Marwah, V. Fortino, et al., Surface PEGylation suppresses pulmonary effects of CuO in allergen-induced lung inflammation, Part. Fibre Toxicol. 16 (1) (2019) 28.

[36] J. Jeong, Y. Han, C.A. Poland, W.S. Cho, Response-metrics for acute lung inflammation pattern by cobalt-based nanoparticles, Part. Fibre Toxicol. 12 (2015) 13.

[37] H.A. Jones, Inflammation imaging, Proc. Am. Thorac. Soc. 2 (6) (2005) 545–548. 13-4.

[38] T. Kiss, T. Bluth, A. Braune, R. Huhle, A. Denz, M. Herzog, et al., Effects of positive end-expiratory pressure and spontaneous breathing activity on regional lung inflammation in experimental acute respiratory distress syndrome, Crit. Care Med. 47 (4) (2019) e358–e365.

[39] T.B. Kothe, M.W. Kemp, A. Schmidt, E. Royse, F. Salomone, M.W. Clarke, et al., Surfactant plus budesonide decreases lung and systemic

inflammation in mechanically ventilated preterm sheep, Am. J. Physiol. Lung Cell. Mol. Physiol. 316 (5) (2019) L888–l93.

[40] L. Li, V.T. Chow, N.S. Tan, Targeting vascular leakage in lung inflammation, Oncotarget 6 (23) (2015) 19338–19339.

[41] L. Li, J. Wei, S. Li, A.M. Jacko, N.M. Weathington, R.K. Mallampalli, et al., The deubiquitinase USP13 stabilizes the anti-inflammatory receptor IL-1R8/Sigirr to suppress lung inflammation, EBioMedicine 45 (2019) 553–562.

[42] B. Lopez, T.M. Maisonet, V.A. Londhe, Alveolar NF-κB signaling regulates endotoxin-induced lung inflammation, Exp. Lung Res. 41 (2) (2015) 103–114.

[43] M.J. McVey, B.E. Steinberg, N.M. Goldenberg, Inflammasome activation in acute lung injury, Am. J. Physiol. Lung Cell. Mol. Physiol. 320 (2) (2021) L165–l78.

[44] F. Meng, I. Mambetsariev, Y. Tian, Y. Beckham, A. Meliton, A. Leff, et al., Attenuation of lipopolysaccharide-induced lung vascular stiffening by lipoxin reduces lung inflammation, Am. J. Respir. Cell Mol. Biol. 52 (2) (2015) 152–161.

[45] D.K. Meyerholz, J.C. Sieren, A.P. Beck, H.A. Flaherty, Approaches to evaluate lung inflammation in translational research, Vet. Pathol. 55 (1) (2018) 42–52.

[46] A. Moeller, K.H. Carlsen, P.D. Sly, E. Baraldi, G. Piacentini, I. Pavord, et al., Monitoring asthma in childhood: lung function, bronchial responsiveness and inflammation, Eur. Respir. Rev. 24 (136) (2015) 204–215.

[47] G. Nocentini, S. Cuzzocrea, R. Bianchini, E. Mazzon, C. Riccardi, Modulation of acute and chronic inflammation of the lung by GITR and its ligand, Ann. N. Y. Acad. Sci. 1107 (2007) 380–391.

[48] X. Pan, K. Xu, Y. Li, X. Wang, X. Peng, M. Li, et al., Interleukin-35 expression protects against cigarette smoke-induced lung inflammation in mice, Biomed. Pharmacother. 110 (2019) 727–732.

[49] A. Patel, A. Woods, Y. Riffo-Vasquez, A. Babin-Morgan, M.C. Jones, S. Jones, et al., Lung inflammation does not affect the clearance kinetics of lipid nanocapsules following pulmonary administration, J. Control. Release 235 (2016) 24–33.

[50] J.L. Pauly, L.A. Smith, M.H. Rickert, A. Hutson, G.M. Paszkiewicz, Review: is lung inflammation associated with microbes and microbial toxins in cigarette tobacco smoke? Immunol. Res. 46 (1–3) (2010) 127–136.

[51] G.R. Polglase, S.K. Barton, J.M. Melville, V. Zahra, M.J. Wallace, M.L. Siew, et al., Prophylactic erythropoietin exacerbates ventilation-induced lung inflammation and injury in preterm lambs, J. Physiol. 592 (9) (2014) 1993–2002.

[52] F. Puttur, L.G. Gregory, C.M. Lloyd, Airway macrophages as the guardians of tissue repair in the lung, Immunol. Cell Biol. 97 (3) (2019) 246–257.

Chapter 2

Autoimmunity and inflammation

Abhitinder Kumar[a], Viney Chawla[a,*], Pooja A. Chawla[b], Nitish Bhatia[c], Manish Pal Singh[d], and Gurpreet Singh[e]

[a]University Institute of Pharmaceutical Sciences and Research, Baba Farid University of Health Sciences, Faridkot, Punjab, India, [b]Department of Pharmaceutical Chemistry and Analysis, ISF College of Pharmacy, Moga, Punjab, India, [c]Department of Pharmacology, Khalsa College of Pharmacy, Amritsar, Punjab, India, [d]Department of Pharmacology, Agra Public Pharmacy College, Agra, Uttar Pradesh, India, [e]Department of Pharmaceutical Sciences, Guru Nanak Dev University, Amritsar, Punjab, India

1 Introduction

Tolerance, or the inability to respond to autoantigens, has long been known to exist in mature B-cell compartments. Clonal deletion of self-reactive B cells by apoptosis, either by the cytokines directly or de novo from hematopoietic stem cells of pluripotency origin, early lymphoid progenitors to rescue cells from death produced by receptor editing, receptor downregulated mediated anergy, proceeded by apoptosis, often induced by T cells, and suppressive regulation, acting indirectly via regulatory T cells. The anergy or elimination of primordial, autoantigen reactive B cells is ensured by a succession of antigen receptor specificity checkpoints throughout B-cell maturation and receptor fitness. Defects in genes encoding molecules used to purge the initial B-cell repertoires could undermine the B-cell tolerance, enabling autoantibody and B-cell-mediated immunological disorder to arise. When helper T-cell tolerance to a portion of a self-antigen is broken, the surviving low or no autoreactive B cells induct a T-cell-dependent germinal center-type response. It stimulates these B cells to live longer and express AiD, which triggers IgV-region hypermutation and Ig class switching [1,2].

2 Autoimmunity: Multidirectional pathways

The immune system's ability to differentiate between foreign and self was not absolute, and in some circumstances, it might be misdirected against the exact thing it is supposed to protect. As a result, abnormal self-reactions have been associated with more than 80 inflammatory conditions, commonly referred to as autoimmune diseases. Autoimmunity can range from self-reactivity of low level required for immune-system homeostasis and lymphocyte selection to an autoimmunity of intermediate level characterized by minor tissue infiltrates and circulating autoantibodies with no clinical implications, to pathological autoimmunity resulting in immune-mediated organ injury. Autoimmune ailments affect a large percentage of the population (7%–9%). Systemic disorders such as systemic lupus erythematosus (SLE), Sjögren's syndrome, and rheumatoid arthritis are classed differently from organ-specific diseases such as inflammatory bowel disease (IBD), type 1 diabetes (T1D), multiple sclerosis (MS), and myasthenia gravis (RA).

Clinical variability, polygenic character, and multifactorial contributions are common in autoimmune disorders, which typically require both environmental and genetic components [3]. Both adaptive and innate immune actions involved in autoimmune illnesses are linked to mutations of monogenic origin that cause hyperactivation of the innate immune response without the adaptive immune system's participation [4]. In general, genetic vulnerability is the consequence of the combined impacts of numerous common risk variations, each of which has a tiny effect size that is insufficient on its own [5,6]. These variants likely remained due to the survival edge in relation to enhanced infection reactions, and they show significant inequality between ethnic groups, but not unexpectedly. A number of autoimmunity-related loci, including more than 100 for RA, multiple sclerosis, and IBD [5], have been identified. The overlaps of loci between diseases, which often include genes related to the immune system, suggest general mechanistic pathways, even though the particular risk alone within the locus may vary according to illness. Some influential major histocompatibility complex (MHC) haplotypes have the most substantial associations in most common autoimmune disorders among known genetic predisposing factors, but a large number of additional genes, including IL23R, CTLA4, TYK2, and PTPN22, have been frequently involved. In addition to rare, autoimmune distributors in FOXP3, AIRE, IFIH1, TREX1, DNASE1, C1Q, or C4A,

*Corresponding author

11

rare monogenic mutations have been identified, many of which have given evidence to understand autonomy pathogenesis. Most of the risks are unknown, however, because of the unbalance of liaisons, incomplete sequence information, and extensive heterogeneity. In addition, in low-defined noncoding regions, most risk variants have defied efforts to determine their outcomes on gene function.

The major tolerance mechanisms of T cells in the thymus and B cells in the liver and bone marrow are exercised centrally; the current view is that the mechanism of negative selection removes high-fidelity self-reactive T cells. Earlier studies and more defining follow-up studies have demonstrated considerable flaw in this process [7]. An analysis by peptide-MHC tetramers showed that in disease-free subjects not previously infected with these viruses, the avidity and recurrence of CD8+T cells that are specially designed for various virus-derived Peptides are within the same range as T cells that recognize self-peptides, whereas the frequency of CD8+ T cells specific to SMCY, a Y-encoded antigen, is just two-thirds in males versus females [8]. Incomplete elimination of CD8+ T SMCY-specific cells was also seen in the male mouse. In addition, in the thymus and peripheries of mice transgenic to ubiquitous Cre expression, only ~60% removal from the recombinase-specific CD4 + T cells and, impressively, no deletion when the pancreas, lungs, and intestines are limited to the Cre expression [9].

As a result, it is considered that the repertoire with an effectiveness proportionate to self-antigenic expression in the thymus is negative, but that self-reactive T cells are not fully eradicated [9,10].

The APECED syndrome (autoimmune polyendocracy-candidiasis-ectodermal dystrophy), a rarely occurring autosomal recessive disease arising out of mutations in the AIRE (autoimmuna regulator) gene, is an excellent example of autoimmunity produced by insufficient central elimination of autoreactive T cells [11,12]. AIRE functions as a transcription regulator that inducts super enhancers and mediates the diverse manifestation of peripherally tissue-controlled self-molecules in individual medullary epithelial cells in a stochastic manner [13]. AIRE also controls chemokine gene expression, which influences the quantity and physiology of thymic dendritic cells (DCs), as well as the generation of regulatory T cells (Treg cells) [14]. Curably, B cells express AIRE as well which have migrated into the thymus, and help to select the repertoire of T cells [15]. APECED is characterized by T-cell-mediated damage of numerous endocrine organs with significant phenotype heterogeneity, implying the involvement of extra genes that predispose to the disease as well as environmental variables [16,17]. Like T cells, certain self-reactive B cells are immune to central tolerance. In humans, there are larger groups of early immature B cells (about 55%–75%), which subsequently decrease to roughly 40% for peripheral transitional B cells and immature bone marrow B cells, and culminate to approximately 20% for adult naive B cells [18,19].

These reductions take place at different control points during development, beginning with receptor editing and apoptosis and ending with anergy initiation before or shortly after migration to the periphery. Despite these limitations, multispecific self-reactive B cells in the peripheral repertoire can detect multispecific autoantibodies of natural origin in individuals and mice of sound health. Autoantibodies of natural origin are nonpathogenic and are encoded by germline immunoglobulin M (IgM). They can be used as carriers for removal of cell debris or as a defense mechanism to prevent germs from spreading to key organs. However, it has been postulated that poly-specific B cells may undergo somatic overmutation and class change in order to make higher affinity IgG harmful autoantibodies. A high incidence of multispecific B-cell clones is found in individuals suffering from rheumatoid arthritis, Sjögren's syndrome, SLE, or multiple sclerosis [19,20]. However, how these cell types contribute to these various traits is unknown. The inhibitory molecules FcRIIb, VISTA, LAG-3, CTLA-4, PD-1, TIM, TIGIT and different Siglec proteins are produced on the T-cell and B-cell surface to control extreme immune reactions, both antiself and normal. Because a lack of some of these elements leads to autoimmune disease, autoreactive cells remain in the peripheral repertoire even if they are generally under control [21–26]. T-cell anergy is a condition in which the T-cell antigen receptor (TCR) is activated in the absence of a costimulatory signals [27]. When inflammation is absent, the recent thymic emigrants are more prone to anergy [28].

The anergic state is regulated by negative regulators of proximal TCR signaling, as well as functioning transcriptional silencing, specifically at the encoding locus of the cytokine IL-2, and regulatory proteins activation. Treg cells have the ability to convert anergic CD4+ T cells with specific gene expression patterns and characteristic phenotype, encourage anergy in pathogenic CD4+ T cells, and prevent autoimmunity [29]. T-cell anergy, on the other side, is a temporary state that can be restored during the presence of inflammation. Anergic B-cells make up about 5%–7% of peripheral B cells, and transitional T3 B-cells in the spleen may be anergic rather than blocked during development [30]. Because anergic B cells have such a short half-life, the proportion of freshly forming B cells that experience anergy is thought to be significantly higher, possibly up to 50% (5 days, compared to 40 days for follicular B cells). The anergic B cells exhibit lower activation, low antibody production because of impaired signal transduction, proliferation, and increased basal intracellular Ca2+ levels after stimulation [31]. Low-level antigen contacts and a negative feedback network controlled in part by inositol phosphatase SHIP-1 and the tyrosine kinase Lyn, tyrosine phosphatase SHP-1 regulate the anergic state, and animals with a conditional deficit in any of these components develop systemic autoimmunity [32,33]. Anergic B-cells, on the other hand, are not destroyed and may operate as a reservoir for self-reactive substances. Reversal of IgM anergic B-cells during inflammatory conditions was linked to autoimmune disorders in people with SLE, rheumatoid arthritis, and type 1 diabetes. One theory is that self-reactive B cells compete inadequately with cognate T-cells, which are necessary for survivability of the B-cell in germinal centers. B cells that express high-density membrane antigens recognize receptor that may also be destroyed via a mechanism involving the cell-surface type death receptor Fas (CD95). Autoreactive T cells and B cells transferred to the periphery may potentially remain dormant and buried behind anatomical barriers due to a lack of knowledge of tissue-specific antigens. This is particularly true for immunologically privileged tissues including the brain, testis, and eye. Antigen sequestration in peripheral tissues can be disrupted by infectious agents or other types of tissue injury, allowing 'ignorant' autoreactive cells to engage and illness to develop.

Self-reactive lymphocytes that have been exported can be activated through a variety of processes. The identification of cryptic determinants that are not well manifested in the bone marrow or thymus can improve in the periphery [34] during inflammation. Mutations, chemical changes, and posttranslational modifications all contribute to the identification of new self-antigens, or the various selfpeptides covalent cross-linking to form hybrid epitopes act as another trigger of immune response [35,36]. Molecular mimicry can activate nontolerant cells when foreign antigens are sufficiently similar in sequence or structure to self-antigens [37,38]. Another way microbes might cause autoimmunity is by capturing viral antigens along with self-antigens by B-cells directing self-antigens presentation, T-cell engagement, and illness [39]. Several cell types suppress adaptive and innate immune responses; among them, the FOXP3+ CD25+ CD4+ Treg cell subset is thought to be of major importance [40,41]. Treg cells can be produced in the thymus (natural or thymic T reg cells) or in the peripheral blood (induced Treg cells). Thymic Treg cell proliferation is restricted by IL-2 generation and thymic DCs' antigen presentation, as well as IL-2 feedback competition from mature T reg cells returning to the thymus [42,43]. T reg cells inhibit all main subsets of immunocytes, as evidenced by in vivo imaging, which demonstrated T reg cells clustering with activated self-reactive T-cells in secondary lymphoid tissue, and cell-to-cell linking interaction, which is required for the suppressive function [44]. The inhibition of DC maturation and function is caused by inhibitory chemicals (IL-10, CTLA-4, IL-35, and TGF), cytolysis, metabolic resistance, or alteration of DC maturation and function [45,46]. FOXP3 is necessary for Treg cell proliferation and function, and mutations in the FOXP3 gene cause IPEX syndrome (immunodysregulation, polyendocrinopathy, enteropathy) in humans and scurvy in mice. The certain types of superenhancers activation is required for Treg cell development, according to research [47]. Targeted PP2A modification in Treg cells results in a severe multiorgan autoimmune disease. PP2A is a serine threonine phosphatase which is critical in metabolic-checkpoint kinase complex mTORC1 pathway regulation [48].

The adaptive immune system has long been a focus of autoimmune disease research. The discovery that innate cells contain a wide range of sensors for self and foreign ligands has shifted the focus to the innate immune system, which is activated before adaptive responses are triggered [49–51]. As a result, autoimmune disease etiology has been linked to cytosolic and endosomal sensors that identify self and foreign nucleic acids. The category of endosomal sensors is exemplified by TLR3 (a type of double-stranded RNA), TLR7 and TLR8 (both RNA molecules with a single strand), and TLR9 (DNA). On the other hand, cytosolic sensors are exemplified by helicases RIG-I (which is an uncapped 5′-triphosphate RNA and MDA5 for long double-stranded RNA), as well as multiple DNA sensors, the most important of which appears to be the cGAS-cGAMP-STING pathway [52,53]. Proinflammatory cytokines (IL-1, IL-6, IL-12, and TNF) and Type I interferons are produced in response to those sensors' responses.

The microbiota, a population of bacteria that live in mutually beneficial coexistence with their hosts on mucosal surfaces and on the skin, influences many physiological responses, ranging from organism evolution, longevity, metabolism to immune system maturation and functioning. According to the findings, changes in this ecosystem, known as "dysbiosis," can lead to a variety of clinical illnesses, including autoimmune disorders that influence not only the gut, the microbiota's most important niche, but also a number of distant organs [54,55]. The earliest IBDs to be linked to dysbiosis were ulcerative colitis and Crohn's disease. Initial studies found significant taxonomic changes in the gut microbiota of the population suffering from these diseases, including decreases in the virulent Bacteroides and Clostridia. Clostridia clusters IV, XVIII, and XIVa break down dietary fibers to produce simpler fatty acids, primarily butyrate possessing antiinflammatory characteristics, promoting peripheral T reg cell growth, and are necessary nutrients for colonocytes [56–58]. Microbiota complex change have been linked to the etiology of T1D in both nonobese diabetic humans and mice. Between seroconversion and diagnosis, studies have discovered declines in butyrate-producing bacteria and microbiota diversity [59].

Only about 2% of the mammalian genome codes for cellular proteins, while the rest is transcribed as noncoding RNA, including long noncoding RNAs (lncRNAs), with 200 nucleotides or more and microRNAs (miRNAs) with 18–23 nucleotides, which have significant effects on both the innate and adaptive immune systems. lncRNAs are cell-specific RNAs that function through interaction with proteins, DNA, or RNA, whereas miRNAs attach to their mRNA targets and silence genes mostly through transcript destruction and translational repression [60–62].

3 Autoimmunity and inflammation: Role of A20

Because of A20 ubiquitin-regulatory actions and susceptibility gene designation for inflammatory disease by genome-wide association studies, A20 has recently gained a lot of attention (GWASs). Its been known for a long time as an antiapoptotic signaling protein and an inhibitor of nuclear factor NF-kB. A20 is a key gatekeeper in tissue homeostasis, as well as new findings provide insight on the physiological and molecular mechanisms of controlling inflammation by A20 through modulating signaling pathways. The molecular level mechanisms through which A20 modulates its numerous functions are yet unknown and are the matter of much research. A20's capability to modulate ubiquitin-dependent signaling pathways has proved crucial to a number of its physiological functions. NF-kB signaling pathways are regulated by several proteins, including A20; in addition ubiquitination may restrict these actions. The discovery of a ubiquitin-editing enzyme, i.e., A20 with a carboxyterminal zinc finger (ZnF) domain which supports E3 ubiquitin ligase activity and an amino-terminal deubiquitinating (DUB) activity driven by its ovarian tumor (OTU) domain, was the first evidence of A20's involvement in ubiquitin-dependent signaling [63,64].

A20's first deubiquitinase substrate was revealed to be receptor interacting protein (RIP)1. The E3 ubiquitin ligases cellular inhibitor of apoptosis protein (cIAP)1 and 2 polyubiquitinate RIP1 at lysine63 in response to TNF receptor (TNFR) activation (K63). A20 blocks RIP1 from interacting with the NF-kB key modulator by removing these K63-linked polyubiquitin chains (NEMO). A20 then targets RIP1 for proteasomal degradation by attaching K48-linked polyubiquitin chains to it. The sequential ubiquitin and deubiquitination-mediated degradation of RIP165 by A20 inhibits TNF-induced NF-kB activation. TLR4 and nucleotide-binding oligomerization domain-containing protein 2 (NOD2) can inhibit NF-kB activity by deubiquitinating TNF receptor-associated factor (TRAF)6 and RIP2, respectively [65,66]. It has been demonstrated to decrease feedback of the IL-17 receptor signaling crescade by deleting polyubiquitin chains linked to K63 from TRAF6. A20 also acts as a DUB for K63-polyubiquitinated mucosa-associated lymphoid tissue lymphoma translocation protein (MALT)1, a scaffolding protein implicated in NF-kB activation downstream of T- and B-cell antigen receptors, inhibiting T- and B-cell-induced NF-kB signaling

[67]. In addition to its function as a regulator of NF-kB signaling, A20 acts as an apoptotic inhibitor protein in a range of cells. These processes include ubiquitin-dependent pathways. Adaptor proteins, which compose the death-inducing signaling complex, help death receptors cause apoptosis (DISC). A20 was identified to be a component of the DISC, with possible physical interaction with caspase-8 [68].

Caspase-8 is polyubiquitinated by a cullin3-based E3 ligase during the induction of apoptosis by stimulation of the TNF-related apoptosis-inducing ligand (TRAIL) death receptor. In hyperexpression studies, A20 suppressed apoptotic signaling via deubiquitination and caspase-8 inhibition, indicating that A20 suppresses apoptotic signaling via deubiquitination and caspase-8 inhibition. A20 is also known to enhance K63-linked polyubiquitination of RIP1 via unknown ZnF4-dependent pathways. This permits RIP1 to bind to the protease domain of caspase-8, limiting TRAIL-induced apoptosis by suppressing caspase-8 dimerization and cleavage. A separate finding discovered that A20 suppresses TNF-mediated apoptosis through proteasomal degradation of the upstream apoptosis signal-regulating kinase (ASK)1, hence decreasing c-Jun N-terminal kinase (JNK) [69,70].

4 Inflammation and autoimmunity: Granulocyte colony-stimulating factor (G-CSF) role

G-CSF is yet another type of CSF that should be investigated as a potential pharmacological target in inflammatory conditions, despite the fact that there is limited data on its dilution in inflammation models and no reports of clinical studies commencing. G-CSF, on the other hand, is difficult to detect in the bloodstream, yet its levels rise substantially in stressful situations like illness [71]. Because the G-CSF receptor is expressed more prominently on neutrophils than on other types of cells, G-CSF is most likely to play a role in inflammation and autoimmune disorders involving neutrophils. The structure of the G-CSF receptor is similar to that of the type I cytokine receptors. In an indeterminate complex, each G-CSF molecule binds to both receptors. Various nonreceptor kinases are activated when the extracellular region of the G-CSF receptor is ligated, resulting in the activation of numerous signaling cascades. Neutropenia is shown in G-CSF-deficient mice, suggesting that G-CSF, like GM-CSF, may play a role in controlling neutrophil numbers and activity during inflammation. G-CSF is a component of the 'CSF network' idea, and it may be produced in vitro by stimulating a variety of cell types with stimuli similar to those that cause GM-CSF to be produced. It was discovered that giving mice G-CSF aggravated collagen-induced arthritis. G-CSF-deficient mice were resistant to inflammatory arthritis, and a neutralizing antibody specific for G-CSF reduced collagen-induced arthritis in mice. The ability to establish protocols to suppress a specific disease without jeopardizing the defense system of the host by bringing about excessive neutropenia or stopping the production of essential neutrophil mediators would be a critical question in any clinical research of G-CSF blocking. Apart from the usual role of G-CSF to restore neutrophil counts and mobilize hematopoietic stem cells after chemotherapy, a number of current studies have shown that G-CSF treatment can help stroke patients and those with dementia [72,73].

5 Conclusions

An efficient immune system is capable of instant recognition and removal of foreign antigens through multiple mechanisms. Autoimmune disorders like inflammation, systemic lupus erythematosus, inflammatory bowel disease, gout, rheumatoid arthritis, and diabetes arise out of abnormal T-cell mediation. This chapter has discussed the different aspects of autoimmunity and inflammation with special emphasis on the role of some mediators.

References

[1] M.S. Anderson, M.A. Su, AIRE expands: new roles in immune tolerance and beyond, Nat. Rev. Immunol. 16 (4) (2016) 247–258, https://doi.org/10.1038/nri.2016.9.

[2] M.S. Anderson, J.L. Casanova, More than meets the eye: monogenic autoimmunity strikes again, Immunity 42 (6) (2015) 986–988, https://doi.org/10.1016/j.immuni.2015.06.004.

[3] S.A. Apostolidis, N. Rodríguez-Rodríguez, A. Suárez-Fueyo, N. Dioufa, E. Ozcan, J.C. Crispín, M.G. Tsokos, G.C. Tsokos, Phosphatase PP2A is requisite for the function of regulatory T cells, Nat. Immunol. 17 (5) (2016) 556–564, https://doi.org/10.1038/ni.3390.

[4] M.K. Atianand, K.A. Fitzgerald, Long non-coding rnas and control of gene expression in the immune system, Trends Mol. Med. 20 (11) (2014) 623–631, https://doi.org/10.1016/j.molmed.2014.09.002.

[5] K. Bansal, H. Yoshida, C. Benoist, D. Mathis, The transcriptional regulator Aire binds to and activates super-enhancers, Nat. Immunol. 18 (3) (2017) 263–273, https://doi.org/10.1038/ni.3675.

[6] G.N. Barber, STING-dependent cytosolic DNA sensing pathways, Trends Immunol. 35 (2) (2014) 88–93, https://doi.org/10.1016/j.it.2013.10.010.

[7] A.C. Bellail, J.J. Olson, X. Yang, Z.J. Chen, C. Hao, A20 ubiquitin ligase-mediated polyubiquitination of RIP1 inhibits caspase-8 cleavage and TRAIL-induced apoptosis in glioblastoma, Cancer Discov. 2 (2) (2012) 140–155, https://doi.org/10.1158/2159-8290.CD-11-0172.

[8] M.J.M. Bertrand, S. Milutinovic, K.M. Dickson, W.C. Ho, A. Boudreault, J. Durkin, J.W. Gillard, J.B. Jaquith, S.J. Morris, P.A. Barker, cIAP1 and cIAP2 facilitate cancer cell survival by functioning as E3 ligases that promote RIP1 ubiquitination, Mol. Cell 30 (6) (2008) 689–700, https://doi.org/10.1016/j.molcel.2008.05.014.

[9] A.L. Blasius, B. Beutler, Intracellular toll-like receptors, Immunity 32 (3) (2010) 305–315, https://doi.org/10.1016/j.immuni.2010.03.012.

[10] D.L. Boone, E.E. Turer, E.G. Lee, R.C. Ahmad, M.T. Wheeler, C. Tsui, P. Hurley, M. Chien, S. Chai, O. Hitotsumatsu, E. McNally, C. Pickart, A. Ma, The ubiquitin-modifying enzyme A20 is required for termination of Toll-like receptor responses, Nat. Immunol. 5 (10) (2004) 1052–1060, https://doi.org/10.1038/ni1110.

[11] C. Bouneaud, P. Kourilsky, P. Bousso, Impact of negative selection on the T cell repertoire reactive to a self-peptide: a large fraction of T cell clones escapes clonal deletion, Immunity 13 (6) (2000) 829–840, https://doi.org/10.1016/S1074-7613(00)00080-7.

[12] S. Ceeraz, P.A. Sergent, S.F. Plummer, A.R. Schned, D. Pechenick, C.M. Burns, R.J. Noelle, VISTA deficiency accelerates the development of fatal murine lupus nephritis, Arthritis Rheum. 69 (4) (2017) 814–825, https://doi.org/10.1002/art.40020.

[13] Q. Chen, L. Sun, Z.J. Chen, Regulation and function of the cGAS-STING pathway of cytosolic DNA sensing, Nat. Immunol. 17 (10) (2016) 1142–1149, https://doi.org/10.1038/ni.3558.

[14] J.M. Chiller, G.S. Habicht, W.O. Weigle, Cellular sites of immunologic unresponsiveness, Proc. Natl. Acad. Sci. U. S. A. 65 (3) (1970) 551–556, https://doi.org/10.1073/pnas.65.3.551.

[15] T. Delong, T.A. Wiles, R.L. Baker, B. Bradley, G. Barbour, R. Reisdorph, M. Armstrong, R.L. Powell, N. Reisdorph, N. Kumar, C.M. Elso, M. DeNicola, R. Bottino, A.C. Powers, D.M. Harlan, S.C. Kent, S.I. Mannering, K. Haskins, Pathogenic CD4 T cells in type 1 diabetes recognize epitopes formed by peptide fusion, Science 351 (6274) (2016) 711–714, https://doi.org/10.1126/science.aad2791.

[16] H.A. Doyle, M.J. Mamula, Autoantigenesis: the evolution of protein modifications in autoimmune disease, Curr. Opin. Immunol. 24 (1) (2012) 112–118, https://doi.org/10.1016/j.coi.2011.12.003.

[17] M. Düwel, V. Welteke, A. Oeckinghaus, M. Baens, B. Kloo, U. Ferch, B.G. Darnay, J. Ruland, P. Marynen, D. Krappmann, A20 negatively regulates T cell receptor signaling to NF-κB by cleaving Malt1 ubiquitin chains, J. Immunol. 182 (12) (2009) 7718–7728, https://doi.org/10.4049/jimmunol.0803313.

[18] C.G. Fathman, N.B. Lineberry, Molecular mechanisms of CD4+ T-cell anergy, Nat. Rev. Immunol. 7 (8) (2007) 599–609, https://doi.org/10.1038/nri2131.

[19] T.J. Friesen, Q. Ji, P.J. Fink, Recent thymic emigrants are tolerized in the absence of inflammation, J. Exp. Med. 213 (6) (2016) 913–920, https://doi.org/10.1084/jem.20151990.

[20] Y. Furusawa, Y. Obata, S. Fukuda, T.A. Endo, G. Nakato, D. Takahashi, Y. Nakanishi, C. Uetake, K. Kato, T. Kato, M. Takahashi, N.N. Fukuda, S. Murakami, E. Miyauchi, S. Hino, K. Atarashi, S. Onawa, Y. Fujimura, T. Lockett, H. Ohno, Commensal microbe-derived butyrate induces the differentiation of colonic regulatory T cells, Nature 504 (7480) (2013) 446–450, https://doi.org/10.1038/nature12721.

[21] A. Getahun, N.A. Beavers, S.R. Larson, M.J. Shlomchik, J.C. Cambier, Continuous inhibitory signaling by both SHP-1 and SHIP-1 pathways is required to maintain unresponsiveness of anergic B cells, J. Exp. Med. 213 (5) (2016) 751–769, https://doi.org/10.1084/jem.20150537.

[22] M. Gutierrez-Arcelus, S.S. Rich, S. Raychaudhuri, Autoimmune diseases-connecting risk alleles with molecular traits of the immune system, Nat. Rev. Genet. 17 (3) (2016) 160–174, https://doi.org/10.1038/nrg.2015.33.

[23] O. Hitotsumatsu, R.C. Ahmad, R. Tavares, M. Wang, D. Philpott, E.E. Turer, B.L. Lee, N. Shiffin, R. Advincula, B.A. Malynn, C. Werts, A. Ma, The ubiquitin-editing enzyme A20 restricts nucleotide-binding oligomerization domain containing 2-triggered signals, Immunity 28 (3) (2008) 381–390, https://doi.org/10.1016/j.immuni.2008.02.002.

[24] K. Honda, D.R. Littman, The microbiota in adaptive immune homeostasis and disease, Nature 535 (7610) (2016) 75–84, https://doi.org/10.1038/nature18848.

[25] K.A. Hunt, V. Mistry, N.A. Bockett, T. Ahmad, M. Ban, J.N. Barker, J.C. Barrett, H. Blackburn, O. Brand, O. Burren, F. Capon, A. Compston, S.C.L. Gough, L. Jostins, Y. Kong, J.C. Lee, M. Lek, D.G. MacArthur, J.C. Mansfield, et al., Negligible impact of rare autoimmune-locus coding-region variants on missing heritability, Nature 498 (7453) (2013) 232–235, https://doi.org/10.1038/nature12170.

[26] K. Iwai, Diverse ubiquitin signaling in NF-κB activation, Trends Cell Biol. 22 (7) (2012) 355–364, https://doi.org/10.1016/j.tcb.2012.04.001.

[27] A. Iwasaki, R. Medzhitov, Control of adaptive immunity by the innate immune system, Nat. Immunol. 16 (4) (2015) 343–353, https://doi.org/10.1038/ni.3123.

[28] Z. Jin, Y. Li, R. Pitti, D. Lawrence, V.C. Pham, J.R. Lill, A. Ashkenazi, Cullin3-based polyubiquitination and p62-dependent aggregation of caspase-8 mediate extrinsic apoptosis signaling, Cell 137 (4) (2009) 721–735, https://doi.org/10.1016/j.cell.2009.03.015.

[29] L.A. Kalekar, S.E. Schmiel, S.L. Nandiwada, W.Y. Lam, L.O. Barsness, N. Zhang, G.L. Stritesky, D. Malhotra, K.E. Pauken, J.L. Linehan, M.G. O'Sullivan, B.T. Fife, K.A. Hogquist, M.K. Jenkins, D.L. Mueller, CD4+ T cell anergy prevents autoimmunity and generates regulatory T cell precursors, Nat. Immunol. 17 (3) (2016) 304–314, https://doi.org/10.1038/ni.3331.

[30] Y. Kitagawa, N. Ohkura, Y. Kidani, A. Vandenbon, K. Hirota, R. Kawakami, K. Yasuda, D. Motooka, S. Nakamura, M. Kondo, I. Taniuchi, T. Kohwi-Shigematsu, S. Sakaguchi, Guidance of regulatory T cell development by Satb1-dependent super-enhancer establishment, Nat. Immunol. 18 (2) (2017) 173–183, https://doi.org/10.1038/ni.3646.

[31] Y.T. Koh, J.C. Scatizzi, J.D. Gahan, B.R. Lawson, R. Baccala, K.M. Pollard, B.A. Beutler, A.N. Theofilopoulos, D.H. Kono, Role of nucleic acid-sensing TLRs in diverse autoantibody specificities and anti-nuclear antibody-producing B cells, J. Immunol. 190 (10) (2013) 4982–4990, https://doi.org/10.4049/jimmunol.1202986.

[32] A. Koh, F. De Vadder, P. Kovatcheva-Datchary, F. Bäckhed, From dietary fiber to host physiology: short-chain fatty acids as key bacterial metabolites, Cell 165 (6) (2016) 1332–1345, https://doi.org/10.1016/j.cell.2016.05.041.

[33] C. Lamagna, Y. Hu, A.L. DeFranco, C.A. Lowell, B cell-specific loss of lyn kinase leads to autoimmunity, J. Immunol. 192 (3) (2014) 919–928, https://doi.org/10.4049/jimmunol.1301979.

[34] K.E. Lawlor, I.K. Campbell, D. Metcalf, K. O'Donnell, A. Van Nieuwenhuijze, A.W. Roberts, I.P. Wicks, Critical role for granulocyte colony stimulating factor in inflammatory arthritis, Proc. Natl. Acad. Sci. U. S. A. 101 (31) (2004) 11398–11403, https://doi.org/10.1073/pnas.0404328101.

[35] F.P. Legoux, J.B. Lim, A.W. Cauley, S. Dikiy, J. Ertelt, T.J. Mariani, T. Sparwasser, S.S. Way, J.J. Moon, CD4+ T cell tolerance to tissue-restricted self antigens is mediated by antigen-specific regulatory T cells rather than deletion, Immunity 43 (5) (2015) 896–908, https://doi.org/10.1016/j.immuni.2015.10.011.

[36] Y. Lei, A.M. Ripen, N. Ishimaru, I. Ohigashi, T. Nagasawa, L.T. Jeker, M.R. Bösl, G.A. Holländer, Y. Hayashi, R. De Waal Malefyt, T. Nitta, Y. Takahama, Aire-dependent production of XCL1 mediates medullary accumulation of thymic dendritic cells and contributes to

regulatory T cell development, J. Exp. Med. 208 (2) (2011) 383–394, https://doi.org/10.1084/jem.20102327.

[37] M.O. Li, A.Y. Rudensky, T cell receptor signalling in the control of regulatory T cell differentiation and function, Nat. Rev. Immunol. 16 (4) (2016) 220–233, https://doi.org/10.1038/nri.2016.26.

[38] Z. Liu, M.Y. Gerner, N. Van Panhuys, A.G. Levine, A.Y. Rudensky, R.N. Germain, Immune homeostasis enforced by co-localized effector and regulatory T cells, Nature 528 (7581) (2015) 225–230, https://doi.org/10.1038/nature16169.

[39] M.S. MacAuley, P.R. Crocker, J.C. Paulson, Siglec-mediated regulation of immune cell function in disease, Nat. Rev. Immunol. 14 (10) (2014) 653–666, https://doi.org/10.1038/nri3737.

[40] D. Malhotra, J.L. Linehan, T. Dileepan, Y.J. Lee, W.E. Purtha, J.V. Lu, R.W. Nelson, B.T. Fife, H.T. Orr, M.S. Anderson, K.A. Hogquist, M.K. Jenkins, Tolerance is established in polyclonal CD4 + T cells by distinct mechanisms, according to self-peptide expression patterns, Nat. Immunol. 17 (2) (2016) 187–195, https://doi.org/10.1038/ni.3327.

[41] D. Mathis, C. Benoist, Aire, Annu. Rev. Immunol. 27 (2009) 287–312, https://doi.org/10.1146/annurev.immunol.25.022106.141532.

[42] E. Meffre, The establishment of early B cell tolerance in humans: lessons from primary immunodeficiency diseases, Ann. N. Y. Acad. Sci. 1246 (1) (2011) 1–10, https://doi.org/10.1111/j.1749-6632.2011.06347.x.

[43] A. Mehta, D. Baltimore, MicroRNAs as regulatory elements in immune system logic, Nat. Rev. Immunol. 16 (5) (2016) 279–294, https://doi.org/10.1038/nri.2016.40.

[44] F. Melchers, A.R. Rolink, B cell tolerance—How to make it and how to break it, Curr. Top. Microbiol. Immunol. 305 (2006) 1–23, https://doi.org/10.1007/3-540-29714-6_1.

[45] H. Morikawa, S. Sakaguchi, Genetic and epigenetic basis of Treg cell development and function: from a FoxP3-centered view to an epigenome-defined view of natural Treg cells, Immunol. Rev. 259 (1) (2014) 192–205, https://doi.org/10.1111/imr.12174.

[46] D. Nemazee, Mechanisms of central tolerance for B cells, Nat. Rev. Immunol. 17 (5) (2017) 281–294, https://doi.org/10.1038/nri.2017.19.

[47] R. Newton, B. Priyadharshini, L.A. Turka, Immunometabolism of regulatory T cells, Nat. Immunol. 17 (6) (2016) 618–625, https://doi.org/10.1038/ni.3466.

[48] B.E. Oftedal, A. Hellesen, M.M. Erichsen, E. Bratland, A. Vardi, J. Perheentupa, E.H. Kemp, T. Fiskerstrand, M.K. Viken, A.P. Weetman, S.J. Fleishman, S. Banka, W.G. Newman, W.A.C. Sewell, L.S. Sozaeva, T. Zayats, K. Haugarvoll, E.M. Orlova, J. Haavik, et al., Dominant mutations in the autoimmune regulator AIRE are associated with common organ-specific autoimmune diseases, Immunity 42 (6) (2015) 1185–1196, https://doi.org/10.1016/j.immuni.2015.04.021.

[49] T. Okazaki, S. Chikuma, Y. Iwai, S. Fagarasan, T. Honjo, A rheostat for immune responses: the unique properties of PD-1 and their advantages for clinical application, Nat. Immunol. 14 (12) (2013) 1212–1218, https://doi.org/10.1038/ni.2762.

[50] M.B.A. Oldstone, Molecular mimicry and autoimmune disease, Cell 50 (6) (1987) 819–820, https://doi.org/10.1016/0092-8674(87)90507-1.

[51] H. Park, A.B. Bourla, D.L. Kastner, R.A. Colbert, R.M. Siegel, Lighting the fires within: the cell biology of autoinflammatory diseases, Nat. Rev. Immunol. 12 (8) (2012) 570–580, https://doi.org/10.1038/nri3261.

[52] A.M. Paterson, A.H. Sharpe, Taming tissue-specific T cells: CTLA-4 reins in self-reactive T cells, Nat. Immunol. 11 (2) (2010) 109–111, https://doi.org/10.1038/ni0210-109.

[53] A. Pincetic, S. Bournazos, D.J. Dilillo, J. Maamary, T.T. Wang, R. Dahan, B.M. Fiebiger, J.V. Ravetch, Type I and type II Fc receptors regulate innate and adaptive immunity, Nat. Immunol. 15 (8) (2014) 707–716, https://doi.org/10.1038/ni.2939.

[54] S. Prasad, S.R. Starck, N. Shastri, Presentation of cryptic peptides by MHC class I is enhanced by inflammatory stimuli, J. Immunol. 197 (8) (2016) 2981–2991, https://doi.org/10.4049/jimmunol.1502045.

[55] C. Procaccini, F. Carbone, D. Di Silvestre, F. Brambilla, V. De Rosa, M. Galgani, D. Faicchia, G. Marone, D. Tramontano, M. Corona, C. Alviggi, A. Porcellini, A. La Cava, P. Mauri, G. Matarese, The proteomic landscape of human ex vivo regulatory and conventional T cells reveals specific metabolic requirements, Immunity 44 (2) (2016) 406–421, https://doi.org/10.1016/j.immuni.2016.01.028.

[56] A.W. Roberts, G-CSF: a key regulator of neutrophil production, but that's not all! Growth Factors 23 (1) (2005) 33–41, https://doi.org/10.1080/08977190500055836.

[57] W.E. Ruff, M.A. Kriegel, Autoimmune host-microbiota interactions at barrier sites and beyond, Trends Mol. Med. 21 (4) (2015) 233–244, https://doi.org/10.1016/j.molmed.2015.02.006.

[58] N.S.R. Sanderson, M. Zimmermann, L. Eilinger, C. Gubser, N. Schaeren-Wiemers, R.L.P. Lindberg, S.K. Dougan, H.L. Ploegh, L. Kappos, T. Derfuss, Cocapture of cognate and bystander antigens can activate autoreactive B cells, Proc. Natl. Acad. Sci. U. S. A. 114 (4) (2017) 734–739, https://doi.org/10.1073/pnas.1614472114.

[59] A.T. Satpathy, H.Y. Chang, Long noncoding RNA in hematopoiesis and immunity, Immunity 42 (5) (2015) 792–804, https://doi.org/10.1016/j.immuni.2015.05.004.

[60] H. Schmitt, S. Sell, J. Koch, M. Seefried, S. Sonnewald, C. Daniel, T. H. Winkler, L. Nitschke, Siglec-H protects from virus-triggered severe systemic autoimmunity, J. Exp. Med. 213 (8) (2016) 1627–1644, https://doi.org/10.1084/jem.20160189.

[61] P.M. Smith, M.R. Howitt, N. Panikov, M. Michaud, C.A. Gallini, M. Bohlooly-Y, J.N. Glickman, W.S. Garrett, The microbial metabolites, short-chain fatty acids, regulate colonic T reg cell homeostasis, Science 341 (6145) (2013) 569–573, https://doi.org/10.1126/science.1241165.

[62] I. Solaroglu, V. Jadhav, J.H. Zhang, Neuroprotective effect of granulocyte-colony stimulating factor, Front. Biosci. 12 (2) (2007) 712–724, https://doi.org/10.2741/2095.

[63] O. Takeuchi, S. Akira, Pattern Recognition Receptors and Inflammation, Cell 140 (6) (2010) 805–820, https://doi.org/10.1016/j.cell.2010.01.022.

[64] A.N. Theofilopoulos, D.H. Kono, R. Baccala, The multiple pathways to autoimmunity, Nat. Immunol. 18 (7) (2017) 716–724, https://doi.org/10.1038/ni.3731.

[65] H. Wardemann, S. Yurasov, A. Schaefer, J.W. Young, E. Meffre, M. C. Nussenzweig, Predominant autoantibody production by early human B cell precursors, Science 301 (5638) (2003) 1374–1377, https://doi.org/10.1126/science.1086907.

[66] B.M. Weist, N. Kurd, J. Boussier, S.W. Chan, E.A. Robey, Thymic regulatory T cell niche size is dictated by limiting IL-2 from antigen-bearing dendritic cells and feedback competition, Nat. Immunol. 16 (6) (2015) 635–641, https://doi.org/10.1038/ni.3171.

[67] I.E. Wertz, K.M. O'Rourke, H. Zhou, M. Eby, L. Aravind, S. Seshagiri, P. Wu, C. Wiesmann, R. Baker, D.L. Boone, A. Ma, E.V. Koonin, V.M. Dixit, De-ubiquitination and ubiquitin ligase domains of A20 downregulate NF-κB signalling, Nature 430 (7000) (2004) 694–699, https://doi.org/10.1038/nature02794.

[68] M. Won, K.A. Park, H.S. Byun, K.C. Sohn, Y.R. Kim, J. Jeon, J.H. Hong, J. Park, J.H. Seok, J.M. Kim, W.H. Yoon, I.S. Jang, H.M. Shen, Z.G. Liu, G.M. Hur, Novel anti-apoptotic mechanism of A20 through targeting ASK1 to suppress TNF-induced JNK activation, Cell Death Differ. 17 (12) (2010) 1830–1841, https://doi.org/10.1038/cdd.2010.47.

[69] K.W. Wucherpfennig, J.L. Strominger, Molecular mimicry in T cell-mediated autoimmunity: viral peptides activate human T cell clones specific for myelin basic protein, Cell 80 (5) (1995) 695–705, https://doi.org/10.1016/0092-8674(95)90348-8.

[70] T. Yamano, J. Nedjic, M. Hinterberger, M. Steinert, S. Koser, S. Pinto, N. Gerdes, E. Lutgens, N. Ishimaru, M. Busslinger, B. Brors, B. Kyewski, L. Klein, Thymic B cells are licensed to present self antigens for central T cell tolerance induction, Immunity 42 (6) (2015) 1048–1061, https://doi.org/10.1016/j.immuni.2015.05.013.

[71] Y. Yarkoni, A. Getahun, J.C. Cambier, Molecular underpinning of B-cell anergy, Immunol. Rev. 237 (1) (2010) 249–263, https://doi.org/10.1111/j.1600-065X.2010.00936.x.

[72] W. Yu, N. Jiang, P.J.R. Ebert, B.A. Kidd, S. Müller, P.J. Lund, J. Juang, K. Adachi, T. Tse, M.E. Birnbaum, E.W. Newell, D.M. Wilson, G.M. Grotenberg, S. Valitutti, S.R. Quake, M.M. Davis, Clonal deletion prunes but does not eliminate self-specific αβ CD8 + T lymphocytes, Immunity 42 (5) (2015) 929–941, https://doi.org/10.1016/j.immuni.2015.05.001.

[73] J. Zikherman, R. Parameswaran, A. Weiss, Endogenous antigen tunes the responsiveness of naive B cells but not T cells, Nature 489 (7414) (2012) 160–164, https://doi.org/10.1038/nature11311.

Chapter 3

Regulatory pathways of inflammation

Jyoti Upadhyay[a], Manvi Suri[a], Jeevan Patra[a], Nidhi Tiwari[b], Mohd Nazam Ansari[c], and Neeraj Mahindroo[d]

[a]School of Health Sciences and Technology, University of Petroleum and Energy Studies, Dehradun, Uttarakhand, India, [b]Institute of Nuclear Medicine and Allied Sciences, Defence Research and Development Organization, New Delhi, Delhi, India, [c]Department of Pharmacology & Toxicology, College of Pharmacy, Prince Sattam Bin Abdulaziz University, Al-Kharj, Saudi Arabia, [d]School of Pharmacy, MIT World Peace University, Pune, Maharashtra, India

1 Introduction

The process of inflammation is triggered by a number of factors like toxicants, degraded cells, and pathogens [1]. Inflammation may be acute or chronic and is characterized by an individual body's reaction to infection, injury, trauma, and other insults. Inflammatory cells reaction and vascular wall responses are two main features that define inflammations, and their actions are facilitated by plasma proteins in the circulation and numerous substances produced locally by inflammatory cells or blood vessel walls [2]. The inflammation process happens because of both infectious and noninfectious agents that give signals to leukocytes to produce cytokines and further stimulates intracellular inflammatory signaling pathways like MAPKs (mitogen-activated protein kinases), NF-κB (nuclear factor kappa B), and JAK-STAT (Janus kinase-signal transducer and activator of transcription) [1]. Although inflammation is a protective response, it can also be damaging, such as hypersensitivity reactions, and can be life-threatening at times. Acute inflammation is an early onset effect occurring for a shorter duration of time (i.e., from minutes to days) and causes cellular edema and emigration of neutrophils. Chronic inflammation is a later onset effect occurring for a longer period (i.e., from weeks to years) that causes fibrosis and proliferation of blood vessels. Inflammation can be identified by five classic clinical signs, i.e., warmth, erythema, edema, pain, and loss of functions [2].

2 Cytokine response to inflammation

Cytokines are small proteins (molecular weight range 4–8000 Da), also known as monokines and lymphokines, to represent their cellular origin. The word cytokines is the best description as it describes cells are produced by all nucleated cells. They are principally involved in host cell response to any infection or disease. Unlike hormones, which are expressed in response to homeostasis in our daily life cycle, the cytokine genes are expressed only in response to noxious stimuli. Thus, it becomes clear that cytokine gene expression is similar to cell stressors and can be triggered by noxious agents like ultraviolet rays, hyperosmolarity, heat shock, or MAPKs activation by foreign surface adherence. MAPKs activation phosphorylates transcription factors for the expression of genes. So during injury or infection, the MAPK pathway is also used by inflammatory products for inducing gene expression of cytokines [3]. Currently, there are 18 cytokines known by the name interleukins (IL). Tumor necrosis factors (TNF) are other cytokines that retained their biological activity. Some cytokines are proinflammatory agents that act directly by promoting inflammation whereas cytokines, which are antiinflammatory, suppress the proinflammatory cytokines. IL-4, 10, and 13 activate B-lymphocytes. However, they also act as antiinflammatory agents act by inhibiting gene expression for proinflammatory cytokines like TNF, IL-1, and chemokines. Another example of cytokine is IF-ϒ active against viral infection. It is also a stimulator of the cytotoxic T cell pathway. However, IF-ϒ is known as proinflammatory cytokines as it induces nitric oxide (NO) and enhances TNF activity [3,4].

3 Proinflammatory and antiinflammatory cytokines

Cytokines primarily function by two mechanisms; either they induce inflammation (proinflammatory) or suppress inflammation (antiinflammatory). This concept is generally built on the coding of genes responsible for the production of mediators upregulated in inflammation. Examples of genes responsible for proinflammation include type II phospholipase A2 (PLA2), inducible nitrogen oxide (NO) synthase, and cyclooxygenase-2 (COX-2). These proinflammatory genes code for enzymes that increase the generation of prostaglandins (PGs), platelet-activating factor (PAF), NO, and leukotrienes (LTs). Chemokines are another category of proinflammatory cytokines, which are

Recent Developments in Anti-Inflammatory Therapy. https://doi.org/10.1016/B978-0-323-99988-5.00018-8

small peptides (molecular weight 8000 Da), that smooth the leukocyte passage from the systemic circulation into the body tissues. IL-8, a prototype chemokine, is a neutrophil attractant. It also causes neutrophils degranulation and tissue damage. TNF and IL-1 are activators of adhesion molecules in the endothelium region essential for leukocytes' adhesion at the surface of the endothelium before moving into the tissues. Thus, proinflammatory cytokine-associated inflammation is a series of reactions involving the formation of gene products not observed in healthy individuals. TNF and IL-1 are produced at the inflammatory site and the severity of inflammation is determined by the cytokines level. Pain at the site of inflammation is caused by elevated levels of prostaglandins (PGE2) which are stimulated by TNF and IL-1 [4]. IL-1 lowers the pain threshold due to increased production of PGE2. Some studies reported that when IL-1 is injected into healthy subjects, it induces fever, myalgias, headache, and arthralgia that is cured by administering COX-2 inhibitors. The important function of IL-1 is the initiation of COX-2 and PLA2 gene expression. It causes the initiation of transcription of COX-2 and has a lesser effect on the COX-1 enzyme production. Moreover, if the reaction is triggered, there is an elevation of COX-2 production. As a result, PGE2 is produced on a larger scale in cells when activated by IL-1. That is why most of the biological events of IL-1 are due to the elevated level of PGE2 [5]. Primarily, two types of IL-1 receptor proteins are present, i.e., IL-1 receptor (IL-1Rs) and IL-1 receptor accessory protein (IL-1R-AcP) [6,7]. The extracellular domains of these two receptors are the Ig member's superfamily and consisted of 3 Ig G domains sharing significant homology. Two distinct IL-1 genes have been identified, i.e., type I IL-1RI and type II IL-1RII situated on the long arm of chromosome 2 [8]. There are 50 IL receptors per cell that have been identified and a signal transduction of IL-1 was detected in cells expressing 10-IL type I receptors per cell. Remarkably, the cytosolic domain of type I IL-1 receptors has 45% homology in amino acid sequence with the cytosolic domain of the Toll 6 gene of Drosophila [8]. Toll-like receptors (TLRs) are mammalian receptors, which are transmembrane proteins. Endotoxin and peptidoglycan are the two ligands for these TLRs [9]. The type II IL-1 receptor consisted of a small cytosolic domain having 29 amino acids. They perform a function as a "decoy" molecule and are known as the "IL-1 Decoy" receptor, especially for IL-1β. IL-1β binds with this receptor with high affinity, thus preventing signal transduction of the Type I IL-1 receptor that makes this receptor (IL-1RII) a functionally negative receptor [10]. Fig. 1 represents the action of IL-1 which causes activation of signal transduction by binding with IL-1RI and the IL-1R-AcP receptor protein, whereas IL-1Ra (IL-1 receptor antagonist) causes signal transduction inhibition.

IL-1 when bind with the cell receptors within few minutes induces a cascade of biochemical events [11–14]. These are cell-specific biochemical events involving phosphorylation of enzyme proteins, activation of phosphatases within 5 min [15], and release of ceramides [16]. In some of the cells, IL-1 acts as a growth factor, and signal transduction includes serine or threonine phosphorylation of the MAP p42/44 [17]. MAPK 38, another member of the MAPK family, gets phosphorylated in fibroblasts [18] whereas p54aMAPK in hepatocytes [19]. Another biological effect produced by IL-1 in cells is the translocation of activating protein-1 (AP-1) and NF-kB [20]. Fig. 2 represents the functions of the IL receptor antagonist.

4 Regulation of innate immune system inflammatory response

Innate immunity includes the first line of defense against any pathogenic infection by distinguishing self and nonself components. It relies upon the pattern recognition receptors (PRRs) of the host communicated by immune cells like dendritic cells (DCs), macrophages to rapidly identify the signals from invading microbes or injured cells and respond to them. Pattern recognition receptors including TLRs, RLRs (retinoic acid-inducible gene I like receptors), and NLRs (nucleotide-binding domain and leucine-rich repeat-containing molecules), mediate PAMPs (pathogen-associated molecular pattern) [21]. This cellular recognition induces a series of intracellular signaling events that terminate in the initiation of transcriptional factors like AP-1 (activator protein-1), IRF (interferon regulatory protein), and NF-κB that stimulates several downstream genes encoding a wide range of chemokines, cytokines, interferons, complement factors, and antimicrobial peptides [22]. TLRs transduce downstream signaling with the help of the MyD88-dependent or -independent pathway. The TIR domain containing the adapter-inducing interferon-β (TRIF)-dependent pathway causes stimulation of the MAPK, NF-κB, and IRF pathway and produces proinflammatory cytokines and interferons [23–26]. The phagocyte activation through TLRs in innate immune response also activates Mst1-Mst2-Rac signals and promotes microbial killing [27].

RLR is the family of RNA helicases present in the cytoplasm is found to be important for virus recognition and plays an active role in regulating viral replication process and dissemination. The two important proteins that recognize viral dsRNA are RIG-I (retinoic acid-inducible gene-I) [28] and MDA5 (melanoma differentiation-associated protein-5) [29]. They also recruit CARDIF, an adaptor protein causing IRF activation and type I IFN production. Along with these RLRs, DNA sensors like AIM-2 (Absent in melanoma 2) [30]; cGAS (cGMP-AMP synthase

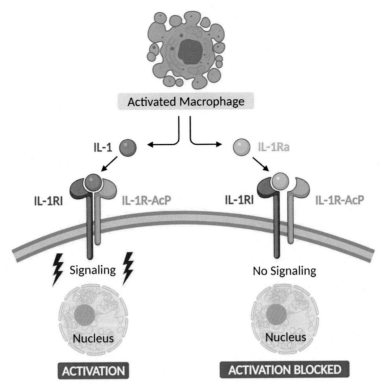

FIG. 1 The action of IL-1 and IL-1 Ra causing activation and inhibition of signal transduction.

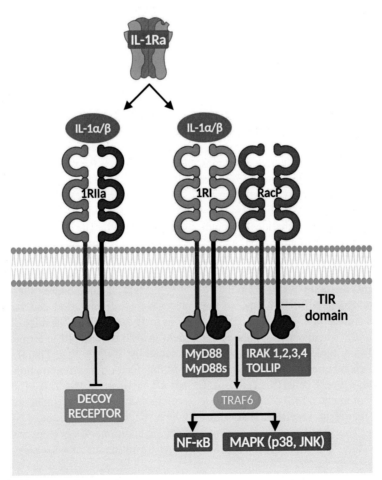

FIG. 2 Functions of the interleukin receptor-1 antagonist.

in the cytosol) [31]; DDX41 [32]; LRRFIP1 [33]; Rad50 [34]; DAI (DNA-dependent activator of IRFs), as well as RNA sensors IFIT1 (IFN-induced protein with tetratrico-peptide repeats 1), play a major role in activating antiviral immune responses, especially through the adaptor protein STING (stimulator of interferon genes) [35].

NLRs are intracellular PRR which includes CIITA (Class II major histocompatibility complex, trans-activator); NODs (nucleotide-binding oligomerization domains); IPAF (ICE protease-activating factor); NLRPs (LRR- and pyrin-domain (PYD)-containing protein) and NAIPs (neuronal apoptosis inhibitory protein) [36]. NOD 1 and 2 recognize muramyl dipeptide and meso-DAP (meso-diaminopimelic acid) of microbes and trigger host cell defense against microbial infection by activating the NF-κB and MAPK pathways. NOD 1 and 2 are also involved in recruiting ATG16L1 at the site of bacterial entrance in the plasma membrane and induce autophagy, a method critical for limiting bacterial invasion [37].

PRR signal activation is important for establishing anti-microbial host resistance and regulation of homeostasis at tissue level. Dysregulation of innate immune response can lead to inflammation and pathogenesis of various auto-immune disorders, cancer, inflammatory diseases, and so on. Therefore, regulations of the inflammatory pathways are required to achieve the best signal output, which effec-tively eliminates the invading bacteria, and to avoid harmful autoimmune diseases.

5 NF-κB pathway

NF-κB is a dimeric transcription factor produced by homo-/hetero-dimerization of proteins of the Rel family involving p50 and p60. Their activation mediates inflammation by gene regulation encoding for adhesion components, proin-flammatory cytokines, chemokines, inducible enzymes (like COX-2, NO synthase), and growth factors [38]. An extracellular event stimulates this pathway, most often by proinflammatory cytokines like IL-1 and TNF; stress; bac-terial components like LPS (lipopolysaccharides) through TLR. NF-κB performs a major role in inflammation. An ele-vated level of the NF-κB DNA binding capacity in synovial fluid precedes murine collagen-induced arthritis devel-opment [39]. p50 and p65 are heterodimers that act as a con-stitutive factor in IL-6 production in the fibroblast of the synovium. In synoviocytes collagenase, expression is acti-vated by homodimer p50 [40], whereas p65 regulates the ICAM-1 (intercellular adhesion molecule) expression and cell surface glycoprotein in endothelial cells [41]. For deter-mining the *in vivo* role of NF-κB on T cells, Chen et al. [42] studied the inhibitory effect of mutated I-kB overexpression on NF-κB induction particularly in T cells, a study con-ducted on transgenic mice. This study represents the role of NF-κB activation in Th1-dependent delayed

hypersensitivity reactions [43]. Activation of NF-κB increases the level of adhesive components like ICAM-1, VCAM-1 (vascular cell adhesion molecule), E-selectin, whereas its inhibition causes reduction of transmigration and adhesion of leukocytes [44]. Therefore, NF-κB performs a major function in inflammation initiation. Sup-pressing the actions of NF-κB was found to be an effective treatment for several inflammatory diseases. I-kB gene transfer can potentially block the NF-κB pathway. Some animal studies reported that inhibition of I-kB by adenovirus encoding reduces the early onset of alcohol-induced liver disorders like focal necrosis, steatosis [45]. Another study reported that NF-κB pathway inhibition by overexpression of the IKK (inhibitor of nuclear factor-κB (IκB) kinase) negative dominant form leads to decreased DNA binding capacity and nuclear translocation and reduced expression of various proinflammatory cytokines, VCAM-1, IL-8, E-selectin, and ICAM-1 in endothelial cells [46]. Transfer of the IKK wild-type adenoviral gene into the synovial joints of healthy rats indicates NF-κB initiation with inflam-mation of the synovial joint and paw swelling [47]. Transfer of an IKK negative dominant form gene into the synovial joints of treated rats can considerably improve arthritis and lower NF-B activity in the synovial joints. These studies investigate the importance of the NF-κB pathway in inflam-mation and its suppression could resolve the process of inflammation.

5.1 NF-κB pathway regulation

From the above studies, it was observed that the I-kB gene is an important major target of the NF-κB pathway. IL-1, LPS, and TNF stimulate the expression of this gene in many of the cells [48]. This is the reason why the I-kB gene is considered a negative regulator of the NF-κB pathway. A20 is another cytoplasmic protein expressed in lymphoid tissues found to impede NF-κB induction caused by TNF and apoptosis in cell lines [49]. The binding of A20 protein to TRAF (TNF receptor-associated factor-2) an IKK, inhibitor and ABIN can potentially regulate the TNF receptor signal mechanism [50]. It was observed that the deficiency of A20 protein in mice causes the development of cachexia and severe inflammation and have hypersensitivity reac-tions to TNF and LPS. The mice die prematurely. Cells defi-cient in A20 protein fail to terminate the NF-κB responses induced by TNF *in vivo*. Therefore, A20 protein can be a limiting factor for inflammation as it terminates *in vivo* NF-κB activation by TNF [50]. Simultaneously, A20 protein inhibits NF-κB induction by TNF but not IL-1, which suggests that IL-1 and TNF can be differently regu-lated. In addition, A20 protein can be used as a gene therapy target for inflammatory diseases.

6 Smad pathway

Smads are a family of proteins with a similar structure that are the main transducer of signals for receptors of the superfamily transforming growth factor-beta (TGF-β) important for regulations of cell growth and development. TGF-β acts as an antiinflammatory factor or as an immunosuppressive agent. It is secreted from a specific category of T cells and from other classes of nonlymphoid cells [51]. It also regulates cellular proliferation, activation of immune cells and differentiation and is involved in immune system-related impairments associated with cancer, autoimmune disorders, fibrotic complications, and opportunistic infections. TGF-β is important for oral tolerance and suppression of immune reactions against antigens ingested orally [52].

6.1 Smad pathway regulation

TGF-β serves as a substrate for type I and II TGF receptors where the cytoplasmic domain contains serine/threonine kinase activity. Type I TGF receptors identifies and phosphorylates the Smad proteins (Smad 2 and 3 associated with 4) forming complexes and contributes to DNA binding and enrollment of transcription factor. Apart from the Smad agonist (Smad 2, 3, and 4), inhibitory Smad (Smad 6 and Smad 7) binds to the receptor protein and interferes with the binding of Smad 2 and 3. TGF induces the expression of Smad 7, which seems to be an antagonist of the Smad pathway [53,54].

Several murine models have been investigated to observe the dysregulation of the TGF pathway leading to inflammation. Like TGFβ1, gene deletion causes inflammation in systemic circulation and death [55]. Type II dominant-negative TGF receptor expression causes autoimmune disorders and hyperactivity in CD4$^+$ regulatory T cells [56]. Inhibitory Smad 7 overexpression and dysregulation of Smad 3 [57] cause inflammation of airways and mucosal surfaces.

7 JAK/STAT pathway

Several cytokines and chemokines modulate the immune reactions and inflammation process. They cause the activation and homodimerization of cognate receptors further activating JAK kinases, intracellular tyrosine kinases [57]. An activated form of JAK phosphorylates cytoplasmic domain receptors and generates docking sites for signaling proteins. The JAK/STAT pathway was initially activated by interferon, hormonal factors, and growth factors and activates the JAK or STAT proteins. Like proinflammatory cytokines, IL-6 binds to the IL-6 receptor and gp 130 that further activates JAK1 and STAT 3. Interferon employs JAK 1 and 2 and activates STAT1. IL-10, an antiinflammatory cytokine, also induces STAT 3 [58]. STAT 4 and 6 are important for the development of Th1 and Th 2, as they are activated by IL-12 and 6 [59].

Some of the studies reported that the abnormal expression of IL-6 cytokines was found to be associated with neoplasia, septic shock, and autoimmune disorders [60]. STAT3 activation was reported in chronic inflammation indicating elevated levels of IL-6. STAT3 protein phosphorylation was observed in inflammatory bowel disease and rheumatoid arthritis patients as well as in mice models. In addition, the level of STAT1 was found to be elevated in the epithelial cells of asthmatic patients [61]. An elevated level of STAT4 in transgenic mice was found to be associated with ulcerative colitis [62]. In Crohn's disease, Th1 activated responses predominate, driven by IL-12 and STAT4 [63]. It was observed that STAT activation has a major role in inflammatory diseases. To determine the *in vivo* precise function of STAT3, the disruption of STAT3 gene in a cell or tissue-specific manner was done by the Cre-loxP recombination method. T cell proliferation was impaired in STAT3 deficient T cells because of the deficiency of IL-6 associated apoptosis prevention [64]. This is consistent with the defensive action of anti-IL-6 receptor monoclonal antibodies against arthritis and colitis inflammatory diseases mediated by T cells [65]. STAT3 activation induces an antiapoptosis effect by the induction of cyclin D, pim-1, c-myc, and Bcl-X [66].

7.1 JAK/STAT pathway regulation (SOCS family)

Cytokine signal transduction by the JAK/STAT pathway is maintained by JAK kinase inhibitors and is referred to as SOCS (suppressor of cytokine signaling) or CIS (cytokine-inducible SH2 proteins) [67]. The CIS1 gene is the first gene identified to be an inhibitor of the STAT5 regulatory pathway [68]. CIS1 acts on cytokine receptors, the phosphorylated tyrosine residues with the help of the SH2 domain mask the docking sites of STAT5. The SOCS family consists of eight members of associated proteins sharing a common group of SH2 sites monitored by a small motif SOCS box [69]. The activity of the JAK tyrosine kinase protein was inhibited by SOCS 1 and 3. SOCS 1 binds to the activated loop of JAK *via* the SH2 domain, whereas SOCS3 binds directly to cytokine receptors. They both have the same kinase inhibitor region (KIR), crucial for JAK inhibition [70]. A study conducted on the SOCS1 knockout (KO) mice model reported the importance of SOCS1 in T cell activation and suppression of IFN-ϒ signals. The SOCS KO mice are normal at the time of birth. They exhibited stunted growth and died within 3 weeks after birth, identified with severe lymphopenia, peripheral T cell activation, liver cell necrosis, fatty acid degeneration, and macrophage infiltration observed in major organs [71]. In the SOCS3 KO mice model, the mice die during embryonic development either by impairment in placental functions or dysregulation of erythropoiesis development [72]. Several studies indicated that cytokine-inducible SH2 proteins are activated by cytokines like IL-6 and IL-10, interferons, and negatively maintained STAT and cytokine functions [73]. Hence, it was observed that TNF, IL-1, and LPS [74] could induce SOCS3 and it was highly expressed in lamina propria as well as epithelial cells in the colon of the mice inflammatory bowel disease model. This was also observed in humans suffering from ulcerative colitis and Crohn's disease [75].

8 MAPK pathway

MAPK consisted of ubiquitous protein proline-directed serine/threonine kinases that activate the intracellular pathway by signal transduction involving acute responses to endogenous proteins and hormones. MAPK is regulated by a cascade of phosphorylation of protein kinases. MAPK is a member of the extracellular signal-regulated kinases (ERK) family [76]. MAP kinases are essential constituents of pathways involved in the maintenance of embryogenesis, cellular proliferation and differentiation, and apoptosis. ERK 1 and ERK 2 are proteins having molecular weights 43 and 41 kDa. They possess threonine and tyrosine phosphoacceptor regions, which are activated to kinases by phosphorylation. Both ERK 1 and 2 are expressed widely, although they have variable relative abundance in cells. Like in various neuroendocrine cells, both are expressed equally, while in several immune cells ERK2 is chiefly expressed. A large number of cellular perturbations and ligands cause their stimulation with cell specificity [77]. Their activity had been measured with two substrate proteins, i.e., MBP (myelin basic protein) and MAP2 (microtubule-associated protein-2); therefore, they are known as MBP and MAP2 K [78]. The MAPK name was assigned as they were first detected in the 1980s, as mitogen stimulates tyrosine phosphoproteins [79]. ERK 1 and 2 are activated in fibroblasts by cytokines, growth factors, stresses, G-protein coupled receptor ligands, and other transforming agents. In highly differentiated cells and post-mitotic neurons, they are significantly expressed [80].

8.1 MAPK pathway regulation

The MAPK pathway functions have been investigated by correlating the activities with particular cellular and biochemical responses. The dominant inhibitory action of the Ras mutant was found to be associated with ERKs, initially involving the proliferation of fibroblasts initially and long-term potentiation in neurons [81]. Protein kinase mutants have defective catalytic activity and are found to infer with functions of kinase cascades. The selective inhibitor of the MAPK pathway targets p38 a and b or MEK 1/2 isoforms, implicated in a wide array of biological cascades [82]. MEK 1/2 isoforms cause the activation of ERK 1/2. Some *in vitro* studies indicate that both of these isoforms abundantly activate ERK1/2 [83]. The phosphorylation of MEK1/2 in a single cascade is performed by Raf isoform proteins. Raf is a family of protein kinases with several isoforms (Raf-1 (or C-Raf), A-Raf, B-Raf) [84,85]. Several proteins influence the phosphorylation of Raf-1 including protein kinase C, p21 (Rac/Cdc 42) induced protein kinase PAK, and protein kinase B (Akt). p 38α was present as a tyrosine phosphoprotein in cytokine-treated cell extracts [86]. This protein acts as the target for the drug pyridinyl imidazole which suppresses TNF-α production and is known as CSBP.

Fig. 3 represents the functions of TNF, IL-6, and TGF-β and their role in the activation of the TRAF, JAK, and Smad pathways.

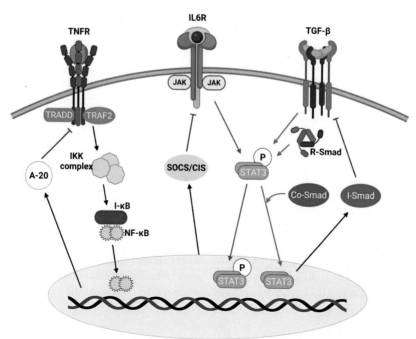

FIG. 3 Functions of TNF, IL-6, and TGF-β and their role in the activation of the TRAF, JAK, and Smad pathway.

9 Conclusions

Several inflammatory mediators regulate the signaling pathway mechanism. The proinflammatory and antiinflammatory cytokines have been discovered recently and can be used in the regulation of inflammation by modulating their effect. We have also discussed about how cells regulate the inflammatory signaling pathway. Some evidence suggested that inflammatory receptor agonists and antagonists are essential for regulating the inflammatory responses and some new therapeutic targets, as well as agents, will emerge from these advanced studies.

References

[1] L. Chen, H. Deng, H. Cui, J. Fang, Z. Zuo, J. Deng, Y. Li, X. Wang, L. Zhao, Inflammatory responses and inflammation-associated diseases in organs, Oncotarget 9 (6) (2018) 7204.

[2] Robbins and Cotran. Pathologic Basis of Disease, eighth ed., Elsevier, 2012.

[3] C.A. Dinarello, Proinflammatory cytokines, Chest 118 (2000) 503 508.

[4] A. Schweizer, U. Feige, A. Fontana, et al., Interleukin-1 enhances pain reflexes: mediation through increased prostaglandin E2 levels, Agents Actions 25 (1988) 246–251.

[5] J.W. Smith, W.J. Urba, B.D. Curti, et al., Phase II trial of interleukin-1 alpha in combination with indomethacin in melanoma patients [abstract], Proc. Am. Soc. Clin. Oncol. Annu. Meet. 10 (1991) 293.

[6] J.E. Sims, J.G. Giri, S.K. Dower, The two interleukin-1 receptors play different roles in IL-1 activities, Clin. Immunol. Immunopathol. 72 (1994) 9–14.

[7] S.A. Greenfeder, P. Nunes, L. Kwee, et al., Molecular cloning and characterization of a second subunit of the interleukin-1 receptor complex, J. Biol. Chem. 270 (1995) 13757–13765.

[8] A. Heguy, C.T. Baldari, G. Macchia, et al., Amino acids conserved in interleukin-1 receptors and the Drosophila Toll protein are essential for IL-1R signal transduction, J. Biol. Chem. 267 (1992) 2605–2609.

[9] J.E. Sims, S.L. Painter, I.R. Gow, Genomic organization of the type I and type II IL-1 receptors, Cytokine 7 (1995) 483–490.

[10] C.A. Dinarello, IL-18: a Th1-inducing, proinflammatory cytokine and new member of the IL-1 family, J. Allergy Clin. Immunol. 103 (1999) 11–24.

[11] G.P.A. Vigers, L.J. Anderson, P. Caffes, et al., Crystal structure of the type I interleukin-1 receptor complexed with interleukin1b, Nature 386 (1997) 190–194.

[12] R.J. Evans, J. Bray, J.D. Childs, et al., Mapping receptor binding sites in the IL-1 receptor antagonist and IL-1b by site directed mutagenesis: identification of a single site in IL-1ra and two sites in IL-1b, J. Biol. Chem. 270 (1994) 11477–11483.

[13] H. Schreuder, C. Tardif, S. Trump-Kallmeyer, et al., A new cytokine-receptor binding mode revealed by the crystal structure of the IL-1 receptor with an antagonist, Nature 386 (1997) 194–200.

[14] H. Wesche, C. Korherr, M. Kracht, et al., The interleukin-1 receptor accessory protein is essential for IL-1-induced activation of interleukin-1 receptor-associated kinase (IRAK) and stress-activated protein kinases (SAP kinases), J. Biol. Chem. 272 (1997) 7727–7731.

[15] S. Mathias, A. Younes, C.-C. Kan, et al., Activation of the sphingomyelin signaling pathway in intact EL4 cells and in a cell-free system by IL-1b, Science 259 (1993) 519–522.

[16] A. Huwiler, J. Pfeilschifter, Interleukin-1 stimulates de novo synthesis of mitogen-activated protein kinase in glomerular mesangial cells, FEBS Lett. 350 (1994) 135–138.

[17] N.W. Freshney, L. Rawlinson, F. Guesdon, et al., Interleukin-1 activates a novel protein cascade that results in the phosphorylation of hsp27, Cell 78 (1994) 1039–1049.

[18] M. Kracht, O. Truong, N.F. Totty, et al., Interleukin-1a activates two forms of p54a mitogen-activated protein kinase in rabbit liver, J. Exp. Med. 180 (1994) 2017–2027.

[19] K. Muegge, T.M. Williams, J. Kant, et al., Interleukin-1 costimulatory activity on the interleukin-2 promoter via AP-1, Science 246 (1989) 249–251.

[20] M.E. Kotas, R. Medzhitov, Homeostasis, inflammation, and disease susceptibility, Cell 160 (2015) 816–827.

[21] A. Wack, E. Terczyńska-Dyla, R. Hartmann, Guarding the frontiers: the biology of type III interferons, Nat. Immunol. 16 (2015) 802–809.

[22] A. Iwasaki, R. Medzhitov, Control of adaptive immunity by the innate immune system, Nat. Immunol. 16 (2015) 343–353.

[23] T. Kawai, S. Akira, Toll-like receptors and their crosstalk with other innate receptors in infection and immunity, Immunity 34 (2011) 637–650.

[24] Z. Ma, E. Zhang, D. Yang, M. Lu, Contribution of Toll-like receptors to the control of hepatitis B virus infection by initiating antiviral innate responses and promoting specific adaptive immune responses, Cell. Mol. Immunol. 12 (2015) 273–282.

[25] J.Y. Li, Y. Liu, X.X. Gao, X. Gao, H. Cai, TLR2 and TLR4 signaling pathways are required for recombinant Brucella abortus BCSP31-induced cytokine production, functional upregulation of mouse macrophages, and the Th1 immune response in vivo and in vitro, Cell. Mol. Immunol. 11 (2014) 477–494.

[26] L.M. Stuart, A. Lacy-Hulbert, De-Mst-ifying microbicidal killing, Nat. Immunol. 16 (2015) 1107–1118.

[27] A. Pichlmair, O. Schulz, C.P. Tan, T.I. Näslund, P. Liljeström, F. Weber, et al., RIG-I-mediated antiviral responses to single-stranded RNA bearing 5'-phosphates, Science 314 (2006) 997–1001.

[28] H. Kato, O. Takeuchi, S. Sato, M. Yoneyama, M. Yamamoto, K. Matsui, et al., Differential roles of MDA5 and RIG-I helicases in the recognition of RNA viruses, Nature 441 (2006) 101–105.

[29] V. Hornung, A. Ablasser, M. Charrel-Dennis, F. Bauernfeind, G. Horvath, D.R. Caffrey, et al., AIM2 recognizes cytosolic dsDNA and forms a caspase-1-activating inflammasome with ASC, Nature 458 (2009) 514–518.

[30] J. Wu, L. Sun, X. Chen, F. Du, H. Shi, C. Chen, et al., Cyclic GMP-AMP is an endogenous second messenger in innate immune signaling by cytosolic DNA, Science 339 (2013) 826–830.

[31] Z. Zhang, B. Yuan, M. Bao, N. Lu, T. Kim, Y.J. Liu, The helicase DDX41 senses intracellular DNA mediated by the adaptor STING in dendritic cells, Nat. Immunol. 12 (2011) 959–965.

[32] P. Yang, H. An, X. Liu, M. Wen, Y. Zheng, Y. Rui, et al., The cytosolic nucleic acid sensor LRRFIP1 mediates the production of type I interferon via a beta-catenin-dependent pathway, Nat. Immunol. 11 (2010) 487–494.

[33] A.G. Bowie, Rad50 and CARD9, missing links in cytosolic DNA stimulated inflammation, Nat. Immunol. 15 (2014) 534–536.

[34] A. Pichlmair, C. Lassig, C.A. Eberle, M.W. Górna, C.L. Baumann, T.R. Burkard, et al., IFIT1 is an antiviral protein that recognizes 5'-triphosphate RNA, Nat. Immunol. 12 (2011) 624–630.

[35] I. Rauch, J.L. Tenthorey, R.D. Nichols, K. Al Moussawi, J.J. Kang, C. Kang, et al., NAIP proteins are required for cytosolic detection of specific bacterial ligands in vivo, J. Exp. Med. 213 (2016) 657–665.

[36] S.T. Shibutani, T. Saitoh, H. Nowag, C. Münz, T. Yoshimori, Autophagy and autophagy-related proteins in the immune system, Nat. Immunol. 16 (2015) 1014–1024.

[37] A.S. Baldwin Jr., The NF-κB and I kappa B proteins: new discoveries and insights, Annu. Rev. Immunol. 14 (1996) 649–683.

[38] Z.N. Han, D.L. Boyle, A.M. Manning, G.S. Firestein, AP-1 and NF-κB regulation in rheumatoid arthritis and murine collagen-induced arthritis, Autoimmunity 28 (1998) 197–208.

[39] M.P. Vincenti, C.I. Coon, C.E. Brinckerhoff, Nuclear factor kappaB/p50 activates an element in the distal matrix metalloproteinase 1 promoter in interleukin-1 beta-stimulated synovial fibroblasts, Arthritis Rheum. 41 (1998) 1987–1994.

[40] A. Rahman, K.N. Anwar, A.L. True, A.B. Malik, Thrombin-induced p65 homodimer binding to downstream NF-κB site of the promoter mediates endothelial ICAM-1 expression and neutrophil adhesion, J. Immunol. 162 (1999) 5466–5476.

[41] M.A. Aronica, A.L. Mora, D.B. Mitchell, et al., Preferential role for NF-κB/Rel signaling in the type 1 but not type 2 T cell-dependent immune response in vivo, J. Immunol. 163 (1999) 5116–5124.

[42] C.C. Chen, C.L. Rosenbloom, D.C. Anderson, A.M. Manning, Selective inhibition of E-selectin, vascular cell adhesion molecule-1, and intercellular adhesion molecule-1 expression by inhibitors of I kappaB-alpha phosphorylation, J. Immunol. 155 (1995) 3538–3545.

[43] T. Uesugi, M. Froh, G.E. Arteel, B.U. Bradford, E. Gabele, M.D. Wheeler, et al., Delivery of I kappaB super-repressor gene with adenovirus reduces early alcohol-induced liver injury in rats, Hepatology 34 (2001) 1149–1157.

[44] W. Oitzinger, R. Hofer-Warbinek, J.A. Schmid, Y. Koshelnick, B.R. Binder, R. de Martin, Adenovirus-mediated expression of a mutant I kappaB kinase 2 inhibits the response of endothelial cells to inflammatory stimuli, Blood 97 (2001) 1611–1617.

[45] P.P. Tak, D.M. Gerlag, K.R. Aupperle, et al., Inhibitor of nuclear factor kappa B kinase beta is a key regulator of synovial inflammation, Arthritis Rheum. 44 (2001) 1897–1907.

[46] J.E. Thompson, R.J. Phillips, H. Erdjument-Bromage, P. Tempst, S. Ghosh, I kappaB-beta regulates the persistent response in a biphasic activation of NF-κB, Cell 80 (1995) 573–582.

[47] J.T. Cooper, D.M. Stroka, C. Brostjan, A. Palmetshofer, F.H. Bach, C. Ferran, A20 blocks endothelial cell activation through a NF-κB-dependent mechanism, J. Biol. Chem. 271 (1996) 18068–18073.

[48] K. Heyninck, D. De Valck, W. Vanden Berghe, et al., The zinc finger protein A20 inhibits TNF-induced NF-κB-dependent gene expression by interfering with an RIP- or TRAF2-mediated transactivation signal and directly binds to a novel NF-κB-inhibiting protein ABIN, J. Cell Biol. 145 (1999) 1471–1482.

[49] E.G. Lee, D.L. Boone, S. Chai, et al., Failure to regulate TNF-induced NF-κB and cell death responses in A20-deficient mice, Science 289 (2000) 2350–2354.

[50] J.J. Letterio, A.B. Roberts, Regulation of immune responses by TGF, Annu. Rev. Immunol. 16 (1998) 137–161.

[51] M.W. Babyatsky, G. Rossiter, D.K. Podolsky, Expression of transforming growth factor and in colonic mucosa in inflammatory bowel disease, Gastroenterology 110 (1996) 975–984.

[52] J. Massague, D. Wotton, Transcriptional control by the TGF/Smad signaling system, EMBO J. 19 (2000) 1745–1754.

[53] J. Massague, TGF signal transduction. Ann Rev, Biochemist 67 (1998) 753–791.

[54] M.M. Shull, I. Ormsby, A.B. Kier, et al., Targeted disruption of the mouse transforming growth factor-1 gene results in multifocal inflammatory disease, Nature 359 (1992) 693–699.

[55] X. Yang, J.J. Letterio, R.J. Lechleider, Targeted disruption of Smad3 results in impaired mucosal immunity and diminished T cell responsiveness to TGF, EMBO J. 18 (1999) 1280–1291.

[56] L. Gorelik, R.A. Flavell, Abrogation of TGF signaling in T cells leads to spontaneous T cell differentiation and autoimmune disease, Immunity 12 (2000) 171–181.

[57] M.H. Kaplan, Y.L. Sun, T. Hoey, M.J. Grusby, Impaired IL-12 responses and enhanced development of Th2 cells in STAT4-deficient mice, Nature 382 (1996) 174–177.

[58] K. Takeda, T. Tanaka, W. Shi, Essential role of STAT6 in IL-4 signalling, Nature 380 (1996) 627–630.

[59] T. Hirano, S. Akira, T. Taga, T. Kishimoto, Biological and clinical aspects of interleukin-6, Immunol. Today 11 (1990) 443–449.

[60] D. Sampath, M. Castro, D.C. Look, M.J. Holtzman, Constitutive activation of an epithelial signal transducer and activator of transcription (STAT) pathway in asthma, J. Clin. Invest. 103 (1999) 1353–1361.

[61] S. Wirtz, S. Finotto, S. Kanzler, et al., Cutting edge: chronic intestinal inflammation in STAT-4 transgenic mice: characterization of disease and adoptive transfer by TNF- plus IFN-producing CD4+ T cells that respond to bacterial antigens, J. Immunol. 162 (1999) 1884–1888.

[62] T. Parrello, G. Monteleone, S. Cucchiara, et al., Up-regulation of the IL-12 receptor beta 2 chain in Crohn's disease, J. Immunol. 165 (2000) 7234–7239.

[63] K. Takeda, T. Kaisho, N. Yoshida, J. Takeda, T. Kishimoto, S. Akira, STAT3 activation is responsible for IL-6-dependent T cell proliferation through preventing apoptosis: generation and characterization of T cell-specific STAT3-deficient mice, J. Immunol. 161 (1998) 4652–4660.

[64] R. Atreya, J. Mudter, S. Finotto, Blockade of interleukin-6 trans signaling suppresses T-cell resistance against apoptosis in chronic intestinal inflammation: evidence in Crohn disease and experimental colitis in vivo, Nat. Med. 6 (2000) 583–588.

[65] T. Shirogane, T. Fukada, J.M. Muller, D.T. Shima, M. Hibi, T. Hirano, Synergistic roles for pim-1 and c-myc in STAT3-mediated cell cycle progression and antiapoptosis, Immunity 11 (1999) 709–719.

[66] D.L. Krebs, D.J. Hilton, SOCS proteins: negative regulators of cytokine signaling, Stem Cells 19 (2001) 378–387.

[67] A. Matsumoto, Y. Seki, M. Kubo, et al., Suppression of STAT5 functions in liver mammary glands and T cells in cytokine-inducible SH2-containing protein 1 transgenic mice, Mol. Cell. Biol. 19 (1999) 6396–6407.

[68] T. Naka, M. Narazaki, T. Hirata, et al., Structure and function of a new STAT-induced STAT inhibitor, Nature 387 (1997) 924–929.

[69] A. Sasaki, H. Yasukawa, A. Suzuki, et al., Cytokine-inducible SH2 protein-3 (CIS3/SOCS3) inhibits Janus tyrosine kinase by binding through the N-terminal kinase inhibitory region as well as SH2 domain, Genes Cells 4 (1999) 339–351.

[70] W.S. Alexander, R. Starr, J.E. Fenner, et al., SOCS1 Is a critical inhibitor of interferon gamma signaling and prevents the potentially fatal neonatal actions of this cytokine, Cell 98 (1999) 597–608.

[71] A.W. Roberts, L. Robb, S. Rakar, et al., Placental defects and embryonic lethality in mice lacking suppressor of cytokine signaling 3, Proc. Natl. Acad. Sci. U. S. A. 98 (2001) 9324–9329.

[72] M.A. Cassatella, S. Gasperini, C. Bovolenta, et al., Interleukin-10 (IL-10) selectively enhances CIS3/SOCS3 mRNA expression in

human neutrophils: evidence for an IL-10-induced pathway that is independent of STAT protein activation, Blood 94 (1999) 2880–2889.

[73] Y.R. Boisclair, J. Wang, J. Shi, K.R. Hurst, G.T. Ooi, Role of the suppressor of cytokine signaling-3 in mediating the inhibitory effects of interleukin-1beta on the growth hormone-dependent transcription of the acid-labile subunit gene in liver cells, J. Biol. Chem. 275 (2000) 3841–3847.

[74] A. Suzuki, T. Hanada, K. Mitsuyama, et al., CIS3/SOCS3/SSI3 plays a negative regulatory role in STAT3 activation and intestinal inflammation, J. Exp. Med. 193 (2001) 471–481.

[75] R. Seger, D. Seger, F.J. Lozeman, N.G. Ahn, L.M. Graves, J.S. Campbell, L. Ericsson, M. Harrylock, A.M. Jensen, E.G. Krebs, Human T-cell mitogen-activated protein kinase kinases are related to yeast signal transduction kinases, J. Biol. Chem. 267 (1992) 25628–25631.

[76] T.S. Lewis, P.S. Shapiro, N.G. Ahn, Signal transduction through MAP kinase cascades, Adv. Cancer Res. 74 (1998) 49–139.

[77] N.G. Ahn, E.G. Krebs, Evidence for an epidermal growth factor-stimulated protein kinase cascade in Swiss 3T3 cells. Activation of serine peptide kinase activity by myelin basic protein kinases in vitro, J. Biol. Chem. 265 (1990) 11495–11501.

[78] A.J. Rossomando, D.M. Payne, M.J. Weber, T.W. Sturgill, Evidence that pp42, a major tyrosine kinase target protein, is a mitogen-activated serine/threonine protein kinase, Proc. Natl Acad. Sci. U. S. A. 86 (1989) 6940–6943.

[79] T.G. Boulton, S.H. Nye, D.J. Robbins, N.Y. Ip, E. Radziejewska, S.D. Morgenbesser, R.A. DePinho, N. Panayotatos, M.H. Cobb, G.D. Yancopoulos, ERKs: a family of protein-serine/threonine kinases that are activated and tyrosine phosphorylated in response to insulin and NGF, Cell 65 (1991) 663–675.

[80] C.M. Atkins, J.C. Selcher, J.J. Petraitis, J.M. Trzaskos, J.D. Sweatt, The MAPK cascade is required for mammalian associative learning, Nat. Neurosci. 1 (1998) 602–609.

[81] G. Pearson, F. Robinson, T.B. Gibson, B. Xu, M. Karandikar, K. Berman, M.H. Cobb, Mitogen-activated protein (MAP) kinase pathways: regulation and physiological functions, Endocr. Rev. 22 (2) (2021) 153–183.

[82] C.N. Prowse, J.C. Hagopian, M.H. Cobb, N.G. Ahn, J. Lew, Catalytic reaction pathway for the mitogen-activated protein kinase ERK2, Biochemistry 39 (2000) 6258–6266.

[83] T. Force, J.V. Bonventre, G. Heidecker, U. Rapp, J. Avruch, J.M. Kyriakis, Enzymatic characteristics of the c-Raf-1 protein kinase, Proc. Natl. Acad. Sci. U. S. A. 91 (1994) 1270–1274.

[84] C. Hagemann, U.R. Rapp, Isotype-specific functions of Raf kinases, Exp. Cell Res. 253 (1999) 34–46.

[85] J. Han, J.-D. Lee, L. Bibbs, R.J. Ulevitch, A MAP kinase targeted by endotoxin and hyperosmolarity in mammalian cells, Science 265 (1994) 808–811.

[86] J.C. Lee, J.T. Laydon, P.C. McDonnell, T.F. Gallagher, S. Kumary, D. Green, D. McNulty, M.J. Blumenthal, J.R. Heys, S.W. Landvatter, J.E. Strickler, M.M. McLaughlin, I.R. Siemens, S.M. Fisher, G.P. Livi, J.R. White, J.L. Adams, P.R. Young, A protein kinase involved in the regulation of inflammatory cytokine biosynthesis, Nature 372 (1994) 739–746.

Chapter 4

Advanced nanomedicine-based therapeutics for targeting airway inflammatory diseases

Yinghan Chan[a], Jun Sing Lim[b], Xiangmei Cui[b], Sin Wi Ng[a], Xin Wei Lim[e], Dinesh Kumar Chellappan[c], and Kamal Dua[d]

[a]*School of Pharmacy, International Medical University (IMU), Kuala Lumpur, Malaysia,* [b]*School of Medicine, Faculty of Medicine and Health Sciences, Royal College of Surgeons in Ireland (RCSI), Dublin, Ireland,* [c]*Department of Life Sciences, School of Pharmacy, International Medical University (IMU), Kuala Lumpur, Malaysia,* [d]*Discipline of Pharmacy, Graduate School of Health, University of Technology Sydney, Sydney, NSW, Australia,* [e]*School of Health Sciences, Faculty of Biology, Medicine and Health, University of Manchester, Manchester, United Kingdom*

1 Introduction

Inflammation is the body's natural defense mechanism to protect against harmful stimuli including pathogens, irritants, and damaged cells. As such, acute inflammation is a process beneficial in the resolution and healing of injury by the immobilization of the injured region while mobilizing the rest of the immune system to the site of injury. On the other hand, chronic inflammation is a major health concern, as chronically inflamed tissues typically recruit immune cells from the systemic circulation to amplify the inflammatory response, which results in self-targeted aggressiveness that destructs normal tissues in a misdirected attempt at initiating the healing process [1–3]. With respect to the respiratory system, chronic airway inflammatory diseases such as asthma, chronic obstructive pulmonary disease (COPD), cystic fibrosis, and lung cancer are among the most notable causes of global morbidity and mortality, posing a huge and significant socioeconomic burden in terms of the cost incurred due to prolonged treatment and hospitalization, as well as reduced productivity. Such a burden has also severely impacted the livelihoods of individuals suffering from these diseases [4,5]. As reported by the World Health Organization (WHO), there are approximately 235 million individuals who suffer from asthma, and there are more than 3 million deaths occur each year due to COPD itself [6]. Besides, lung cancer has also claimed 1.8 million lives among 2.21 million suffering individuals in the year 2020 [7]. To make matters worse, such figures are projected to grow rapidly in the coming years, raising the concerns that a large population will be shredded because of these diseases [8].

Typically, pharmacotherapy is essential for the management of chronic airway inflammatory diseases, in which the developing fields of science and medical research have contributed to the discovery and development of various therapeutic agents. Nevertheless, most of these agents are unable to completely cure and/or reverse the progression of the disease and the quality of life of patients remains poor [9–11]. For example, controlling the symptoms is the only available option in the management of asthma, whereas in patients who are poorly controlled, administration of more than one type of therapeutic agents may be required, thereby exposing them to a higher risk of adverse drug reactions. These include the development of dyspepsia, dizziness, tremors, as well as sore throat, which are associated with an extended use of bronchodilators and corticosteroids [12,13]. Besides, in cases of COPD and pulmonary fibrosis, although the use of drugs including pirfenidone and nintedanib displayed a certain extent of therapeutic effects, they failed to restore lung tissues to their normal state and had no significant positive effects on disease mortality [13,14]. On the other hand, despite displaying remarkable antiinflammatory activities that can potentially modulate various inflammatory pathways involved in the pathogenesis of airway inflammatory diseases, some of these chemical moieties, especially those extracted from herbs and plants, have poor water solubility, which leads to low oral bioavailability and poor absorption, thereby limiting their clinical application [8,15,16]. Thus, there is a pressing need for researchers to identify and develop novel strategies that can be employed as alternatives to current conventional therapeutics for effective management and treatment of airway inflammatory diseases.

Recent Developments in Anti-Inflammatory Therapy. https://doi.org/10.1016/B978-0-323-99988-5.00007-3

Nanomedicine is a field of multidisciplinary research with an integration of traditional sciences including materials science, physics, chemistry, and biology, in which the application of nanomedicine-based strategies for airway inflammatory diseases has attracted great interest and has grown rapidly over the recent years [17]. Nanomedicine-based strategy utilizes colloid systems of sizes within the nanoscale range for enhancing the diagnosis, treatment, and prevention of diseases, in which nanocarriers can be constructed on various nanomaterials including lipids, polymers, and metals that enable the encapsulation of diverse chemical moieties [18–20]. As an advanced strategy, the use of nanocarriers for targeted drug delivery has demonstrated promising outcomes as the alternatives to conventional therapeutic approaches, which can be attributed to their capability in improving the biodistribution and bioavailability of therapeutic agents due to enhanced solubility of hydrophobic moieties, minimizing clearance, reducing premature degradation of unstable compounds, as well as locating target tissues to enhance therapeutic effects while minimizing off-target adverse effects [13,19,20]. Hence, such an approach may prove useful in the management of airway inflammatory diseases and could facilitate the eventual clinical translation of novel therapeutics that can effectively treat these diseases and improve patients' quality of life.

In this chapter, we provide a brief overview of the underlying inflammatory mechanisms of several airway inflammatory diseases. We then discuss the advantages and perspectives of the application of nanomedicine-based strategies as advanced therapeutics to address the limitations of conventional therapeutics in the management of airway inflammatory diseases, supported by various findings from research that has been conducted in the recent years.

2 Inflammatory mechanisms of airway inflammatory diseases

2.1 Asthma

Asthma is defined as a heterogeneous disease and is commonly characterized by chronic pulmonary inflammation. A classic asthma diagnosis would typically include a history of intermittent respiratory symptoms such as coughing, wheezing, shortness of breath, and chest tightness with fluctuating periods of intensity associated with triggers [21]. In broad terms, there are multiple types of asthma, including intrinsic and atopic asthma, with intrinsic asthma being prevalent in older age groups, and the latter is associated with childhood and younger age groups; it is the most common phenotype of asthma [22]. According to the WHO, asthma had affected approximately 262 million people and there had been 461,000 asthma-related deaths worldwide in 2019 alone. With such a huge prevalence

worldwide and being the most common chronic disease in children, asthma is often under-treated and under-diagnosed, which led to the rising asthma-related morbidities and mortalities [23]. The multifactorial etiology of asthma spans from the characteristic triggers that cause episodic bronchoconstriction, to a positive family history of atopy [21,24]. The Center for Disease Control and Prevention (CDC) describes triggers as substances or conditions that could potentially initiate an asthmatic attack [24]. Triggers range from allergens such as dust mites, tobacco smoke, and disinfectants and other conditions such as infections, physical exercise, and strong emotional response, that could vary from person to person [24,25]. A person with a strong personal or family history of atopic disease, including seasonal rhinoconjunctivitis and eczema, which subsequently develops similar respiratory symptoms, would result in a high clinical suspicion for asthma as well [21,23].

The pathogenesis of asthma is well documented and is characterized by exposure to environmental triggers, leading to repeated episodes of airway inflammation involving eosinophilic infiltration, neutrophils, mast cells, and CD4$^+$ lymphocytes, associated with rearrangement in vascularization patterns and disruption of the innervation and airway smooth muscles [26,27]. The inflammation results in tissue damage and exacerbation of transient respiratory symptoms including edema and airway narrowing, which then resolve initially. As the disease progresses, resolution of inflammation becomes incomplete, and abnormal tissue repair and remodeling becomes increasingly frequent, which lead to a decline in lung function over time [28]. Generally, inflammation occurs in the smooth muscle layer of the large conducting airways with the majority involving the submucosal layer; however, as the disease progresses, it could involve the smaller airways and alveoli with inflammation predominantly involving areas outside of the smooth muscles [26,29].

Generally, the pathogenesis of atopic asthma involves the two arms of the immune response of the human body, namely, the innate and adaptive immune responses [27]. Initiation of the inflammatory cascade for atopic asthma begins with an allergen contaminated with pathogen-associated molecular patterns (PAMP), which allows the pattern-recognition receptors (PRR) on the surface of antigen-presenting cells (APC), such as dendritic cells (DC), to bind and subsequently internalizes and degrades the antigens via the endogenous proteosome pathway, which releases the antigenic peptides that bind to the major histocompatibility complex (MHC) class II in the DC rough endoplasmic reticulum and is transported to the DC cell surface for presentation. The activated DC upregulates costimulatory molecules through intermediate messengers such as interleukin (IL)-1b and tumor necrosis factor (TNF)-α, and migrate to the local draining lymph nodes to prime a T-cell response specific to the antigen, thereby activating the adaptive immune response [27,30]. The migrating speed and chemotaxis of DC into the dermal afferent lymph nodes are regulated by a chemokine receptor (CCR)-7 that is expressed by DC itself through two pathways: the activation of G_i protein-dependent mitogen-activated protein kinases (MAPK), including extracellular signal-regulated protein kinase (ERK)1/2, c-Jun N-terminal kinase (JNK), and p38, as well as Rho/Pyk2/cofilin influencing the actin filaments in the DC cytoskeleton [31]. After entering the local lymph nodes, DC presents peptide–MHC complexes to the naïve $CD4^+$ T-helper cells, which bind the complex with T-cell receptors (TCRs) and initiates the adaptive immune response signaling cascade. Th2, as a subset of the $CD4^+$ T cells, becomes activated and releases proinflammatory cytokines including IL-4, IL-5, IL-10, and IL-13, with IL-4 promoting interactions between T cells and B cells, leading to B-cell class switching to produce mainly immunoglobulin (Ig) E (IgE) antibodies against the antigens that are released into the circulation [27]. These IgE antibodies cross-link on the surface of mast cells by binding to the high-affinity Fcε antibody receptor-1 (FcεR-1), which results in increased responsiveness of mast cells toward the allergens [27,32]. As the disease becomes increasingly severe and chronic, Th1 cells that could secrete TNF-α and interferon (IFN)-γ are recruited, which could lead to progressive lung-tissue damage, as observed in severe asthmatics [33].

Mast cells are leukocytes that mature in bone-marrow tissue and circulate as immature precursor forms, with their development tightly linked to the interaction between the stem cell factor (SCF) and Kit receptor. SCF is produced by marrow stromal cells, but also lung epithelium, airway smooth muscles (ASM), and fibroblasts, where it serves as a regulator to control the native population of mast cells in the body and is upregulated in asthma [26,32]. Mast cells are strategically located in proximity to the ASM, where their activation leads to local effects on the lungs as seen in asthma [32]. In the context of inflammation, IL-1β and TNF-α that are upregulated by immune cells such as DC activate ASM cells, lead to the production of a variety of proinflammatory cytokines such as CC-chemokine ligand 11 (CCL11 or eotaxin-1), CCL-5, C-X-C motif ligand (CXCL)-8, CXCL-10, and monocyte chemoattractant protein 1 (MCP-1), alongside with GM-CSF, IL-1, IL-6, and IL-8, which aid in mast cell recruitment and retention, as well as recruitment of eosinophils into the inflammatory infiltrate [1,26,27,32]. The cross-linkage of IgE on mast cells results in the degranulation of mast cells, releasing preformed mediators such as histamine, tryptases, chymase, and heparin, which are also detected in bronchoalveolar lavage (BAL) samples from asthmatic patients from an allergen inhalation challenge. Lipid mediators of inflammation such as leukotriene B4 (LTB4) and prostaglandin D2 (PGD2) are also synthesized and play a role in local bronchoconstriction, edema, and recruitment of other inflammatory cells to the site of inflammation. Mast cells may also interact with T cells through the PGD2 receptor, CrTh2 on Th2 cells, and the LTB4 receptor, BLT; the latter is implicated in mast cell-induced $CD8^+$ T-cell recruitment [27,32].

Apart from that, eosinophils are also recruited into the affected lung tissues by mediators, such as IL-5, CCL-5, or Regulated upon Activation, Normal T-cell Expressed and Secreted (RANTES), and MCP-1 [27], released by mast cells. Other factors such as eotaxins 1, 2, and 3 that are secreted by the mesenchymal, epithelial, and endothelial cells locally, alongside MCP-3 and MCP-4, also attract eosinophils [34,35]. Mast cells also aid the maturation of eosinophils from cytokines such as IL-3, IL-5, and granulocyte-macrophage colony-stimulating factor (GM-CSF), which results in the degranulation of eosinophils to release major basic protein (MBP) and eosinophil peroxidase (EPO). EPO produces superoxide radicals that are damaging to the lung tissue, alongside factors such as IL-4, IL-13, and eicosanoids such as prostacyclins and leukotrienes, thereby leading to the clinical hallmarks of asthma [26]. Throughout the inflammatory phase, the ASM epithelium releases a variety of chemokines and factors, such as platelet-derived growth factor (PDGF), fibroblast growth factor (FGF), and transforming growth factor (TGF)-β, that recruits other inflammatory cells such as neutrophils [27]. As the inflammation persists and progresses to a chronic stage, mast cells and eosinophils contribute to fibrogenesis and ASM remodeling, as both contain matrix metalloproteinases (MMP)-3 and MMP-9, which result in increased thickness of the airways and increased ASM with the integration of new matrix proteins, collagen fibers, and proteoglycans, and increased vascularization along the airway wall [26,27]. The new vessels friable due to vascularization can lead to increased vascular permeability and edema. Growth factors such as epidermal growth factor (EGF) and amphiregulin, usually contribute to epithelial repair; however, in asthma, the repair process of epithelial cells is impaired, partly due to the presence of TGF-β affecting the epithelial repair response [26].

2.2 Chronic obstructive pulmonary disease

COPD is a common, preventable disease characterized by irreversible airway obstruction accompanied by systemic inflammation and persistent respiratory symptoms most commonly due to exposure to toxic gases and particles that cause airway or alveolar abnormalities, usually resulting in the destruction of smaller airways and mucociliary dysfunction [36,37]. Cigarette smoke (CS) is the greatest risk factor for developing COPD, with the amount and duration of smoke (pack-years) linked to disease severity, where the

American Lung Association quotes that an approximate 85%–90% of COPD cases are caused by cigarette smoking, with increased mortality rates among men and women when compared to their nonsmoking counterparts [37,38]. Other risk factors include genetic factors (alpha-1-antitrypsin deficiency), significant exposure to air pollution, second-hand smoke or occupational exposure to noxious gases, and a history of childhood respiratory tract infections [38]. COPD is characterized by chronic, progressive inflammatory response of the airways, often involving the lung parenchyma and pulmonary vasculature, with patterns of inflammation depending on the different subtypes of COPD. The most common earliest symptom presented by patients is usually exertional dyspnea, with the three essential features of COPD being intermittent worsening episodes of dyspnea, chronic cough, and excessive sputum production [37,39].

As the leading causative factor of COPD, CS contains over 4500 different substances that include toxins, heavy metals, mutagens, and carcinogens, which are deposited along the entire respiratory tract from the upper airways to the smaller alveoli, according to particulate size [40]. This deposition causes an imbalance of oxidants and antioxidants produced by the body, which results in the initiation of various genetic expressions of inflammatory molecules, increased mucus secretion, and deactivation of antiproteases, ultimately contributing to bronchial cell apoptosis and destruction of local respiratory tissues [40,41]. As with asthma, COPD also involves both arms of the immune response linked via dendritic cell activation [36]. Starting from the innate immunity pathway, CS could activate PRR directly and purinergic receptors to commence the inflammatory response, which is also contributed by the necrotic apoptotic cells releasing DAMPs, thereby recruiting inflammatory cells [1]. It was found that CS may damage the epithelial cells by inhibiting vascular endothelial growth factor (VEGF) and hepatocyte growth factor in patients with COPD, resulting in apoptosis of alveolar cells and the emphysema phenotype. Damaged alveolar epithelial cells then release TGF-β, which leads to local fibrosis and airway remodeling [36,41]. Irritants within CS activate alveolar surface macrophages and airway epithelial cells to release chemotactic factors such as CCL2 that attracts monocytes, CXCL-1 and CXCL-8 that attract neutrophils, and CXCL-9, -10, and -11 that attract Th1 and cytotoxic T cells [1]. DAMPs released by damaged tissue lead to the secretion of proinflammatory cytokines such as IL-1β and IL-18. These cytokines further activate neutrophils, macrophages, and Th1 and Th17 cell types via the formation of nucleotide-binding oligomerization domain-like receptor P3 (DLRP3) and inflammasomes, as seen in type 1 airway inflammation [41].

During the innate immunity phase, alveolar macrophages and neutrophils play a central role in promoting inflammation. Alveolar macrophages are recruited as a response to the chemokines CCL2 and CXCL-1, and produce reactive oxygen species (ROS), MMP-9, and cathepsins K, L, and S, which collectively damage the alveolar tissue, and have a more prominent elastolytic activity in smokers when compared to their nonsmoking counterparts. Granulocyte production is increased by CS, mediated by GM-CSF and granulocyte CSF formed by the lung macrophages, leading to increased numbers of granulocytes and hence, neutrophils, in the circulation. The accumulation of ROS-induced phosphatidylinositol-3,4,5-triphosphate and various neutrophil chemotactic factors, for instance, LTB4, CXCL-1, CXCL-5, and CXCL-8, leads to chemotaxis of neutrophils toward the affected area [36]. Neutrophils are activated by relatively large quantities of myeloperoxidase (MPO) and the human neutrophil lopocalin in the sputum supernatant and secrete serine proteases such as neutrophil elastase (NE), cathepsin G, and proteinase 3, which contribute directly to the destruction of alveoli and promote the secretion of mucus via activation of airway goblet cells [41]. Resistance to corticosteroids is observed in COPD patients, with impaired mechanisms in reducing the production of CXCL-8, TNF-α, and MMP-9 from alveolar macrophages as compared to healthy subjects, due to reduction in histone deacetylase (HDAC) activity in macrophages. This abnormal macrophage activity also impairs phagocytosis of bacterial and apoptotic cells, resulting in chronic bacterial colonization of lower airways and increased risk of community-acquired pneumonia in COPD patients [36].

The deviation of inflammation toward adaptive inflammation occurs when DAMPs and antigens from damaged tissue and necrotic cells are recognized by DCs, which are presented to T cells while the normal immune tolerance generated by regulatory T cells (T_{reg}), myeloid suppressor cells, and M2 macrophages is impaired in COPD patients [41]. The persistent inflammation might also be due to a self-sustaining mechanism; however, this is yet to be clarified, and other mechanisms such as memory T cells, bacterial colonization, or autoimmunity may contribute to the perpetual cycle of inflammation leading to augmented airway remodeling and destruction of lung parenchyma in COPD. Studies have found a greater proportion of $CD8^+$ T cells compared to $CD4^+$ T cells in the lung parenchyma; however, both cell lines are increased, especially $CD4^+$ Th17 T lymphocytes that produce IL-17A and IL-22, which may play a role in neutrophilic inflammation. IL-17A is elevated in end-stage COPD patients and may also contribute to lymphoid neogenesis induced by CS [36,39].

2.3 Cystic fibrosis

Unlike asthma and COPD, cystic fibrosis (CF) is a multisystem disease involving other organ systems aside from the respiratory tract, for instance, digestive and male reproductive systems and sweat glands [42]. Mutations in the cystic fibrosis transmembrane conductance regulator (CFTR) gene that is involved in ion transport cause disorder in the transport of chloride ions and other CFTR-affected ions, particularly, sodium and bicarbonate, thereby leading to increased viscosity in the secretions of the lungs, pancreas, liver, intestine, and reproductive tract. As such, in terms of the respiratory system, CF is a form of obstructive airway disease and it could be demonstrated in pulmonary function tests, in addition to symptoms such as continuous productive cough and the hyperinflation of lung fields in CXR. Respiratory symptoms are prominent in CF beginning from infancy, with 35% of infants tested positive in neonatal screening tests having respiratory symptoms [43].

The CFTR gene is located on chromosome 7 and pathogenic mutations on both copies of the gene cause clinical CF symptoms, with mutations on one copy of the gene being known as CFTR-related disorder with symptoms generally limited to one organ system. There are more than 2000 different types of mutations that could occur on the CFTR gene as described by the CF Mutation Database, with the most common being the deletion of the DNA base pairs coding for the amino acid phenylalanine, also known as F508del. Mutations in the CFTR gene are also categorized into five types (I—V) with each category describing the different types of the disease process as seen in CF patients [44]. At the time of birth, the lung is typically not inflamed and over the period of months to years, signs of recurrent infections with respiratory viruses, *Haemophilus influenza*, and *Staphylococcus aureus* dominate the infectious picture in early life, which is followed by chronic inflammation of the lungs. Although CF has an aggressive neutrophilic inflammatory response, this however fails to remove these infectious agents, and as the disease progresses, pulmonary infections by other pathogens such as Gram-negative species and *Pseudomonas aeruginosa* become increasingly common [45].

There are multiple hypotheses regarding the pathogenesis of CF and the role of the CFTR gene in the disease process, and the airway surface fluid (ASL) depletion hypothesis has been the most supported hypothesis over the past decade [46]. In healthy lungs, the mucus clearance (MC) system is responsible for particulate entrapment in the mucus layer and removal of such particulates via the beating of cilia and coughing [45]. The maintenance of the mucus layer is a coordinated response between chloride ion (Cl^-) secretion mediated by CFTR channel proteins and sodium (Na^+) absorption from epithelial sodium channels (ENaC), which allows the cilia to beat effectively and aid in mucus mobility across the airway epithelium. The absence of CFTR in CF patients leads to decreased Cl^- presence in the airway epithelium and low salt (NaCl)

formation, which in turn reduces water moving into the lumen of the airways via osmosis. The lack of the CFTR protein also results in the dysregulation of ENaC, causing excessive Na^+ reabsorption and when combined with the former situation, the resultant ASL becomes dry and dehydrated, and suppresses airway ciliary action [46]. Thus, the MC system becomes ineffective in removing particulates and the persistent secretions from goblet cells result in the formation of mucus plaques in the airway and increase the oxygen diffusion pathway toward airway epithelial cells resulting in tissue hypoxia. This hypoxic state generates a favorable environment for the growth of bacteria, especially those that secrete biofilm such as *Pseudomonas* species in alginate form, as the anaerobic state promotes biofilm generation. The formation of biofilm coupled with the thickened mucus impedes the penetration and migration of neutrophils and other antimicrobial agents, leading to a chronic infectious state. Further insults to the airway epithelia such as infections also contribute to ASL volume depletion, which further perpetuates the vicious cycle [47]. Once an infection is established, recurrent infections become more likely, and inflammatory mechanisms seem to persist even after the eradication of infection to the point where the presence of mucus alone can trigger an inflammatory response, as seen in ferret models [48].

Inflammation in CF is predominantly mediated by neutrophils, where they generate and maintain the destructive inflammatory state. Functioning and necrotic neutrophils alike release chemoattractants, proteases, and reactive oxygen species in the airway which damage pulmonary structures. Particularly, levels of IL-17A producing neutrophils are linked to pulmonary exacerbations of CF. In CF patients, neutrophils are present in pathological amounts that could undergo necrosis instead of apoptosis, forming neutrophil extracellular traps (NETs). NETs are usually present in normal lung tissues, and they aid in the entrapment of bacterial agents in acute infections; however, when present in a chronic situation, NETs contribute adversely to the local lung microenvironment. Pathological microbes such as *P. aeruginosa* also develop resistance to NET-mediated extermination over time; therefore, NETs become increasingly inefficient. Yet they contribute to the inflammatory pathways by activating macrophages to release proinflammatory mediators and stimulate Th17 lymphocytes to further increase neutrophil chemotaxis toward the affected area. The imbalance between proinflammatory and antiinflammatory metabolites in CF contributes to the chronic inflammatory state, and as such, antiinflammatory metabolites such as resolvin D1 (RVD1) became the focus of research in CF inflammatory mechanisms. RVD1 has been shown to reduce bacterial burden and neutrophil influx; thus, it is implicated to play a role as a therapeutic target in CF [48].

2.4 Lung cancer

Lung cancer or bronchogenic carcinoma refers to the development of tumors from uncontrollable growth of cells in the tissue originating in the lung parenchyma or the bronchi [49]. Such behavior is a result of genetic alteration that facilitates the activation of oncogenes and deactivation of tumor suppressor genes [50]. There are currently two types of lung carcinoma, namely, small-cell lung cancer (SCLC) and non-small cell lung cancer (NSCLC), with the latter accounting for most lung cancer cases worldwide (85%) [51]. The greatest risk factor for lung cancer is exposure to cigarette smoking (CS), with the majority of rise in incidence being attributable to CS, especially in males who smoke [49]. Lung cancer is associated with 25% of overall cancer mortality and is the most common cause of cancer mortality, with 83,550 deaths for men and 70,500 deaths for women in 2018, and it has caused an estimated 1.8 million deaths worldwide in 2020. In the United States, the 5-year survival rate for lung cancer is poor, with only 18% between 2003 and 2009, and even more so in advanced disease, where the 5-year survival rate is only 5% and is a more common presentation as the discovery of lung cancer is often at its late stage [52,53].

Chronic inflammatory processes are shown to increase the risk of tumorigenesis and promote the advancement of tumor in all stages, from invasion to metastasis [50,54–56]. As oncogenes and tumor suppressor genes are implicated in tumorigenesis, they play a role in inflammation by regulating inflammatory mediators and inducing neovascularization. The same genetic alterations that result in tumorigenesis by oncogene activation and inactivation of tumor suppressor genes also aid in creating a favorable microenvironment for tumors and promoting immune escape by reducing antitumor activity [50]. As discussed earlier, CS contains mutagens and irritants that lead to widespread pulmonary inflammation and induces repeated insults to the lung parenchyma, facilitating a mutagenic environment [55]. Therefore, the persistent chronic inflammation present in COPD also increases the risk of developing malignant tissue within the lungs as it was shown that low-grade emphysema is a risk factor for lung cancer. Other independent risk factors include exposure to asbestos, silicon, and infections such as tuberculosis [55,57].

Macrophages are largely involved in the inflammatory infiltrate seen in cancers and are involved in tumor initiation and progression. Likewise, tumor cells produce macrophage differentiation factors such as CCL2 and macrophage colony-stimulating factor (M-CSF) for macrophage recruitment and differentiation, especially into M2-like tumor-associated macrophages (TAM). Besides, tumor cells secrete transcription factors such as nuclear factor kappa B (NF-κB), signal transducer and activator of transcription 3 (STAT3), and hypoxia-inducible factor-1 alpha (HIF1α), which aid in a variety of tumor functions including proliferation, neoangiogenesis, migration, and invasion. Simultaneously, these transcription factors also affect the influx and activation of inflammatory cells via the generation of inflammatory mediators and production of a tumor-friendly chronic inflammatory state. TAMs are dysfunctional macrophages associated with reduced production of ROS and proinflammatory cytokines, with downregulation of MHC class II affecting antigen presentation, resulting in a local immunosuppressive state that is also contributed by the ability of TAM to activate the immune checkpoint PD-L1, thus promoting immune evasion of tumor cells [50].

In adaptive immune response, T-lymphocytes are also seen in the inflammatory infiltrate in most cases. However, these T-lymphocytes commonly represent a dysfunctional cohort with aberrations in the T-cell receptor (TCR), rendering it unable to recognize MHC antigen complexes, hence interfering with the innate ability of T cells to interact and eliminate tumor cells. Conversely, the presence of CD3$^+$ and CD8$^+$ and B-type tumor infiltrating lymphocytes (TIL) bears a more favorable prognosis as it is associated with increased tumor cell apoptosis. The high numbers of T lymphocytes in tumor cell infiltrate without significant T-cell cytotoxicity may be attributable to the relative lymphocyte anergy found in intratumoral cells [55]. The lymphocyte anergy is speculated to be due to alterations in TCR, loss of signal transducing protein, modified costimulatory factors, and altered reduction in MHC class II molecules from APCs, while cancer cells downregulate the surface expression of MHC class I molecules and secrete antiinflammatory mediators such as TGF-β and forkhead box protein P3 (FoxP3), of which the latter is overexpressed in lung cancer cells and is involved in the regulation of immune tolerance [55,58]. Furthermore, the presence of altered MHC class I surface expression by cancer cells may prevent the activation of T lymphocytes. However, natural killer (NK) cells are able to detect and facilitate the direct lysis of tumor cells via the secretion of perforins and granzymes. Nevertheless, multiple studies have shown that NK cell functioning was suppressed in cigarette smokers when compared to noncigarette smokers, and NK cells in lung cancer tissue was found to have reduced expression of NK cell-activation markers such as NKGD2D and NKp46. Most NK cells are also found in the peritumoral stroma and do not interact with tumor cells directly [55].

Apart from that, myeloid-derived suppressor cells (MDSC) are a subset of immature myelomonocytic cells that are involved in autoimmunity, and MDSC expansion may be driven by inflammatory factors secreted by tumor cells such as cyclooxygenase 2 (COX-2), prostaglandins, IL-1β, M-CSF, and VEGF. The modus operandi of MDSC is by the nitration of TCR, thereby rendering them dysfunctional in the recognition and processing of tumor antigens. MDSC also modulates the expansion of FoxP3$^+$ Tregs, thus further promoting the state of immunosuppression and allowing the immune evasion of tumor cells through indirect inhibition of T-cell activation and affecting cell-mediated immunity. The role of MDSC in innate immunity is the promotion of macrophage differentiation into M2-like TAMs, which are involved in angiogenesis and tissue remodeling, contributing to the progression of cancer [55,57].

3 Advantages and perspectives for the use of nanomedicine-based strategies in airway inflammatory diseases

Nanotechnology represents a rapidly developing field of scientific research, which primarily involves the know-how of manufacturing as well as the study of properties, structure, and behavior of materials within the nanoscale range, known as nanomaterials. Specifically, nanomedicine is a branch of medicine that employs the science of nanotechnology, in which the application of nanomedicine for clinical purposes can have a significant impact on human health through improvement in disease diagnosis, prevention, and treatment [59–61]. Nanomedicines are primarily intended to enhance the efficacy of therapeutics by enabling efficient and targeted delivery of loaded therapeutic moieties to specific sites in a sustained and controlled manner, while minimizing accumulation in healthy body sites to avoid off-target toxicity [13,62]. Nanomedicines have also attracted increasing attention as the nanomaterials used in drug-loaded carriers typically possess unique physical, chemical, electrical, and optical properties, which significantly differ from those of their macroscale counterparts. Besides, nanoencapsulation of therapeutic compounds can protect them from premature degradation in biological environments and can provide increased solubilization for poorly water-soluble compounds [17,63,64]. Furthermore, recent technological advancements in nanotechnology have enabled nanocarriers to be custom engineered to achieve specific pharmacokinetic and pharmacodynamic properties, such as solubility, drug release profile, immunogenicity, bioavailability, as well as diffusivity depending on their intended applications, thereby allowing personalized therapeutics [17,65]. Thus, nanomedicine has been poised to revolutionize the biomedical field soon and is by far the most studied technology in drug-delivery research. In the following sections, we further elaborate the advantages of employing nanomedicine-based strategies in airway inflammatory diseases and provide an insight into the perspectives in designing efficient and multifunctional nanoparticles for drug delivery in airway inflammatory diseases.

3.1 Improvement in pharmacokinetic properties

Over the years, various chemical and biological agents with profound antiinflammatory effects, as well as immunomodulatory agents, such as cytokines, growth factors, antioxidants, and small interfering RNAs (siRNAs), have presented great potential in preventing and/or alleviating airway inflammatory diseases in multiple studies [65–67]. Furthermore, given the significant roles of chronic inflammation and oxidative stress in the pathogenesis of airway inflammatory diseases, many plants and herbs have also been shown to be beneficial as they are the rich source of antioxidative compounds and have demonstrated remarkable antiinflammatory activities [8,68–70]. For example, natural compounds such as resveratrol in grapes and red wine, garlic, as well as curcumin, were found to exhibit antitumor effects by the inhibition of COX enzymes or VEGF, and by targeting proinflammatory signaling pathways including NF-κB, MAPK, and JNK [56]. Despite that, these agents are often unable to achieve therapeutic success due to several pharmacokinetic drawbacks, which include low solubility, rapid clearance, and poor in vivo stability. Thus, the application of nanoparticles has been proposed by researchers as a feasible solution to overcome these drawbacks and to improve the therapeutic efficacies of these potential agents in the management of airway inflammatory diseases [71,72].

3.1.1 Solubility

Solubility is defined as the degree to which a pure substance can be dissolved in a solvent to form a homogeneous solution, in which the distribution of atoms, molecules, and ions is uniform throughout the solution. Solubility is a major parameter to achieve the desired concentration of drugs in systemic circulation for eliciting a pharmacological effect [73–75]. As such, drugs with poor water solubility often require higher doses for achieving therapeutic plasma concentrations upon their administration. Therefore, conventional dosage forms may result in under- or overmedication and incidences of undesirable side effects, thereby affecting patient compliance and reduced overall therapeutic efficacy [74,75].

Due to the significance of inflammation in the pathogenesis of various chronic airway diseases, compounds with remarkable antiinflammatory properties have attracted great interest for the management of these diseases. In this respect, many bioactive compounds obtained from natural plant sources, such as curcumin, celastrol, quercetin, luteolin, and triptolide, have been found to possess excellent antioxidative and antiinflammatory effects that are beneficial in the treatment of multiple airway inflammatory diseases [76–78]. However, as observed in most studies, these plant-derived natural compounds often have poor solubility and permeability, resulting in low systemic bioavailability, which limits their successful clinical translation for use as therapeutics in airway inflammatory diseases [73,75,79,80]. Ideally, drug molecules should possess well-balanced properties where sufficient hydrophilicity is essential for the molecules to solubilize in aqueous biological liquids, and with sufficient lipophilicity for the molecules to penetrate through biological membranes [73].

Nanomedicine represents a versatile technology that gained rising interest among formulation scientists and researchers for developing poorly water-soluble compounds into viable dosage forms. Overall, the technique of delivering drug molecules using various nanocarriers appeared as a potential strategy for enhancing systemic bioavailability and therapeutic efficacy of poorly water-soluble compounds, as this technique can facilitate the delivery of drug molecules to their physiological target while preserving their integrity and bioactivity [79]. Drug molecules can be either conjugated, complexed, encapsulated, entrapped, adsorbed, and attached to the nanocarriers for this purpose [81]. Studies have affirmed that once a therapeutic agent is encapsulated within a nanocarrier, its pharmacokinetic properties, biodistribution, and in vivo behavior will be dictated by the physicochemical properties of the nanocarrier rather than the therapeutic agent itself [82]. Apart from that, due to the submicron size of nanoparticles, there will be a significant increase in surface area and the surface-to-volume ratio, which can be positively exploited to enhance dissolution rate and offer opportunities for modulating the behavior of nanocarriers [83–85]. To date, many different types of drug delivery systems have been identified to improve solubility and subsequent bioavailability of hydrophobic compounds, in which every type of nanocarrier has its distinct characteristics as well as advantages and disadvantages [86,87]. These will be further explored and discussed later in this chapter within the context of airway inflammatory diseases.

3.1.2 Bio-circulation and therapeutic action

Apart from poor solubility, certain therapeutic agents used in the management of airway inflammatory diseases have also displayed short biological half-life that is insufficient to achieve the optimal concentration in the systemic circulation needed for an effective therapeutic response [17,20]. Generally, if the half-life of a therapeutic agent is too short, more frequent dosing is required to maintain desired exposures, which may pose challenges to achieve an optimal efficacy, safety, as well as patient compliance. On the other hand, if the half-life of a therapeutic agent is too long, the period over accumulation and subsequent elimination will be prolonged, which may pose challenges to the management of adverse reactions [88]. Therefore, the half-life of therapeutic agents is another key parameter in the design and development of advanced therapeutics to ensure

effective therapeutic action and enhancement of treatment outcomes in airway inflammatory diseases.

Ideally, the drug level in systemic circulation should be maintained within the therapeutic window, which is between the minimum toxic concentration and the minimum effective concentration. Utilization of advanced drug-delivery systems has been proven advantageous to optimize the circulation half-life of therapeutic agents. This is attributed to the ability of these nanocarriers to achieve a sustained and controlled drug-release profile, which subsequently prolongs therapeutic action and improves therapeutic efficacy [89,90]. Nanocarriers that exhibit a sustained release pattern of a drug can improve patient compliance; at the same time, it also brings about other benefits in the treatment of a disease, such as reduction of required dosage and frequency of administration, maintenance of drug circulation time greater than the biological half-life of the drug, as well as the generation of steady-state and fixed therapeutic action due to persistent biological concentration of the drug within the therapeutic window [89,91]. As the half-life and bio-circulation of a compound are profoundly influenced by the compound's release from a nanocarrier, modulation of the structure and composition of a nanocarrier and its method of preparation can produce varying effects on the overall therapeutic action. Other factors that can influence the release of therapeutic compounds from nanocarriers include pH, temperature, desorption of adsorbed or surface-bound drugs, diffusion of drugs through the nanoparticle matrix, as well as the swelling and erosion of the nanoparticle matrix [87,90]. Hence, nanocarriers developed for therapeutic use in airway inflammatory diseases must be carefully designed and evaluated to ensure an efficient drug-release profile and maintenance of drug half-life over a reasonable period for maximal therapeutic efficacy.

Nonetheless, the presence of the host mononuclear phagocyte system (MPS) poses a great challenge to an effective delivery of drug-loaded nanoparticles. This is attributed to the recognition of nanoparticles as foreign objects by cells of the MPS, which consists of dendritic cells, granulocytes, monocytes, and tissue-resident macrophages, leading to their early clearance from systemic circulation and/or release of loaded drugs at off-target sites [92–94]. A technique known as PEGylation, which is referred to as the process of coating the nanoparticle surface with a synthetic polymeric nanomaterial known as polyethylene glycol (PEG), has been well established as an efficient strategy to overcome this challenge. PEGylation typically confers "stealth" behavior to nanocarriers, which can effectively diminish their recognition and uptake by cells of the MPS, resulting in further enhancement of the bio-circulation time and therapeutic action of drug-loaded nanoparticles, as well as improved site-selective delivery of drugs [93,95,96]. Double PEGylation of nanoparticles has also been demonstrated as a promising strategy to remarkably improve pharmacodynamic and pharmacokinetic properties of drugs, which offers additional benefits on top of those offered by drug-delivery systems [96].

3.1.3 *In vivo stability*

Biopharmaceutical drugs, or biologics, offer the benefits of high specificity and potency as compared to other small-molecule drugs in the treatment of diseases. This is attributed to their macromolecular nature that provides structural complexity, which is often a prerequisite for specificity. However, the structural complexity of biopharmaceutical drugs has rendered their formulation and intracellular delivery challenging [97]. In terms of airway inflammatory diseases, siRNA is an example of a biologic that has potential therapeutic benefits via the post-transcriptional modulation of target gene expressions. Typically, siRNAs can "silence" specific genes to influence the expression of proinflammatory cytokines and chemokines, thereby modifying the molecular mechanisms underlying the pathogenesis of airway inflammatory diseases [98]. Nevertheless, these are often highly fragile and relatively unstable in vivo. Namely, the loss of bioactivity due to environmental triggers such as temperature and moisture, as well as chemical and enzymatic degradation that can occur in storage and/or in the body, puts a substantial pressure on formulation scientists and researchers to develop an efficient biopharmaceutical drug [99]. In addition, despite intranasal delivery of siRNAs being the preferred route due to reduced invasiveness and systemic toxicities, as well as increased specificity for the respiratory system, several biological barriers such as the respiratory cilia and mucus layer have hindered their effective delivery for target gene suppression [100]. Thus, nanoencapsulation of these biologics within advanced drug-delivery systems may be a feasible strategy to improve the delivery of these agents. Like those discussed previously, nanocarriers can enhance the half-life of biologics and their retention time in systemic circulation while facilitating their absorption, as well as to protect these sensitive cargoes from degradation in hostile biological environments, thereby enhancing therapeutic outcomes [101,102]. In short, nanocarriers can act as the solution to various drawbacks of conventional biologics' delivery, resulting in enhanced patient acceptability and eventual clinical success.

3.2 Pulmonary drug delivery

Due to their submicron-sized diameter, nanotherapeutics can be administered through different routes such as oral administration, intravenous injection, and pulmonary inhalation. Generally, pulmonary delivery via inhalation is the means of delivering therapeutic agents directly into the lungs with preferential deposition and retention within diseased lung regions with specificity and it is particularly useful for the management of airway inflammatory disease. In contrast to other routes of administration, pulmonary inhalation presented a multitude of advantages in the treatment and management of these diseases [103,104]. Namely, drug delivery via pulmonary inhalation offers direct administration to the lungs, resulting in high drug concentrations in the diseased tissues with low systemic concentrations. The pulmonary route of drug delivery also evades the hepatic first-pass metabolism and gastrointestinal proteolysis. This is further associated with high pulmonary efficacy and improved drug bioavailability within the lung, thereby minimizing the risks of systemic adverse reactions, as a lower dosage is needed to produce therapeutic effects [104–106]. Apart from improving the biodistribution of therapeutic agents for site-specific delivery, pulmonary inhalation also takes advantage of the extremely large alveolar surface area, a dense capillary network, and a thin biological barrier that contributes to efficient drug absorption, and rapid onset of action [106,107]. In short, an efficient drug-delivery system for pulmonary inhalation is designed to be specifically retained in the diseased area of the lung and does not penetrate in its active form into the systemic circulation to protect other body parts from potential toxicity [107].

Advanced drug-delivery systems for pulmonary inhalation are often suspended in liquid or dry powder aerosol droplets, whereby the deposition of these droplets in the lung after inhalation is influenced by their particulate properties, such as particle size, shape, density, surface charge, and surface composition. Specifically, particle size is the major determinant of the fate and biodistribution of inhaled nanotherapeutics, in which drugs can be deposited in different areas of the lung depending on their particle size (Fig. 1) [13,106]. Upon inhalation, particles with sizes between 5 and 10 μm travel through the oropharynx and upper respiratory tracts at high velocity. These particles may collide with the respiratory wall via a mechanism known as impaction, which leads to their deposition in the nasal cavity or oropharynx regions [13,108]. Generally, particle deposition via impaction increases with increasing particle size. As such, larger particles can be easily deposited in the upper airways [109]. However, particles larger than 5–6 μm are easily eliminated via exhalation and are rarely deposited in the airways. Next, through sedimentation, particles with sizes between 3 and 5 μm can be delivered into the trachea, whereas particles with sizes between 1 and 3 μm can be deposited in the bronchus-bronchiole regions [13]. Especially in the smaller airways, the deposition of particles in these airway regions is primarily affected by gravitational force as there is a high residence time of inhaled air. The breathing pattern can also influence the sedimentation of particles, in which a slower

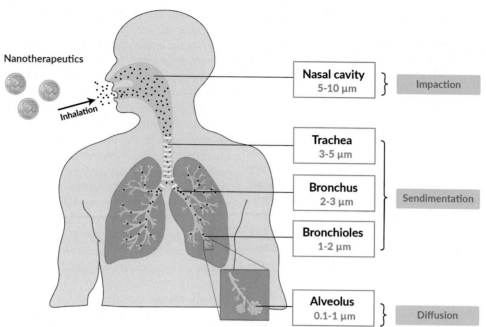

Nanotherapeutics

Inhalation

Nasal cavity 5-10 μm	Impaction
Trachea 3-5 μm	
Bronchus 2-3 μm	Sendimentation
Bronchioles 1-2 μm	
Alveolus 0.1-1 μm	Diffusion

FIG. 1 Size-dependent deposition of inhaled nanotherapeutics within the lung. *(No permission required.)*

breathing pattern enables a longer timespan for the sedimentation of inhaled particles [108,109]. Lastly, particles at the nanoscale, typically those with particle sizes of less than 1 μm can be delivered to the lower respiratory tract including the alveolus. In these airway regions, particles are mainly deposited via diffusion as the air velocity is negligible. Typically, diffusional deposition of particles decreases with increasing particle size and increasing respiratory rate [13,106,108,109]. Hence, the evident correlation between particles' size and their retention in the airway must be carefully considered during the design of nanocarriers to achieve an optimal pulmonary delivery and maximal therapeutic effects in the treatment of airway inflammatory diseases.

3.3 Passive and active targeting

As mentioned earlier, the targeted delivery of nanotherapeutics is aimed at retaining their loaded active therapeutic moieties within their desired site of action while limiting their accumulation in healthy tissues and organs. Such a goal can be achieved by both passive and active targeting of therapeutic agents [110]. The strategy of passive targeting refers to the exploitation of specific pathophysiological characteristics of the diseased cells and their surrounding microenvironments by drug-loaded nanocarriers to accumulate in their targeted sites. Particularly, a passive targeting strategy via the enhanced permeability and retention (EPR) effect is useful in the treatment of lung cancer, in which particles with sizes between 10 and 1000 nm can preferentially accumulate within tumor tissues instead of normal tissues [111,112]. Generally, the

endothelial gap of angiogenic tumor vasculature is usually larger as compared to that of normal vasculature due to the nonresponsiveness of tumor cells to cell signaling processes involved in regulating vasculogenesis. Therefore, it enables the entry of these macromolecules into tumor tissues through their leaky vasculature and abnormally wide pores. In addition, tumor tissues have limited lymphatic drainage and reduced molecule clearance, which could further result in higher drug retention [111–113]. Thus, nanocarriers can be designed to deliver therapeutic agents to targeted sites via the EPR effect, in which a high concentration of these agents can be deposited within diseased tissues while minimizing any off-target side effects, leading to more effective therapy. Nevertheless, the efficiency of passive targeting is limited as the conditions attributed to the EPR effect are not observed in all diseased tissues that commonly develop specific mechanisms involved in the resistance of conventional therapeutic approaches [110].

On the other hand, active targeting refers to the strategy where the surface of nanocarriers is functionalized with targeting moieties such as proteins, antibodies, aptamers, peptides, carbohydrates, and glycoproteins that present great affinity to their cellular binding partners such as cell-surface receptors, tumor antigens, and tumor vasculature [110]. Typically, such a strategy can contribute to the specific localization of drug-loaded nanocarriers in diseased cells instead of healthy cells; at the same time, it reduces nonspecific interactions between the nanocarrier and the cell plasma membrane [113,114]. Therefore, an active targeting strategy can be employed to complement the EPR-based passive targeting strategy to further enhance the deposition of therapeutic agents within their targeted tissues. Apart from targeting ligands, hydrophilic molecules such as PEG can also be functionalized on the surface of nanocarriers to extend their bio-circulation time via the avoidance of recognition and clearance by the reticuloendothelial system (RES) [94]. Nonetheless, the targeting efficiency of ligands may vary depending on their molecular weight, valency, targeting affinity, density, and their biocompatibility with the nanocarriers. Thus, to ensure an effective targeting of nanocarriers and perfect optimization of their intended therapeutic effects in the treatment of airway inflammatory diseases, it is of utmost importance that these targeting ligands are carefully designed based on the specificity of overexpressed antigens on the surface of diseased cells, while considering their biocompatibility with nanomaterials [113,115,116].

4 Advanced drug-delivery systems as advanced therapeutics in airway inflammatory diseases

As discussed, nanomedicine-based delivery of therapeutic agents offers a platform to carry diversified cargos including hydrophobic drugs to their desired sites with high specificity and efficiency. Therefore, the utilization of advanced drug-delivery systems provides highly focused and fine-tuned treatment of diseases at the molecular level, thereby enhancing the therapeutic outcomes of conventional drugs as they become more effective with minimal adverse effects. Besides, advanced drug-delivery systems are highly capable of modulating the biodistribution of therapeutic agents by releasing them in a controlled manner over a prolonged period and retaining them in specific sites within the body [117,118]. Many types of advanced drug-delivery systems have been developed and are already in use today, which include liposomes, polymeric nanoparticles, carbon nanotubes, mesoporous silica nanoparticles, and gold nanoparticles (Fig. 2). However, the characteristics and behavior of each type of nanocarrier may differ from one another depending on its structure, composition, and technique of fabrication. In the following sections, we provide an insight into the major features and characteristics that are specific to a few of the commonly employed nanocarriers in the management of airway inflammatory diseases. Besides, we further present how these advanced drug-delivery systems could contribute to enhanced therapeutic outcomes in airway inflammatory diseases by highlighting a few studies conducted in this area of research. Notably, most findings from these studies corroborate our earlier discussions,

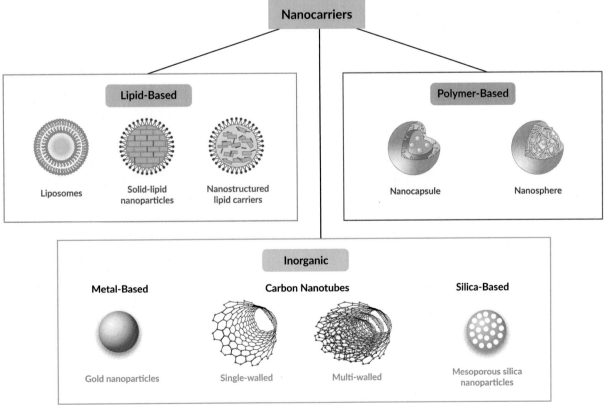

FIG. 2 Various advanced drug-delivery systems that are employed in the treatment of airway inflammatory diseases. *(No permission required.)*

which affirmed that the utilization of advanced nanomedicine-based strategies is indeed a feasible approach and can be developed as the next-generation therapeutics in airway inflammatory diseases.

4.1 Lipid-based delivery systems

4.1.1 Liposomes

Liposomes are small, artificial, and sphere-shaped vesicles that are composed of cholesterol and other natural nontoxic phospholipids. In terms of their structure, liposomes typically consist of one or more concentric lipid bilayers that enclose discrete aqueous spaces. They are the most common and well-studied nanocarriers employed for targeted drug delivery, which can be attributed to their unique ability to entrap both hydrophilic and hydrophobic agents, thereby enabling a wide range of therapeutic agents to be encapsulated [119,120]. Typically, hydrophobic agents are loaded within the bilayer membrane whereas hydrophilic agents are loaded within the aqueous center of its structure [121]. Given that phospholipids are the major components of biological cell membranes, both cell membranes and liposomes can coexist during the release mechanism [122]. Generally, the application of liposomes as an advanced drug-delivery system offers multiple benefits, which include their high degree of biocompatibility, biodegradability, capacity for self-assembly, as well as their ability to encapsulate large payloads and macromolecules, such as DNA, RNA, and proteins. Besides, liposomes can be easily engineered with specific physiochemical and biophysical properties to modify their biological behavior depending on their intended application. Like most advanced drug-delivery systems, encapsulation of therapeutic agents within liposomes helps to shield them from early inactivation and premature degradation, resulting in prolonged therapeutic action [119–122]. In addition, liposomal formulations are often less toxic, and they present much improved pharmacological parameters as compared to free drugs. Despite that, the properties and behavior of liposomes can be altered by their composition, size, surface charge, bilayer rigidity, method of preparation, number of lamellae, as well as surface modification [122]. Therefore, liposomal formulations must be carefully evaluated regarding the practicability for their intended application prior to clinical translation.

The potential of liposomes as drug-loaded nanocarriers for the management of airway inflammatory diseases have been investigated by many researchers. In a study by Ng et al., curcumin, a natural bioactive ingredient derived from *Curcuma longa*, was loaded into liposomes, and their anti-inflammatory effects on lipopolysaccharide (LPS)-induced BCi-NS1.1 cell lines were evaluated. Although the antiinflammatory and antioxidative effects of curcumin have been

well documented in multiple studies, it has poor solubility, which had limited its application in the medical field. Therefore, encapsulation of curcumin in liposomes may present as a feasible strategy to enhance its absorption and therapeutic efficacy. In this study, the researchers reported that the nanoformulation effectively suppressed the expressions of proinflammatory cytokines, including TNF-α, IL-1β, IL-6, and IL-8 via the modulation of NF-κB and STAT3 signaling pathways. Notably, treatment with unloaded liposomes resulted in slight reduction of IL-6 and IL-8 expressions, indicating the intrinsic antiinflammatory activity of the nanocarrier attributed to phosphatidylcholine in its components. As such, the nanoformulation can lead to a synergistic activity in inhibiting proinflammatory signaling responses involved in the pathogenesis of airway inflammatory diseases [123]. Hydroxycitrate, a component of the fruit rind of *Garcinia cambogia*, is a citrate analog that exhibits inhibitory effects on the enzyme ATP citrate lyase, which can ultimately reduce the levels of proinflammatory mediators, including ROS, NO, and PGE2 which are involved in the pathogenesis of various airway inflammatory diseases. Despite that, hydroxycitrate has low membrane permeability, which requires a large concentration to elicit an optimal biological effect. To overcome this issue, Vassallo et al. had loaded hydroxycitrate into liposomes as an attempt to enhance its bioavailability and reduce the concentration required to produce a biological effect. It was reported that the liposomal formulation resulted in higher intracellular accumulation of hydroxycitrate in macrophages by approximately 4 times, whereas the amount of hydroxycitrate needed to downregulate ROS, NO, and PGE2 was reduced by ten times, which suggests that liposomes can potentially be employed to enhance the effects of hydroxycitrate in targeting the citrate pathway involved in inflammatory processes underlying the development of airway inflammatory diseases [124]. Apart from that, research by Honmane et al. had attempted to improve the oral bioavailability of salbutamol sulfate, a β2-adrenergic agonist used in the treatment of asthma, by incorporating it into liposomes and further loaded into dry powder inhalers (DPI) for pulmonary inhalation. It was shown that the liposomal DPI had prolonged in vitro drug release of up to 14 h, which improved the retention of drug in the lungs while avoiding the first-pass hepatic metabolism of salbutamol sulfate. These phenomena suggested that liposomes are feasible for the pulmonary delivery of salbutamol sulfate, and such a formulation can reduce the dosing frequency and the associated adverse effects of salbutamol sulfate [125]. Likewise, Chen et al. presented that liposomes sustained the release of salbutamol sulfate in the respiratory tract and lungs for up to 48 h. Notably, the in vivo antiasthmatic effect persisted for up to 18 h in contrast to free salbutamol sulfate, which only persisted for less than 8 h [126]. Taken together, these studies indicate that liposomes can be a promising platform for the delivery of various therapeutic agents to their targeted sites, which enhances the biological activities and therapeutic outcomes of the loaded therapeutic agents in the management of airway inflammatory diseases.

4.1.2 Solid lipid nanoparticles

Solid lipid nanoparticles (SLNs) are a newer types of nanocarriers constructed on a solid lipid matrix, such as highly purified triglycerides, complex glyceride mixtures, or waxes that are stabilized by multiple surfactants, such as soybean lecithin, Poloxamer 188, and sodium glycocholate, so that they remain in a solid state at both storage and body temperatures [120]. SLNs are developed as an improvement to liposomes, in which they can achieve a sustained drug-release pattern due to their solid matrix [127]. Other major characteristics of SLNs include great tolerability, biocompatibility and biodegradability, protection of the incorporated drugs from environmental, chemical, photochemical, and oxidative degradation, reduced drug leakage, as well as high physical stability of the incorporated drugs. Over the years, the use of SLNs as nanocarriers for therapeutic applications has become increasingly common due to their small size and large surface area, as well as their potential to improve the performances of therapeutic agents [120,127,128]. Additionally, SLNs are favored as they offer the feasibility of carrying both hydrophilic and lipophilic drugs, with higher entrapment efficiency for hydrophobic drugs as they do not contain an aqueous core like liposomes [129,130]. The drug-loading capacity in SLNs is mainly dependent on the solubility of drug in molten lipid, miscibility of drug and melted lipid, chemical and physical structure of the solid lipid matrix, as well as the polymorphic state of the lipid material. Ideally, higher concentration of the drug should be soluble in the melted lipid for a higher drug loading capacity. At the same time, drug solubility should be significantly higher than desired, as solubility typically decreases when the lipid melt is cooled and further reduced in solid lipids [130].

In terms of airway inflammatory diseases, there have been several studies conducted to investigate the potential of SLNs in enhancing therapeutic outcomes. A study by Castellani et al. has developed SLNs for the encapsulation of grape-seed extract for the reduction of oxidative stress and inflammation. The nanoformulation was rapidly internalized by airway epithelial cells and was retained for a reasonable time for the optimal exertion of its antioxidative and antiinflammatory effects. This corresponded to the observation where there was a significant reduction in the production of ROS and downregulation of NF-κB nuclear translocation with a prolonged retention time in vivo as compared with free grape-seed extract, indicating the high stability and long-term persistence of SLNs in releasing their cargoes within targeted sites [131]. In another work, Ji et al. encapsulated naringenin in SLNs to improve its physical stability and pulmonary bioavailability. Naringenin is a flavonoid that exhibits antioxidative and antiinflammatory effects, which may be beneficial for the treatment of airway inflammatory diseases. However, it is a poorly water-soluble compound with poor oral bioavailability, which has restricted its therapeutic application. The researchers showed that the naringenin-loaded SLNs were nontoxic and had a sustained drug-release profile. In vivo study also revealed that the nanoformulation produced a remarkable improvement in the relative bioavailability, which was 2.53-fold greater in comparison to the free naringenin suspension upon pulmonary administration. These findings supported the potential of SLNs as an advanced drug-delivery system for enhancing the solubility and bioavailability of poorly water-soluble drugs, thus improving their therapeutic efficacy [132]. Similarly, SLNs have been shown to enhance the therapeutic effects of curcumin in an ovalbumin-induced allergic rat model of asthma. In the study by Wang et al., curcumin-loaded SLNs demonstrated a sustained drug-release profile, resulting in a significantly higher plasma concentration as compared to free curcumin. Therefore, the nanoformulation remarkably suppressed airway hyperresponsiveness and the infiltration of inflammatory cells, as well as downregulated the expressions of Th2 cytokines, such as IL-4 and IL-13, in the bronchoalveolar lavage fluid in contrast to the asthmatic group and free curcumin-treated group [133]. Apart from that, Melo et al. had evaluated the immunomodulatory potential of 15-deoxy-delta(12,14)-prostaglandin J2 (15d-PGJ2)-loaded SLNs. 15d-PGJ2 is a PPAR-γ agonist that can exert antiinflammatory activity, which may be beneficial in the treatment of airway inflammatory diseases. However, its high affinity to serum proteins led to the need for higher concentrations to induce an antiinflammatory response. The researchers reported that SLN-encapsulated 15d-PGJ2 was able to reduce neutrophil migration to an inflammatory site at a concentration 33 times lower as compared to free 15d-PGJ2 in the models of carrageenan, LPS, and methylated bovine serum albumin-induced inflammation. The level of IL-10 was also increased, whereas the levels of IL-1β and IL-17 were decreased, indicating that SLNs can exert antiinflammatory effects using only a low concentration of 15d-PGJ2 [134]. In short, the delivery of therapeutic agents using SLNs can offer additional advantages on top of those presented by liposomes, which can result in further enhancement of positive therapeutic outcomes in the management of airway inflammatory diseases.

4.1.3 Nanostructured lipid carriers

Nanostructured lipid carriers (NLCs) are regarded as the second generation of SLNs, as NLCs were mainly developed to overcome the shortcomings of SLNs. While SLNs are composed of solid lipids, NLCs consists of an unstructured lipid matrix that results from a blend of solid and liquid lipids, such as ethyl oleate, glyceryl dioleate, glyceryl tricaprylate, and isopropyl myristate [120,135]. A major advantage of NLCs over SLNs is that NLCs offer increased drug-loading capacity while preventing drug expulsion to achieve long-term drug stability, which can be attributed to their highly unordered structures that offer firmer inclusion of the drug molecules within the matrix [135,136]. In contrast to NLCs, SLNs have a perfect crystal lattice structure that offers much lesser space for the accommodation of drug molecules within the lipid core, resulting in reduced drug-loading capacity and drug expulsion from the system. Besides, higher drug-entrapment efficiency in NLCs can also be associated with a higher solubility of drugs in liquid lipids as compared with solid lipids [137]. Another advantage of NLCs as compared to SLNs is the modulation of the drug-release pattern. A biphasic release pattern is often exhibited by NLCs, whereby the drug is released in a burst manner initially, followed by a constant rate of sustained drug release. The initial burst-release pattern is attributed to the drug-enriched casing formed by the liquid lipid located in the outer layers of NLCs. Generally, it is possible to modify the drug-release profile of NLCs by varying the ratio of liquid lipid to solid lipid [138–140]. Other benefits of NLCs include feasibility for surface modification, site-specific targeting, capability to encapsulate both hydrophilic and hydrophobic therapeutic agents, as well as low toxicity [120].

The advantages of NLCs in improving the efficacy of therapeutic moieties have been proven in a study by Patil-Gadhe and Pokharkar. It was found that montelukast-loaded NLCs had a sustained drug-release profile over 24 h with an improvement in maximum concentration (C_{max}) and area under the plasma concentration-time curve over the last 24 h (AUC_{0-24}) by 9- and 60-fold, respectively. Besides, as compared with free montelukast aqueous solution, the nanoformulation demonstrated 143-fold improvement in bioavailability, 4-fold decrease in elimination rate, prolonged half-life, as well as increased mean residence time, which collectively implied that NLCs can be employed to enhance the therapeutic effects of montelukast in the management of asthma [141]. The same researchers have also successfully formulated NLCs loaded with rosuvastatin for the treatment of COPD, in which there was an increased deposition of rosuvastatin in the lungs of up to 97%. The nanoformulation also presented an approximate 1.14-fold increase in the lung concentration of rosuvastatin and improved drug half-life following intratracheal instillation as compared to free rosuvastatin. These findings can be attributed to the lipid composition of NLC as well as its ability to avoid macrophage clearance, thereby improving its targeting and subsequent therapeutic efficacy [142].

Apart from asthma and COPD, NLCs have also been broadly explored as a delivery system for therapeutic agents that are used in the treatment of lung cancer. In a study by Wang et al., NLCs were loaded with both paclitaxel and doxorubicin as an attempt to increase synergism between the two drugs for the treatment of lung cancer. A decrease in tumor weight and volume was reported in vivo, which was demonstrated by an enhanced tumor inhibition rate of up to 84% in mice with NCL-H460 lung cancer cells as compared to a tumor inhibition rate of only 26% in mice given free paclitaxel and free doxorubicin. Besides, cytotoxicity studies carried out on NCL-H460 lung cancer cell lines using the nanoformulation showed a 9-fold decrease in half maximal inhibitory concentration (IC_{50}) when compared to free paclitaxel and free doxorubicin, further proving the enhanced antitumor activity of the drugs when encapsulated within NLCs [143]. Likewise, Somayeh et al. showed that there was an increased cytotoxic effect on A549 lung cancer cell lines with the use of sunitinib-loaded NLCs. The nanoformulation exhibited an IC_{50} value of 2.17 μg/mL as compared to 3.14 μg/mL in free sunitinib, and upon modification of SUN-NLCs with biotin, an IC_{50} value of 1.66 μg/mL can be obtained. The addition of biotin also improved tumor targeting, thereby allowing an increase in the cellular uptake of sunitinib, which can improve therapeutic outcomes in lung cancer [144]. In short, NLCs can be utilized as an advanced drug-delivery system for improving the efficacy of various therapeutic agents in the treatment of airway inflammatory diseases. Nevertheless, the surface charges of NLCs and the components attached on their surface for active targeting may trigger an immune response in the human biological system [145]. Hence, nanoformulations designed with NLCs as nanocarriers should undergo toxicity tests to ensure their safety prior to clinical use.

4.2 Polymer-based delivery systems

Polymeric nanoparticles (PNPs) have received considerable attention in drug-delivery research and have been widely regarded as a promising tool for improving therapeutic outcomes in the treatment of various human diseases [146]. As an advanced drug-delivery system, PNPs possess several advantages, such as easy preparation and synthesis, superior biocompatibility, as well as biomimetic character. Another major feature of PNPs is their highly water-soluble property that contributes to enhanced bio-circulation and efficient drug delivery to targeted sites within the body. PNPs also exhibit higher storage stability by protecting their cargoes against the external environment, which can be translated to longer shelf-life that leads to lower therapeutic cost in a clinical setting [147,148]. Moreover, recent technological advancements in polymer chemistry have enabled modulation to the physicochemical characteristics and surface chemistry of polymeric nanomaterials, thereby allowing the fabrication of customized PNPs that can achieve both sustained drug release and site-specific localization depending on their intended therapeutic application [149].

Although PNP is a collective term that can be generally used to describe any type of nanosized particles fabricated using polymeric nanomaterials, it is specifically referred to two distinct systems depending on their structural organization and composition. Namely, a nanocapsule is a reservoir system in which the therapeutic moieties are retained in an aqueous or lipid core and is contained by a narrow, solidified polymeric envelope that controls the drug-release profile from the core [146,150]. As such, the therapeutic moieties loaded within the core of nanocapsules can be protected from unwanted degradation by the polymeric coat, and the polymeric coat can be further functionalized to specifically recognize its targeted site [150,151]. On the other hand, a nanosphere is referred to as a matrix system that is formed by a continuous network of dense, spherical polymeric matrix. In nanospheres, the therapeutic moieties are entrapped within the spherical center or are adsorbed on the mass surface. One advantage of the nanosphere system over the nanocapsule system is that therapeutic moieties can be uniformly distributed and evenly dispersed within the polymeric matrix [146,151].

4.2.1 Natural polymers

Naturally occurring polymers are commonly utilized in the design of advanced drug-delivery systems due to their abundance, biocompatibility, biodegradability, and low toxicity. These may include polysaccharide-based polymers, such as chitosan, alginate, hyaluronic acid, and cyclodextrin, or protein-based polymers such as albumin, collagen, and gelatin [152]. In general, polysaccharides have numerous functional groups and a wide range of molecular weights with differing chemical and structural compositions, contributing to their diversity in terms of their physical properties and structure. Therefore, these functional groups on the molecular chains of polysaccharides can be subjected to chemical modifications that lead to the generation of various polysaccharide derivatives [153]. As most polysaccharides consist of hydrophilic groups such as carboxyl, hydroxyl, and amino groups, they exhibit bio-adhesive properties due to the formation of noncovalent bonds with biological tissues, which results in increased retention time and improved absorption of drugs at the targeted sites [154,155]. As for protein-based polymers, they are natural macromolecules that can be obtained from various plants and animal sources. As renewable resources, they can be easily derived and processed at a relatively low cost. Besides, they are water-soluble, biodegradable, biocompatible, nonantigenic, and have greater stability [156,157]. Drugs encapsulated in protein-based polymeric nanocarriers are also able to exert their functions at a minimum dose, thus minimizing drug resistance and other adverse effects. Moreover, the amphiphilicity of protein-based polymers, along with their versatility, allow them to interact well and form covalent linkages with multiple drugs and ligands [157].

Chitosan is the most widely used natural polymer for drug delivery due to its capability to blend with a vast range of polymers and ease of surface modification, along with lower toxicity and its nonimmunogenic property. Besides, the cationic property of chitosan enables it to interact with negatively charged components, such as nucleic acids and cell-surface macromolecules [152]. Generally, the properties of chitosan are dictated by the level of substitution of the acetamido group with amine groups, referred to as the degree of deacetylation. The molecular weight of chitosan also influences its biological and physiological properties. For instance, high molecular-weight chitosan demonstrates lower solubility and slower degradation as compared to chitosan with a lower molecular weight [152,154]. While chitosan is insoluble in most organic solvents and under neutral conditions, it can be solubilized in acidic media due to its high crystallinity and abundance of amino groups. As such, chitosan derivatives have been developed for the improvement of their solubility and processing [158].

In terms of airway inflammatory diseases, there have been several studies that demonstrated the potential of chitosan as an effective nanocarrier to enhance therapeutic outcomes. For example, one study by Yang et al. had evaluated the therapeutic efficacy of bacillus Calmette-Guerin-polysaccharide nucleic acid (BCG-PSN) and ovalbumin-loaded chitosan nanoparticles on airway inflammation. BCG-PSN can exert an immunomodulatory effect by regulating Tregs and inhibiting the production of antigen-specific IgE, which can significantly reduce airway eosinophilic inflammation and alleviate airway hyperresponsiveness. Desensitization by allergen-specific immunotherapy also represents an effective means for asthma therapy and has been proven to relieve symptoms, decrease asthma deterioration, and attenuate airway hyperresponsiveness. However, BCG-PSN is currently only employed as an adjuvant whereas desensitization therapy is slow in efficacy and requires gradual dosage increment of allergens, which may lead to adverse reactions. In this study, the simultaneous encapsulation of BCG-PSN and ovalbumin into chitosan nanoparticles remarkably suppressed the level of eosinophils and immune cells in the bronchoalveolar lavage fluid and downregulated IL-4, while the levels of IL-10 and IFN-γ were increased. The proliferation rate of T cells was also significantly reduced with an increased proportion of CD4+CD25+Foxp3+. Notably, the antiinflammatory and airway hyperresponsiveness-alleviating effects of the nanoformulation were more pronounced in vivo as compared to

BCG-PSN or ovalbumin alone, indicating that there is a promising application prospect for chitosan nanoparticles to improve therapeutic outcomes in asthma [159]. In another work, Lee et al. employed thiolated chitosan nanoparticles to enhance the capacity of theophylline in alleviating allergic asthma. It was found that thiolated chitosan had enhanced mucoadhesiveness as compared to unmodified chitosan, which can be attributed to the formation of disulphide bonds between the thiol groups and the cysteine-rich subdomains of mucus glycoproteins, thereby deeming it an excellent candidate for the delivery of therapeutic agents to the mucus-rich bronchial epithelium. The increased mucoadhesiveness of thiolated chitosan nanoparticles led to greater reduction in eosinophils in the bronchoalveolar lavage fluid as compared to unmodified chitosan and theophylline alone. At the same time, theophylline induced the apoptosis of inflammatory cells to a greater extent when delivered with thiolated chitosan nanoparticles. Besides, mucus hypersecretion was also greatly suppressed by the nanoformulation, further affirming that thiolated chitosan nanoparticles can enhance the antiinflammatory effects of theophylline for the treatment of allergic lung inflammation [160]. Apart from that, Lee et al. had investigated the potential of hyaluronic acid-decorated glycol chitosan nanoparticles for the delivery of doxorubicin and celecoxib in NSCLC. Doxorubicin is an anthracycline antibiotic that inhibits the synthesis of DNA and cell growth through the disruption of topoisomerase I and II, as well as RNA polymerase, whereas celecoxib is a nonsteroidal antiinflammatory drug that inhibits the COX-2 enzyme. However, doxorubicin has been associated with multidrug resistance and low target selectivity, while the hydrophobic nature of celecoxib has hindered its effective clinical use. The nanoformulation demonstrated a pH-sensitive controlled drug-release profile in vitro and the drugs were effectively delivered into NSCLC cells via CD44-mediated endocytosis. In vivo, the nanoformulation remarkably suppressed tumor growth with an enhanced drug retention in the tumor tissues. Besides this, there were significant reductions in the expression of COX-2, MMP-2, and NF-κB without any evidence of hepatotoxicity. These suggest that the hyaluronic acid-decorated glycol chitosan nanoparticles can effectively deliver both anticancer and antiinflammatory drugs to targeted sites by exploiting the acidic condition of the tumor microenvironment and active targeting through the recognition of the CD44 receptor on NSCLC cells [161].

4.2.2 Synthetic polymers

The major disadvantages of the natural-based polymers, such as high degree of variability, complex structures, as well as a complicated and expensive extraction process have led to the advent of synthetic-based polymers. As such, the use of synthetic-based polymers as advanced drug-delivery

systems offers several advantages over natural-based polymers. Typically, synthetic-based polymers can be easily fabricated using reproducible protocols, resulting in the production of near-exact polymers with negligible batch-to-batch variation [162]. Besides, synthetic-based polymers offer researchers a versatile platform to engineer tailor-made nanomaterials with varying compositions and modifiable properties depending on their intended applications, thereby yielding a wide array of possibilities with the fabrication of different nanocarriers. Polymers for a specific application can also be fabricated by copolymerizing or blending several different polymers, leading to the generation of copolymers that inherit the intrinsic characteristics of the monomers [162,163].

Poly(lactic-glycolic acid) (PLGA) is an example of copolymer synthesized from poly(lactic acid) (PLA) and poly(glycolic acid) (PGA) via ring-opening copolymerization. It is a biodegradable polymer that degrades via the hydrolysis of ester bonds to its monomeric anions, namely glycolate and lactate, forming nontoxic degradation products that can be safely eliminated from the body [164]. As a copolymer of PLA and PGA, the degradation rate of PLGA is heavily dependent on its polymeric content, specifically the PLA-to-PGA ratio. For instance, as PLA has higher hydrophobicity due to the presence of methyl side groups as compared to PGA, PLGA containing a higher content of PLA is less hydrophilic, resulting in reduced water absorption and slower rate of degradation [164,165]. Unlike pure PLA and PGA, PLGA can also be solubilized in a wide range of organic solvents; therefore, it can be easily processed into various shape and size. At the same time, it allows the encapsulation of drugs and biomolecules of any size [166,167]. In short, the versatility of PLGA provides researchers with an opportunity to design drug-delivery systems with tailor-made properties, which can effectively facilitate the delivery of payload to the desired site at an appropriate duration for achieving an optimal therapeutic action.

Over the years, PLGA nanoparticles have been employed as potential tools to enhance therapeutic outcomes of airway inflammatory diseases in several studies. A study conducted by Roy et al. has formulated chrysin-loaded PLGA nanoparticles for ameliorating asthma progression in an in vivo model of ovalbumin-sensitized mice. Like most natural compounds, despite the antiinflammatory and antiallergic activities possessed by chrysin, its pharmaceutical application is limited due to poor solubility and bioavailability. Although free chrysin has negligible therapeutic effects, its encapsulation within PLGA nanoparticles remarkably reduced serum IgE, ovalbumin-induced lung histological alteration, and Th2 cytokines such as IL-4, IL-5, and IL-13 in bronchoalveolar lavage fluid. The expressions of proinflammatory cytokines such as TNF-α, IL-1β, IL-6, and IL-18, as well as their upstream signaling pathways including TLR, NF-κB, and NLRP3, were also downregulated, with a more pronounced effect as compared to free chrysin and of similar extent to the glucocorticoid dexamethasone. Thus, this study demonstrated the potential of PLGA nanoparticles in augmenting the therapeutic response of chrysin for ameliorating asthma [168]. PLGA nanoparticles were also employed for the encapsulation of alpha-1-antitrypsin (α1AT) in a study by Pirooznia et al. α1AT is a glycoprotein that inhibits serine protease and a broad group of other proteases that can shield the lungs from cellular inflammatory enzymes. For example, CF patients given α1AT demonstrated reduced sputum neutrophil numbers and the concentration of IL-8. The inhibitory effect of α1AT on IL-8 to reduce neutrophil recruitment to the lungs is also beneficial in the treatment of COPD as neutrophils are regarded as the primary causes of COPD pathogenesis. Despite that, α1AT is usually administered intravenously, which presents several drawbacks including high costs and undesirable immune reactions. As such, the pulmonary route is an alternative for the direct local delivery of α1AT to the lungs while avoiding prolonged systemic circulation. The researchers demonstrated that the nanoformulation was able to reach deep into the lungs for maximal therapeutic benefits while varying the lactide-to-glycolide ratio of PLGA can result in differing drug-release profiles. Namely, PLGA at the 75:25 ratio had an extended drug-release profile that allowed high local drug concentrations for the effective treatment of airway inflammatory diseases [169].

PEG is another example of a synthetic-based polymer that has been widely employed in drug-delivery applications. It is a hydrophilic polyether synthesized from ethylene oxide, and it can be fabricated in a wide range of molecular weights. Its popularity can be ascribed to the favorable characteristics of PEG, namely its nontoxicity, nonimmunogenicity, and nonionic properties, as well as great biocompatibility [170,171]. Besides, PEG helps to reduce the aggregation of particles via steric stabilization, resulting in nanocarriers with increased physical stability [172]. The high solubility of PEG in organic solvents also allows a wide range of functional groups to be attached to the terminal sites of PEG, thereby offering a plethora of opportunities in drug-delivery applications [171]. As discussed earlier, PEG is also widely known for its "stealth" behavior, in which therapeutic drugs, proteins, peptides, and oligonucleotides can be directly conjugated with PEG, or can be attached to the surface of various advanced drug-delivery systems, which is collectively known as the technique of PEGylation, to improve drug bioavailability and cellular uptake. This is the typical approach to achieve greater site-specific targeting, as the high level of hydration of the polyether backbone of PEG prevents nonspecific protein adsorption through steric repulsion. Shielding of drug-delivery systems also helps to avoid rapid recognition by the immune system, thereby increasing bio-circulation time in the body [93,94,171].

The benefits of PEG as an advanced drug-delivery system in the management of airway inflammatory diseases have been presented in several studies. One of them is a study by Matsuo et al. that developed betamethasone disodium 21-phosphate-loaded PEG–PLA nanoparticles for the evaluation of antiinflammatory activity in a murine model of asthma. It was reported that the nanoformulation reduced the number of infiltrating cells as well as the levels of IL-4 and IL-13 in bronchoalveolar lavage fluid. Such antiinflammatory effects were sustained for 7 days upon administration, in which a single intravenous injection was able to induce a pronounced and long-lasting therapeutic effect in vivo. The application of PEG–PLA nanoparticles also facilitated dose reduction of steroids, which is useful to avoid systemic adverse effects while preserving the positive effects of the steroids. The prolonged biocirculation of the nanoformulation can be associated with the "stealth" behavior conferred by PEG, thereby achieving greater benefits at the site of airway inflammation as compared to free steroids [173]. Another work by Wang et al. had employed PEG-PLGA nanoparticles to overcome the low water solubility of bavachinin, an essential small molecule obtained from the traditional Chinese herb *Psoralea corylifolia*, for the treatment of asthma. It was revealed that the nanoformulation had selectively accumulated within the inflamed lungs of asthmatic mice, which can be attributed to the EPR effect in which there may be vasculature leakage in the lungs due to chronic inflammation. Besides, the Th1/Th2 balance in the lung tissues was modulated, in which the differentiation of Th2 cells was remarkably suppressed while Th1 cell differentiation was increased. The mRNA expressions of Th2 cytokines, including IL-4, IL-5, IL-9, IL-13, and IL-33, were also downregulated, while IFN-γ was upregulated, which can lead to the alleviation of airway hyperresponsiveness and airway infiltration of inflammatory cells. These findings affirmed the potential of PEG-PLGA nanoparticles in enhancing the therapeutic effects of bavachinin, with great biocompatibility and specific targeting capability to the inflamed lung tissues for the treatment of asthma [174]. PEG nanoparticles have also been utilized for airway gene therapy in a study by da Silva et al. The researchers had developed DNA-PEG nanoparticles to encapsulate methionine serum thymus factor, a thymulin analog gene, for lung delivery in the management of asthma. Although intratracheal administration of thymulin plasmid alone reduced certain inflammatory aspects in the lungs as compared to saline-treated control, there was a significant reduction of collagen deposition and smooth muscle hypertrophy when the thymulin plasmid was delivered within the DNA-PEG nanoparticles. These were consistent to the findings in which VEGF and TGF-β were downregulated with a more pronounced effect in DNA-PEG nanoparticles in contrast to thymulin plasmid alone, which effectively prevented the airway remodeling process in asthmatic lungs. Airway inflammation was also attenuated, signified by increased IFN-γ that stimulates Th1 cells and inhibits Th2-induced effector functions, which further inhibited eosinophil recruitment and the secretion of eotaxin and IL-13. Such findings can be attributed to the prolonged retention of thymulin plasmid in the lungs for up to 27 days post administration due to increased stability under physiological conditions and shielding of the nanoparticles by surface PEG, thereby improving gene transfer and overall therapeutic efficacy in asthma [175].

4.3 Inorganic drug-delivery systems

4.3.1 Carbon nanotubes

Carbon nanotubes (CNTs) are tube-shaped nanocarriers consisting of hexagonally arranged atoms, resembling that of graphite. They are formed through the rolling of either a single layer of graphene sheet, known as single-walled carbon nanotubes (SWCNTs), or through rolling multiple layers of graphene sheets, known as multiwalled carbon nanotubes (MWCNTs) [176]. Generally, SWCNTs have a better defined wall structure as compared to MWCNTs in which structural defects are more likely, resulting in less stable nanostructures. However, no conclusive evidence has been provided by researchers in terms of the advantages of SWCNTs relative to MWCNTs in drug-delivery applications [176,177]. Nevertheless, CNTs are intrinsically poorly soluble compounds due to the hydrophobic character of their graphene side walls along with a strong interaction between individual tubes [176,178]. One solution to this drawback is by the technique of functionalization through the introduction of functional groups on the surface of CNTs via chemical synthesis. This can result in improved practicability in drug-delivery applications as a wide range of therapeutic and diagnostic moieties can also be easily conjugated; these may include proteins, peptides, nucleic acids, as well as other macromolecules [176–178]. One attractive feature that functionalized CNTs offer as nanocarriers is the possibility of crossing biological barriers and penetrating individual cells effectively to release their payloads at their targeted sites, which can lead to improved therapeutic action. Other advantages of functionalized CNTs include their unique physical, mechanical, and thermal properties, stiffness and toughness, high aspect ratio of length to diameter, great biocompatibility, as well as exceptionally high drug-loading capacity attributed to their high surface area [179,180].

There are a few studies that demonstrated that functionalized CNTs may be potentially feasible to be employed in the management of lung cancer. ABT737 is a small molecule that has Bcl-2 targeting activities, but it exhibits low target efficacy at systemically tolerable doses, whereas high doses that are sufficient to trigger mitochondrial apoptosis may result in adverse effects. A study by Kim et al. has reported that PEGylated CNTs improved mitochondrial targeting of ABT737 to lung cancer cells by promoting internalization into early endosomes via clathrin-mediated endocytosis. This led to an increased release of ABT737 from CNTs in the cytosol, leading to the generation of reactive oxygen species and Bcl-2-mediated apoptosis [181]. Another study by Salas-Treviño et al. has evaluated the efficacy of hyaluronate and carboplatin-conjugated oxidized MWCNTs (oxMWCNTs-HA-CPT) as a treatment in an in vitro lung cancer model. It was found that oxMWCNTs-HA-CPT were endocytosed in a higher proportion by TC-1 and NIH/3T3 tumor cell lines as compared to normal cells, which led to significantly higher cytotoxicity in these tumor cells [182]. Besides, Cirillo et al. have proposed in their study that chitosan-coated MWCNTs can be used as a pH-responsive vehicle for delivering methotrexate to lung-cancer tissues. It was found that methotrexate was released from the nanocarrier at a higher and faster rate within the acidic environment as compared to neutral environments, thereby allowing a tumor-targeted delivery of the therapeutic agent for the selective killing of tumor cells. This was signified by a 44% increase in the amount of death cells by the nanoformulation as compared to the free drug. Chitosan-coated MWCNTs were also found to be highly biocompatible in both healthy MRC-5 cells and H1299 tumor cells, with drug toxicity greatly minimized in healthy MRC-5 cells and the anticancer activity of methotrexate enhanced in H1299 lung-cancer cells [183].

Nevertheless, the clinical use of CNTs in other airway inflammatory diseases other than lung cancer is still debatable. In vivo studies have shown that exposure of CNTs can potentially cause harm to the lungs and result in various adverse effects, which may include exacerbation of preexisting respiratory diseases, fibrosis of the lungs, adverse immune reactions, as well as DNA damage [184,185]. Although no human studies have been conducted regarding the use of CNTs, the potential toxicities of CNTs as reported in various preclinical studies could suggest that although they may be useful in the treatment of lung cancer, they may not be an appropriate pulmonary delivery platform for allergic airway inflammatory diseases. As such, the mechanisms of their pathological effects should be further investigated to develop various modifications and improvements that can prevent such toxicities prior to the translation of CNTs as an effective nanocarrier for the treatment of airway inflammatory diseases.

4.3.2 Gold nanoparticles

Gold nanoparticles (AuNPs) represent another example of inorganic nanocarriers that are composed of a gold atom core surrounded by negative reactive groups on the surface. Over the years, AuNPs have been intensively employed for medical imaging, disease theranostics, and drug-delivery applications. This can be attributed to their unique biochemical, optical, sensing, and electronic properties, as well as other advantages such as high functionality, stability, and biocompatibility [186,187]. One unique characteristic of AuNPs is the presence of surface plasmon resonance (SPR) bands, in which the interaction of light with the surface electrons of AuNPs induces a collective oscillation of electrons, resulting in the absorption of light and scattering of heat energy. The SPR effect can be modified to produce varying absorption spectra, through the fine-tuning of the size and shape of AuNPs, depending on their desired application [86,187]. In addition, AuNPs can be conjugated with a wide range of biomarkers, such as oligonucleotides and antibodies, for the detection of target biomolecules. Studies have also shown their tendency to accumulate in specific cells and to exert their optical scattering effect [186]. Thus, AuNPs have great potential to be employed in various imaging applications, such as computed tomography, Raman spectroscopy, and dark-field light scattering [188].

AuNPs are also widely utilized for the delivery of drugs and genes due to their modifiable physicochemical properties and their high surface-loading capacity. The wide surface area of AuNPs enables dense binding of targeting moieties, drugs, and other macromolecules while achieving targeted delivery into specific sites via active and/or passive targeting mechanisms [186,189,190]. Nevertheless, it has been shown that nonsurface-modified AuNPs may present reduced colloidal stability. Therefore, modification of AuNPs with polymers, namely PEG and chitosan, can enhance their colloidal stability and mechanical strength for traveling through the complex physiological conditions of diseased tissues, leading to improved practicability with enhanced therapeutic outcomes. Polymers can also act as an adjuvant to improve the interaction and permeation of AuNPs across biological membranes by modulating their surface physical adsorption and electrostatic interactions [86,186].

The potential of AuNPs in enhancing therapeutic effects in airway inflammatory diseases was investigated in a study by Geiser et al. The researchers had evaluated the distribution of inhaled AuNPs in whole lungs and in bronchoalveolar lavage macrophages in a transgenic mouse model of COPD (Scnn1b mice) as compared to that of wild-type mice. There was a rapid binding of AuNPs to the alveolar epithelium, namely, to the primary surface-covering alveolar type I epithelial cells. Particularly, in contrast to wild-type mice, the uptake of AuNPs by surface macrophages was reduced and delayed with an increased AuNP uptake by type I epithelial cells in Scnn1b mice, signifying the reduced clearance of the nanoparticles. This can lead to a prolonged retention time of deposited AuNPs on the epithelial surface due to increased uptake by the alveolar epithelium, thus deeming them as a favorable nanocarrier for enhancing therapeutic targeting of the lung parenchyma for the treatment of COPD [191]. In another work, Crous and Abrahamse constructed a nanobioconjugate using AuNPs with the photosensitizer aluminum (III) phthalocyanine chloride tetrasulfonic acid (AlPcS$_4$Cl) and anti-CD133 antibodies for the photodynamic therapy of lung cancer. It was demonstrated that anti-CD133-conjugated AuNPs effectively enhanced the uptake of AlPcS$_4$Cl in lung cancer stem cells as compared to free AlPcS$_4$Cl. The improved intracellular accumulation of the photosensitizer can be attributed to the nano-size and stability of AuNPs, as well as the targeting affinity of anti-CD133 antibodies for lung cancer stem cells. Therefore, there was a remarkable increase in cytotoxicity and apoptosis with a significant reduction in cell proliferation and viability, resulting in significant destruction of lung cancer stem cells to the point of eradication. Taken together, these findings indicate that the delivery of AlPcS$_4$Cl can be enhanced by the utilization of AuNPs and active targeting by conjugated antibodies, thereby improving the efficacy and outcomes of photodynamic therapy on lung cancer cells [192]. In terms of diagnosis, an array of sensors based on AuNPs has been developed by Peng et al. as a novel diagnostic method of lung cancer. Given that the chemical analysis of the breath of lung cancer patients has revealed dramatic increase in several volatile organic compounds such as acetaldehyde, functionalizing AuNPs with ligands such as dodecanethiol, decanethiol, hexanethiol, and methoxy-toluenethiol has provided broad cross-selective absorption sites in AuNPs for the detection of exhaled volatile organic compounds with robustness and organic specificity. As a result, the AuNPs-based sensor array can produce a rapid and highly sensitive detection system as compared to conventional diagnostics such as gas-chromatography/mass spectrometry, mainly attributed to the ability of these functionalized AuNPs to monitor and distinguish the overall composition of volatile organic compounds in the breath between those of lung cancer patients and healthy individuals. Thus, such a simple, noninvasive breath test can be developed using AuNPs as a diagnostic tool for lung cancer [193].

5 Conclusions and future directions

Airway inflammatory diseases such as asthma, COPD, and lung cancer have been associated with poor clinical outcomes, leading to increased worldwide morbidity and mortality, as well as heavy clinical and socioeconomic burden every year. Despite the rising prevalence of airway inflammatory diseases, specific therapeutic agents that can be used to effectively treat these diseases are currently not available;

most of the conventional agents are only symptomatic and are unable to reverse the progression of the diseases. As advancements in medical research has led to more accurate and precise elucidation of underlying disease pathogenesis, studies that aim to develop advanced therapeutics with respect to the pathophysiological mechanisms of airway inflammatory diseases have been actively performed by many researchers, with several chemical and biological agents proven to be beneficial thus far. Nevertheless, some of these agents are poorly water soluble or are easily degraded in vivo, which results in poor bioavailability that limits their clinical translation as effective therapeutics in airway inflammatory diseases. Besides, certain agents are unable to achieve specific delivery to the injured sites within the lungs, thereby requiring a higher dosage to achieve the optimal concentration needed to elicit an effective therapeutic response. This may result in adverse reactions and could significantly affect patients' compliance to therapy.

Nanomedicine is a rapidly emerging field of technology that offers benefits in the management of various diseases. Generally, the application of drug-delivery systems can facilitate targeted delivery to specific sites within the body while improving the bioavailability of the encapsulated drugs, resulting in an enhanced therapeutic outcome. Therefore, it offers tremendous potential as a safe, effective, and alternative therapeutic approach for airway inflammatory diseases as compared to conventional treatment approaches. In recent years, several studies have been performed using various advanced drug-delivery systems that have shown promising outcomes in the therapy of these diseases. However, these are mainly preclinical studies focusing on cell lines and animal models of airway inflammatory diseases. More clinical studies should be carried out as the findings obtained in human studies may significantly deviate from those obtained in preclinical studies due to the presence of a complex biological environment within the human body that may affect nanoparticle interactions. Moreover, the specific mechanisms underlying the observed effects brought upon by the application of advanced drug-delivery systems must also be investigated to elucidate a clear safety parameter for their use in the clinical setting. In short, it is anticipated that nanomedicines will shift the paradigm of therapeutics in airway inflammatory diseases and bridge the translational bench-to-bedside gap in the future. As such, multidisciplinary approaches for knowledge exchange between researchers, clinicians, and academia are perhaps the best platform to address the multiple challenges faced during the development of advanced nanomedicine-based therapeutics of airway inflammatory diseases, to ensure their ultimate success, which can significantly improve public health and the overall well-being of society.

Declaration of competing interests

The authors declare that they have no known competing financial interests or personal relationships that could have appeared to influence the work reported in this chapter.

References

[1] P. Aghasafari, U. George, R. Pidaparti, A review of inflammatory mechanism in airway diseases, Inflamm. Res. 68 (1) (2019) 59–74, https://doi.org/10.1007/s00011-018-1191-2.

[2] Y. Chan, R. MacLoughlin, F.C. Zacconi, M.M. Tambuwala, R.M. Pabari, S.K. Singh, T. de Jesus Andreoli Pinto, G. Gupta, D.K. Chellappan, K. Dua, Advances in nanotechnology-based drug delivery in targeting PI3K signaling in respiratory diseases, Nanomedicine 16 (16) (2021) 1351–1355, https://doi.org/10.2217/nnm-2021-0087.

[3] D. Furman, J. Campisi, E. Verdin, P. Carrera-Bastos, S. Targ, C. Franceschi, L. Ferrucci, D.W. Gilroy, A. Fasano, G.W. Miller, A.H. Miller, A. Mantovani, C.M. Weyand, N. Barzilai, J.J. Goronzy, T.A. Rando, R.B. Effros, A. Lucia, N. Kleinstreuer, G.M. Slavich, Chronic inflammation in the etiology of disease across the life span, Nat. Med. 25 (12) (2019) 1822–1832, https://doi.org/10.1038/s41591-019-0675-0.

[4] Y. Chan, S.W. Ng, H.S. Liew, L.J.W. Pua, L. Soon, J.S. Lim, K. Dua, D.K. Chellappan, Introduction to chronic respiratory diseases: A pressing need for novel therapeutic approaches, in: Medicinal Plants for Lung Diseases, Springer Science and Business Media LLC, 2021, pp. 47–84, https://doi.org/10.1007/978-981-33-6850-7_2.

[5] S.D. Shukla, K. Swaroop Vanka, A. Chavelier, M.D. Shastri, M.M. Tambuwala, H.A. Bakshi, K. Pabreja, M.Q. Mahmood, R.F. O'Toole, Chronic respiratory diseases: An introduction and need for novel drug delivery approaches, in: Targeting Chronic Inflammatory Lung Diseases Using Advanced Drug Delivery Systems, Elsevier BV, 2020, pp. 1–31, https://doi.org/10.1016/b978-0-12-820658-4.00001-7.

[6] Chronic Respiratory Diseases. (n.d.). World Health Organization. Retrieved August 20, 2021, from https://www.who.int/health-topics/chronic-respiratory-diseases.

[7] Cancer, World Health Organization, 2021. https://www.who.int/news-room/fact-sheets/detail/cancer.

[8] Y. Chan, S.W. Ng, K. Dua, D.K. Chellappan, Plant-based chemical moieties for targeting chronic respiratory diseases, in: Targeting Cellular Signalling Pathways in Lung Diseases, Springer Science and Business Media LLC, 2021, pp. 741–781, https://doi.org/10.1007/978-981-33-6827-9_34.

[9] B.-F. Lin, B.-L. Chiang, Y. Ma, J.-Y. Lin, M.-L. Chen, Traditional herbal medicine and allergic asthma, Evid. Based Complement. Alternat. Med. 2015 (2015) 1–2, https://doi.org/10.1155/2015/510989.

[10] F. Liu, N.-X. Xuan, S.-M. Ying, W. Li, Z.-H. Chen, H.-H. Shen, Herbal medicines for asthmatic inflammation: from basic researches to clinical applications, Mediators Inflamm. 2016 (2016) 1–12, https://doi.org/10.1155/2016/6943135.

[11] F.P.R. Santana, N.M. Pinheiro, M.I.B. Mernak, R.F. Righetti, M.A. Martins, J.H.G. Lago, F.D.T.Q.S. dos Lopes, I.F.L.C. Tibério, C.M. Prado, Evidences of herbal medicine-derived natural products effects in inflammatory lung Diseases, Mediators Inflamm. 2016 (2016) 1–14, https://doi.org/10.1155/2016/2348968.

[12] A.L. Durham, G. Caramori, K.F. Chung, I.M. Adcock, Targeted anti-inflammatory therapeutics in asthma and chronic obstructive lung disease, Transl. Res. 167 (1) (2016) 192–203, https://doi.org/10.1016/j.trsl.2015.08.004.

[13] J. Yhee, J. Im, R. Nho, Advanced therapeutic strategies for chronic lung disease using nanoparticle-based drug delivery, J. Clin. Med. 82 (2016), https://doi.org/10.3390/jcm5090082.

[14] N.J. Gross, P.J. Barnes, New therapies for asthma and chronic obstructive pulmonary disease, Am. J. Respir. Crit. Care Med. 195 (2) (2017) 159–166, https://doi.org/10.1164/rccm.201610-2074PP.

[15] H.M. Ahmed, S. Nabavi, S. Behzad, Herbal drugs and natural products in the light of nanotechnology and nanomedicine for developing drug formulations, Mini-Rev. Med. Chem. 21 (3) (2021) 302–313, https://doi.org/10.2174/1389557520666200916143240.

[16] B.V. Bonifácio, P.B. da Silva, A. dos Santos, M. Ramos, K. Maria Silveira Negri, T. Maria Bauab, M. Chorilli, Nanotechnology-based drug delivery systems and herbal medicines: A review, Int. J. Nanomedicine 9 (1) (2013) 1–15, https://doi.org/10.2147/IJN.S52634.

[17] M. Doroudian, R. MacLoughlin, F. Poynton, A. Prina-Mello, S.C. Donnelly, Nanotechnology based therapeutics for lung disease, Thorax 74 (10) (2019) 965–976, https://doi.org/10.1136/thoraxjnl-2019-213037.

[18] Y. Chan, S.W. Ng, M. Mehta, K. Anand, S. Kumar Singh, G. Gupta, D.K. Chellappan, K. Dua, Advanced drug delivery systems can assist in managing influenza virus infection: A hypothesis, Med. Hypotheses 144 (2020), 110298, https://doi.org/10.1016/j.mehy.2020.110298.

[19] S.W. Ng, Y. Chan, X.Y. Ng, K. Dua, D.K. Chellappan, Neuroblastoma: Current advancements and future therapeutics, in: Advanced Drug Delivery Systems in the Management of Cancer, Elsevier BV, 2021, pp. 281–297, https://doi.org/10.1016/b978-0-323-85503-7.00001-8.

[20] W. Zhong, X. Zhang, Y. Zeng, D. Lin, J. Wu, Recent applications and strategies in nanotechnology for lung diseases, Nano Res. 14 (7) (2021) 2067–2089, https://doi.org/10.1007/s12274-020-3180-3.

[21] C.H. Fanta, Asthma in adolescents and adults: evaluation and diagnosis, in: UpToDate, 2020. https://www.uptodate.com/contents/asthma-in-adolescents-and-adults-evaluation-and-diagnosis.

[22] P.G. Holt, P.D. Sly, Interaction between adaptive and innate immune pathways in the pathogenesis of atopic asthma: operation of a lung/bone marrow axis, Chest 139 (5) (2011) 1165–1171, https://doi.org/10.1378/chest.10-2397.

[23] Asthma, World Health Organization, 2021. https://www.who.int/news-room/fact-sheets/detail/asthma.

[24] Common Asthma Triggers. (n.d.). Centers for Disease Control and Prevention. Retrieved August 20, 2021, from https://www.cdc.gov/asthma/triggers.html.

[25] S. Corbridge, T.C. Corbridge, Asthma in adolescents and adults, AJN, Am. J. Nurs. 110 (5) (2010) 28–38, https://doi.org/10.1097/01.naj.0000372069.78392.79.

[26] S.T. Holgate, Pathogenesis of asthma, Clin. Exp. Allergy 38 (6) (2008) 872–897, https://doi.org/10.1111/j.1365-2222.2008.02971.x.

[27] J.R. Murdoch, C.M. Lloyd, Chronic inflammation and asthma, Mutat. Res./Fund. Mol. Mech. Mutagen. 690 (1–2) (2010) 24–39, https://doi.org/10.1016/j.mrfmmm.2009.09.005.

[28] P.G. Holt, P.D. Sly, Viral infections and atopy in asthma pathogenesis: new rationales for asthma prevention and treatment, Nat. Med. 18 (5) (2012) 726–735, https://doi.org/10.1038/nm.2768.

[29] M. Kraft, R.J. Martin, S. Wilson, R. Djukanovic, S.T. Holgate, Lymphocyte and eosinophil influx into alveolar tissue in nocturnal asthma, Am. J. Respir. Crit. Care Med. 159 (1) (1999) 228–234, https://doi.org/10.1164/ajrccm.159.1.9804033.

[30] D. Alvarez, E.H. Vollmann, U.H. von Andrian, Mechanisms and consequences of dendritic cell migration, Immunity 29 (3) (2008) 325–342, https://doi.org/10.1016/j.immuni.2008.08.006.

[31] L. Riol-Blanco, N. Sánchez-Sánchez, A. Torres, A. Tejedor, S. Narumiya, A.L. Corbí, P. Sánchez-Mateos, J.L. Rodríguez-Fernández, The chemokine receptor CCR7 activates in dendritic cells two signaling modules that independently regulate chemotaxis and migratory speed, J. Immunol. 174 (7) (2005) 4070–4080, https://doi.org/10.4049/jimmunol.174.7.4070.

[32] D.S. Robinson, The role of the mast cell in asthma: induction of airway hyperresponsiveness by interaction with smooth muscle? J. Allergy Clin. Immunol. 114 (1) (2004) 58–65, https://doi.org/10.1016/j.jaci.2004.03.034.

[33] N.A. Barrett, K.F. Austen, Innate cells and T helper 2 cell immunity in airway inflammation, Immunity 31 (3) (2009) 425–437, https://doi.org/10.1016/j.immuni.2009.08.014.

[34] E.W. Gelfand, D. Simon, H.U. Simon, A. Thomas, W.W. Busse, P. Nair, G.M. Gauvreau, J.A. Denburg, E.R. Bivins-Smith, D.B. Jacoby, B.P. Davis, M.E. Rothenberg, P. Khoury, A.D. Klion, R. Lotfi, N. Spada, M.T. Lotze, R.P. Schleimer, A. Kato, N. Levy, Eosinophils in human disease, in: Eosinophils in Health and Disease, Elsevier Inc., 2013, pp. 431–536, https://doi.org/10.1016/B978-0-12-394385-9.00013-4.

[35] S.T. Holgate, Asthma: Clinical aspects and mucosal immunology, in: Mucosal Immunology, fourth edition, Vols. 2–2, Elsevier Inc., 2015, pp. 1833–1856, https://doi.org/10.1016/B978-0-12-415847-4.00096-3.

[36] P.J. Barnes, Inflammatory mechanisms in patients with chronic obstructive pulmonary disease, J. Allergy Clin. Immunol. 138 (1) (2016) 16–27, https://doi.org/10.1016/j.jaci.2016.05.011.

[37] M.K. Han, M.T. Dransfield, F.J. Martinez, Chronic obstructive pulmonary disease: definition, clinical manifestations, diagnosis, and staging, in: UpToDate, 2020. https://www.uptodate.com/contents/chronic-obstructive-pulmonary-disease-definition-clinical-manifestations-diagnosis-and-staging.

[38] COPD Causes and Risk Factors, American Lung Association, 2021. https://www.lung.org/lung-health-diseases/lung-disease-lookup/copd/what-causes-copd.

[39] P.T. King, Inflammation in chronic obstructive pulmonary disease and its role in cardiovascular disease and lung cancer, Clin. Transl. Med. (2015), https://doi.org/10.1186/s40169-015-0068-z.

[40] Lugg, S.T., Scott, A., Parekh, D., Naidu, B., & Thickett, D.R. (2021). Cigarette smoke exposure and alveolar macrophages: mechanisms for lung disease. Thorax, thoraxjnl-2020-216296. doi:https://doi.org/10.1136/thoraxjnl-2020-216296.

[41] M. Hikichi, K. Mizumura, S. Maruoka, Y. Gon, Pathogenesis of chronic obstructive pulmonary disease (COPD) induced by cigarette smoke, J. Thorac. Dis. 11 (2019) S2129–S2140, https://doi.org/10.21037/jtd.2019.10.43.

[42] J.P. Katkin, Cystic fibrosis: clinical manifestations of pulmonary disease, in: UpToDate, 2021. https://www.uptodate.com/contents/cystic-fibrosis-clinical-manifestations-of-pulmonary-disease.

[43] J.P. Katkin, Cystic fibrosis: clinical manifestations and diagnosis, in: UpToDate, 2020. https://www.uptodate.com/contents/cystic-fibrosis-clinical-manifestations-and-diagnosis.

[44] J.P. Katkin, Cystic fibrosis: genetics and pathogenesis, in: UpToDate, 2020. https://www.uptodate.com/contents/cystic-fibrosis-genetics-and-pathogenesis.

[45] S.H. Donaldson, R.C. Boucher, Pathophysiology of cystic fibrosis, Annal. Nestle 64 (3) (2006) 101–109, https://doi.org/10.1159/000095374.

[46] M.T. Clunes, R.C. Boucher, Cystic fibrosis: the mechanisms of pathogenesis of an inherited lung disorder, Drug Discov. Today: Disease Mech. 4 (2) (2007) 63–72, https://doi.org/10.1016/j.ddmec.2007.09.001.

[47] R.C. Boucher, New concepts of the pathogenesis of cystic fibrosis lung disease, Eur. Respir. J. 23 (1) (2004) 146–158, https://doi.org/10.1183/09031936.03.00057003.

[48] E.A. Roesch, D.P. Nichols, J.F. Chmiel, Inflammation in cystic fibrosis: an update, Pediatr. Pulmonol. 53 (S3) (2018) S30–S50, https://doi.org/10.1002/ppul.24129.

[49] A.L. Dougall, Cancer: Lung, in: Cambridge Handbook of Psychology, Health and Medicine, second edition, Cambridge University Press, 2014, pp. 605–606, https://doi.org/10.1017/CBO9780511543579.138.

[50] E.M. Conway, L.A. Pikor, S.H.Y. Kung, M.J. Hamilton, S. Lam, W.L. Lam, K.L. Bennewith, Macrophages, inflammation, and lung cancer, Am. J. Respir. Crit. Care Med. 193 (2) (2016) 116–130, https://doi.org/10.1164/rccm.201508-1545CI.

[51] K.W. Thomas, M.K. Gould, Overview of the initial evaluation, diagnosis, and staging of patients with suspected lung cancer, in: UpToDate, 2020. https://www.uptodate.com/contents/overview-of-the-initial-evaluation-diagnosis-and-staging-of-patients-with-suspected-lung-cancer.

[52] P.M. de Groot, C.C. Wu, B.W. Carter, R.F. Munden, The epidemiology of lung cancer, Trans. Lung Cancer Res. 7 (3) (2018) 220–233, https://doi.org/10.21037/tlcr.2018.05.06.

[53] A.M. Patel, S.G. Peters, Clinical manifestations of lung cancer, Mayo Clin. Proc. 68 (3) (1993) 273–277, https://doi.org/10.1016/s0025-6196(12)60049-4.

[54] X. Hua, J. Chen, Y. Wu, J. Sha, S. Han, X. Zhu, Prognostic role of the advanced lung cancer inflammation index in cancer patients: a meta-analysis, World J. Surg. Oncol. 17 (1) (2019), https://doi.org/10.1186/s12957-019-1725-2.

[55] D.S. O'Callaghan, D. O'Donnell, F. O'Connell, K.J. O'Byrne, The role of inflammation in the pathogenesis of non-small cell lung cancer, J. Thorac. Oncol. 5 (12) (2010) 2024–2036, https://doi.org/10.1097/JTO.0b013e3181f387e4.

[56] S. Zappavigna, A.M. Cossu, A. Grimaldi, M. Bocchetti, G.A. Ferraro, G.F. Nicoletti, R. Filosa, M. Caraglia, Anti-inflammatory drugs as anticancer agents, Int. J. Mol. Sci. 21 (7) (2020) 2605, https://doi.org/10.3390/ijms21072605.

[57] D.W. Kamp, E. Shacter, S.A. Weitzman, Chronic inflammation and cancer: the role of the mitochondria, Oncology 25 (5) (2011) 400–410.

[58] L. Lu, J. Barbi, F. Pan, The regulation of immune tolerance by FOXP3, Nat. Rev. Immunol. 17 (11) (2017) 703–717, https://doi.org/10.1038/nri.2017.75.

[59] Y. Chan, X.H. Wu, B.W. Chieng, N.A. Ibrahim, Y.Y. Then, Superhydrophobic Nanocoatings as intervention against biofilm-associated bacterial infections, Nanomaterials 11 (4) (2021) 1046, https://doi.org/10.3390/nano11041046.

[60] S. Hua, S.Y. Wu, Editorial: advances and challenges in nanomedicine, Front. Pharmacol. 9 (2018), https://doi.org/10.3389/fphar.2018.01397.

[61] Y.Y. Tan, P.K. Yap, G.L. Xin Lim, M. Mehta, Y. Chan, S.W. Ng, D.N. Kapoor, P. Negi, K. Anand, S.K. Singh, N.K. Jha, L.C. Lim, T. Madheswaran, S. Satija, G. Gupta, K. Dua, D.K. Chellappan, Perspectives and advancements in the design of nanomaterials for targeted cancer theranostics, Chem. Biol. Interact. 329 (2020), 109221, https://doi.org/10.1016/j.cbi.2020.109221.

[62] Y. Chan, P. Prasher, R. Löbenberg, G. Gupta, S.K. Singh, B.G. Oliver, D.K. Chellappan, K. Dua, Applications and practice of advanced drug delivery systems for targeting toll-like receptors in pulmonary diseases, Nanomedicine 16 (10) (2021) 783–786, https://doi.org/10.2217/nnm-2021-0056.

[63] Y. Chan, M. Mehta, K.R. Paudel, T. Madheswaran, J. Panneerselvam, G. Gupta, Q.P. Su, P.M. Hansbro, R. MacLoughlin, K. Dua, D.K. Chellappan, Versatility of liquid crystalline nanoparticles in inflammatory lung diseases, Nanomedicine 16 (18) (2021) 1545–1548, https://doi.org/10.2217/nnm-2021-0114.

[64] Y. Chan, S.W. Ng, M. Mehta, G. Gupta, D.K. Chellappan, K. Dua, Sugar-based nanoparticles for respiratory diseases: a new paradigm in the nanoworld, Future Med. Chem. 12 (21) (2020) 1887–1890, https://doi.org/10.4155/fmc-2020-0206.

[65] A.J. Omlor, J. Nguyen, R. Bals, Q.T. Dinh, Nanotechnology in respiratory medicine, Respir. Res. 16 (1) (2015), https://doi.org/10.1186/s12931-015-0223-5.

[66] M. Passi, S. Shahid, S. Chockalingam, I.K. Sundar, G. Packirisamy, Conventional and nanotechnology based approaches to combat chronic obstructive pulmonary disease: implications for chronic airway diseases, Int. J. Nanomedicine 15 (2020) 3803–3826, https://doi.org/10.2147/IJN.S242516.

[67] L.R. Stolzenburg, A. Harris, The role of microRNAs in chronic respiratory disease: recent insights, Biol. Chem. 399 (3) (2018) 219–234, https://doi.org/10.1515/hsz-2017-0249.

[68] S. Afzal, H.I. Ahmad, A. Jabbar, M.M. Tolba, S. AbouZid, N. Irm, F. Zulfiqar, M.Z. Iqbal, S. Ahmad, Z. Aslam, S. Ahmed, Use of medicinal plants for respiratory Diseases in Bahawalpur, Pakistan, Biomed. Res. Int. 2021 (2021) 1–10, https://doi.org/10.1155/2021/5578914.

[69] M. Mehta, P. Sharma, S. Kaur, D.S. Dhanjal, B. Singh, M. Vyas, G. Gupta, D.K. Chellappan, S. Nammi, T.G. Singh, K. Dua, S. Satija, Plant-based drug delivery systems in respiratory diseases, in: Targeting Chronic Inflammatory Lung Diseases Using Advanced Drug Delivery Systems, Elsevier BV, 2020, pp. 517–539, https://doi.org/10.1016/b978-0-12-820658-4.00024-8.

[70] W. Younis, H. Asif, A. Sharif, H. Riaz, I.A. Bukhari, A.M. Assiri, Traditional medicinal plants used for respiratory disorders in Pakistan: a review of the ethno-medicinal and pharmacological evidence, Chin. Med. 13 (1) (2018), https://doi.org/10.1186/s13020-018-0204-y.

[71] F.d.M. Garcia, Nanomedicine and therapy of lung diseases, Einstein (São Paulo) 12 (4) (2014) 531–533, https://doi.org/10.1590/S1679-45082014MD3113.

[72] Y. Xu, H. Liu, L. Song, Novel drug delivery systems targeting oxidative stress in chronic obstructive pulmonary disease: a review,

J. Nanobiotechnol. 18 (2020), https://doi.org/10.1186/S12951-020-00703-5.

[73] A.-R. Coltescu, M. Butnariu, I. Sarac, The importance of solubility for new drug molecules, Biomed. Pharmacol. J. 13 (2) (2020) 577–583, https://doi.org/10.13005/bpj/1920.

[74] K.T. Savjani, A.K. Gajjar, J.K. Savjani, Drug solubility: importance and enhancement techniques, ISRN Pharm. 1–10 (2012), https://doi.org/10.5402/2012/195727.

[75] M. Sharma, R. Sharma, D.K. Jain, Nanotechnology based approaches for enhancing oral bioavailability of poorly water soluble antihypertensive drugs, Scientifica 2016 (2016) 1–11, https://doi.org/10.1155/2016/8525679.

[76] M. Ghasemian, S. Owlia, M.B. Owlia, Review of anti-inflammatory herbal medicines, Adv. Pharm. Sci. 2016 (2016) 1–11, https://doi.org/10.1155/2016/9130979.

[77] L. Possebon, I. de Souza Lima Lebron, L. Furlan da Silva, J. Tagliaferri Paletta, B.G. Glad, M. Sant'Ana, M.M. Iyomasa-Pilon, H. Ribeiro Souza, S. de Souza Costa, G. Pereira da Silva Rodriguesa, M.L. de Pereira, A. de Haro Moreno, A.P. Girol, Anti-inflammatory actions of herbal medicines in a model of chronic obstructive pulmonary disease induced by cigarette smoke, Biomed. Pharmacother. 99 (2018) 591–597, https://doi.org/10.1016/j.biopha.2018.01.106.

[78] J. Wieczfinska, P. Sitarek, T. Kowalczyk, E. Skała, R. Pawliczak, The anti-inflammatory potential of selected plant-derived compounds in respiratory Diseases, Curr. Pharm. Des. 26 (24) (2020) 2876–2884, https://doi.org/10.2174/1381612826666200406093257.

[79] S.H. Thilakarathna, H.P. Vasantha Rupasinghe, Flavonoid bioavailability and attempts for bioavailability enhancement, Nutrients 5 (9) (2013) 3367–3387, https://doi.org/10.3390/nu5093367.

[80] J. Zhao, J. Yang, Y. Xie, Improvement strategies for the oral bioavailability of poorly water-soluble flavonoids: an overview, Int. J. Pharm. 570 (2019), 118642, https://doi.org/10.1016/j.ijpharm.2019.118642.

[81] A.C. Santos, I. Pereira, M. Pereira-Silva, L. Ferreira, M. Caldas, M. Magalhães, A. Figueiras, A.J. Ribeiro, F. Veiga, Nanocarriers for resveratrol delivery: impact on stability and solubility concerns, Trends Food Sci. Technol. 91 (2019) 483–497, https://doi.org/10.1016/j.tifs.2019.07.048.

[82] J. Wang, Y. Li, G. Nie, Y. Zhao, Precise design of nanomedicines: perspectives for cancer treatment, Natl. Sci. Rev. 6 (6) (2019) 1107–1110, https://doi.org/10.1093/nsr/nwz012.

[83] A.R. Bilia, V. Piazzini, L. Risaliti, G. Vanti, M. Casamonti, M. Wang, M.C. Bergonzi, Nanocarriers: A successful tool to increase solubility, stability and optimise bioefficacy of natural constituents, Curr. Med. Chem. 26 (24) (2019) 4631–4656, https://doi.org/10.2174/0929867325666181101110050.

[84] S. Kalepu, V. Nekkanti, Improved delivery of poorly soluble compounds using nanoparticle technology: a review, Drug Deliv. Transl. Res. 6 (3) (2016) 319–332, https://doi.org/10.1007/s13346-016-0283-1.

[85] E.M. Merisko-Liversidge, G.G. Liversidge, Drug nanoparticles: formulating poorly water-soluble compounds, Toxicol. Pathol. 36 (1) (2008) 43–48, https://doi.org/10.1177/0192623307310946.

[86] D. Lombardo, M.A. Kiselev, M.T. Caccamo, Smart nanoparticles for drug delivery application: development of versatile nanocarrier platforms in biotechnology and nanomedicine, J. Nanomater. 2019 (2019) 1–26, https://doi.org/10.1155/2019/3702518.

[87] S.A.A. Rizvi, A.M. Saleh, Applications of nanoparticle systems in drug delivery technology, Saudi Pharm. J. 26 (1) (2018) 64–70, https://doi.org/10.1016/j.jsps.2017.10.012.

[88] D.A. Smith, K. Beaumont, T.S. Maurer, L. Di, Relevance of half-life in drug design, J. Med. Chem. 61 (10) (2018) 4273–4282, https://doi.org/10.1021/acs.jmedchem.7b00969.

[89] E. Blanco, H. Shen, M. Ferrari, Principles of nanoparticle design for overcoming biological barriers to drug delivery, Nat. Biotechnol. 33 (9) (2015) 941–951, https://doi.org/10.1038/nbt.3330.

[90] J.H. Lee, Y. Yeo, Controlled drug release from pharmaceutical nanocarriers, Chem. Eng. Sci. 125 (2015) 75–84, https://doi.org/10.1016/j.ces.2014.08.046.

[91] J. Emami, M.A. Shetabboushehri, J. Varshosaz, A. Eisaei, Preparation and characterization of a sustained release buccoadhesive system for delivery of terbutaline sulfate, Res. Pharm. Sci. 8 (4) (2013) 219–231.

[92] H.H. Gustafson, D. Holt-Casper, D.W. Grainger, H. Ghandehari, Nanoparticle uptake: the phagocyte problem, Nano Today 10 (4) (2015) 487–510, https://doi.org/10.1016/j.nantod.2015.06.006.

[93] Z. Hussain, S. Khan, M. Imran, M. Sohail, S.W.A. Shah, M. de Matas, PEGylation: a promising strategy to overcome challenges to cancer-targeted nanomedicines: a review of challenges to clinical transition and promising resolution, Drug Deliv. Transl. Res. 721–734 (2019), https://doi.org/10.1007/s13346-019-00631-4.

[94] J.S. Suk, Q. Xu, N. Kim, J. Hanes, L.M. Ensign, PEGylation as a strategy for improving nanoparticle-based drug and gene delivery, Adv. Drug Deliv. Rev. 99 (2016) 28–51, https://doi.org/10.1016/j.addr.2015.09.012.

[95] S.Y. Fam, C.F. Chee, C.Y. Yong, K.L. Ho, A.R. Mariatulqabtiah, W.S. Tan, Stealth coating of nanoparticles in drug-delivery systems, Nano 10 (4) (2020) 787, https://doi.org/10.3390/nano10040787.

[96] U. Saxena, M. Rajadurai, S. Basaveni, S. Yellanki, R. Medishetti, A. Sevilimedu, P. Kulkarni, Double PEGylation significantly improves pharmacokinetic properties of irinotecan containing nanoparticles in a zebrafish model, Curr. Nanomed. 173–181 (2019), https://doi.org/10.2174/2468187308666180925143701.

[97] S. Mitragotri, P.A. Burke, R. Langer, Overcoming the challenges in administering biopharmaceuticals: formulation and delivery strategies, Nat. Rev. Drug Discov. 13 (9) (2014) 655–672, https://doi.org/10.1038/nrd4363.

[98] M. Zoulikha, Q. Xiao, G.F. Boafo, M.A. Sallam, Z. Chen, W. He, Pulmonary delivery of siRNA against acute lung injury/acute respiratory distress syndrome, Acta Pharm. Sin. B (2021), https://doi.org/10.1016/j.apsb.2021.08.009.

[99] J. Wahlich, A. Desai, F. Greco, K. Hill, A.T. Jones, R.J. Mrsny, G. Pasut, Y. Perrie, F.P. Seib, L.W. Seymour, I.F. Uchegbu, Nanomedicines for the delivery of biologics, Pharmaceutics 11 (5) (2019) 210, https://doi.org/10.3390/pharmaceutics11050210.

[100] J. McCaskill, R. Singhania, M. Burgess, R. Allavena, S. Wu, A. Blumenthal, N.A. McMillan, Efficient biodistribution and gene silencing in the lung epithelium via intravenous liposomal delivery of siRNA, Mol. Therapy Nucl. Acids 2 (2013), e96, https://doi.org/10.1038/mtna.2013.22.

[101] J. Chen, Y. Tang, Y. Liu, Y. Dou, Nucleic acid-based therapeutics for pulmonary Diseases, AAPS Pharm. SciTech 19 (8) (2018) 3670–3680, https://doi.org/10.1208/s12249-018-1183-0.

[102] Y.-D. Kim, T.-E. Park, B. Singh, S. Maharjan, Y.-J. Choi, P.-H. Choung, R.B. Arote, C.-S. Cho, Nanoparticle-mediated delivery of

siRNA for effective lung cancer therapy, Nanomedicine 10 (7) (2015) 1165–1188, https://doi.org/10.2217/nnm.14.214.

[103] C.F. Anderson, M.E. Grimmett, C.J. Domalewski, H. Cui, Inhalable nanotherapeutics to improve treatment efficacy for common lung diseases, WIREs Nanomed. Nanobiotechnol. 12 (1) (2020), https://doi.org/10.1002/wnan.1586.

[104] J.M. Borghardt, C. Kloft, A. Sharma, Inhaled therapy in respiratory disease: the complex interplay of pulmonary kinetic processes, Can. Respir. J. 2018 (2018) 1–11, https://doi.org/10.1155/2018/2732017.

[105] D. Chenthamara, S. Subramaniam, S.G. Ramakrishnan, S. Krishnaswamy, M.M. Essa, F.-H. Lin, M.W. Qoronfleh, Therapeutic efficacy of nanoparticles and routes of administration, Biomater. Res. (2019), https://doi.org/10.1186/s40824-019-0166-x.

[106] R. Iyer, C. Hsia, K. Nguyen, Nano-therapeutics for the lung: state-of-the-art and future perspectives, Curr. Pharm. Des. 21 (36) (2015) 5233–5244, https://doi.org/10.2174/1381612821666150923095742.

[107] A. Kuzmov, T. Minko, Nanotechnology approaches for inhalation treatment of lung diseases, J. Control. Release 219 (2015) 500–518, https://doi.org/10.1016/j.jconrel.2015.07.024.

[108] M. Paranjpe, C. Müller-Goymann, Nanoparticle-mediated pulmonary drug delivery: A review, Int. J. Mol. Sci. 15 (4) (2014) 5852–5873, https://doi.org/10.3390/ijms15045852.

[109] J. Heyder, Deposition of inhaled particles in the human respiratory tract and consequences for regional targeting in respiratory drug delivery, Proc. Am. Thorac. Soc. 1 (4) (2004) 315–320, https://doi.org/10.1513/pats.200409-046TA.

[110] J. Majumder, T. Minko, Targeted nanotherapeutics for respiratory diseases: Cancer, fibrosis, and coronavirus, Adv. Therapeut. 4 (2) (2021) 2000203, https://doi.org/10.1002/adtp.202000203.

[111] S.K. Golombek, J.-N. May, B. Theek, L. Appold, N. Drude, F. Kiessling, T. Lammers, Tumor targeting via EPR: strategies to enhance patient responses, Adv. Drug Deliv. Rev. 130 (2018) 17–38, https://doi.org/10.1016/j.addr.2018.07.007.

[112] Y. Shi, R. van der Meel, X. Chen, T. Lammers, The EPR effect and beyond: strategies to improve tumor targeting and cancer nanomedicine treatment efficacy, Theranostics 10 (17) (2020) 7921–7924, https://doi.org/10.7150/thno.49577.

[113] D. Rosenblum, N. Joshi, W. Tao, J.M. Karp, D. Peer, Progress and challenges towards targeted delivery of cancer therapeutics, Nat. Commun. 9 (1) (2018), https://doi.org/10.1038/s41467-018-03705-y.

[114] Y. Zhang, J. Cao, Z. Yuan, Strategies and challenges to improve the performance of tumor-associated active targeting, J. Mater. Chem. B 8 (18) (2020) 3959–3971, https://doi.org/10.1039/d0tb00289e.

[115] A.G. Arranja, V. Pathak, T. Lammers, Y. Shi, Tumor-targeted nanomedicines for cancer theranostics, Pharmacol. Res. 115 (2017) 87–95, https://doi.org/10.1016/j.phrs.2016.11.014.

[116] U. Chitgupi, Y. Qin, J.F. Lovell, Targeted nanomaterials for phototherapy, Nanotheranostics 1 (1) (2017) 38–58, https://doi.org/10.7150/ntno.17694.

[117] J.Y.C. Edgar, H. Wang, Introduction for design of nanoparticle based drug delivery systems, Curr. Pharm. Des. 23 (14) (2017), https://doi.org/10.2174/1381612822666161025154003.

[118] B. Mukherjee, Editorial (thematic issue: "Nanosize drug delivery system"), Curr. Pharm. Biotechnol. 1221–1221 (2014), https://doi.org/10.2174/138920101415140804121008.

[119] A. Akbarzadeh, R. Rezaei-Sadabady, S. Davaran, S.W. Joo, N. Zarghami, Y. Hanifehpour, M. Samiei, M. Kouhi, K. Nejati-Koshki, Liposome: classification, preparation, and applications, Nanoscale Res. Lett. (2013), https://doi.org/10.1186/1556-276x-8-102.

[120] B. García-Pinel, C. Porras-Alcalá, A. Ortega-Rodríguez, F. Sarabia, J. Prados, C. Melguizo, J.M. López-Romero, Lipid-based nanoparticles: application and recent advances in cancer treatment, Nano 9 (4) (2019) 638, https://doi.org/10.3390/nano9040638.

[121] L. Sercombe, T. Veerati, F. Moheimani, S.Y. Wu, A.K. Sood, S. Hua, Advances and challenges of liposome assisted drug delivery, Front. Pharmacol. 6 (2015), https://doi.org/10.3389/fphar.2015.00286.

[122] E. Beltrán-Gracia, A. López-Camacho, I. Higuera-Ciapara, J.B. Velázquez-Fernández, A.A. Vallejo-Cardona, Nanomedicine review: clinical developments in liposomal applications, Cancer Nanotechnol. 10 (1) (2019), https://doi.org/10.1186/s12645-019-0055-y.

[123] Z.Y. Ng, J.-Y. Wong, J. Panneerselvam, T. Madheswaran, P. Kumar, V. Pillay, A. Hsu, N. Hansbro, M. Bebawy, P. Wark, P. Hansbro, K. Dua, D.K. Chellappan, Assessing the potential of liposomes loaded with curcumin as a therapeutic intervention in asthma, Colloids Surf. B Biointerfaces 172 (2018) 51–59, https://doi.org/10.1016/j.colsurfb.2018.08.027.

[124] A. Vassallo, V. Santoro, I. Pappalardo, A. Santarsiero, P. Convertini, M. De Luca, G. Martelli, V. Infantino, C. Caddeo, Liposome-mediated inhibition of inflammation by hydroxycitrate, Nano 10 (10) (2020) 2080, https://doi.org/10.3390/nano10102080.

[125] S. Honmane, A. Hajare, H. More, R.A.M. Osmani, S. Salunkhe, Lung delivery of nanoliposomal salbutamol sulfate dry powder inhalation for facilitated asthma therapy, J. Liposome Res. 29 (4) (2019) 332–342, https://doi.org/10.1080/08982104.2018.1531022.

[126] Z. Yang, X. Chen, W. Huang, B.C. Kwan Wong, L. Yin, I. Wong, Liposomes prolong the therapeutic effect of anti-asthmatic medication via pulmonary delivery, Int. J. Nanomedicine 7 (2012) 1139, https://doi.org/10.2147/ijn.s28011.

[127] M. Harms, C.C. Müller-Goymann, Solid lipid nanoparticles for drug delivery, J. Drug Deliv. Sci. Technol. 21 (1) (2011) 89–99, https://doi.org/10.1016/S1773-2247(11)50008-5.

[128] V. Mishra, K. Bansal, A. Verma, N. Yadav, S. Thakur, K. Sudhakar, J. Rosenholm, Solid lipid nanoparticles: emerging colloidal Nano drug delivery systems, Pharmaceutics 10 (4) (2018) 191, https://doi.org/10.3390/pharmaceutics10040191.

[129] Y. Duan, A. Dhar, C. Patel, M. Khimani, S. Neogi, P. Sharma, N. Siva Kumar, R.L. Vekariya, A brief review on solid lipid nanoparticles: part and parcel of contemporary drug delivery systems, RSC Adv. 10 (45) (2020) 26777–26791, https://doi.org/10.1039/d0ra03491f.

[130] R.K. Shirodkar, L. Kumar, S. Mutalik, S. Lewis, Solid lipid nanoparticles and nanostructured lipid carriers: emerging lipid based drug delivery systems, Pharm. Chem. J. 53 (5) (2019) 440–453, https://doi.org/10.1007/s11094-019-02017-9.

[131] S. Castellani, A. Trapani, A. Spagnoletta, L. di Toma, T. Magrone, S. Di Gioia, D. Mandracchia, G. Trapani, E. Jirillo, M. Conese, Nanoparticle delivery of grape seed-derived proanthocyanidins to airway epithelial cells dampens oxidative stress and inflammation, J. Transl. Med. 16 (1) (2018), https://doi.org/10.1186/s12967-018-1509-4.

[132] C. Wu, P. Ji, T. Yu, Y. Liu, J. Jiang, J. Xu, Y. Zhao, Y. Hao, Y. Qiu, W. Zhao, Naringenin-loaded solid lipid nanoparticles: preparation,

[133] W. Wang, R. Zhu, Q. Xie, A. Li, Y. Xiao, K. Li, H. Liu, D. Cui, Y. Chen, S. Wang, Enhanced bioavailability and efficiency of curcumin for the treatment of asthma by its formulation in solid lipid nanoparticles, Int. J. Nanomedicine 7 (2012) 3667–3677, https://doi.org/10.2147/IJN.S30428.

[134] N.F. de Melo, C.G. de Macedo, R. Bonfante, H.B. Abdalla, C.M.G. da Silva, T. Pasquoto, R. Lima, L.F. Fraceto, J.T. Clemente-Napimoga, M.H. Napimoga, 15d-PGJ2-loaded solid lipid nanoparticles: physicochemical characterization and evaluation of pharmacological effects on inflammation, PLoS One 11 (8) (2016), https://doi.org/10.1371/JOURNAL.PONE.0161796.

[135] A. Beloqui, M.Á. Solinís, A. Rodríguez-Gascón, A.J. Almeida, V. Préat, Nanostructured lipid carriers: promising drug delivery systems for future clinics, Nanomedicine 12 (1) (2016) 143–161, https://doi.org/10.1016/j.nano.2015.09.004.

[136] F.-Q. Hu, S.-P. Jiang, Y.-Z. Du, H. Yuan, Y.-Q. Ye, S. Zeng, Preparation and characterization of stearic acid nanostructured lipid carriers by solvent diffusion method in an aqueous system, Colloids Surf. B Biointerfaces 45 (3–4) (2005) 167–173, https://doi.org/10.1016/j.colsurfb.2005.08.005.

[137] V.R. Salvi, P. Pawar, Nanostructured lipid carriers (NLC) system: A novel drug targeting carrier, J. Drug Deliv. Sci. Technol. 51 (2019) 255–267, https://doi.org/10.1016/j.jddst.2019.02.017.

[138] A. Beloqui, A. del Pozo-Rodríguez, A. Isla, A. Rodríguez-Gascón, M.Á. Solinís, Nanostructured lipid carriers as oral delivery systems for poorly soluble drugs, J. Drug Deliv. Sci. Technol. 42 (2017) 144–154, https://doi.org/10.1016/j.jddst.2017.06.013.

[139] S. Khan, S. Baboota, J. Ali, S. Khan, R. Narang, J. Narang, Nanostructured lipid carriers: an emerging platform for improving oral bioavailability of lipophilic drugs, Int. J. Pharm. Invest. 5 (4) (2015) 182, https://doi.org/10.4103/2230-973X.167661.

[140] R. Tiwari, K. Pathak, Nanostructured lipid carrier versus solid lipid nanoparticles of simvastatin: comparative analysis of characteristics, pharmacokinetics and tissue uptake, Int. J. Pharm. 415 (1–2) (2011) 232–243, https://doi.org/10.1016/j.ijpharm.2011.05.044.

[141] A. Patil-Gadhe, V. Pokharkar, Montelukast-loaded nanostructured lipid carriers: part I Oral bioavailability improvement, Eur. J. Pharm. Biopharm. 88 (1) (2014) 160–168, https://doi.org/10.1016/j.ejpb.2014.05.019.

[142] A. Patil-Gadhe, V. Pokharkar, Pulmonary targeting potential of rosuvastatin loaded nanostructured lipid carrier: optimization by factorial design, Int. J. Pharm. 501 (1–2) (2016) 199–210, https://doi.org/10.1016/j.ijpharm.2016.01.080.

[143] Y. Wang, H. Zhang, J. Hao, B. Li, M. Li, W. Xiuwen, Lung cancer combination therapy: co-delivery of paclitaxel and doxorubicin by nanostructured lipid carriers for synergistic effect, Drug Deliv. 23 (4) (2016) 1398–1403, https://doi.org/10.3109/10717544.2015.1055619.

[144] S. Taymouri, M. Alem, J. Varshosaz, M. Rostami, V. Akbari, L. Firoozpour, Biotin decorated sunitinib loaded nanostructured lipid carriers for tumor targeted chemotherapy of lung cancer, J. Drug Deliv. Sci. Technol. 50 (2019) 237–247, https://doi.org/10.1016/j.jddst.2019.01.024.

[145] M. Haider, S.M. Abdin, L. Kamal, G. Orive, Nanostructured lipid carriers for delivery of chemotherapeutics: A review, Pharmaceutics 12 (3) (2020) 288, https://doi.org/10.3390/pharmaceutics12030288.

[146] A. Zielińska, F. Carreiró, A.M. Oliveira, A. Neves, B. Pires, D.N. Venkatesh, A. Durazzo, M. Lucarini, P. Eder, A.M. Silva, A. Santini, E.B. Souto, Polymeric nanoparticles: production, characterization, toxicology and ecotoxicology, Molecules 3731 (2020), https://doi.org/10.3390/molecules25163731.

[147] K.O. Paredes, J. Ruiz-Cabello, D.I. Alarcón, M. Filice, The state of the art of investigational and approved nanomedicine products for nucleic acid delivery, in: Nucleic Acid Nanotheranostics: Biomedical Applications, Elsevier, 2019, pp. 421–456, https://doi.org/10.1016/B978-0-12-814470-1.00015-0.

[148] H.K.S. Yadav, A.A. Almokdad, shaluf, S. I. M., & Debe, M. S., Polymer-based nanomaterials for drug-delivery carriers, in: Nanocarriers for Drug Delivery, Elsevier BV, 2019, pp. 531–556, https://doi.org/10.1016/b978-0-12-814033-8.00017-5.

[149] X.Y. Lu, D.C. Wu, Z.J. Li, G.Q. Chen, Polymer nanoparticles, in: Progress in Molecular Biology and Translational Science, vol. 104, Elsevier B.V, 2011, pp. 299–323, https://doi.org/10.1016/B978-0-12-416020-0.00007-3.

[150] P.P.D. Kondiah, Y.E. Choonara, P.J. Kondiah, T. Marimuthu, P. Kumar, L.C. du Toit, G. Modi, V. Pillay, Nanocomposites for therapeutic application in multiple sclerosis, in: Applications of Nanocomposite Materials in Drug Delivery, Elsevier, 2018, pp. 391–408, https://doi.org/10.1016/B978-0-12-813741-3.00017-0.

[151] B. Iyisan, K. Landfester, Polymeric nanocarriers, in: Biological Responses to Nanoscale Particles, Springer Science and Business Media LLC, 2019, pp. 53–84, https://doi.org/10.1007/978-3-030-12461-8_3.

[152] A. George, P.A. Shah, P.S. Shrivastav, Natural biodegradable polymers based nano-formulations for drug delivery: A review, Int. J. Pharm. 561 (2019) 244–264, https://doi.org/10.1016/j.ijpharm.2019.03.011.

[153] F.R. Wurm, C.K. Weiss, Nanoparticles from renewable polymers, Front. Chem. (2014), https://doi.org/10.3389/fchem.2014.00049.

[154] T. Miao, J. Wang, Y. Zeng, G. Liu, X. Chen, Polysaccharide-based controlled release systems for therapeutics delivery and tissue engineering: from bench to bedside, Adv. Sci. 5 (4) (2018) 1700513, https://doi.org/10.1002/advs.201700513.

[155] J. Yao, F.Z. Dahmani, H. Xiong, Y. Xiao, Y. Li, C. Xu, Polysaccharides-based polymeric nanoparticles for drug delivery and tumor therapy, in: The World Scientific Encyclopedia of Nanomedicine and Bioengineering II, vol. 9, World Scientific, 2017, pp. 195–223, https://doi.org/10.1142/9789813202566_0008.

[156] S. Nagarajan, S. Radhakrishnan, S.N. Kalkura, S. Balme, P. Miele, M. Bechelany, Overview of protein-based biopolymers for biomedical application, Macromol. Chem. Phys. 220 (14) (2019), https://doi.org/10.1002/macp.201900126.

[157] D. Verma, N. Gulati, S. Kaul, S. Mukherjee, U. Nagaich, Protein based nanostructures for drug delivery, J. Pharm. 1–18 (2018), https://doi.org/10.1155/2018/9285854.

[158] J.K. Kim, H.J. Kim, J.-Y. Chung, J.-H. Lee, S.-B. Young, Y.-H. Kim, Natural and synthetic biomaterials for controlled drug delivery, Arch. Pharm. Res. 37 (1) (2014) 60–68, https://doi.org/10.1007/s12272-013-0280-6.

[159] W. Yang, Z. Dong, Y. Li, Y. Zhang, H. Fu, Y. Xie, Therapeutic efficacy of chitosan nanoparticles loaded with BCG-polysaccharide nucleic acid and ovalbumin on airway inflammation in asthmatic mice, Eur. J. Clin. Microbiol. Infect. Dis. 40 (8) (2021) 1623–1631, https://doi.org/10.1007/s10096-021-04183-9.

[160] D.-W. Lee, S.A. Shirley, R.F. Lockey, S.S. Mohapatra, Thiolated chitosan nanoparticles enhance anti-inflammatory effects of intranasally delivered theophylline, Respir. Res. (2006), https://doi.org/10.1186/1465-9921-7-112.

[161] R. Lee, Y.J. Choi, M.S. Jeong, Y.I. Park, K. Motoyama, M.W. Kim, S.-H. Kwon, J.H. Choi, Hyaluronic acid-decorated glycol chitosan nanoparticles for pH-sensitive controlled release of doxorubicin and celecoxib in nonsmall cell lung cancer, Bioconjug. Chem. 31 (3) (2020) 923–932, https://doi.org/10.1021/acs.bioconjchem.0c00048.

[162] K.K. Bansal, J.M. Rosenholm, Synthetic polymers from renewable feedstocks: an alternative to fossil-based materials in biomedical applications, Ther. Deliv. 11 (5) (2020) 297–300, https://doi.org/10.4155/tde-2020-0033.

[163] S. Bhatia, Natural polymers vs synthetic polymer, in: Natural Polymer Drug Delivery Systems, Springer Science and Business Media LLC, 2016, pp. 95–118, https://doi.org/10.1007/978-3-319-41129-3_3.

[164] S. Rezvantalab, N.I. Drude, M.K. Moraveji, N. Güvener, E.K. Koons, Y. Shi, T. Lammers, F. Kiessling, PLGA-based nanoparticles in Cancer treatment, Front. Pharmacol. 9 (2018), https://doi.org/10.3389/fphar.2018.01260.

[165] F. Danhier, E. Ansorena, J.M. Silva, R. Coco, A. Le Breton, V. Préat, PLGA-based nanoparticles: an overview of biomedical applications, J. Control. Release 161 (2) (2012) 505–522, https://doi.org/10.1016/j.jconrel.2012.01.043.

[166] P. Gentile, V. Chiono, I. Carmagnola, P. Hatton, An overview of poly(lactic-co-glycolic) acid (PLGA)-based biomaterials for bone tissue engineering, Int. J. Mol. Sci. 15 (3) (2014) 3640–3659, https://doi.org/10.3390/ijms15033640.

[167] H.K. Makadia, S.J. Siegel, Poly lactic-co-glycolic acid (PLGA) as biodegradable controlled drug delivery carrier, Polymers 3 (3) (2011) 1377–1397, https://doi.org/10.3390/polym3031377.

[168] S. Roy, K. Manna, T. Jha, K.D. Saha, Chrysin-loaded PLGA attenuates OVA-induced allergic asthma by modulating TLR/NF-κB/NLRP3 axis, Nanomedicine 30 (2020), 102292, https://doi.org/10.1016/j.nano.2020.102292.

[169] N. Pirooznia, S. Hasannia, A. Lotfi, M. Ghanei, Encapsulation of Alpha-1 antitrypsin in PLGA nanoparticles: In Vitro characterization as an effective aerosol formulation in pulmonary diseases, J. Nanobiotechnol. 10 (2012) 20, https://doi.org/10.1186/1477-3155-10-20.

[170] M.S. Hamid Akash, K. Rehman, S. Chen, Natural and synthetic polymers as drug carriers for delivery of therapeutic proteins, Polym. Rev. 55 (3) (2015) 371–406, https://doi.org/10.1080/15583724.2014.995806.

[171] D. Hutanu, Recent applications of polyethylene glycols (PEGs) and PEG derivatives, Mod. Chem. Appl. (2014), https://doi.org/10.4172/2329-6798.1000132.

[172] K. Knop, R. Hoogenboom, D. Fischer, U.S. Schubert, Poly(ethylene glycol) in drug delivery: pros and cons as well as potential alternatives, Angew. Chem. Int. Ed. 49 (36) (2010) 6288–6308, https://doi.org/10.1002/anie.200902672.

[173] Y. Matsuo, T. Ishihara, J. Ishizaki, K. Miyamoto, M. Higaki, N. Yamashita, Effect of betamethasone phosphate loaded polymeric nanoparticles on a murine asthma model, Cell. Immunol. 260 (1) (2009) 33–38, https://doi.org/10.1016/j.cellimm.2009.07.004.

[174] K. Wang, Y. Feng, S. Li, W. Li, X. Chen, R. Yi, H. Zhang, Z. Hong, Oral delivery of Bavachinin-loaded PEG-PLGA nanoparticles for asthma treatment in a murine model, J. Biomed. Nanotechnol. 14 (10) (2018) 1806–1815, https://doi.org/10.1166/jbn.2018.2618.

[175] A.L. da Silva, S.V. Martini, S.C. Abreu, C.d.S. Samary, B.L. Diaz, S. Fernezlian, V.K. de Sá, V.L. Capelozzi, N.J. Boylan, R.G. Goya, J.S. Suk, P.R.M. Rocco, J. Hanes, M.M. Morales, DNA nanoparticle-mediated thymulin gene therapy prevents airway remodeling in experimental allergic asthma, J. Control. Release 180 (1) (2014) 125–133, https://doi.org/10.1016/j.jconrel.2014.02.010.

[176] W. Zhang, Z. Zhang, Y. Zhang, The application of carbon nanotubes in target drug delivery systems for cancer therapies, Nanoscale Res. Lett. 6 (2011) 1–22, https://doi.org/10.1186/1556-276X-6-555.

[177] R. Aboofazeli, Carbon nanotubes: A promising approach for drug delivery, Iranian J. Pharmaceut. Res. 9 (1) (2010) 1–3.

[178] M. Roldo, Carbon nanotubes in drug delivery: just a carrier? Ther. Deliv. 7 (2) (2016) 55–57, https://doi.org/10.4155/tde.15.89.

[179] S.K.S. Kushwaha, S. Ghoshal, A.K. Rai, S. Singh, Carbon nanotubes as a novel drug delivery system for anticancer therapy: a review, Braz. J. Pharm. Sci. 49 (4) (2013) 629–643, https://doi.org/10.1590/S1984-82502013000400002.

[180] C.-M. Tîlmaciu, M.C. Morris, Carbon nanotube biosensors, Front. Chem. 3 (2015), https://doi.org/10.3389/fchem.2015.00059.

[181] S.-W. Kim, Y. Kyung Lee, J. Yeon Lee, J. Hee Hong, D. Khang, PEGylated anticancer-carbon nanotubes complex targeting mitochondria of lung cancer cells, Nanotechnology 28 (46) (2017), 465102, https://doi.org/10.1088/1361-6528/aa8c31.

[182] D. Salas-Treviño, O. Saucedo-Cárdenas, M.J. de Loera-Arias, H. Rodríguez-Rocha, A. García-García, R. Montes-de-Oca-Luna, E.I. Piña-Mendoza, F.F. Contreras-Torres, G. García-Rivas, A. Soto-Domínguez, Hyaluronate functionalized Multi-Wall carbon nanotubes filled with carboplatin as a novel drug Nanocarrier against murine lung Cancer cells, Nano 9 (11) (2019) 1572, https://doi.org/10.3390/nano9111572.

[183] G. Cirillo, O. Vittorio, D. Kunhardt, E. Valli, F. Voli, A. Farfalla, M. Curcio, U.G. Spizzirri, S. Hampel, Combining carbon nanotubes and chitosan for the vectorization of methotrexate to lung cancer cells, Materials 12 (18) (2019) 2889, https://doi.org/10.3390/ma12182889.

[184] J.C. Bonner, Carbon nanotubes as delivery systems for respiratory disease: do the dangers outweigh the potential benefits? Expert Rev. Respir. Med. 5 (6) (2011) 779–787, https://doi.org/10.1586/ers.11.72.

[185] S. Luanpitpong, L. Wang, Y. Rojanasakul, The effects of carbon nanotubes on lung and dermal cellular behaviors, Nanomedicine 9 (6) (2014) 895–912, https://doi.org/10.2217/nnm.14.42.

[186] H. Katas, N.Z. Moden, C.S. Lim, T. Celesistinus, J.Y. Chan, P. Ganasan, S.I. Abdalla, S., Biosynthesis and potential applications of silver and gold nanoparticles and their chitosan-based nanocomposites in nanomedicine, J. Nanotechnol. 2018 (2018) 1–13, https://doi.org/10.1155/2018/4290705.

[187] A.K. Khan, R. Rashid, G. Murtaza, A. Zahra, Gold nanoparticles: synthesis and applications in drug delivery, Trop. J. Pharm. Res. 13 (7) (2014) 1169–1177, https://doi.org/10.4314/tjpr.v13i7.23.

[188] Y.-C. Yeh, B. Creran, V.M. Rotello, Gold nanoparticles: preparation, properties, and applications in bionanotechnology, Nanoscale 4 (6) (2012) 1871–1880, https://doi.org/10.1039/c1nr11188d.

[189] H. Daraee, A. Eatemadi, E. Abbasi, S. Fekri Aval, M. Kouhi, A. Akbarzadeh, Application of gold nanoparticles in biomedical and drug delivery, Artif. Cells, Nanomed. Biotechnol. 410–422 (2014), https://doi.org/10.3109/21691401.2014.955107.

[190] H. Jahangirian, K. Kalantari, Z. Izadiyan, R. Rafiee-Moghaddam, K. Shameli, T.J. Webster, A review of small molecules and drug delivery applications using gold and iron nanoparticles, Int. J. Nanomedicine 14 (2019) 1633–1657, https://doi.org/10.2147/ijn.s184723.

[191] M. Geiser, O. Quaile, A. Wenk, C. Wigge, S. Eigeldinger-Berthou, S. Hirn, M. Schäffler, C. Schleh, W. Möller, M.A. Mall, W.G. Kreyling, Cellular uptake and localization of inhaled gold nanopar-ticles in lungs of mice with chronic obstructive pulmonary disease, Part. Fibre Toxicol. 10 (1) (2013) 19, https://doi.org/10.1186/1743-8977-10-19.

[192] A. Crous, H. Abrahamse, Effective gold nanoparticle-antibody-mediated drug delivery for photodynamic therapy of lung Cancer stem cells, Int. J. Mol. Sci. 21 (11) (2020) 3742, https://doi.org/10.3390/ijms21113742.

[193] G. Peng, U. Tisch, O. Adams, M. Hakim, N. Shehada, Y.Y. Broza, S. Billan, R. Abdah-Bortnyak, A. Kuten, H. Haick, Diagnosing lung cancer in exhaled breath using gold nanoparticles, Nat. Nano-technol. 4 (10) (2009) 669–673, https://doi.org/10.1038/nnano.2009.235.

Chapter 5

Modulation of intestinal microbiome: Promising therapies in the treatment of inflammatory bowel disease

Koushik Das, Shashi Upadhyay, and Shalini Oli
Department of Allied Health Science, School of Health Science, University of Petroleum and Energy Studies, Dehradun, India

1 Introduction

IBD is a term that refers to a group of immune-mediated gastrointestinal illnesses such as UC and CD [1]. The immunological disorder, changes in genetics, and the impact of environmental factors such as nutrition, socioeconomic development, lifestyle, and intestinal dysbiotic microbiota play a key role in the etiology of IBD [2]. Corticosteroids, thiopurines, aminosalicylates, biological treatments, and folic acid antagonists are examples of traditional drugs that aid in the regulation of inflammation and the prevention of disease recurrence [3]. So far, the traditional remedies are ineffective and the patient may become susceptible to them. IBD (an immune-mediated disease) can be treated by therapies with many targets of altering the microorganism that reside in the human body, especially the intestine [4]. This treatment in that area of keen interest now became traditional treatments that are failing to replenish the normal microflora of patients' anguish from IBD, inspite of proper care and nutrition [5]. In IBD patients, probiotics and FMT are utilized to reestablish the normal microbiota while also removing additional microbial interference.

2 Intestinal microbiota

In this section, we will discuss how gut microbiota interacts with the vertebrate host and thus influencing the health and disease status of the host. The GIT contains the most diverse microbiota in the human body [6]. GIT contains many microbial species (more than 1000) such as viruses, bacteria, and fungi [7]. The microbiota contains symbiotic and commensal communities of microbes, which are skilled to influence directly or indirectly the complete physiology of the human body, it also includes the immunological, nervous, and endocrine systems [8]. Lifestyle, xenobiotics, diet, and genetics alter the makeup of gut microbiota [9].

Therefore, we can conclude that there will be a tremendous impact because of the intricate bidirectional relationship between gut microbes and vertebrate hosts on human physiology. IBD and several other diseases are caused due to this complex interaction [10]. Microbiota is the term used for bacterial species within GIT although it contains bacteria, fungi, archaea, and viruses, 96% of the entire population of microbes residues in GIT [7]. IBD development is often implicated by fungal and viral dysbiosis [5,11].

Microbiota and immune cells are detached from each other by the development of physical and chemical barriers to prevent inappropriate activation on a surface with good interaction with microbes such as GIT [7]. Yet the barriers are not invincible and they encounter nervous, endocrine, and immune systems [12]. There is two hypothetically developed mechanism to identify PRR (the presence of pattern recognition receptors) which detects microbial-associated molecular (MAMPS/DAMPS) patterns in host cells and they also regulate the metabolic activity of microbes over diverse mammalian metabolic systems [13]. Polycarbohydrates A of *Bacteroides fragilis* is highly beneficial as it helps in the stimulation of variation and regulatory action of T lymphocytes (Tregs) in the human gut [14]. Inflammation in the intestine can be maintained by the presence of Tregs as its serves as an environment controller [15]. The intestine is protected from pathobionts and is given through IgA (produced in plasma), which is beneficially affected through epithelium-associated bacteria such as segmented filamentous bacteria (SFB) and Muciopirillum [16]. Short-chain fatty acids (SCFAs) are one of the key researched categories of microbiota—drives metabolites that have defensive effects toward the mammalian host which are extracted from nutritional fibers fermentation [17]. There are mainly three types of scfas namely butyrate propionate and acetate which helps in maintaining the reliability of intestinal epithelium, and also influences immune and host metabolic functions [18].

Recent Developments in Anti-Inflammatory Therapy. https://doi.org/10.1016/B978-0-323-99988-5.00021-8

3   Intestinal dysbiosis

Dysbiosis has been discovered to be the expressing agent of both local and systemic disorders affecting our gastrointestinal tract, which also includes CD and UC [19]. The intestinal microbiome and microbial alteration into the IBD are summarized in Table 1. Pathogenic microorganisms such as Ruminococcus gnavus-Firmicutes, Fusobacteria species, and proteobacteria, [28] are increased in IBD patients due to a reduction in microbial composition (25%); their diversity and richness, and there is also a reduction in useful microbes such as Faecalibacterium prausnitzii (Firmicutes) Lachnospiraceae (Firmicutes), Sulterella (Proteobacteria), Roseburia (Firmicutes), and Bifidobacterium species (Actinobacteria) [20,29]. From the total bacterial population, F. Prausnitzii represents almost 5% and is a key component of healthy intestinal microbiota in humans [30]. Besides providing energy to colonocytes this bacterium also contributes to maintaining a situation in the gut through the synthesis of butyrate [31]. IBD often leads to the disruption of microorganisms in the intestine that collaborate to maintain intestinal epithelial integrity. Inflammation is the main cause of the occurrence of dysbiosis in IBD. However, perturbation and provocative responses in microbes configuration in the ileum and additional intestinal sites are the most common symptom of dysbiosis. Nonaffected areas of diseased subjects were having a less dysbiotic environment [32,33].

Dysbiosis has been postulated as a cause of IBD. Where environmental factors play a major role in the occurrence of IBD, according to the pathophysiology of IBD (Fig. 1). Breastfeeding in early life and parental smoking in pregnancy have been found to be inversely proportional and associated with the disease consequence in CD respectively [34]. Microbial therapies that are probiotics, FMT, and antibiotics [35] are used in the treatment of UC. There is still debate and investigation going on regarding the mechanism, which influences dysbiosis in IBD. The existence of a certain type of bacterial species and the alliance between the development of inflammation are looked upon as major factors [36]. Intestinal inflammation, mucosal, and augmented vascular permeability is caused by a reduction in stringent anaerobes such as Clostridium groups IV and XI Va which in company with facultative aerobic or aerobic bacteria expands which increases its oxygen concentration [37]. Immunosuppressive pursuit is shown by prompting Treg cells in IL-10, TGF-b, or butyrate-dependent manner which is produced from various straining of Clostridium species (e.g., IV, XI Va, and XVIII) which do not have virulence factor and also lack toxicity [36]. Antiinflammatory factors are reduced due to microbial inequity in IBD, which favors inflammation and the growth of the proinflammatory system. Infection plays a key role in the growth of dysbiotic conditions. Therapeutic strategies must be developed based on strong interdependent interactions between inflammation and dysbiosis or vice versa. Dysbiosis plays an important role in this disease pathogenesis, and the therapies, which aim at restoring microbial balance, may be used as an effective measure to cure inflammatory diseases such as IBD.

TABLE 1 Changes of gut microbiota in patients with IBD.

Microorganisms (S)	Commensal (C) or pathogenic (P) microorganisms[a]	DC	UC
Candida albicans	P	↑	↑
Clostridium species (clusters IV and XIVa)	C	↓↑	↓
Verrucomicrobia	C	↓	↓
Roseburia species	C	?	↓
Proteobacteria	P	↑	↑
Firmicutes	C	↓	↓
Pseudomonas	P	↓	↓
Bacteroides	C	↑	↑↓
Saccharomyces cerevisiae	C	↓	↓
Ruminococcus gnavus	P	↑	↑
Fusobacterium	P	↑	↑

CD, Crohn's disease; UC, Ulcerative colitis.
[a]Changes were identified in majority of the species under the indicated genus of microorganisms [5,20–27].

4   Transplantation of fecal microbiota

Persistent Clostridium difficile infection (CDI) is cured with the help of FMT, it is incredibly successful and safe, with a 90% success rate [38]. Intestinal microbiota balance restoration is regarded as one of the main mechanisms propose to define the efficiency of FMT in the cure of CDI [39].

Irritable bowel syndrome (IBS) [40], metabolic syndrome, and other gut-related diseases both local and systemic illnesses are treated using FMT [41,42]. Firstly, we will elucidate how FMT is transported to recipients and how donors for microbiota are chosen. Therefore, the most significant scientific findings are FMT as a treatment for IBD will be presented and discussed (Table 2).

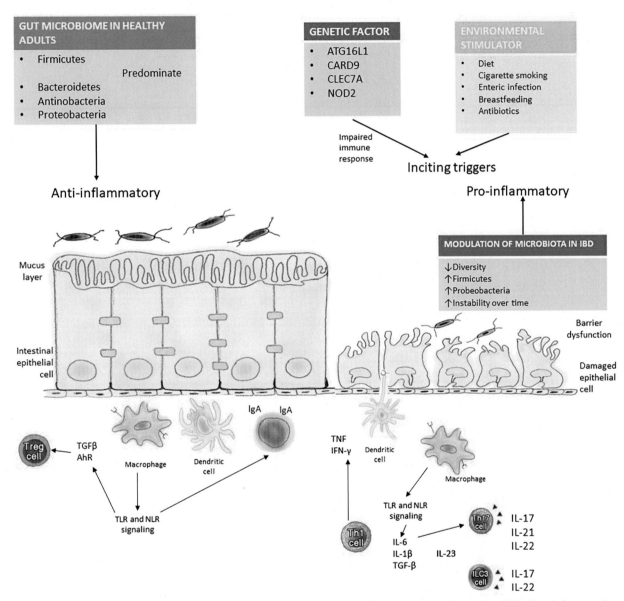

FIG. 1 Interaction of intestinal microbiome with environmental, genetic, and immune factors during the pathogenesis of IBD. Genetic factors and environmental changes induce an impaired immune response with intestinal microbiota, resulting in a proinflammatory condition. NOD-like receptors (NLRs) and Toll-like receptors (TLR) on dendritic cells, macrophages and epithelial cells in association with microbiota trigger the differentiation of TH17 cells, type 3 innate lymphoid cells (ILC3s), and TH1 cells, which in-turn release proinflammatory cytokines and results in inflammation, epithelial barrier dysfunction, and bacterial translocation. Instability of intestinal microbiome composition with time is evident in IBD patients, which is associated with a reduction of *Firmicutes* species and an increase of *Proteobacteria* species. In healthy individuals, bacteria detected by TLRs and NLRs stimulate the production of IgA-secreting B cells and differentiation of T regulatory (Treg) cells under the influence of TGF-b and AhR signaling. IgA produced from B cells prevents pathogenic bacteria and induces the production of antiinflammatory cytokine, IL-10 through Treg cells and thus regulates intestinal homeostasis.

TABLE 2 Transplantation of fecal microbiota in patients with IBD.

Diagnosis	Number of patients (P) or studies (S)[a,b]	Curative routine[c]	FMT route	Results	Authors
UC	n = 50 (P)	60 g of feces/500 mL of saline; two doses (days 0 and 21)	Naso-duodenal tube	No statistical difference between control and treated patients	Rossen et al. [43]
CD	n = 30 (P)	150–200 mL[d]; one dose	Endoscopy	86.7% and 76.7% of clinical improvement and remission, respectively at 4 weeks	Cui et al. [44]
UC	n = 70 (P)	50 g of feces/300 mL of water; once weekly for 6 weeks.	Enema	24% of clinical remission	Maoyedi et al. [45]
CD	n = 9 (P)	30 g of feces/100 or 200 mL of saline; one dose	Nasogastric tube	77.77% of clinical remission at week 2, 55.55% of clinical remission at week 6 and 12	Suskind et al. [46]
CD	n = 19 (P)	50 g of feces/250 mL of saline; one dose	Colonoscopy	58% of clinical response (control group not included)	Vaughn et al. [47]
UC	n = 85 (P)	150 mL[d]; once a day, 5 days per week for 8 weeks	Enema	27% of clinical and endoscopic remission or response	Paramsothy et al. [48]
UC	n = 41 (S)	N.A	N.A.	33% of clinical remission	Paramsothy et al. [49]
CD	n = 11 (S)	N.A.	N.A.	52% of clinical remission	Paramsothy et al. [49]

CD, Crohn's disease; N.A, not applicable; UC, Ulcerative colitis.
[a]Both total number of patients for clinical trials and number of studies for systematic analysis or meta-analysis were included.
[b]Includes the number of control patients.
[c]Feces may have undergone additional steps for FMT samples preparation.
[d]Initial solution concentration is not available.

5 FMT donor screening

Microbiota donors must be chosen carefully after looking for several aspects. Putative screening of the donor must be done to detect the presence of intestinal parasites (C. difficle) and viruses (e.g., Norovirus) before doing gut microbial sequencing [50]. HIV, Hepatitis, and HTLV like transmissible infectious agents, and the presence of inflammatory markers must be detected along with electrolytes, kidney, liver function tests (LFT), and count of blood [50]. The donor should not be taking antimicrobial or should have no history of gastrointestinal tract infection and other important active chronicity [50,51]. The following criteria must be used to select a healthy donor; there should be no first-degree relatives with colorectal cancer in the family history; before donating, take a probiotic for at least 3 months; GIT injections in household members, severity in family history obesity, malnutrition, and neural developmental disorder [50,51]. The above criteria are difficult to fulfill which creates a bridge between the donor and the recipient stopping broader consumption of this therapy. People have started doing it at home without appropriate donors and medical guidance resulting in grave difficulty [52]. Enema was the most followed procedure for FMT but there are so many alternatives such as a colonoscopy, self-administered enemas, capsule, and nasogastric tube [53]. The most popular enemas are colonoscopy and retention enema which are the used directions of FMT administered [54].

6 FMT in IBD

The two most frequent kinds of IBD are CD and UC. FMT's role in ulcerative colitis has received increased attention. The FMT-induced reduction was discovered in 33% of patients in a meta-analysis of 307 adult patients from 24 UC cohort studies. Out of 24 UC patients, Clinical reduction was about 23% [55], six pediatric cohort study was observed. Fabulous results were found under three randomized controlled trials concerning FMT usage against UC treatment. Remission was influenced in 24% of the patients getting FMT treatment, while 5% remission was reduced in the case of the placebo group when 70 UC patients were treated, 36 of them were using FMT and 34 placeboes, for a total of 6 weeks, once a week [49]. FMT groups and placebo both were receiving immunosuppressive therapy or concomitant antiinflammatory therapy such as corticosteroids, anti-TNF therapy, or mesalamine [49]. In Australia when the patient took an enema 5 days a week for 8 weeks, they observe about a 27% reduction rate in UC sick persons, cured with FMT, and 8% in placebo patients [45]. Regardless of the kind of treatment, the patients were given immunosuppressant drugs such as 5-amino salicylates, methotrexate, thiopurines, and oral prednisone with a minimal dosage [45]. Patients treated with their chronicity fecal microbiota have the same kind of reduction rate as that of UC patients treated with FMT from healthy donors [48].

No clinical trial results are available to suggest that FMT plays a key role in CD is rarer than UC. Small or uncontrolled studies were taken into consideration to take all the benefits of FMT in CD. About 58% of patients showed improvement when FMT was performed through colonoscopy [43]. Increased level of Tregs in lamina propria of in recipients is followed by an increase in microbial diversity suggesting negligible inflammation and separation of microbial equilibrium [43], CD patients showed clinical improvement and remission when treated with FMT [47]. Patient's body weight increases after using FMT 12 club time internal works compulsory for the persons who took immunosuppressive treatments such as cyclosporine, infliximab, or tacrolimus. Before FMT probiotics and antibiotics were stopped before 30 or 60 days respectively. Young patients with CD also showed satisfactory results after treatment with FMT. Nasogastric was used to give FM T49 individuals of age group 12–19 years who were having mild to adequate symptoms and work continuously given for 12 weeks [44]. After using it for 2 weeks FMT the clinical scores were as such, seven out of nine patients were in remission and after using it for 6–12 weeks five of nine were in remission. Immunomodulatory were allowed to use during their treatment either placebo or FMT cure [44].

7 Limitations in FMT studies

The investigation related to this study discussed here enlightened hopeful outcomes concerning FMT utilization to persuade lessening in UC and also, a slighter extent in CD patients. Dissimilarity in the root of the interval of intaking, adding with constitution and load within FMT, can clarify the study, in terms of the analysis and differentiation. In addition, a major downside is an insufficiency toward complete guidelines, which are followed around the world in terms of assessing and standardizing presumed microbiota contributors (Age, health status, and gender). Altogether by means of production approaches, dosing routine and to access the engraftment of transplantation.

Furthermore, clinical investigations, ostensibly for budgetary reasons, do not thoroughly study the microbiological structure of fecal donors considering 16 S RNA sequencing and the similarities to the microbiota of the recipient. Hence, the findings of likeness or resemblance amid the gut microbial framework of receivers and donors. Each piece of information accomplishes the engraftment of FMT. Firstly, appropriate recognizing of microbial community and the entire microbial load is needed which is relocated to an unwell subject from a healthy donor, and only then is it feasible to forecast the effect of FMT in IBD or additional sicknesses. Mainly, clinical trials or screening were controlled through the collateral usage of the immunomodulatory drug, it is reasonable to presume about an FMT scan which functions of adjuvant treatment relatively better than an insulated approach to approve the involvement of FMT in IBD, control therapeutic studies through a large number of patients and a more standard fecal sample could be directed. Advanced techniques that focus on existing gut microbiota rebalance employing different microbial species could be a better option for whole FMT.

8 FMT Adverse effects

Generally, FMT possesses slight to mild self-limited adverse effects, near about 10%. Most of the problems such as abdominal discomfort or pain and diarrhea are associated with GIT [46,52]. Although, a reduced amount of noticeable severe adverse events may comprise colectomy, IBD flares, small bowel obstruction, CDI and other infections, pancreatic disease, and even lead to death as currently revised [56]. However, a few pieces of evidence revealed no difference between FMT and control groups regarding undesirable incidents of displeasing events [57]. Regardless of the chances of incidence of unfavorable or side effects, FMT is contemplated as being safe IBD. A detailed selection of donors all together with a greater knowledge of physiopathology in IBD can promote the progress of approaches or methods to ignore undesirable consequences.

9 Probiotics

Currently, Food additives containing probiotics are utilized, and medicinal ingredients and supplements for nutrition are "live microorganisms that, when fed in an adequate amount, provide a health benefit on the host," according to the World Health Organization (WHO) [58]. Moreover, According to research deceased microorganism and their organically active compound may have big things that provide protective roles, concluding that the "probiotic" definition should be reexplored and reviewed or another categorization is implemented [59].

The elementary machinery related to probiotics is reliant on the microbial strain. The consequences of probiotic combinations may be both complementary (Also called additives) or synergistic [60]. Antimicrobial compounds (e.g., bacteriocins, short-chain fatty acids (SCFAs), lactic acids, hyper oxides, and bile acids) that reduce harmful microorganisms are delivered by probiotic strains to the gut epithelium [61]. Resulting, cellular apparatuses (for example, DNA, cellular lining) are delivered in the epithelium of the gastrointestinal tract, which activates the immunological reactions via inducing the cytokines which cause inflammation, produces the immunoglobulins synthesis, aside from rectifying lymphocyte and activity of macrophages [62]. The use of Bifidobacterium infantis 35624 in human volunteers or takes interest in this context by increasing the number of IL-10 and FoxP3+ cells (Treg) in the blood [61,63]. Moreover, immunological tolerance is assumed because of this progress, no harmony is present in this stuff [64].

The other advantages associated with probiotics include assistance in optimal digestion and absorption processes, competition with potential pathogens for adhesion sites and nutrients, site-specific alteration of pH, neutralization of metabolic toxins, etc. [65]. In vitro Assays and animal models Illustrate the fact that probiotics lower apoptosis, tissue repair enhance the mucus, rebalancing tight junctions in the gut epithelium, hence lowering the permeableness of the intestinal and improving the barrier's function and protection [40]. Generally most consumed strains, in probiotics of Lactobacillus (e.g., *rhamnosus, reuteri, casei Plantarum, acidophilus, gasseri, paracasei, ghallinarum, johnsonii and crispatus)* and Bifidobacterium (e.g., *string infantis, animalis, longum, bifidium, lactis, adolescentis, and breve)* in probiotic formulations, but multispecies perspectives have been progressively applied [66]. Other strains used comprise Lactococcus, Streptococcus species, nonpathogenic *Escherichia coli* (strain Nissle), Clostridium spp., and Enterococcus spp. [67].

New bacteria species and genera have also been investigated in preclinical trials, with promising results. These microorganisms are shown as younger-generation prebiotics that add complexity to conventional probiotics in a venture toward reproducing hard or mimic FMT treatments. *Eubacterium hallii, Akkermansia muciniphila, Clostridium clusters*, IV, XIVa, and XVIII, prausmitzii, *B. fragilis*, and *Bacteroides uniformis* are included in the new generation probiotics [68]. Using these probiotic bacteria is the new challenge concerning technological restrictions. Above all, as described earlier, *Clostridium clusters* IV and XIVa are described as differentiated promoters, crucial for immune tolerance [69]. Actually, in IBD patients these bacteria are reduced in the gut [70]. The Treg quantity in IBD patients is enhanced in the gut, but not enough to grow to confine the inflammatory expansion. Because the gut microbiota is made up of more than one bacteria, some preparations and researchers combine yeasts with bacterial

strains or utilize single-drug formulations. In this reference, the most frequently used yeast strain is *Saccharomyces boulardii*, having various properties related to antiinflammation [71].

10 Principles for the development of novel probiotic

Probiotics being pharmaceutical or nutraceutical products should achieve a standard level to remain accessible for commercial use. Other than productivity, the security properties of a given medication are the major concern of researchers and administrative offices [72]. Yeast and bacterial strains or their resulting products have different levels of protocols based on their specific purpose and should encounter the necessities, bordered, and commonly restructured guiding principles designed through regulatory supports [72]. They may be regarded as food (medical food, food ingredient, and nutritional supplement), biological product, or drug (new drug) [73].

Besides in FMT, safety is supremacy, considering some patients under immune suppressive therapy enhance the vulnerability toward infectious complications, together with sepsis [74]. Probiotics must have human beginning, deductively demonstrated favorable impacts, be cautious indeed in high-risk populaces, unable to cause sensitivities, and must hold great innovation properties (e.g., attainable culture and large-scale populace) [75].

At the first glance, various in vitro assessments can be employed to identify the potentiality of probiotics, microbicide activity, adherence toward epithelium, capable of minimizing the number of infective bacteria, and use of antibiotic-resistant, stomach acids, digestive enzyme, bile suits, and pH [63]. In spite of the fact that not mandatory, investigates and thinks about ought to too recognize the unfavorable impacts and medicate intuition of probiotics as they have been utilized as a treatment in a few afflictions [76]. For case, the probiotic loci strain Nissl 1917 affects the pharmacokinetics of concurrently taken antiarrhythmic sedate amiodarone by quickening the bioavailability of the drug [77]. Hence, their supposed protection must be ignored, also the probable dangers not ignored.

11 Probiotics in IBD

In IBD treatment, probiotics are generally utilized efficiently for preventing dysbiosis in patients experiencing continued antibiotics or immunosuppressant therapies [78]. Furthermore, such microorganisms are applied through adjuvant therapy in an effort to converse the dysbiotic environment connected to exacerbation and IBD incidence [79]. Despite the fact that the increasing number of clinical and also experimental studies on probiotics in IBD is significant, low sample numbers, therapeutic regimens lack of regular practices, and reduced disease characterization narrowed the related decisions of probiotics' effectiveness in this situation.

In probiotics explanation (*L. Plantarum, L. casei, L. Subsp. Bulgarcies*, and *L. acidophilus*), *one of streptococcus* (*S. Salivarius* subsp.). In UC, thermophilus targeted as an alternate induces and maintains remission, whereas, in CD, it has very little or no impact. The multispecies of probiotics are used as adjuvants, VS#3, which consists of four Lactobacillus strains and three Bifidobacterium sp. (*B. logum, B. Breve*, and *B. infantics*), enhanced the patients' clinical symptoms, who had active UC (mild to moderate) after receiving 3.6×10^{12} CFO dose [80]. The observation was further strengthened by the result obtained from the treatment of UC patients with VSL#3 alone, twice a day at the same dose as described earlier [81].

Patients receiving single-drug treatment with Mesalazine (1500 mg/day) or E. coli Nissle 1917 with no pathogenicity ($5-50 \times 109$/day) had similar remission rates in UC [82]. While using meticulous statistical techniques, the systematic review revealed about the advantages and effects of both E. coli Nissle or VSL#3 on UC are delicate and indeterminate. No positive association in CD confirms the requirements of the upcoming random regulatory trials to escalate the significance level of these discoveries. [83]. The usage of in milk, which is fermented, Bifidobacterium (consisting of *B. bifidum, B. breve*, and *L. acidophilus*) as the adjuvant therapy for treatments of 20 patients (included, placebo) having mild to medium active UC, after 12 weeks it revealed noticeable development in the clinical and endoscopic activity directories (10 billion bacteria per day) [84]. Appealingly, there were higher SCFAs concentrations found in feces in the group which is probiotic-treated in comparison with a placebo-treated group. Although according to a recent study, usage of an identical approach (B. breve, L. acidophilus containing fermented milk) displayed no effectiveness for the treatment or manage the suspension of UC in 195 patients [85]. Indeed, a single *B. bifidium* strain-containing probiotic was sufficient to increase faeces SCFA levels in healthy volunteers [86]; even the preventive role in UC or CD is unknown. Despite discrepancies about the number of patients used in the above mentioned studies, an increased number of Bifidobacteria in the faeces of probiotics-treated patients was confirmed. Compared to the immunosuppressants drug-treated group was treated alone in a 12-month relapse-free treatment mechanism, but was prolonged in patients having UC, treated with Lactobacillus GG (per day 18×10^9 viable bacteria) alone or A complaint with mesalazine [87]. Likewise, a structural evaluation of the clinical trials which were performed randomly, revealed the use of distinct Bifidobacterium and bacteria, producing lactic acid, as adjuvant therapy improves illness period and regulation reduction in terms of clinical features in UC [88].

As declared earlier, probiotics have meager or no direct effects on CD. Moreover, results were obtained as positive outcomes to urge suspension through combining prebiotics and probiotics (defined as symbiotic) [88]. In expansion to it, one open-label test considers comprising four children with gentle to modestly dynamic CD incorporates an outstanding progression or enhancement in clinical perspectives after treating through Lactobacillus GG (10^{10} CFU/tablet 2 times a day for 6 months) [89]. In spite of the fact that the lesser number of tests and the nonattendance of appropriate control (patients or beneath normal treatment) disrupt the exactness of the consideration.

Probiotics are ineffective in controlling the reduction of CD [90]. Eventually, probiotics are conceivable potential choices in actuating and keeping up mellow to direct UC, in spite of the fact that show up to have no impacts in DC (Table 3). The outcomes should be respected as basic proof also extra-random double-blind placebo, multicellular trials should be conducted to improve the outcome validity.

12 Limitations of probiotics studies

The major problem in designing protocols for treatment is the different therapeutic treatments (consistent doses and frequency of administration). However, they are different based on the bacterial strains, studies have revealed that after consuming 100 ML or 100 g of probiotic-containing products, about 10^8 to 10^{10} Colony Forming Units/day are consumed [93]. Consequently, there is divergence related to clinical trials which draw related conclusions.

The pathway of administration, in contrast to FMT therapy, is not the possible dilemma, seeing that the mainstream study utilizes the oral route of administration, as a major one. However, another main method for the delivery of probiotics is, enemas [70]. Quality control is the second important problem concerning probiotic inventions. Quality control, is considered the second important problem of the probiotic formulation.

A number of varying data are explained among the product and tag information, consisting of lower strain quality and contamination, among others, as discussed earlier [94]. However, the same strain can show distinct efficiency in dissimilar batches, and shows lower standardization in bacterial cell culture procedure utilized during the studies and manufacturing. Hence, improvements and guidelines on regulation are exceedingly uplifted for delivering enough data on the blueprint of novel studies, besides avoiding undesirable and contrary conclusions.

For clinicians and researchers, therapy related to immunosuppression is a recent challenge. Extended use of immunosuppressants can cause dysbiosis, determining the presumptive factor is critical which causes a patient's sensitivity toward probiotic treatments [95]. Collectively, these aspects denote crucial boundaries in studies set up, on the

TABLE 3 Probiotics-mediated treatment of patients with IBD.

Diagnosis	Number of patients (P) or studies (S)[a,b]	Curative routine	Probiotic	Results	Authors
CD	n = 4 (P)	Oral; 10^{10} CFU/dose; twice a day for 6 months	Lactobacillus GG	75% of clinical improvement at weeks 4 and 12	Gupta et al. [90]
UC	n = 20 (P)	Oral; 10^9 bacteria/day; once a week for 12 weeks	Fermented milk (B, breve, B. bifidum and L. acidophilus)	70% of clinical responsiveness and 40% of clinical remission	Kato et al. [85]
UC	n = 327 (P)	Oral; 5–50×10^9 viables bacteria; once a day for 12 months	Escherichia coli Nissle 1917	No difference between probiotic-and mesalazine-treated groups	Kruis et al. [83]
UC	n = 187 (P)	Oral; 9×10^9 viable bacteria/dose; twice a day for 12 months	Lactobacillus GG	No difference between probiotic and mesalazine-treated groups	Zocco et al. [88]
CD	n = 10 (P)	Oral; 75×10^9 bacteria/day; once a day for 13($\pm$4.5) months	B. breve, L. casei and B. longum	70% of clinical improvement and 60% of clinical remission	Fujimori et al. [91]
UC	n = 147 (P)	ORAL; 3.6×10^{12} CFU/dose; twice a day for 12 weeks	VSL# 3[c]	51.9% of clinical improvement and 42.9% of clinical remission at 12 weeks	Sood et al. [82]
UC	n = 144 (P)	ORAL; 3.6×10^{12} CFU/day; once a day for 8 weeks	VSL# 3[c]	53.4% of clinical improvement and 47.3% of clinical remission	Tursi et al. [92]
UC	n = 5 (S); n = 441 (P)	ORAL; 3.6×10^{12} CFU/da y[d]	VSL# 3[c]	53.4% of clinical responsiveness and 43.8% of clinical remission	Mardini and Grigorian [81]

CD, Crohn's disease; UC: Ulcerative colitis.
[a]Both total number of patients for clinical trials and number of studies for systematic analysis or meta-analysis were included.
[b]Includes the number of control patients.
[c]VSL#3 is composed by L. casei, L. plantarum, L. acidophilus, L. delbrueckii subsp. bulgaricus, B. longum, B. breve, B. infantis and Streptococcus sulivarius subsp. thermophiles.
[d]Length of treatments not available.

contrary, clinical findings in the literature could be the consequence of research that was inadequately designed and standardized.

13   Conclusions and further directions

Probiotics and FMT treatment have decent applications in IBD as well as in the medical field. Compared with other therapies, which have been developed recently, the emerging challenges regarding safety enhancement, trustability, standardization of probiotics, and FMT are substantial. Hence, more multicenter studies should be performed to improve the sample parameters (characteristics of IBD, genotypic also phenotypic features of patients,

therapeutic regimen standardization, etc.). Thus, further powerful outcomes will be derived.

Acknowledgments

This chapter is supported by SEED grant (UPES/R&D-HS/12032021/03 to KD) from the University of Petroleum and Energy Studies, Dehradun, India.

References

[1] L. Mao, A. Kitani, W. Strober, I.J. Fuss, The role of NLRP3 and IL-1beta in the pathogenesis of inflammatory bowel disease, Front. Immunol. 9 (2018) 2566, https://doi.org/10.3389/fimmu.2018.02566.

[2] P.J. Basso, M.T. Fonseca, G. Bonfa, V.B. Alves, H. Sales-Campos, V. Nardini, et al., Association among genetic predisposition, gut microbiota, and host immune response in the etiopathogenesis of inflammatory bowel disease, 2014.

[3] H. Sales-Campos, P.J. Basso, V.B. Alves, M.T. Fonseca, G. Bonfa, V. Nardini, et al., Classical and recent advances in the treatment of inflammatory bowel diseases, Braz. J. Med. Biol. Res. 48 (2015) 96–107, https://doi.org/10.1590/1414-431X20143774.

[4] M. Alipour, D. Zaidi, R. Valcheva, J. Jovel, I. Martinez, C. Sergi, et al., Mucosal barrier depletion and loss of bacterial diversity are primary abnormalities in paediatric ulcerative colitis, J. Crohns Colitis 10 (2016) 462–471, https://doi.org/10.1093/ecco-jcc/jjv223.

[5] J.D. Lewis, E.Z. Chen, R.N. Baldassano, A.R. Otley, A.M. Griffiths, D. Lee, et al., Inflammation, antibiotics, and diet as environmental stressors of the gut microbiome in pediatric Crohn's disease, Cell Host Microbe 18 (2015) 489–500, https://doi.org/10.1016/j.chom.2015.09.008.

[6] L.V. Hooper, J.I. Gordon, Commensal host-bacterial relationships in the gut, Science 292 (2001) 1115–1118, https://doi.org/10.1126/science.1058709.

[7] P.J. Turnbaugh, R.E. Ley, M. Hamady, C.M. Fraser-Liggett, R. Knight, J.I. Gordon, The human microbiome project, Nature 449 (2007) 804–810, https://doi.org/10.1038/nature06244.

[8] Y.M. Lei, L. Nair, M.L. Alegre, The interplay between the intestinal microbiota and the immune system, Clin. Res. Hepatol. Gastroenterol. 39 (2015) 9–19, https://doi.org/10.1016/j.clinre.2014.10.008.

[9] L. Wen, A. Duffy, Factors influencing the gut microbiota, inflammation, and type 2 diabetes, J. Nutr. 147 (2017) 1468S–1475S, https://doi.org/10.3945/jn.116.240754.

[10] A. Eck, E.F.J. de Groot, T.G.J. de Meij, M. Welling, P.H.M. Savelkoul, A.E. Budding, Robust microbiota-based diagnostics for inflammatory bowel disease, J. Clin. Microbiol. 55 (2017) 1720–1732, https://doi.org/10.1128/JCM.00162-17.

[11] B.A. Duerkop, M. Kleiner, D. Paez-Espino, W. Zhu, B. Bushnell, B. Hassell, et al., Murine colitis reveals a disease-associated bacteriophage community, Nat. Microbiol. 3 (2018) 1023–1031, https://doi.org/10.1038/s41564-018-0210-y.

[12] L.V. Hooper, D.R. Littman, A.J. Macpherson, Interactions between the microbiota and the immune system, Science 336 (2012) 1268–1273, https://doi.org/10.1126/science.1223490.

[13] P.D. Cani, C. Knauf, How gut microbes talk to organs: the role of endocrine and nervous routes, Mol. Metab. 5 (2016) 743–752, https://doi.org/10.1016/j.molmet.2016.05.011.

[14] C.N. Castro, J. Freitag, L. Berod, M. Lochner, T. Sparwasser, Microbe-associated immunomodulatory metabolites: influence on T cell fate and function, Mol. Immunol. 68 (2 Pt C) (2015) 575–584, https://doi.org/10.1016/j.molimm.2015.07.025.

[15] G.P. Donaldson, S.M. Lee, S.K. Mazmanian, Gut biogeography of the bacterial microbiota, Nat. Rev. Microbiol. 14 (2016) 20–32, https://doi.org/10.1038/nrmicro3552.

[16] R.E. Hoeppli, K.N. MacDonald, P. Leclair, V.C.W. Fung, M. Mojibian, J. Gillies, et al., Tailoring the homing capacity of human Tregs for directed migration to sites of Th1-inflammation or intestinal regions, Am. J. Transplant. 19 (2018) 62–76, https://doi.org/10.1111/ajt.14936.

[17] J.J. Bunker, T.M. Flynn, J.C. Koval, D.G. Shaw, M. Meisel, B.D. McDonald, et al., Innate and adaptive humoral responses coat distinct commensal bacteria with immunoglobulin A, Immunity 43 (2015) 541–553, https://doi.org/10.1016/j.immuni.2015.08.007.

[18] D. Rios-Covian, P. Ruas-Madiedo, A. Margolles, M. Gueimonde, C. G. de Los Reyes-Gavilan, N. Salazar, Intestinal short chain fatty acids and their link with diet and human health, Front. Microbiol. 7 (2016) 185, https://doi.org/10.3389/fmicb.2016.00185.

[19] M. van de Wouw, M. Boehme, J.M. Lyte, N. Wiley, C. Strain, O. O'Sullivan, et al., Short-chain fatty acids: microbial metabolites that alleviate stressinduced brain-gut axis alterations, J. Physiol. 596 (2018) 4923–4944, https://doi.org/10.1113/JP276431.

[20] D.N. Frank, A.L. St Amand, R.A. Feldman, E.C. Boedeker, N. Harpaz, N.R. Pace, Molecular-phylogenetic characterization of microbial community imbalances in human inflammatory bowel diseases, Proc. Natl. Acad. Sci. U. S. A. 104 (2007) 13780–13785, https://doi.org/10.1073/pnas.0706625104.

[21] U. Gophna, K. Sommerfeld, S. Gophna, W.F. Doolittle, S.J.O. Veldhuyzen van Zanten, Differences between tissue-associated intestinal microfloras of patients with Crohn's disease and ulcerative colitis, J. Clin. Microbiol. 44 (11) (2006) 4136–4141.

[22] N.O. Kaakoush, N. Castaño-Rodríguez, H.M. Mitchell, S.M. Man, Global epidemiology of campylobacter infection, Clin. Microbiol. Rev. 2015 (2015).

[23] K. Machiels, M. Joossens, J. Sabino, V.D. Preter, I. Arijs, E. Eeckhaut, V. Ballet, K. Claes, F. Van Immerseel, K. Verbeke, M. Ferrante, J. Verhaegen, P. Rutgeerts, S. Vermeire, A decrease of the butyrate-producing species Roseburia hominis and Faecalibacterium prausnitzii defines dysbiosis in patients with ulcerative colitis, Gut 63 (8) (2014) 1275–1283.

[24] Y. Tahara, et al., Gut microbiota-derived short chain fatty acids induce circadian clock entrainment in mouse peripheral tissue, Sci. Rep. 8 (1) (2018) 1395.

[25] P. Shah, J.V. Fritz, E. Glaab, M.S. Desai, K. Greenhalgh, A. Frachet, M. Niegowska, M. Estes, C. Jäger, C. Seguin-Devaux, A microfluidics-based in vitro model of the gastrointestinal humanmicrobe interface, Nat. Commun. 7 (2016) 11535.

[26] H. Sokol, V. Leducq, H. Aschard, H.-P. Pham, S. Jegou, C. Landman, D. Cohen, G. Liguori, A. Bourrier, I. Nion-Larmurier, J. Cosnes, P. Seksik, P. Langella, D. Skurnik, M.L. Richard, L. Beaugerie, Fungal microbiota dysbiosis in IBD, Gut 66 (6) (2017) 1039–1048.

[27] S. Vrakas, K.C. Mountzouris, G. Michalopoulos, G. Karamanolis, G. Papatheodoridis, C. Tzathas, M. Gazouli, Intestinal bacteria composition and translocation of bacteria in inflammatory bowel disease, PLoS One 12 (1) (2017), e0170034.

[28] A.D. Kostic, R.J. Xavier, D. Gevers, The microbiome in inflammatory bowel disease: current status and the future ahead, Gastroenterology 146 (2014) 1489–1499, https://doi.org/10.1053/j.gastro.2014.02.009.

[29] J.A. Gilbert, R.A. Quinn, J. Debelius, Z.Z. Xu, J. Morton, N. Garg, et al., Microbiome-wide association studies link dynamic microbial consortia to disease, Nature 535 (2016) 94–103, https://doi.org/10.1038/nature18850.

[30] L. Xiao, Q. Feng, S. Liang, S.B. Sonne, Z. Xia, X. Qiu, et al., A catalog of the mouse gut metagenome, Nat. Biotechnol. 33 (2015) 1103–1108, https://doi.org/10.1038/nbt.3353.

[31] P. Louis, H.J. Flint, Diversity, metabolism and microbial ecology of butyrate-producing bacteria from the human large intestine, FEMS Microbiol. Lett. 294 (2009) 1–8, https://doi.org/10.1111/j.1574-6968.2009.01514.x.

[32] H. Sokol, B. Pigneur, L. Watterlot, O. Lakhdari, L.G. Bermudez-Humaran, J.J. Gratadoux, et al., Faecalibacterium prausnitzii is an anti-inflammatory commensal bacterium identified by gut microbiota analysis of Crohn disease patients, Proc. Natl. Acad. Sci. U. S. A. 105 (2008) 16731–16736, https://doi.org/10.1073/pnas.0804812105.

[33] D. Gevers, S. Kugathasan, L.A. Denson, Y. Vazquez-Baeza, W. Van Treuren, B. Ren, et al., The treatment-naive microbiome in new-onset Crohn's disease, Cell Host Microbe 15 (2014) 382–392, https://doi.org/10.1016/j.chom.2014.02.005.

[34] J.D. Forbes, G. Van Domselaar, C.N. Bernstein, Microbiome survey of the inflamed and noninflamed gut at different compartments within the gastrointestinal tract of inflammatory bowel disease patients, Inflamm. Bowel Dis. 22 (2016) 817–825, https://doi.org/10.1097/MIB.0000000000000684.

[35] L. Lindoso, K. Mondal, S. Venkateswaran, H.K. Somineni, C. Ballengee, T.D. Walters, et al., The effect of early-life environmental exposures on disease phenotype and clinical course of crohn's disease in children, Am. J. Gastroenterol. 113 (2018) 1524–1529, https://doi.org/10.1038/s41395-018-0239-9.

[36] E. Elinav, T. Strowig, A.L. Kau, J. Henao-Mejia, C.A. Thaiss, C.J. Booth, et al., NLRP6 inflammasome regulates colonic microbial ecology and risk for colitis, Cell 145 (2011) 745–757, https://doi.org/10.1016/j.cell.2011.04.022.

[37] L. Albenberg, T.V. Esipova, C.P. Judge, K. Bittinger, J. Chen, A. Laughlin, et al., Correlation between intraluminal oxygen gradient and radial partitioning of intestinal microbiota, Gastroenterology 147 (2014) 1055–1063.e8, https://doi.org/10.1053/j.gastro.2014.07.020.

[38] K. Atarashi, T. Tanoue, K. Oshima, W. Suda, Y. Nagano, H. Nishikawa, et al., Treg induction by a rationally selected mixture of Clostridia strains from the human microbiota, Nature 500 (2013) 232–236, https://doi.org/10.1038/nature12331.

[39] M.Y. Khan, A. Dirweesh, T. Khurshid, W.J. Siddiqui, Comparing fecal microbiota transplantation to standard-of-care treatment for recurrent Clostridium difficile infection: a systematic review and meta-analysis, Eur. J. Gastroenterol. Hepatol. 30 (2018) 1309–1317, https://doi.org/10.1097/MEG.0000000000001243.

[40] A. Gagliardi, V. Totino, F. Cacciotti, V. Iebba, B. Neroni, G. Bonfiglio, et al., Rebuilding the gut microbiota ecosystem, Int. J. Environ. Res. Public Health 15 (2018) E1679, https://doi.org/10.3390/ijerph15081679.

[41] S. Mizuno, T. Masaoka, M. Naganuma, T. Kishimoto, M. Kitazawa, S. Kurokawa, et al., Bifidobacterium-rich fecal donor may be a positive predictor for successful fecal microbiota transplantation in patients with irritable bowel syndrome, Digestion 96 (2017) 29–38, https://doi.org/10.1159/000471919.

[42] S. Kunde, A. Pham, S. Bonczyk, T. Crumb, M. Duba, H. Conrad Jr., et al., Safety, tolerability, and clinical response after fecal transplantation in children and young adults with ulcerative colitis, J. Pediatr. Gastroenterol. Nutr. 56 (2013) 597–601, https://doi.org/10.1097/MPG.0b013e318292fa0d.

[43] N.G. Rossen, S. Fuentes, M.J. van der Spek, J.G. Tijssen, J.H. Hartman, A. Duflou, et al., Findings from a randomized controlled trial of fecal transplantation for patients with ulcerative colitis, Gastroenterology 149 (2015) 110–118.e4, https://doi.org/10.1053/j.gastro.2015.03.045.

[44] B. Cui, Q. Feng, H. Wang, M. Wang, Z. Peng, P. Li, et al., Fecal microbiota transplantation through mid-gut for refractory Crohn's disease: safety, feasibility, and efficacy trial results, J. Gastroenterol. Hepatol. 30 (2015) 51–58, https://doi.org/10.1111/jgh.12727.

[45] P. Moayyedi, M.G. Surette, P.T. Kim, J. Libertucci, M. Wolfe, C. Onischi, D. Armstrong, J.K. Marshall, Z. Kassam, W. Reinisch, C.H. Lee, Fecal microbiota transplantation induces remission in patients with active ulcerative colitis in a randomized controlled trial, Gastroenterology 149 (1) (2015) 102–109.e6.

[46] D.L. Suskind, M.J. Brittnacher, G. Wahbeh, M.L. Shaffer, H.S. Hayden, X. Qin, N. Singh, C.J. Damman, K.R. Hager, H. Nielson, S.I. Miller, Fecal microbial transplant effect on clinical outcomes and fecal microbiome in active Crohn's disease, Inflamm. Bowel Dis. 21 (3) (2015) 556–563.

[47] B.P. Vaughn, T. Vatanen, J.R. Allegretti, A. Bai, R.J. Xavier, J. Korzenik, et al., Increased intestinal microbial diversity following fecal microbiota transplant for active Crohn's disease, Inflamm. Bowel Dis. 22 (2016) 2182–2190, https://doi.org/10.1097/MIB.0000000000000893.

[48] S. Paramsothy, M.A. Kamm, N.O. Kaakoush, A.J. Walsh, J. van den Bogaerde, D. Samuel, et al., Multidonor intensive faecal microbiota ransplantation for active ulcerative colitis: a randomised placebo-controlled trial, Lancet 389 (2017) 1218–1228, https://doi.org/10.1016/S0140-6736(17)30182-4.

[49] S. Paramsothy, R. Paramsothy, D.T. Rubin, M.A. Kamm, N.O. Kaakoush, H.M. Mitchell, et al., Faecal microbiota transplantation for inflammatory bowel disease: a systematic review and meta-analysis, J. Crohns Colitis 11 (2017) 1180–1199, https://doi.org/10.1093/ecco-jcc/jjx063.

[50] A. Vrieze, E. Van Nood, F. Holleman, J. Salojarvi, R.S. Kootte, J.F. Bartelsman, et al., Transfer of intestinal microbiota from lean donors increases insulin sensitivity in individuals with metabolic syndrome, Gastroenterology 143 (2012) 913–916.e7, https://doi.org/10.1053/j.gastro.2012.06.031.

[51] S. Paramsothy, T.J. Borody, E. Lin, S. Finlayson, A.J. Walsh, D. Samuel, et al., Donor recruitment for fecal microbiota transplantation, Inflamm. Bowel Dis. 21 (2015) 1600–1606, https://doi.org/10.1097/MIB.0000000000000405.

[52] G. Holleran, F. Scaldaferri, G. Ianiro, L. Lopetuso, D. Mc Namara, M.C. Mele, et al., Fecal microbiota transplantation for the treatment of patients with ulcerative colitis and other gastrointestinal conditions beyond Clostridium difficile infection: an update, Drugs Today 54 (2018) 123–136, https://doi.org/10.1358/dot.2018.54.2.2760765.

[53] E.L. Hohmann, A.N. Ananthakrishnan, V. Deshpande, Case Records of the Massachusetts General Hospital. Case 25-2014. A 37-year-old man with ulcerative colitis and bloody diarrhea, N. Engl. J. Med. 371 (2014) 668–675, https://doi.org/10.1056/NEJMcpc1400842.

[54] J. Allegretti, L.M. Eysenbach, N. El-Nachef, M. Fischer, C. Kelly, Z. Kassam, The current landscape and lessons from fecal microbiota transplantation for inflammatory bowel disease: past, present, and future, Inflamm. Bowel Dis. 23 (2017) 1710–1717, https://doi.org/10.1097/MIB.0000000000001247.

[55] E. Gough, H. Shaikh, A.R. Manges, Systematic review of intestinal microbiota transplantation (fecal bacteriotherapy) for recurrent Clostridium difficile infection, Clin. Infect. Dis. 53 (2011) 994–1002, https://doi.org/10.1093/cid/cir632.

[56] M. Baxter, A. Colville, Adverse events in faecal microbiota transplant: a review of the literature, J. Hosp. Infect. 92 (2016) 117–127, https://doi.org/10.1016/j.jhin.2015.10.024.

[57] S.R. Jeon, J. Chai, C. Kim, C.H. Lee, Current evidence for the management of inflammatory bowel diseases using fecal microbiota transplantation, Curr. Infect. Dis. Rep. 20 (2018) 21, https://doi.org/10.1007/s11908-018-0627-8.

[58] N. Narula, Z. Kassam, Y. Yuan, J.F. Colombel, C. Ponsioen, W. Reinisch, et al., Systematic review and meta-analysis: fecal

microbiota transplantation for treatment of active ulcerative colitis, Inflamm. Bowel Dis. 23 (2017) 1702–1709, https://doi.org/10.1097/MIB.0000000000001228.

[59] C. Hill, F. Guarner, G. Reid, G.R. Gibson, D.J. Merenstein, B. Pot, et al., Expert consensus document. The International Scientific Association for Probiotics and Prebiotics consensus statement on the scope and appropriate use of the term probiotic, Nat. Rev. Gastroenterol. Hepatol. 11 (2014) 506–514, https://doi.org/10.1038/nrgastro.2014.66.

[60] D. Rachmilewitz, K. Katakura, F. Karmeli, T. Hayashi, C. Reinus, B. Rudensky, et al., Toll-like receptor 9 signaling mediates the anti-inflammatory effects of probiotics in murine experimental colitis, Gastroenterology 126 (2004) 520–528, https://doi.org/10.1053/j.gastro.2003.11.019.

[61] F.O. Ruiz, G. Gerbaldo, P. Asurmendi, L.M. Pascual, W. Giordano, I.L. Barberis, Antimicrobial activity, inhibition of urogenital pathogens, and synergistic interactions between lactobacillus strains, Curr. Microbiol. 59 (2009) 497–501, https://doi.org/10.1007/s00284-009-9465-0.

[62] P. Konieczna, C.A. Akdis, E.M. Quigley, F. Shanahan, L. O'Mahony, Portrait of an immunoregulatory Bifidobacterium, Gut Microbes 3 (2012) 261–266, https://doi.org/10.4161/gmic.20358.

[63] P. Markowiak, K. Slizewska, Effects of probiotics, prebiotics, and synbiotics on human health, Nutrients 9 (2017) E1021, https://doi.org/10.3390/nu9091021.

[64] C.A. Haskard, H.S. El-Nezami, P.E. Kankaanpaa, S. Salminen, J.T. Ahokas, Surface binding of aflatoxin B (1) by lactic acid bacteria, Appl. Environ. Microbiol. 67 (2001) 3086–3091, https://doi.org/10.1128/AEM.67.7.3086-3091.2001.

[65] A.M. Castellazzi, C. Valsecchi, S. Caimmi, A. Licari, A. Marseglia, M.C. Leoni, et al., Probiotics and food allergy, Ital. J. Pediatr. 39 (2013) 47, https://doi.org/10.1186/1824-7288-39-47.

[66] C. Caballero-Franco, K. Keller, C. De Simone, K. Chadee, The VSL#3 probiotic formula induces mucin gene expression and secretion in colonic epithelial cells, Am. J. Physiol. Gastrointest. Liver Physiol. 292 (2007) G315–G322, https://doi.org/10.1152/ajpgi.00265.2006.

[67] W.H. Holzapfel, P. Haberer, R. Geisen, J. Bjorkroth, U. Schillinger, Taxonomy and important features of probiotic microorganisms in food and nutrition, Am. J. Clin. Nutr. 73 (Suppl. 2) (2001) 365S–373S, https://doi.org/10.1093/ajcn/73.2.365s.

[68] M. Kechagia, D. Basoulis, S. Konstantopoulou, D. Dimitriadi, K. Gyftopoulou, N. Skarmoutsou, et al., Health benefits of probiotics: a review, ISRN Nutr. 2013 (2013), 481651, https://doi.org/10.5402/2013/481651.

[69] R. El Hage, E. Hernandez-Sanabria, T. Van de Wiele, Emerging trends in "smart probiotics": functional consideration for the development of novel health and industrial applications, Front. Microbiol. 8 (2017) 1889, https://doi.org/10.3389/fmicb.2017.01889.

[70] K. Atarashi, T. Tanoue, T. Shima, A. Imaoka, T. Kuwahara, Y. Momose, et al., Induction of colonic regulatory T cells by indigenous Clostridium species, Science 331 (2011) 337–341, https://doi.org/10.1126/science.1198469.

[71] S. Kang, S.E. Denman, M. Morrison, Z. Yu, J. Dore, M. Leclerc, et al., Dysbiosis of fecal microbiota in Crohn's disease patients as revealed by a customphylogenetic microarray, Inflamm. Bowel Dis. 16 (2010) 2034–2042, https://doi.org/10.1002/ibd.21319.

[72] C. Pothoulakis, Review article: anti-inflammatory mechanisms of action of Saccharomyces boulardii, Aliment. Pharmacol. Ther. 30 (2009) 826–833, https://doi.org/10.1111/j.1365-2036.2009.04102.x.

[73] S. Doron, D.R. Snydman, Risk and safety of probiotics, Clin. Infect. Dis. 60 (Suppl. 2) (2015) S129–S134, https://doi.org/10.1093/cid/civ085.

[74] F.H. Degnan, The US Food and Drug Administration and probiotics: regulatory categorization, Clin. Infect. Dis. 46 (Suppl. 2) (2008) S133–S136. discussion S144–S151. https://doi.org/10.1086/523324.

[75] A.J. Riquelme, M.A. Calvo, A.M. Guzman, M.S. Depix, P. Garcia, C. Perez, et al., Saccharomyces cerevisiae fungemia after Saccharomyces boulardii treatment in immunocompromised patients, J. Clin. Gastroenterol. 36 (2003) 41–43, https://doi.org/10.1097/00004836-200301000-00013.

[76] M. Saarela, G. Mogensen, R. Fonden, J. Matto, T. Mattila-Sandholm, Probiotic bacteria: safety, functional and technological properties, J. Biotechnol. 84 (2000) 197–215, https://doi.org/10.1016/S0168-1656(00)00375-8.

[77] M. Thomsen, S. Clarke, L. Vitetta, The role of adjuvant probiotics to attenuate intestinal inflammatory responses due to cancer treatments, Benef. Microbes (2018), https://doi.org/10.3920/BM2017.0172 (Epub ahead of print).

[78] Z. Matuskova, E. Anzenbacherova, R. Vecera, H. Tlaskalova-Hogenova, M. Kolar, P. Anzenbacher, Administration of a probiotic can change drug pharmacokinetics: effect of E. coli Nissle 1917 on amidarone absorption in rats, PLoS One 9 (2014), e87150, https://doi.org/10.1371/journal.pone.0087150.

[79] T. Zuo, S.C. Ng, The gut microbiota in the pathogenesis and therapeutics of inflammatory bowel disease, Front. Microbiol. 9 (2018) 2247, https://doi.org/10.3389/fmicb.2018.02247.

[80] H. Tamaki, H. Nakase, S. Inoue, C. Kawanami, T. Itani, M. Ohana, et al., Efficacy of probiotic treatment with Bifidobacterium longum 536 for induction of remission in active ulcerative colitis: a randomized, double-blinded, placebo-controlled multicenter trial, Dig. Endosc. 28 (2016) 67–74, https://doi.org/10.1111/den.12553.

[81] H.E. Mardini, A.Y. Grigorian, Probiotic mix VSL#3 is effective adjunctive therapy for mild to moderately active ulcerative colitis: a meta-analysis, Inflamm. Bowel Dis. 20 (2014) 1562–1567, https://doi.org/10.1097/MIB.0000000000000084.

[82] A. Sood, V. Midha, G.K. Makharia, V. Ahuja, D. Singal, P. Goswami, et al., The probiotic preparation, VSL#3 induces remission in patients with mild-to-moderately active ulcerative colitis, Clin. Gastroenterol. Hepatol. 7 (2009) 1202–1209.e1, https://doi.org/10.1016/j.cgh.2009.07.016.

[83] W. Kruis, P. Fric, J. Pokrotnieks, M. Lukas, B. Fixa, M. Kascak, et al., Maintaining remission of ulcerative colitis with the probiotic Escherichia coli Nissle 1917 is as effective as with standard mesalazine, Gut 53 (2004) 1617–1623, https://doi.org/10.1136/gut.2003.037747.

[84] D. Jonkers, J. Penders, A. Masclee, M. Pierik, Probiotics in the management of inflammatory bowel disease: a systematic review of intervention studies in adult patients, Drugs 72 (2012) 803–823, https://doi.org/10.2165/11632710-000000000-00000.

[85] K. Kato, S. Mizuno, Y. Umesaki, Y. Ishii, M. Sugitani, A. Imaoka, et al., Randomized placebo-controlled trial assessing the effect of bifidobacteriafermented milk on active ulcerative colitis, Aliment. Pharmacol. Ther. 20 (2004) 1133–1141, https://doi.org/10.1111/j.1365-2036.2004.02268.x.

[86] K. Matsuoka, Y. Uemura, T. Kanai, R. Kunisaki, Y. Suzuki, K. Yokoyama, et al., Efficacy of bifidobacterium breve fermented milk in maintaining remission of ulcerative colitis, Dig. Dis. Sci. 63 (2018) 1910–1919, https://doi.org/10.1007/s10620-018-4946-2.

[87] G. Gargari, V. Taverniti, S. Balzaretti, C. Ferrario, C. Gardana, P. Simonetti, et al., Consumption of a bifidobacterium bifidum strain for 4 weeks modulates dominant intestinal bacterial taxa and fecal butyrate in healthy adults, Appl. Environ. Microbiol. 82 (2016) 5850–5859, https://doi.org/10.1128/AEM.01753-16.

[88] M.A. Zocco, L.Z. dal Verme, F. Cremonini, A.C. Piscaglia, E.C. Nista, M. Candelli, et al., Efficacy of Lactobacillus GG in maintaining remission of ulcerative colitis, Aliment. Pharmacol. Ther. 23 (2006) 1567–1574, https://doi.org/10.1111/j.1365-2036.2006.02927.x.

[89] M.J. Saez-Lara, C. Gomez-Llorente, J. Plaza-Diaz, A. Gil, The role of probiotic lactic acid bacteria and bifidobacteria in the prevention and treatment of inflammatory bowel disease and other related diseases: a systematic review of randomized human clinical trials, Biomed. Res. Int. 2015 (2015), 505878, https://doi.org/10.1155/2015/505878.

[90] P. Gupta, H. Andrew, B.S. Kirschner, S. Guandalini, Is lactobacillus GG helpful in children with Crohn's disease? Results of a preliminary, openlabel study, J. Pediatr. Gastroenterol. Nutr. 31 (2000) 453–457, https://doi.org/10.1097/00005176-200010000-00024.

[91] S. Fujimori, A. Tatsuguchi, K. Gudis, T. Kishida, K. Mitsui, A. Ehara, T. Kobayashi, Y. Sekita, T. Seo, C. Sakamoto, High dose probiotic and prebiotic cotherapy for remission induction of active Crohn's disease, J. Gastroenterol. Hepatol. 22 (8) (2007) 1199–1204.

[92] A. Tursi, G. Brandimarte, A. Papa, A. Giglio, W. Elisei, G.M. Giorgetti, G. Forti, S. Morini, C. Hassan, M.P. Pistoia, M.E. Modeo, S. Rodino, T. D'Amico, L. Sebkova, N. Sacca, E.D. Giulio, F. Luzza, M. Imeneo, T. Larussa, S.D. Rosa, V. Annese, S. Danese, A. Gasbarrini, Treatment of relapsing mild-to-moderate ulcerative colitis with the probiotic VSL#3 as adjunctive to a standard pharmaceutical treatment: a double-blind, randomized, placebo-controlled study, Am. J. Gastroenterol. 105 (10) (2010) 2218–2227.

[93] A. Bourreille, G. Cadiot, G. Le Dreau, D. Laharie, L. Beaugerie, J.L. Dupas, et al., Saccharomyces boulardii does not prevent relapse of Crohn's disease, Clin. Gastroenterol. Hepatol. 11 (2013) 982–987, https://doi.org/10.1016/j.cgh.2013.02.021.

[94] S. Oliva, G. Di Nardo, F. Ferrari, S. Mallardo, P. Rossi, G. Patrizi, et al., Randomised clinical trial: the effectiveness of Lactobacillus reuteri ATCC 55730 rectal enema in children with active distal ulcerative colitis, Aliment. Pharmacol. Ther. 35 (2012) 327–334, https://doi.org/10.1111/j.1365-2036.2011.04939.x.

[95] S. Kolacek, I. Hojsak, R. Berni Canani, A. Guarino, F. Indrio, R. Orel, et al., Commercial probiotic products: a call for improved quality control. a position paper by the ESPGHAN working group for probiotics and prebiotics, J. Pediatr. Gastroenterol. Nutr. 65 (2017) 117–124, https://doi.org/10.1097/MPG.0000000000001603.

Chapter 6

Advanced therapeutics for renal inflammation

Manish Pal Singh[a], Rashita Makkar[b], Tapan Behl[c], and Kamla Pathak[d]

[a]Anand College of Pharmacy (SGI), Agra, Uttar Pradesh, India, [b]Chitkara College of Pharmacy, Chitkara University, Rajpura, Punjab, India, [c]School of Health Science and Technology, University of Petroleum and Energy Studies, Bidholi, Uttarakhand, India, [d]Faculty of Pharmacy, Uttar Pradesh University of Medical Sciences, Etawah, Uttar Pradesh, India

1 Introduction

1.1 Overview of renal inflammation

Body inflammation is a multifold process for maintaining cellular homeostasis and to escape from tissue injury. Excessive stress on body cells leads to chronic inflammation, which further interrupts cell homeostasis [1]. Inflammation occurring at the kidney cellular site tends to injure the resident cells of the renal system and leads to acute kidney inflammation (AKI) and chronic kidney disease (CKD). Nephritis can be used as an ordinary term for renal inflammation. It can be classified into inflammation occurring in glomeruli (glomerulonephritis) and inflammation present in spaces between renal tubules (interstitial nephritis). The main clinical manifestation of renal inflammation is 'proteinuria,' a pathological condition signalized by immoderate expulsion of blood proteins in urine [2].

The inflammation in kidney can be induced by monoleukocytes and polyleukocytes and migration of other chemotactic factors, which leads to the activation of interleukins (ILs), and other proinflammatory cytokines. In AKI, inflammation initiates due to necrosis of kidney cells and in CKD, it can also be induced by atrophy of the renal tubular cells [3]. T and B lymphocyte cells also play a key factor in the expeditious inflammatory process in AKI [4]. Different pathogenetic pathways contribute to the development of CKD but all of them coincide on a general single pathway, which ultimately leads to fibrosis in renal tubular spaces and causes loss of nephritic function due to renal cell atrophy [5].

1.2 Role of resident kidney cells

The etiology of renal inflammation, especially at the site of glomerulus injury, is directly proportional to the participation of resident renal cells. The more the renal cells are involved the higher is the progression of GN, which is mediated via the upregulation of cytokines into the injury area [6]. Fibroblastic reticular cells in conjunction with the resident renal lymph nodes are involved in the advancement of renal inflammation, as they act by operating the immune T lymphocyte cells which forms an important element for the progression of glomerulonephritis [7]. Additionally, other resident kidney cells such as mesangial cells and podocytes are also important regulators for maintaining renal function. Mesangial cells escape the entomb remnant and prevent the accumulation of proteins from the basement membrane and podocytes, which form the glomerular filtration barrier. The affliction of a couple of cells can be responsible for the development of lupus nephritis [8]. The other resident cells such as renal tubular cells present in the tubulointerstitium, can also be responsible for concatenation of the lupus nephritis. Renal tubular cells mainly upregulate the proinflammatory cytokines such as B-cell activating factor (BAFF), which further interact with tubulointerstitial immune cells and lead to renal inflammation [9].

1.3 Role of infiltrating cells

Leukocyte infiltration is the principal moderator of renal inflammation and is available within the glomerulus or tubulointerstitium. The infiltration of monocytes into the injured area of tissue and their successive divergence into macrophage cells is responsible for tissue injury and repair process of cells. The neutrophils in the renal inflammatory area also encourage the activation of reactive oxygen species (ROS) and proteases, which further lead to the progression of acute inflammation in the kidney [10]. Chemokines are proteins that initiate the attraction of leukocytes into the injury area and the expression of chemokine receptor 5 (CCR5) in the progression of nephritis is well established [11]. However, the glomerular macrophages

Recent Developments in Anti-Inflammatory Therapy. https://doi.org/10.1016/B978-0-323-99988-5.00008-5

have higher susceptibility for nephritis compared to the interstitial macrophages [12]. The interstitial infiltrates are mainly composed of lymphocytes, macrophages, eosinophilis, and plasma cells. They are the key elements for the generation of interstitial fibrosis in acute interstitial nephritis (AIN). In the pathogenesis of AIN, the helper T cells (CD+4) are the predominant type of infiltrating inflammatory components compared to other inflammatory mediators [13].

1.4 Microinflammation process in renal injury

Microinflammation is a mild grade inflammation, which corresponds to sclerosis disease progression in the body [14]. A microinflammation mechanism, directly or indirectly, is involved in the progression of renal failure. It plays a major role in the initiation of different types of kidney disorders, mainly the uremic condition resulting in renal insufficiency. Aggregation of proinflammatory cytokines and advanced glycation end products (AGEs) promotes inflammation in patients with uremia [15]. Renal fibrosis disrupts the endothelial cells in the basement membrane, which causes activation and release of type III and IV collagen, which further stimulates the microinflammation process in CKD [16]. The process of microinflammation in uremic patients can result through imbalance between the ratio of Th22/Treg cells (helper T cell/regulatory T cells), which can further prolong the dialysis period in hemodialysis patients [17]. Renal death cells also initiate necroinflammation in AKI and CKD. Necrotic cells result in damage of the plasma membrane, which activates other innate immune mediators such as danger-associated molecular patterns (DAMPs) and alarmins. The DAMPs and alarmins induce the release of inflammatory cytokine and chemokine and enhance the infiltration of leukocytes into renal cells that promotes necroinflammation [3]. Microinflammation acts as a key element in the development of diabetic nephropathy (DN) and other renal complications in diabetic patients. It directly activates cell adhesion molecules, chemokines, and other proinflammatory cytokines, which causes the progression of diabetic nephropathy and other diabetic vascular complications in diabetic patients [18].

1.5 Role of microbial infection

Microbial infection releases toxins, which can act as microbial antigens. Microbial antigens initiate cellular and innate immunity complex, which further aggravates renal inflammation (Prasad and Patel [19]). Unrestrained population of Gram-negative bacteria can promote the release of proinflammatory cytokines, which further leads to systemic inflammation in CKD [20]. The possible roles of cellular immunity and autoimmunity are the main generators of GN. Involvement of nonrenal bacterial infection can

mediate postinfectious glomerulonephritis (GN), which is mainly initiated through the immune process. In this context, two streptococcal antigens such as glyceraldehyde-3-phosphate dehydrogenase (GAPDH) and pyrogenic exotoxin B (SepB) can be held accountable for GN [21,22]. Another target for glomerular infection is staphylococcal neutral phosphates (NPtase). Affinity of NPtase selectively with the glomerular basement membrane stimulates the complement system, thus triggering a series of events which leads to glomerulonephritis [23,24].

The motive of this chapter is to expound possible targets of renal inflammation and challenges of current antiinflammatory drugs and advanced antiinflammatory drugs for renal inflammation.

2 Therapeutic perspective for renal inflammation

2.1 Physiological targets of antiinflammatory agents

Arachidonic acid (AA) is the main component of cell-membrane phospholipid, which is metabolized by three types of enzyme, namely, cyclooxygenase (COX), lipooxygenase (LOX), and cytochrome P450 (CYP450). Prostaglandins (PGs), thromboxane A_2 (TXA_2), and leukotrienes B_4 (LTB_4) act as inflammatory modulators in renal inflammation [25]. Patients with lupus nephritis can be diagnosed by urinary biomarkers such as urinary prostaglandin D synthase (uPGDS). [26] In addition, accumulation of LTs in kidney cells also contributes inflammatory reactions. The LTB4 helps in the migration of polymorphonuclear nuclear neutrophils (PMNs) in the renal parenchymal cells, which leads to renal inflammation [27]. A diverse number of factors, viz., transforming growth factor-β (TGF-β), connective tissue growth factor (CTGF), and myofibroblast activation also contribute to the growth of renal fibrosis and hence cause advancement of CKD. [28,29]

A hyperglycemia condition in patients also contributes to the activation of inflammatory mediators and further DN. The excess level of glucose can alter intracellular signaling, which promotes leukocyte migration into the renal endothelial cells and causes progression of renal injury [30]. The attachment of leukocytes into the endothelial vascular cells is through adhesion molecules. The vascular cell adhesion protein-1 can (VAP-1) help in the extravasation of leukocytes into the inflammatory region [31]. Cytokines also initiate kidney inflammation through activation of innate and adaptive immune processes. It potentially regulates the immune TH 1 and TH 2 cells for a nephritogenic immune sequence and can cause progression of GN [32]. The different cytokines are involved in activation of T and B immune cells, which further induce autoimmunity and alter renal resident cells, which form the key pathogenesis for LN [33]. The other platelet activating factors (PAFs) such as TXA2 and P-selectin also regulate the alteration of vascular permeability, leukocyte infiltration, and cross talk between leukocytes and endothelial cells for the pathogenesis of AKI [34].

2.2 Receptor targets for antiinflammatory agents

2.2.1 Chemokine ligand/receptor-2 (CCL2/CCR2) inhibitors

Chemokines are the main modulators for the migration of inflammatory cells into the kidney compartment [35]. Chemokine receptor families can be classified into four different subgroups (C, CC, CXC, and CX_3C). An activation of CCR2 can induce the generation of reactive oxygen species (ROS), which initiates the pathogenesis of renal injury [36]. Kang et al. have reported that the action of the RS504393 type of specific antagonist of CCR2 can ameliorate insulin resistance through modulation of fat tissue and prevent nephropathy in diabetic mice (db/db mice). Several investigators have also explored that the antagonism of CCR2 is beneficial for DN as it inhibits proinflammatory cytokines, which reduces the vasopressin level and increases urine output in the diabetic animals [37]. Additionally, the expression of CCL2 can be facilitated by the proteinuria effect specifically in patients with lupus nephritis. However, the antagonism of CCR2 can be effective in diminishing proteinuria in experimental animal models [38]. In this context, another research investigation revealed that the role of CCR2 antagonist RS102895 can prevent diabetic nephropathy in an experimental animal type 2 diabetic model. Study results concluded the preventive action of CCR2 antagonist through upregulation of mRNA expression of vascular endothelial growth factor (VEGF) and downregulation of nephron mRNA expression in the treatment groups of diabetic animals [39].

Chemokines and their receptors are involved in the infiltration of glomerular monocytes, which is essential for progressive inflammation in glomerulonephritis [40]. The activation of the CCR2 receptor can be initiated by the expression of genes, which are activated by the blood clotting factors X (FXa) and which regulate chronic microinflammation in hemodialysis patients. The FXa-initiated CCR2 mRNA expression can be eradicated by JNK (Janus kinase) and tyrosine kinase inhibition. Hence, the antagonism of CCR2 is beneficial for systemic microinflammation in hemodialysis patients [41]. Chemoattractant protein-1, known as chemokine ligand-2 (CCL2), can bind with CCR2 and leads to infiltration of inflammatory cells, which induce the proliferation of glomerular resident cells and induce glomerulonephritis. In this context, the novel antagonist RS-504393 of CCR2 has proven to be beneficial in preventing renal fibrosis [42,43].

2.2.2 Janus kinase (JAK) inhibitors

The Janus kinase-2 (JAK-2) and Signal transducer and activator of transcription-3 (STAT 3) are regulated by different inflammatory processes such as proliferation and infiltration of resident kidney cells, which further regulates gene expression and cytokine-mediated signaling which leads to inflammation of kidney cells and development of renal fibrosis [44]. The selective JAK2/STAT3 inhibitors pose a therapeutic significance in the end stage of renal disease in infants. Tyrphostin AG490, a type of JAK2/STAT3 inhibitor, can cause congenital obstructive nephropathy in children. Due to its prevention of JAK2/STAT3, it can be used in preventing mediated inflammation and renal fibrosis of the cell [45]. The protective action of mefunidone has been established in the treatment of tubulointerstitial fibrosis in an experimental rat model for unilateral ureteral obstruction (UUO). The mechanism of mefunidone is probably due to the inhibition of p-STAT3 and formation of proinflammatory cytokines in treated groups of experimental animals [46].

Another inhibitor agent such as paclitaxel also decreased macrophage infiltration and fibroblast activation through STAT3 inhibition in an experimental adult mice model for UUO [47]. Similarly, the inhibition of JAK2 by AG490 can be associated with the treatment of glomerulosclerosis. The blocking of JAK2 inhibition in mice remarkably reduced the expression of smooth muscle alpha action (α-SMA) and monocyte chemoattractant protein-1 (MCP-1) [48]. The transcription of JAKs/STATs signaling initiates the focal segmental glomerulosclerosis [49]. Additionally, it may also lead to augmentation of considerable proliferation and development of glomerular mesangial cells, which cause progression of diabetic nephropathy [50]. The lipid-lowering agent fluvastatin, has been reported to play a beneficial role in the treatment of diabetic nephropathy. Authors have explored the site of beneficial renoprotective effect of fluvastatin through inhibition phosphorylation of the JAK2/STAT1 pathway (Shi et al. [51]). A novel antagonist of JAK2 polyglutamic acid/peptoid 1 (QM56) protects renal injury through its antiapoptic action as well as it has markedly reduced proliferation of nephrotoxin cells and inflammatory cytokines [52]. Another antagonist CP-690550, also inhibits JAK3/STAT and has significantly reduced circulatory cytokines and have proven to be effective in the treatment of LN [53].

2.3 Drug targeting oxidative stress

Stress due to the generation of ROS and reactive nitrogen species (RNS) regulates the CKD and the inflammatory effect at the renal site. The kidney is a determinant metabolic organ, which prompts high oxidative reactions in mitochondrial cells. Excessive production of oxidative stress (OS) can be directly responsible in hastening the inflammatory process in the kidneys [54]. The formation of ROS through nicotinamide adenine dinucleotide phosphate (NADPH) oxidase isoform Nox4 in renal cells may regulate different inflammatory actions in AKI and CKD [55]. The ROS formation induced by purine metabolism can mediate through xanthine oxidase (XO) enzyme [5]. The reduction of ROS and other mediators of oxidative stress can play a beneficial role in the prevention of renal inflammatory mechanism in renal disorders.

2.3.1 Nox4 inhibitors

Nox4 blocking is expressed as a therapeutic treatment in DN. The novel inhibitor GKT137831 reduced glomerular hypertrophy and urinary albumin excretion in an experimental type I animal model [56]. Similarly, pitavastatin can also be used in diminishing Nox4 mediated oxidative stress in experimental diabetic mice and has shown beneficial effects in the prevention of DN [57]. NADPH oxidases (Noxs) generate ROS, which further stimulates the release of free radicals for renal cell injury. Meng et al. have reported that the inhibition of Nox4 overexpression is beneficial in cisplatin-induced cell inflammation in AKI. However, N-acetyl-L-cysteine (NAC) moderation of ROS suppressed cell injury lead by Nox4 overexpression and they concluding that the Nox4-mediated ROS formation can be an important element in cisplatin-induced nephritis [58]. Finally, the main target of Nox4 inhibition can be to produce preventive action in DN. Nox4 is also involved in the pathogenesis of DN by pathways that regulate enzymes and resides within mitochondria. Regulation of NADPH can be regulated by growth factors such as platelet-derived growth factor (PDGF). It can be suppressed by a novel Nox inhibitor VAS2870, on PDGF-dependent ROS liberation in vascular smooth muscle cells [59].

2.3.2 Xanthine oxidase inhibitors

Activation of xanthine oxidase (XO) contributes to ROS formation in interstitial tubular cells. The stimulation of oxidative stress leads to inflammation in renal interstitial tissues as the formation of ROS causes infiltration of mononuclear leukocyte cells and activation of MCP-1 and intracellular adhesive molecules (ICAM-1) and VCAM-1 within the tissue space of kidney cells [60]. Gondouin et al. have disclosed the possible mechanism of XO-mediated inflammation in patients with hemodialysis, where it can be responsible for inducing CKD-related oxidative stress and generation of ROS in renal cells during inflammation. The XO activity also corresponded with a malondialdehyde oxidation product in hemodialysis patients. Further, they have proposed a clinical significant effect of XO-inhibitor in diminishing oxidative stress in CKD [61]. Omori et al. also revealed that another XO inhibitor, febuxostat, has been

used in CKD treatment. Study results have supported the hypothesis raised about the role of XO inhibitors in reducing oxidative stress and proliferation of inflammatory mediators such as infiltration of macrophage cells, early proinflammatory cytokine expression, and downregulation of expression of TGF-β. In addition, febuxostat can reduce renal interstitial fibrosis in patients with CKD [62].

2.4 Novel targets of renal inflammation treatment

The majority of antiinflammatory drugs act on systemic inflammation and are commonly used in AKI, CKD, and other renal inflammatory-associated disorders. Antiinflammatory agents, which are clinically used in diseases associated with CKD, generally inhibit the direct inflammatory pathways and the released mediators along with inhibition of the innate and autoimmunity in renal disorders [63]. The renin angiotensin system (RAS) is an important regulator of cardiorenal toxicity. Renal inflammation is mainly caused by activation of the RAS system through the angiotensin-converting enzyme (ACE). The involvement of ACE by the formation of angiotensin-active peptides (Ang-II and Ang 1-7) induces an inflammatory mechanism at the renal site [64]. Aliskiren, a direct renin inhibitor, can diminish the formation of angiotensin I and II by blocking renin activity. Aliskiren also reduces proinflammatory mediators and downregulates lipogenic pathways and causes systemic insulin resistance, and can act as a preventive agent in patients with nondiabetic chronic kidney disease (NDCKD) [65]. Additionally, Ang-II formation is directly involved in the progression of renal inflammation. Ang-II induces the generation of TNF-α in renal cells. In addition it is responsible for the upregulation of proinflammatory mediators together with IL-6 and NF-kβ and expression of cytokines and chemokines in renal inflammation [66]. The angiotensin bioactive peptides mainly regulates their physiological function by the expression of angiotensin receptors I and II (AT I and AT II). These receptors synchronize the expression of profibrotic factors, including connective tissue growth factor (CTGF) and initiate renal fibrosis [67].

Remarkably, the lipoperoxidative stress can be a determinant-causing factor in the pathogenesis of CKD. Nuclear transcription factors such as peroxisome proliferator-activated receptors (PPARs) and farnesoid X-receptor (FXR) control lipid metabolism, inflammation, and fibrosis. Activation of PPAR-α by thiazolidinediones can produce an antiinflammatory effect in CKD patients [68]. The modulation of FXR by its ligands controls lipid metabolism, bile acid and carbohydrate metabolism, and other inflammatory mechanisms. The essential endogenous FXR ligands in the body such as cholic acid and chenodeoxycholic acid and synthetic ligands such as GW4064 and α-ethyl-chenodeoxycholic acid can be used effectively in the treatment of renal inflammatory disorders (Shaik et al. [69]). In another investigation, it was reported that the role of free acid oxidation can responsible for the progression of renal fibrosis. By analysis of the study results data, it was confirmed that the imbalance of fatty oxidation is related with the expression of microRNAs, which can reduce the expression of PPAR-α in renal epithelial cells [70]. Toll-like receptors (TLRs) act as a key player in the development of inflammation through the generation of proinflammatory mediators and activation of innate immunity, which can originate insulin resistance in type II diabetic patients. However, the type of TLR 2 and TLR 4 are involved in insulin resistance and progression of DN in diabetic patients [71]. The physiological role of TLR 2 and TLR 4 expression in tubulointerstitial nephritis can be studied by a leptospira experimental animal model. Expression of TLRs leads to p38 mitogen-activated protein kinase (p38 MAPK) and stimulation of proinflammatory cytokines in renal proximal tubule cells [72]. The involvement of other TLRs (TLR 3 and TLR 7) is also responsible for the pathogenesis of glomerulonephritis in viral infections, because viral infection trigger the expression of TLR 3 and TLR 7 by distinguishing viral RNA and stimulate immunity-mediated reaction in glomerular site cells during viral infection [73].

A novel class of other targets has been discovered in the area of renal inflammation. Vitamin D receptor (VDR) activation is significantly involved in the treatment of different types of renal disorders. The therapeutic role of activation of the VDR in suppressing both the innate and adaptive immunity possesses significant involvement in the treatment of lupus nephritis [74,75]. Tan et al. reported that the vitamin D agonist drug paricalcitol reduced renal inflammation by suppressing the infiltration of T cells and macrophages. The mechanism of paricalcitol by blocking the RANTES mRNA and protein expression reduced the migration of lymphocytes and monocytes into the tubular site during renal inflammation. The study results were concluded to achieve the antiinflammatory action of paricalcitol by reducing the infiltration of lymphocytes and macrophages as well as suppressing the expression of RANTES through promoting VDR-arbitrated sequestration of NF-κB signaling [76]. Another target site for a protective role of expression of nuclear factor erythroid-2 related factor (Nrf-2) in the kidneys is inflammation. Nrf-2 is a main transcription factor that can protect cells through different oxidative stress-induced ROS formation and inflammation in AKI [77]. The progression of renal disorders depends upon two regulatory mechanisms, oxidative stress and mitochondrial dysfunction. Activation of the Nrf-2 factor through resveratrol controls inflammation and oxidative stress related to kidney aging [78]. In a different kind

of CKD, including DN leading to end stage renal fibrosis, transforming growth factor-β (TGF-β) is the key element for renal fibrosis. A novel class of noncoding RNA is microRNA (miRNA), and miRNA are dominant regulators for the expression of TGF-β in renal fibrosis, which can lead to progression of diabetic renal disease [79].

3 Novel emergence therapies for renal inflammation

3.1 Antimalarial drug treatment for renal inflammation

Antimalarial agents are ancient therapies and have been used as immunomodulatories in clinical practice for the treatment of various renal inflammatory disorders. Treatment of lupus nephritis and other inflammatory renal conditions can be achieved by targeting autoimmunity and causing its suppression. Conventional antimalarial drugs such as hydroxychloroquine and chloroquine can be utilized in the prevention of lupus nephritis for their antiinflammatory action along with their immunosuppressive action. It can also reduce the formation of PGs, cytokine synthesis and causes downregulation of TLR [80]. The immunosuppressive action of antimalarial drugs can be responsible their beneficial role in patients with lupus nephritis. In this context, the novel antimalarial drug artemisinin and its derivatives can be effective in the prevention of systemic lupus erythematosus (SLE) through suppressing T-cell activation and inhibiting the NF-κB signal transduction pathway [81]. Another study was carried out to evaluate the efficacy of artemisinin in the treatment of tubulointerstitial inflammation and renal fibrosis. Study results indicated significant effect of drug through the inhibition of the NF-κB/NLRP3 signaling pathway [82]. Xia et al. revealed that the derivative of dihydroartemisinin can be used as a substitute therapy in the prevention of IgA nephropathy. The authors have confirmed that dihydroartemisinin acts through inhibition of the mammalian target of rapamycin/ribosomal protein S6 kinase beta-1 (mTOR/S6K1) signaling pathway, cell proliferation, and inducing cell autophagy in in vitro IgAN mesangial cell model [83]. Furthermore, another class of antimalarial agents can be also used as therapeutic moderators for renal inflammatory disorders. For example, mefloquine and quinacrine-like antimalarial agents can be used for the treatment of AKI. The antimalarial drug quinacrine can protect renal inflammation in a glycerol-induced AKI animal model via the inhibition of the phospholipase A2 enzyme, which is a key element for renal inflammation through the activation of arachidonic acid pathways of the cell membrane [84]. Mefloquine can also be used in the treatment of IgA nephropathy patients due to their immunosuppressive effect [85].

3.2 Management of renal inflammation by immunosuppressants

Body immunity (innate and autoimmunity) is the dominant contestant for the development of renal inflammation. For example, TLR target site incitement depends upon body immune system activation. The autoimmune injury of tissues mainly depends upon the proliferation of the autoreactive lymphocyte population [86]. The role of immunosuppressive drugs in the management in renal inflammatory disorders can be effective. In the past, for the treatment of lupus nephritis corticosteroids therapy or its combination with some other immunosuppressive agents such as cyclophosphamide was used. Some of the recent emerging therapy agents include mycophenolate, an immunosuppressive drug, which can be used in the prevention of lupus nephritis [87]. During maintenance therapy with older immunosuppressive drugs such as cyclophophosphamide, adverse effects such as higher risk of opportunistic infections, premature gonadal failure, and malignancy can also be induced [88]. Mycophenolate can produce beneficial effect in patients with lupus nephritis with less risk factor as comparable to cyclophosphamide. [89]

The induction regimen of immunosuppressants such as calcineurin inhibitors can be beneficial in the treatment of lupus nephritis and it is also safer in pregnancy and lactation. The pharmacodynamic stance of calcineurin inhibitors such as tacrolimus and cyclosporin act as a multitarget regimen for lupus nephritis as it diminishes the activation of T cells. Both immunosuppressive agents inhibit T-cell activation via suppression of calcium and calmodulin-dependent phosphatase calcineurin [90]. In a controlled trial study for the treatment of lupus nephritis patients, the mycophenolate is no lesser than cyclophosphamide for induction regimen but is superior to azathioprine as maintenance therapy [91]. A novel mineralocorticoid receptor (MR) antagonist such as apararenone can be effective in controlling type 2 diabetic condition in patients and is beneficial in the treatment of CKD. The activation of MR in tissue injury further stimulates the synthesis of macrophages and T cells [92]. The aldosterone inhibitor spironolactone also shows preventive effect in the management of renal fibrosis. Aldosterone expresses the activation of MR and induces kidney inflammation through the generation of ROS and it can also contribute individually in preventing MR effects via the stimulation of angiotensin II receptor and G protein-coupled receptor 30 [93]. Cha et al. revealed the protective effect of spironolactone in diabetic animal models. Investigators have also explored the significant role of spironolactone in DN through inhibited NF-KB signaling pathway in diabetic animals [94].

3.3 Depletion of B-lymphocytes through monoclonal antibodies

Plasma cells (B-lymphocytes) are the key elements of the adaptive immunity system. Autoimmune disorder occurs when the adaptive immunity targets against 'soul antigens,' which cannot be eliminated through immune effector process. The immune action encourages and prolongs inflammation development. Therefore, B-cell-based target therapies can offer the therapeutic prevention of renal inflammatory diseases such as lupus nephritis [95]. The monoclonal antibody-targeted therapies can be beneficial for the depletion of B cells under different nephritis conditions. A novel B-cell target agent rituximab can be used in B-cells' depletion along with circulating CD20 in the condition of autoimmune disorder. In addition, it can down regulate the activation of costimulatory T-lymphocyte cells [96]. Additionally, CD22 is another cell surface B-cell marker, which helps in the stimulation of B cells and complexes with T cells [97]. The anti-CD22 monoclonal antibody can be a beneficial therapeutic target for the depletion of B cells along with suppression of autoimmune disorder. Epratuzumab is the class of target agent, which helps in diminishing circulation of B cells in patients with lupus nephritis. It has also been significantly used in treatment of refractory lymphoma in combination with rituximab [98,99]. In the current study, upon interpretation the level of overexpression of biomarkers BAFF and B-cell infiltration in patients with lupus nephritis was found. The BAFF inhibitor can be used as a treatment approach in the treatment of renal functional impairment in patients with systemic lupus erythematosus (SLE) disease [100,101].

3.4 Modulation of gut microbiota

A manifold of bacterial population available in the gut microbial flora can cross talk between renal inflammation, proteinuria, and progression of CKD. Different inflammatory mediators and immune activators can augment through the alteration of gut microbiota. The gut microbiota release uremic toxins, which are responsible for the development of CKD [102]. Because of this modulation of gut microbiota through probiotics, prebiotics and synbiotics can be used as an emerging approach for the treatment of renal inflammatory disorders. Probiotics are a type of living bacterial preparation, which give better health benefits to the host living cells. The probiotics consist of various types of bacterial species such as *Bifidobacteria* sp., *Lactobacilli*, and *Streptococci* [103]. Utilization of probiotics is beneficial for the treatment of patients with SLE and other renal inflammatory disorders. The oral consumption of *Lactobacillus acidophilus* in hemodialysis patients leads to reduced plasma uremic

TABLE 1 Patents on therapeutic candidates for renal inflammatory disorders.

Patent name (Patent no.)	Invention description	Drugs/therapeutic candidates	Reference
US Patent (12/667,450)	Invention related for expression of TLR-2 by specific antagonist such as monoclonal or polyclonal antibodies and it can beneficial for treatment of renal inflammatory condition such as glomerulonephritis	C07K16/2896 (immunoglobulins)	Heffernan et al. [107]
US Patent (13/301,898)	Application of bcl2-protein inhibitors in the treatment of systemic lupus erythematosus, lupus nephritis or Sjogren's syndrome	A61K45/06 (mixtures of active ingredients)	Elmore et al. [108]
Japanese Patent (JP2019501935A)	Invention related for human suffering from C3 nephropathy and it treatment by effective amount of an C5aR antagonist	A61K31/451 (noncondensed piperidines)	Petrus et al. [109]
Japanese Patent (JP2019528039A)	Invention described the use of anti-C5 antibodies in the renal disorders for example, a typical hemolytic uremic syndrome	C07K16/18 (immunoglobulins)	Ratusek et al. [110]
Spanish Patent (ES2352453T3)	Application of triazoles as inhibitor of kinase proteins useful in the treatment of glomerulonephritis condition and other autoimmune disorders	C07D249/14 (heterocyclic compounds)	Davies et al. [111]
US Patent (9,643,956)	Invention related for solid form of ASK1 inhibitor, which can be used for diabetic renal disease and chronic renal disorder	C07D401/14 (heterocyclic compounds)	Andres et al. [112]
US Patent (8,828,396)	Application of immunoglobulin's (anti-CD40 antibodies) into the treatment of lupus erythematosus	C07K16/2878 (immunoglobulins)	Heusser et al. [113]

toxins such as dimethylamine [104]. The prebiotics are the undigestible food materials, which helps in the growth of one or more bacteria in the colon. Prebiotic agents such as inulin, fructo-oligosaccharides, galacto-oligosaccharides, soya-oligosaccharides, xylo-oligosaccharides, and pyro-dextrins can help in the development of bacterial growth of *Bifidobacteria* and *Lactobacilli* sp. [105]. Synbiotics is a combined formulation of probiotic and prebiotic therapy. The beneficial bacteria such as *L. fermentum* can reduce dysbiosis and improve gut barrier function, which is helpful in the treatment of patients with SLE [106].

Various patents on therapeutic candidates for renal inflammatory disorders are given in Table 1.

4 Conclusions and future prospects for renal inflammation therapies

The balance between death signals and antagonistic survival signals decide the fate of resident renal cells during inflammation. The treatment strategies employed in the management of renal inflammation must be appreciated as they undoubtedly prevent renal apoptosis. Table 1 capturing patents on therapeutic approaches emphasizes the sustainability of the therapeutic strategies. Hence, developing new treatment approaches for preventing renal inflammation by gene targeting and other advanced techniques is the need of the hour as the global death rate due to renal

disorders is extremely high and the death and survival rates can be determined through it. The development of new therapies by new interventional techniques will support and encourage the survival rate and preserve renal tissue and its functioning.

References

[1] R. Medzhitov, Inflammation 2010: new adventures of an old flame, Cell 140 (6) (2010) 771–776.

[2] M.D. Milne, The classification and prognosis of nephritis and allied renal diseases, Postgrad. Med. J. 30 (350) (1954) 640.

[3] S.R. Mulay, S.V. Kumar, M. Lech, J. Desai, H.J. Anders, How kidney cell death induces renal necroinflammation, Semin. Nephrol. 36 (3) (2016) 162–173 (WB Saunders).

[4] D. Linfert, T. Chowdhry, H. Rabb, Lymphocytes and ischemia-reperfusion injury, Transplant. Rev. 23 (1) (2009) 1–10.

[5] A.A. Eddy, Progression in chronic kidney disease, Adv. Chronic Kidney Dis. 12 (4) (2005) 353–365.

[6] J.R. Timoshanko, P.G. Tipping, Resident kidney cells and their involvement in glomerulonephritis, Curr. Drug Targets Inflamm. Allergy 4 (3) (2005) 353–362.

[7] V. Kasinath, O.A. Yilmam, M. Uehara, L. Jiang, F. Ordikhani, X. Li, D.J. Salant, R. Abdi, Activation of fibroblastic reticular cells in kidney lymph node during crescentic glomerulonephritis, Kidney Int. 95 (2) (2019) 310–320.

[8] S.K. Kwok, G.C. Tsokos, New insights into the role of renal resident cells in the pathogenesis of lupus nephritis, Korean J. Intern. Med. 33 (2) (2018) 284.

[9] S. Hong, H. Healy, A.J. Kassianos, The emerging role of renal tubular epithelial cells in the immunological pathophysiology of lupus nephritis, Front. Immunol. 11 (2020).

[10] D. Ferenbach, D.C. Kluth, J. Hughes, Inflammatory cells in renal injury and repair, Semin. Nephrol. 27 (3) (2007) 250–259 (WB Saunders).

[11] S. Segerer, M. Mack, H. Regele, D. Kerjaschki, D. Schlöndorff, Expression of the CC chemokine receptor 5 in human kidney diseases, Kidney Int. 56 (1) (1999) 52–64.

[12] M. Frosch, T. Vogl, R. Waldherr, C. Sorg, C. Sunderkötter, J. Roth, Expression of MRP8 and MRP14 by macrophages is a marker for severe forms of glomerulonephritis, J. Leukoc. Biol. 75 (2) (2004) 198–206.

[13] M. Praga, E. González, Acute interstitial nephritis, Kidney Int. 77 (11) (2010) 956–961.

[14] G. Tsirpanlis, S. Chatzipanagiotou, C. Nicolaou, Microinflammation versus inflammation in chronic renal failure patients, Kidney Int. 66 (5) (2004) 2093–2094.

[15] R. Schindler, Causes and therapy of microinflammation in renal failure, Nephrol. Dial. Transplant. 19 (Suppl. 5) (2004) S34–S40.

[16] F. Genovese, P. Boor, M. Papasotiriou, D.J. Leeming, M.A. Karsdal, J. Floege, Turnover of type III collagen reflects disease severity and is associated with progression and microinflammation in patients with IgA nephropathy, Nephrol. Dial. Transplant. 31 (3) (2016) 472–479.

[17] T. Ren, J. Xiong, G. Liu, S. Wang, Z. Tan, B. Fu, R. Zhang, X. Liao, Q. Wang, Z. Guo, Imbalance of Th22/Treg cells causes microinflammation in uremic patients undergoing hemodialysis, Biosci. Rep. 39 (10) (2019).

[18] K. Shikata, H. Makino, Microinflammation in the pathogenesis of diabetic nephropathy, J. Diabetes Investig. 4 (2) (2013) 142–149.

[19] N. Prasad, M.R. Patel, Infection-induced kidney diseases, Front. Med. 5 (2018) 327.

[20] M. Wei, Z. Wang, H. Liu, H. Jiang, M. Wang, S. Liang, K. Shi, J. Feng, Probiotic Bifidobacterium animalis subsp. lactis B i-07 alleviates bacterial translocation and ameliorates microinflammation in experimental uraemia, Nephrology 19 (8) (2014) 500–506.

[21] S.H. Nasr, J. Radhakrishnan, V.D. D'Agati, Bacterial infection–related glomerulonephritis in adults, Kidney Int. 83 (5) (2013) 792–803.

[22] A.S. Markowitz, C.F. Lange, Streptococcal related glomerulonephritis: I. Isolation, immunochemistry and comparative chemistry of soluble fractions from type 12 nephritogenic streptococci and human glomeruli, J. Immunol. 92 (4) (1964) 565–575.

[23] Y. Yousif, K. Okada, S. Batsford, A. Vogt, Induction of glomerulonephritis in rats with staphylococcal phosphatase: new aspects in post-infectious ICGN, Kidney Int. 50 (1) (1996) 290–297.

[24] Y. Fujigaki, Y. Yousif, T. Morioka, S. Batsford, A. Vogt, A. Hishida, M. Miyasaka, Glomerular injury induced by cationic 70-kD staphylococcal protein; specific immune response is not involved in early phase in rats, J. Pathol. 184 (4) (1998) 436–445.

[25] T. Wang, X. Fu, Q. Chen, J.K. Patra, D. Wang, Z. Wang, Z. Gai, Arachidonic acid metabolism and kidney inflammation, Int. J. Mol. Sci. 20 (15) (2019) 3683.

[26] R. Gupta, A. Yadav, R. Misra, A. Aggarwal, Urinary prostaglandin D synthase as biomarker in lupus nephritis: a longitudinal study, Clin. Exp. Rheumatol. 33 (5) (2015) 694–698.

[27] E. Noiri, T. Yokomizo, A. Nakao, T. Izumi, T. Fujita, S. Kimura, T. Shimizu, An in vivo approach showing the chemotactic activity of leukotriene B4 in acute renal ischemic-reperfusion injury, Proc. Natl. Acad. Sci. 97 (2) (2000) 823–828.

[28] A.E. Declèves, K. Sharma, Novel targets of antifibrotic and anti-inflammatory treatment in CKD, Nat. Rev. Nephrol. 10 (5) (2014) 257–267.

[29] Q. Guan, S. Li, S. Gao, H. Chen, C.Y. Nguan, C. Du, Reduction of chronic rejection of renal allografts by anti-transforming growth factor-β antibody therapy in a rat model, Am. J. Physiol. Ren. Physiol. 305 (2) (2013) F199–F207.

[30] S. Rayego-Mateos, J.L. Morgado-Pascual, L. Opazo-Ríos, M. Guerrero-Hue, C. García-Caballero, C. Vázquez-Carballo, S. Mas, A.B. Sanz, C. Herencia, S. Mezzano, C. Gómez-Guerrero, Pathogenic pathways and therapeutic approaches targeting inflammation in diabetic nephropathy, Int. J. Mol. Sci. 21 (11) (2020) 3798.

[31] K. Koskinen, P.J. Vainio, D.J. Smith, M. Pihlavisto, S. Ylä-Herttuala, S. Jalkanen, M. Salmi, Granulocyte transmigration through the endothelium is regulated by the oxidase activity of vascular adhesion protein-1 (VAP-1), Blood 103 (9) (2004) 3388–3395.

[32] P.G. Tipping, S.R. Holdsworth, Cytokines in glomerulonephritis, Semin. Nephrol. 27 (3) (2007) 275–285 (WB Saunders).

[33] C. Adamichou, S. Georgakis, G. Bertsias, Cytokine targets in lupus nephritis: current and future prospects, J. Clin. Immunol. 206 (2019) 42–52.

[34] M.P. Jansen, S. Florquin, J.J. Roelofs, The role of platelets in acute kidney injury, Nat. Rev. Nephrol. 14 (7) (2018) 457–471.

[35] C. Ruster, G. Wolf, The role of chemokines and chemokine receptors in diabetic nephropathy, Front. Biosci. 13 (1) (2008) 944–955.

[36] H.J. Anders, V. Vielhauer, D. Schlöndorff, Chemokines and chemokine receptors are involved in the resolution or progression of renal disease, Kidney Int. 63 (2) (2003) 401–415.

[37] Y.S. Kang, M.H. Lee, H.K. Song, G.J. Ko, O.S. Kwon, T.K. Lim, S.H. Kim, S.Y. Han, K.H. Han, J.E. Lee, J.Y. Han, CCR2 antagonism improves insulin resistance, lipid metabolism, and diabetic nephropathy in type 2 diabetic mice, Kidney Int. 78 (9) (2010) 883–894.

[38] J.A. Moreno, S. Moreno, A. Rubio-Navarro, C. Gómez-Guerrero, A. Ortiz, J. Egido, Role of chemokines in proteinuric kidney disorders, Expert Rev. Mol. Med. 16 (2014).

[39] S.J. Seok, E.S. Lee, G.T. Kim, M. Hyun, J.H. Lee, S. Chen, R. Choi, H.M. Kim, E.Y. Lee, C.H. Chung, Blockade of CCL2/CCR2 signalling ameliorates diabetic nephropathy in db/db mice, Nephrol. Dial. Transplant. 28 (7) (2013) 1700–1710.

[40] A. Zernecke, K.S. Weber, L.P. Erwig, D.C. Kluth, B. Schröppel, A.J. Rees, C. Weber, Combinatorial model of chemokine involvement in glomerular monocyte recruitment: role of CXC chemokine receptor 2 in infiltration during nephrotoxic nephritis, J. Immunol. 166 (9) (2001) 5755–5762.

[41] G. Pertosa, S. Simone, M. Soccio, D. Marrone, L. Gesualdo, F.P. Schena, G. Grandaliano, Coagulation cascade activation causes CC chemokine receptor-2 gene expression and mononuclear cell activation in hemodialysis patients, Clin. J. Am. Soc. Nephrol. 16 (8) (2005) 2477–2486.

[42] Y.S. Kang, J.J. Cha, Y.Y. Hyun, D.R. Cha, Novel CC chemokine receptor 2 antagonists in metabolic disease: a review of recent developments, Expert Opin. Investig. Drugs 20 (6) (2011) 745–756.

[43] K. Kitagawa, T. Wada, K. Furuichi, H. Hashimoto, Y. Ishiwata, M. Asano, M. Takeya, W.A. Kuziel, K. Matsushima, N. Mukaida, H. Yokoyama, Blockade of CCR2 ameliorates progressive fibrosis in kidney, Am. J. Pathol. 165 (1) (2004) 237–246.

[44] J. Tao, L. Mariani, S. Eddy, H. Maecker, N. Kambham, K. Mehta, J. Hartman, W. Wang, M. Kretzler, R.A. Lafayette, JAK-STAT signaling is activated in the kidney and peripheral blood cells of patients with focal segmental glomerulosclerosis, Kidney Int. 94 (4) (2018) 795–808.

[45] M. Gasparitsch, A. Schieber, T. Schaubeck, U. Keller, M. Cattaruzza, B. Lange-Sperandio, Tyrphostin AG490 reduces inflammation and fibrosis in neonatal obstructive nephropathy, PLoS One 14 (12) (2019), e0226675.

[46] C. Liu, W. Mei, J. Tang, Q. Yuan, L. Huang, M. Lu, L. Wu, Z. Peng, J. Meng, H. Yang, H. Shen, Mefunidone attenuates tubulointerstitial fibrosis in a rat model of unilateral ureteral obstruction, PLoS One 10 (6) (2015), e0129283.

[47] L. Zhang, X. Xu, R. Yang, J. Chen, S. Wang, J. Yang, X. Xiang, Z. He, Y. Zhao, Z. Dong, D. Zhang, Paclitaxel attenuates renal interstitial fibroblast activation and interstitial fibrosis by inhibiting STAT3 signaling, Drug Des. Devel. Ther. 9 (2015) 2139.

[48] R. Li, N. Yang, L. Zhang, Y. Huang, R. Zhang, F. Wang, M. Luo, Y. Liang, X. Yu, Inhibition of Jak/STAT signaling ameliorates mice experimental nephrotic syndrome, Am. J. Nephrol. 27 (6) (2007) 580–589.

[49] Y. Liang, Y. Jin, Y. Li, Expression of JAKs/STATs pathway molecules in rat model of rapid focal segmental glomerulosclerosis, Pediatr. Nephrol. 24 (9) (2009) 1661–1671.

[50] M.B. Marrero, A.K. Banes-Berceli, D.M. Stern, D.C. Eaton, Role of the JAK/STAT signaling pathway in diabetic nephropathy, Am. J. Physiol. Ren. Physiol. 290 (4) (2006) F762–F768.

[51] Y.H. Shi, S. Zhao, C. Wang, Y. Li, H.J. Duan, Fluvastatin inhibits activation of JAK and STAT proteins in diabetic rat glomeruli and mesangial cells under high glucose conditions 1, Acta Pharmacol. Sin. 28 (12) (2007) 1938–1946.

[52] A.C. Ucero, S. Berzal, C. Ocaña-Salceda, M. Sancho, M. Orzáez, A. Messeguer, M. Ruiz-Ortega, J. Egido, M.J. Vicent, A. Ortiz, A.M. Ramos, A polymeric nanomedicine diminishes inflammatory events in renal tubular cells, PLoS One 8 (1) (2013), e51992.

[53] È. Ripoll, L. de Ramon, J. Draibe, A. Merino, N. Bolaños, M. Goma, J.M. Cruzado, J.M. Grinyó, J. Torras, JAK3-STAT pathway blocking benefits in experimental lupus nephritis, Arthritis Res. Ther. 18 (1) (2016) 1–12.

[54] K. Daenen, A. Andries, D. Mekahli, A. Van Schepdael, F. Jouret, B. Bammens, Oxidative stress in chronic kidney disease, Pediatr. Nephrol. 34 (6) (2019) 975–991.

[55] M.S. Li, S.E. Adesina, C.L. Ellis, J.L. Gooch, R.S. Hoover, C.R. Williams, NADPH oxidase-2 mediates zinc deficiency-induced oxidative stress and kidney damage, Am. J. Phys. Cell Phys. 312 (1) (2017) C47–C55.

[56] Y. Gorin, R.C. Cavaglieri, K. Khazim, D.Y. Lee, F. Bruno, S. Thakur, P. Fanti, C. Szyndralewicz, J.L. Barnes, K. Block, H.E. Abboud, Targeting NADPH oxidase with a novel dual Nox1/Nox4 inhibitor attenuates renal pathology in type 1 diabetes, Am. J. Physiol. Ren. Physiol. 308 (11) (2015) F1276–F1287.

[57] M. Fujii, T. Inoguchi, Y. Maeda, S. Sasaki, F. Sawada, R. Saito, K. Kobayashi, H. Sumimoto, R. Takayanagi, Pitavastatin ameliorates albuminuria and renal mesangial expansion by downregulating NOX4 in db/db mice, Kidney Int. 72 (4) (2007) 473–480.

[58] X.M. Meng, G.L. Ren, L. Gao, Q. Yang, H.D. Li, W.F. Wu, C. Huang, L. Zhang, X.W. Lv, J. Li, NADPH oxidase 4 promotes cisplatin-induced acute kidney injury via ROS-mediated programmed cell death and inflammation, Lab. Investig. 98 (1) (2018) 63–78.

[59] H. ten Freyhaus, M. Huntgeburth, K. Wingler, J. Schnitker, A.T. Bäumer, M. Vantler, M.M. Bekhite, M. Wartenberg, H. Sauer, S. Rosenkranz, Novel Nox inhibitor VAS2870 attenuates PDGF-dependent smooth muscle cell chemotaxis, but not proliferation, Cardiovasc. Res. 71 (2) (2006) 331–341.

[60] W. Gwinner, H. Scheuer, H. Haller, R.P. Brandes, H.J. Groene, Pivotal role of xanthine oxidase in the initiation of tubulointerstitial renal injury in rats with hyperlipidemia, Kidney Int. 69 (3) (2006) 481–487.

[61] B. Gondouin, N. Jourde-Chiche, M. Sallee, L. Dou, C. Cerini, A. Loundou, S. Morange, Y. Berland, S. Burtey, P. Brunet, R. Guieu, Plasma xanthine oxidase activity is predictive of cardiovascular disease in patients with chronic kidney disease, independently of uric acid levels, Nephron 131 (3) (2015) 167–174.

[62] H. Omori, N. Kawada, K. Inoue, Y. Ueda, R. Yamamoto, I. Matsui, J. Kaimori, Y. Takabatake, T. Moriyama, Y. Isaka, H. Rakugi, Use of xanthine oxidase inhibitor febuxostat inhibits renal interstitial inflammation and fibrosis in unilateral ureteral obstructive nephropathy, Clin. Exp. Nephrol. 16 (4) (2012) 549–556.

[63] A. Machowska, J.J. Carrero, B. Lindholm, P. Stenvinkel, Therapeutics targeting persistent inflammation in chronic kidney disease, Transl. Res. 167 (1) (2016) 204–213.

[64] W. Asghar, A. Aghazadeh-Habashi, F. Jamali, Cardiovascular effect of inflammation and nonsteroidal anti-inflammatory drugs on renin–angiotensin system in experimental arthritis, Inflammopharmacology 25 (5) (2017) 543–553.

[65] M. Renke, S. Lizakowski, L. Tylicki, P. Rutkowski, N. Knap, Z. Heleniak, M. Sławińska-Morawska, E. Aleksandrowicz-Wrona, J. Januszczyk, M. Wójcik-Stasiak, S. Małgorzewicz, Aliskiren attenuates oxidative stress and improves tubular status in non-diabetic patients with chronic kidney disease-placebo controlled, randomized, cross-over study, Adv. Med. Sci. 59 (2) (2014) 256–260.

[66] M. Ruiz-Ortega, M. Ruperez, O. Lorenzo, V. Esteban, J. Blanco, S. Mezzano, J. Egido, Angiotensin II regulates the synthesis of proinflammatory cytokines and chemokines in the kidney, Kidney Int. (Suppl. 62) (2002) S12–S22.

[67] M. Ruiz-Ortega, M. Rupérez, V. Esteban, J. Rodríguez-Vita, E. Sánchez-López, G. Carvajal, J. Egido, Angiotensin II: a key factor in the inflammatory and fibrotic response in kidney diseases, Nephrol. Dial. Transplant. 21 (1) (2006) 16–20.

[68] G. Musso, M. Cassader, S. Cohney, F. De Michieli, S. Pinach, F. Saba, R. Gambino, Fatty liver and chronic kidney disease: novel mechanistic insights and therapeutic opportunities, Diabetes Care 39 (10) (2016) 1830–1845.

[69] F.B. Shaik, D.V. Prasad, V.R. Narala, Role of farnesoid X receptor in inflammation and resolution, Inflamm. Res. 64 (1) (2015) 9–20.

[70] K.W. Chung, E.K. Lee, M.K. Lee, G.T. Oh, B.P. Yu, H.Y. Chung, Impairment of PPARα and the fatty acid oxidation pathway aggravates renal fibrosis during aging, J. Am. Soc. Nephrol. 29 (4) (2018) 1223–1237.

[71] R.H. Aly, A.E. Ahmed, W.G. Hozayen, A.M. Rabea, T.M. Ali, A. El Askary, O.M. Ahmed, Patterns of Toll-like receptor expressions and

inflammatory cytokine levels and their implications in the progress of insulin resistance and diabetic nephropathy in type 2 diabetic patients, Front. Physiol. 11 (2020).

[72] C.C. Hung, C.T. Chang, Y.C. Tian, M.S. Wu, C.C. Yu, M.J. Pan, A. Vandewalle, C.W. Yang, Leptospiral membrane proteins stimulate pro-inflammatory chemokines secretion by renal tubule epithelial cells through toll-like receptor 2 and p38 mitogen activated protein kinase, Nephrol. Dial. Transplant. 21 (4) (2006) 898–910.

[73] P.S. Patole, R.D. Pawar, J. Lichtnekert, M. Lech, O.P. Kulkarni, A. Ramanjaneyulu, S. Segerer, H.J. Anders, Coactivation of Toll-like receptor-3 and-7 in immune complex glomerulonephritis, J. Autoimmun. 29 (1) (2007) 52–59.

[74] S. Yang, A. Li, J. Wang, J. Liu, Y. Han, W. Zhang, Y.C. Li, H. Zhang, Vitamin D receptor: a novel therapeutic target for kidney diseases, Curr. Med. Chem. 25 (27) (2018) 3256–3271.

[75] K. Sumethkul, S. Boonyaratavej, T. Kitumnuaypong, S. Angthararuk, P. Cheewasat, N. Manadee, V. Sumethkul, The predictive factors of low serum 25-hydroxyvitamin D and vitamin D deficiency in patients with systemic lupus erythematosus, Rheumatol. Int. 33 (6) (2013) 1461–1467.

[76] X. Tan, X. Wen, Y. Liu, Paricalcitol inhibits renal inflammation by promoting vitamin D receptor–mediated sequestration of NF-κB signaling, J. Am. Soc. Nephrol. 19 (9) (2008) 1741–1752.

[77] S.M. Hejazian, S.M.H. Khatibi, A. Barzegari, G. Pavon-Djavid, S. Razi, S. Hassannejhad, E. Ahmadian, M. Ardalan, S.Z. Vahed, Nrf-2 as a therapeutic target in acute kidney injury, Life Sci. 118581 (2020).

[78] E.N. Kim, J.H. Lim, M.Y. Kim, T.H. Ban, I.A. Jang, H.E. Yoon, C. W. Park, Y.S. Chang, B.S. Choi, Resveratrol, an Nrf2 activator, ameliorates aging-related progressive renal injury, Aging (Albany NY) 10 (1) (2018) 83.

[79] Q. Cao, X.M. Chen, C. Huang, C.A. Pollock, MicroRNA as novel biomarkers and therapeutic targets in diabetic kidney disease: an update, FASEB Bioadv. 1 (6) (2019) 375–388.

[80] S.J. Lee, E. Silverman, J.M. Bargman, The role of antimalarial agents in the treatment of SLE and lupus nephritis, Nat. Rev. Nephrol. 7 (12) (2011) 718.

[81] X. Mu, C. Wang, Artemisinins—a promising new treatment for systemic lupus erythematosus: a descriptive review, Curr. Rheumatol. Rep. 20 (9) (2018) 1–10.

[82] Y. Wen, M.M. Pan, L.L. Lv, T.T. Tang, L.T. Zhou, B. Wang, H. Liu, F.M. Wang, K.L. Ma, R.N. Tang, B.C. Liu, Artemisinin attenuates tubulointerstitial inflammation and fibrosis via the NF-κB/NLRP3 pathway in rats with 5/6 subtotal nephrectomy, J. Cell. Biochem. 120 (3) (2019) 4291–4300.

[83] M. Xia, D. Liu, X. Tang, Y. Liu, H. Liu, Y. Liu, G. Chen, H. Liu, Dihydroartemisinin inhibits the proliferation of IgAN mesangial cells through the mTOR signaling pathway, Int. Immunopharmacol. 80 (2020), 106125.

[84] A.K. Al Asmari, K.T. Al Sadoon, A.A. Obaid, D. Yesunayagam, M. Tariq, Protective effect of quinacrine against glycerol-induced acute kidney injury in rats, BMC Nephrol. 18 (1) (2017) 1–10.

[85] J.W. Shin, K.H. Jung, S.T. Lee, J. Moon, J.A. Lim, J.I. Byun, K.I. Park, S.K. Lee, K. Chu, Mefloquine improved progressive multifocal leukoencephalopathy in a patient with immunoglobulin A nephropathy, J. Clin. Neurosci. 21 (10) (2014) 1661–1664.

[86] R. Allam, H.J. Anders, The role of innate immunity in autoimmune tissue injury, Curr. Opin. Rheumatol. 20 (5) (2008) 538–544.

[87] T.M. Chan, Treatment of severe lupus nephritis: the new horizon, Nat. Rev. Nephrol. 11 (1) (2015) 46–61.

[88] J.P. Ioannidis, K.A. Boki, M.E. Katsorida, A.A. Drosos, F.N. Skopouli, J.N. Boletis, H.M. Moutsopoulos, Remission, relapse, and re-remission of proliferative lupus nephritis treated with cyclophosphamide, Kidney Int. 57 (1) (2000) 258–264.

[89] M.A. Dooley, Mycophenolate mofetil: what role in the treatment of lupus? Lupus 15 (3) (2006) 179–182.

[90] Y. Peleg, A.S. Bomback, J. Radhakrishnan, The evolving role of calcineurin inhibitors in treating lupus nephritis, Clin. J. Am. Soc. Nephrol. 15 (7) (2020) 1066–1072.

[91] C.C. Mok, Mycophenolate mofetil for lupus nephritis: an update, Expert. Rev. Clin. Immunol. 11 (12) (2015) 1353–1364.

[92] Z. Belden, J.A. Deiuliis, M. Dobre, S. Rajagopalan, The role of the mineralocorticoid receptor in inflammation: focus on kidney and vasculature, Am. J. Nephrol. 46 (4) (2017) 298–314.

[93] N.J. Brown, Contribution of aldosterone to cardiovascular and renal inflammation and fibrosis, Nat. Rev. Nephrol. 9 (8) (2013) 459–469.

[94] D.R. Cha, Y.S. Kang, S.Y. Han, Y.H. Jee, K.H. Han, H.K. Kim, J.Y. Han, Y.S. Kim, Role of aldosterone in diabetic nephropathy, Nephrology (Suppl. 10) (2005) S37–S39.

[95] P. Bhat, J. Radhakrishnan, B lymphocytes and lupus nephritis: new insights into pathogenesis and targeted therapies, Kidney Int. 73 (3) (2008) 261–268.

[96] J.H. Anolik, J. Barnard, A. Cappione, A.E. Pugh-Bernard, R.E. Felgar, R.J. Looney, I. Sanz, Rituximab improves peripheral B cell abnormalities in human systemic lupus erythematosus, Arthritis Rheum. 50 (11) (2004) 3580–3590.

[97] T. Dörner, Crossroads of B cell activation in autoimmunity: rationale of targeting B cells, J. Rheumatol. Suppl. 77 (2006) 3–11.

[98] T. Dörner, J. Kaufmann, W.A. Wegener, N. Teoh, D.M. Goldenberg, G.R. Burmester, Initial clinical trial of epratuzumab (humanized anti-CD22 antibody) for immunotherapy of systemic lupus erythematosus, Arthritis Res. Ther. 8 (3) (2006) 1–11.

[99] J.P. Leonard, M. Coleman, J. Ketas, M. Ashe, J.M. Fiore, R.R. Furman, R. Niesvizky, T. Shore, A. Chadburn, H. Horne, J. Kovacs, Combination antibody therapy with epratuzumab and rituximab in relapsed or refractory non-Hodgkin's lymphoma, J. Clin. Oncol. 23 (22) (2005) 5044–5051.

[100] C.Y. Sun, Y. Shen, X.W. Chen, Y.C. Yan, F.X. Wu, M. Dai, T. Li, C. D. Yang, The characteristics and significance of locally infiltrating B cells in lupus nephritis and their association with local BAFF expression, Int. J. Rheum. Dis. 2013 (2013).

[101] S. Manzi, J. Sánchez-Guerrero, J.T. Merrill, R. Furie, D. Gladman, S. V. Navarra, E.M. Ginzler, D.P. D'Cruz, A. Doria, S. Cooper, Z.J. Zhong, Effects of belimumab, a B lymphocyte stimulator-specific inhibitor, on disease activity across multiple organ domains in patients with systemic lupus erythematosus: combined results from two phase III trials, Ann. Rheum. Dis. 71 (11) (2012) 1833–1838.

[102] A. Nallu, S. Sharma, A. Ramezani, J. Muralidharan, D. Raj, Gut microbiome in chronic kidney disease: challenges and opportunities, Transl. Res. 179 (2017) 24–37.

[103] R.A. Rastall, G.R. Gibson, H.S. Gill, F. Guarner, T.R. Klaenhammer, B. Pot, G. Reid, I.R. Rowland, M.E. Sanders, Modulation of the microbial ecology of the human colon by probiotics, prebiotics and synbiotics to enhance human health: an overview of enabling science and potential applications, FEMS Microbiol. Ecol. 52 (2) (2005) 145–152.

[104] N. Ranganathan, B. Patel, P. Ranganathan, J. Marczely, R. Dheer, T. Chordia, S.R. Dunn, E.A. Friedman, Probiotic amelioration of azotemia in 5/6th nephrectomized Sprague-Dawley rats, Sci. World J. 5 (2005) 652–660.

[105] D.B.A. Silk, A. Davis, J. Vulevic, G. Tzortzis, G.R. Gibson, Clinical trial: the effects of a trans-galactooligosaccharide prebiotic on faecal microbiota and symptoms in irritable bowel syndrome, Aliment. Pharmacol. Ther. 29 (5) (2009) 508–518.

[106] N. de la Visitación, I. Robles-Vera, M. Toral, J. Duarte, Protective effects of probiotic consumption in cardiovascular disease in systemic lupus erythematosus, Nutrients 11 (11) (2019) 2676.

[107] M. Heffernan, L. O'neill, P. Mcguirk, B. Keogh, C. Locher, Compounds and methods for the treatment of renal disease, 2010. US Patent 12/667,450.

[108] S. Elmore, A. Souers, L.C. Wang, T. Ghayur, S.J. Perper, Methods of treatment using selective bcl-2 inhibitors, 2012. US Patent 13/301,898.

[109] B. Petrus, B. Petrus, Methods for treating C3 nephropathy, 2019. Japanese Patent JP2019501935A.

[110] A. Ratusek, C. Romano, W. Olson, Anti-C5 antibodies and their use, 2019. Japanese Patent JP2019528039A.

[111] R.J. Davies, C.J. Forster, M.J. Arnost, J. Wang, Useful triazols as inhibitors of kinase proteins, 2011. Spanish Patent ES2352453T3.

[112] M. Andres, B.J.B. Chan, E.A. Carra, A. Chiu, O.V. Lapina, S.P. Lathrop, G. Notte, V. Smolenskaya, L.H. Yu, Solid forms of an ASK1 inhibitor, 2017. US Patent 9,643,956.

[113] C. Heusser, R.U.S.H. James, K. Vincent, Silent Fc variants of anti-CD40 antibodies, 2014. US Patent 8,828,396.

Chapter 7

Advanced therapeutics for targeting inflammatory arthritis

Vikram Jeet Singh[a], Pooja A. Chawla[a], Bhupinder Kumar[a], and Parteek Prasher[b]

[a]Department of Pharmaceutical Chemistry and Analysis, ISF College of Pharmacy, Moga, Punjab, India, [b]Department of Chemistry, University of Petroleum & Energy Studies, Dehradun, Uttarakhand, India

1 Introduction

The term "arthritis" refers to a rigid, inflamed, and painful joint. It is a complicated and common condition. The pathogenesis of arthritis is not well known at this time. Arthritis is a condition that causes discomfort in the joints. More than a hundred different forms of arthritis and their related diseases have been documented so far. Arthritis is most common in women and the elderly, although it can affect persons of any age, gender, or color, and it is the biggest cause of disability in the United States. A total of 50 million and 3 lakh adult children suffer from some form of arthritis. Arthritis manifests itself in a variety of ways, from joint swelling to pain to stiffness, and it is likely to worsen over time. It can range from minor to severe. Some varieties of arthritis, however, damage the heart, eyes, lungs, kidneys, and skin. Arthritis can be categorized into three different types: (a) Degenerative arthritis is also known as osteoarthritis and is frequently referred to as a "wear-and-tear" deformity. The pathophysiology includes the gradual deterioration of protecting cartilage (at the ends of the bones). The hands, spine, hips, and knees are the most common joints affected by degenerative arthritis. Pain, stiffness, and lack of flexibility, as well as bone spurs and edema, are all frequent symptoms. Obesity, heredity, and obesity-related bone abnormalities are all variables that can raise the risk of osteoarthritis [1]. (b) Inflammatory arthritis—Inflammatory arthritis is an autoimmune condition that affects several types of arthritis. The presence of WBC in the joint (fluid) is a defining hallmark of inflammatory arthritis, as is the development of a scar, instability, and joint abnormalities. One of the most frequent types of inflammatory arthritis is rheumatoid arthritis. It affects the synovial lining between the joints in the hand, wrist, and foot and is persistent. Inflammatory arthritis severity varies from person to person, and pain perception ranges from mild to severe. The condition develops gradually but quickly [2]. (c) Metabolic arthritis, also known as crystalline-induced arthritis, is a kind of arthritis. Gout or pseudogout is a type of metabolic arthritis. Extreme joint pain is caused by the presence of monosodium urate crystals in the joint. Gout is defined by the presence of needlelike urate crystals in the cartilage, whereas pseudogout is defined by the presence of calcium pyrophosphate crystals in the cartilage [1,3].

The epidemiology, pathogenesis, evaluation, and current treatment/management techniques of degenerative arthritis or osteoarthritis were covered in detail in the preceding section.

2 Signs and symptoms

Pain, joint stiffness, muscular weakness, and bone enlargement/swelling are all signs and symptoms of osteoarthritis. The release of the excitatory neurotransmitter glutamate from sensory neurons in the spinal cord is thought to be the cause of pain perception [4]. The decreasing level of surface-active phospholipids in the joints causes joint stiffness [2,5]. Muscle weakness is caused by atherogenic muscle inhibition (reflex inhibition surrounding joints) weakening the quadriceps muscle [6,7]. The degenerative alterations in articular cartilage are to blame for the bone enlargement/swelling.

3 Etiology

Women are more likely than men to get osteoarthritis, which is likely due to hormonal changes (menopause) or weight gain. It mostly affects people in their later years, although it can also affect people in their middle years. Osteoarthritis is caused by a variety of biophysical and biochemical changes, including advanced age, weak muscle, excess weight, lower levels of sex hormones, joint injury/surgery/infection, and congenital disease [8]. The etiology of osteoarthritis, on the other hand, is divided into systemic and local risk factors. Age, gender, food, and hormones are among the systemic causes, while joint injury, obesity, occupation, and physical activity are among the local factors. Systemic factors include decreased tensile strength of cartilage (articular), decreased levels of osteocalcin or hormonal alterations, and a lack of vitamin consumption. Local factors that have a role in osteoarthritis include an elevated body mass index and vigorous exercise involving the knee joints that can promote tissue damage [9]. The genesis of osteoarthritis is depicted in Fig. 1.

4   Epidemiology

Osteoarthritis is a more prevalent type of arthritis that has yet to be fully investigated in terms of management, therapy, and research, falling behind other types of arthritis such as inflammatory, metabolic, and viral arthritis. The multiple etiological causes that cause osteoarthritis have increased the need for joint replacement therapy, which has becoming increasingly unsustainable. It occurs more frequently in people between the ages of 40 and 50, when joint arthroplasty is considered doubtful. It causes a lot of pain and costs a lot of money to treat [10]. According to another study, females (about 68%) are more susceptible than males (approximately 58%) aged 65 and up [11]. Genetic factors play a major role, as 39%–65% of cases are genetically linked while aged 48–70 years, with monozygotic twins accounting for 65% of instances [12]. About a third of persons over 45 years old wanted therapy for osteoarthritis, and 81% of patients had continuous pain or activity limitations [13]. According to various figures, roughly 75 million working days are lost each year in the United Kingdom alone. The majority of people with

osteoarthritis blame joint replacement for their suffering. According to various sources or study data, approximately 5 million hip replacements will be performed in the United States by 2030 [14].

5   Morphological changes during osteoarthritis

Osteoarthritis is characterized by cartilage degradation, joint space narrowing, osteophyte formation, and increased bone density. Trabecular thickness and bone volume have an impact on cartilage deterioration. There is apparently a link between deteriorated articular cartilage and changed subchondral bone, according to the studies [15]. Radin and Paul studied osteoarthritis in depth in 1970, based on tightened subchondral bone and increased bone density [16]. The previous finding revealed that osteophyte development (because of the biomechanical element) is symmetrical, except for varied diameters at the medial patella and lateral tibia [17]. The tightened subchondral bone may be able to take less strain, resulting in greater cartilage stress [18]. Varied investigations have revealed different biochemical markers, inflammatory mediators, and chondropathy of the patella (softening of the articular cartilage due to erosion) [19,20].

6   The pathogenesis of osteoarthritis

6.1   The role of cytokines in osteoarthritis

Cytokines and growth factors play a big role in the matrix-forming/breaking cells, or chondrocytes. In arthritis, the

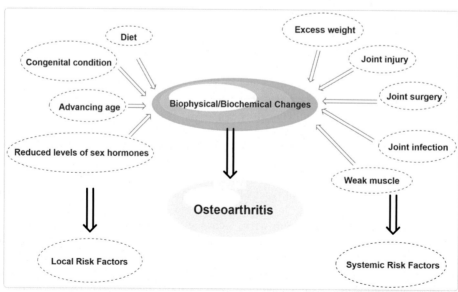

FIG. 1 Etiology of osteoarthritis.

balance between these cells is disrupted. IL1, TNF, cartilage oligomeric matrix protein, TGF, and insulin-like growth factor are some of the cytokines that play a role in articular cartilage. Catabolic cytokines are the first three, while anabolic cytokines are the last three. The enzyme activity is regulated by the proteins IL6/4/10 and IFN [21,22]. Interleukin-l, a proinflammatory cytokine, has stimulatory effects on lymphocytes and macrophages, lytic effects on cartilage, inhibits growth factor function, and reduces matrix component synthesis, including fibroblasts [23–25]. The NF-kb [26,27] also contributes to this stimulatory effect. By triggering lipid peroxidation and ROS, IL-1 is also linked to matrix deterioration [28]. In arthritic patients, IL-1 and TNF drive articular deterioration, which leads to the generation of nitric oxide, which increases oxidative stress and matrix metalloproteinase activity in joints [29–31]. Furthermore, they operate in concert to activate IL-6, worsening the situation in these patients [32]. Synovial fibroblasts and chondrocytes are also degraded when proteolytic enzymes are activated. IFN worsens the situation by exacerbating the inflammatory response [33,34]. The osteophyte grows as a result of an increased level of transforming growth factor-beta caused by tissue injury (Fig. 2) [35].

6.2 Role of proteinases in osteoarthritis

Proteoglycans, particularly aggrecan, provide hydration and flexibility to the cartilage tissues in articular cartilage [36–38]. The aggrecanase enzymes, aggrecanase 1 or ADAMTS-4 and aggrecanase 2 or ADAMTS-5 (a disinterring and metalloprotease with thrombospondin motifs 4 and 5, respectively), were first discovered by DuPont and

were found to be highly expressed during osteoarthritis. These proteases boost the activity of TNF-alpha and IL-1, as well as the expression of transforming growth factor-beta [39–41]. The overexpression of matrix metalloproteinases is also linked to aggrecan breakdown [42]. Matrix metalloproteinases are highly regulated by tissue inhibitors of metalloproteinases (Fig. 2) and play an important role in the development of osteoarthritis activity [43,44]. Overexpression of MMPs (particularly MMP-9/13) is strongly linked to cytokine activity in osteoarthritis, as MMP activity requires calcium and zinc [45].

6.3 Role of reactive oxygen species in osteoarthritis

Activated macrophages and neutrophils produce reactive oxygen species such as superoxide ions, hydrogen peroxide, and nitric oxide during inflammatory processes. This is also aided by chondrocytes responding to interleukin 1. In chondrocytes, reactive oxygen species can decrease hyaluronic acid (an important component of the extracellular matrix), and degrade collagen and aggrecan (Fig. 3) [45–48].

6.4 Role of lipid peroxidation in osteoarthritis

The oxidation of polyunsaturated fats is also involved in the breakdown of the extracellular matrix and collagen. The creation of a highly reactive intermediate, such as aldehyde, mediates these reactions [49]. The pathogenesis of osteoarthritis is depicted in Fig. 4.

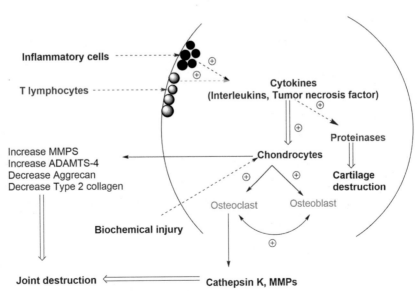

FIG. 2 Role of cytokine and proteinases in osteoarthritis.

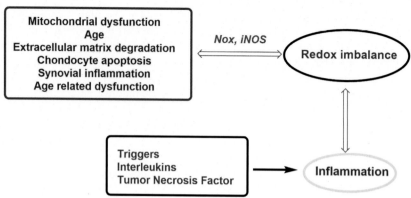

FIG. 3 Role of reactive oxygen species in osteoarthritis.

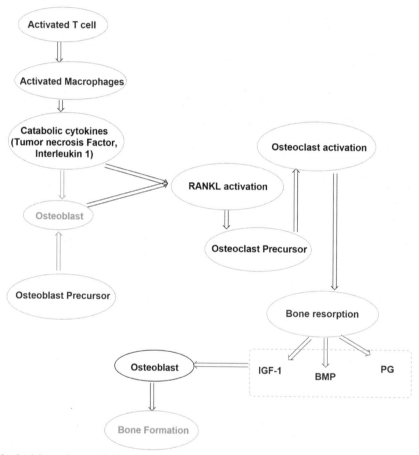

FIG. 4 Summary of pathophysiology of osteoarthritis.

7 Advancements and current strategies in research for management of osteoarthritis

Subjects are given NSAIDs, opiates, and corticosteroids to help with their osteoarthritis symptoms. A recent study found that NSAIDs had just a minor benefit in terms of pain relief and have few side effects [50–52]. In the management of osteoarthritis, more and more strategies have been implemented with time, as detailed in the current section. Table 1 and Fig. 5 summarize the various drugs utilized in the treatment of osteoarthritis.

7.1 Treatment targeting cartilage

Sprifermin, an osteoarthritis medication, has been demonstrated to increase matrix cartilage formation and promote

TABLE 1 Summary of the agent used in osteoarthritis.

S. no.	Drug	Target/condition	Comments	References
1.	Sprifermin	Knee osteoarthritis	Matrix cartilage and induce chondrocyte proliferation	[53,54]
2.	BMP-7	Knee osteoarthritis	Pro-anabolic effect and enhance articular cartilage repair.	[55]
3.	CP-544439, AZD-8955, and WAY-170523	MMPs inhibitors	Anticatabolic effect	[56]
4.	Disodium zoledronate tetrahydrate	Knee osteoarthritis	Reduce the bone turnover	Clinicaltrials.gov, [57]
5.	MIV-711	Cathepsin K	Highly efficacious in the rabbit osteoarthritis model	[58]
6.	Denosumab	Hand osteoarthritis	–	Clinicaltrials.gov
7.	Teriparatide	Parathyroid hormone	Efficacious in decreasing osteoarthritis progression in rat models	Clinicaltrials.gov, [59]
8.	Atorvastatin	HMG-Co A reductase inhibitor	Reduced the symptoms of osteoarthritis	[60]
9.	GSK3196165	Antigranulocyte/macrophage colony-stimulating factor	A phase 2 trial completed, (ClinicalTrials.gov Identifier: NCT02683785)	[61]
10.	PH-797804	Inhibition of upstream initiator of the proinflammatory signaling cascade	Completed phase 2 trial along with naproxen in the knee osteoarthritis subjects	Clinicaltrials.gov
11.	Tanezumab	Antinerve growth factor antibody	Safety is still in question	[62,63]
12.	GZ389988, AR786, ASP7962, ONO-4474, and VM902A	Antagonize the TrkA receptor	–	[64,65]
13.	LEVI-04	p75NTR	Currently under phase 1 trial (Clinicaltrials.gov identifier: NCT03227796)	Clinicaltrials.gov
14.	Capsaicin or resiniferatoxin	TRP vanilloid 1 (TRPV1) channels agonists	Inihibit sensory neuron	[66,67]
15.	A-803467	Nav1.8 blocking agent	Disrupting pain signaling transmission in monoiodoacetate-induced OA	[68]
16.	Difelikefalin	Kappa-specific opioid receptor agonists	Phase 2 trial (clinicaltrials.gov: NCT02944448) and is evaluated for pain relief in subjects with hip/knee osteoarthritis	[69]
17.	Genistein	COX-2, NO, iNOS, and MMP inhibitory effect	–	[70,71]
18.	DHA and omega-3-fatty acid	Anticatabolic activity	Inhibiting matrix degradation and regulating gene expression	[72,73]
19.	Sulforaphane	COX-2, MMP-2, and ADAMTS-5	Protect chondrocytes from oxidative stress induced by inflammatory cytokines	[74,75]
20.	Resveratrol	NF-κB, IL-1β	Chondroprotective effect	[76]
21.	Berberine	MMP-1/5/13, COX-2, and ADMATS-5	Antiinflammatory and anticatabolic effects	[77,78]

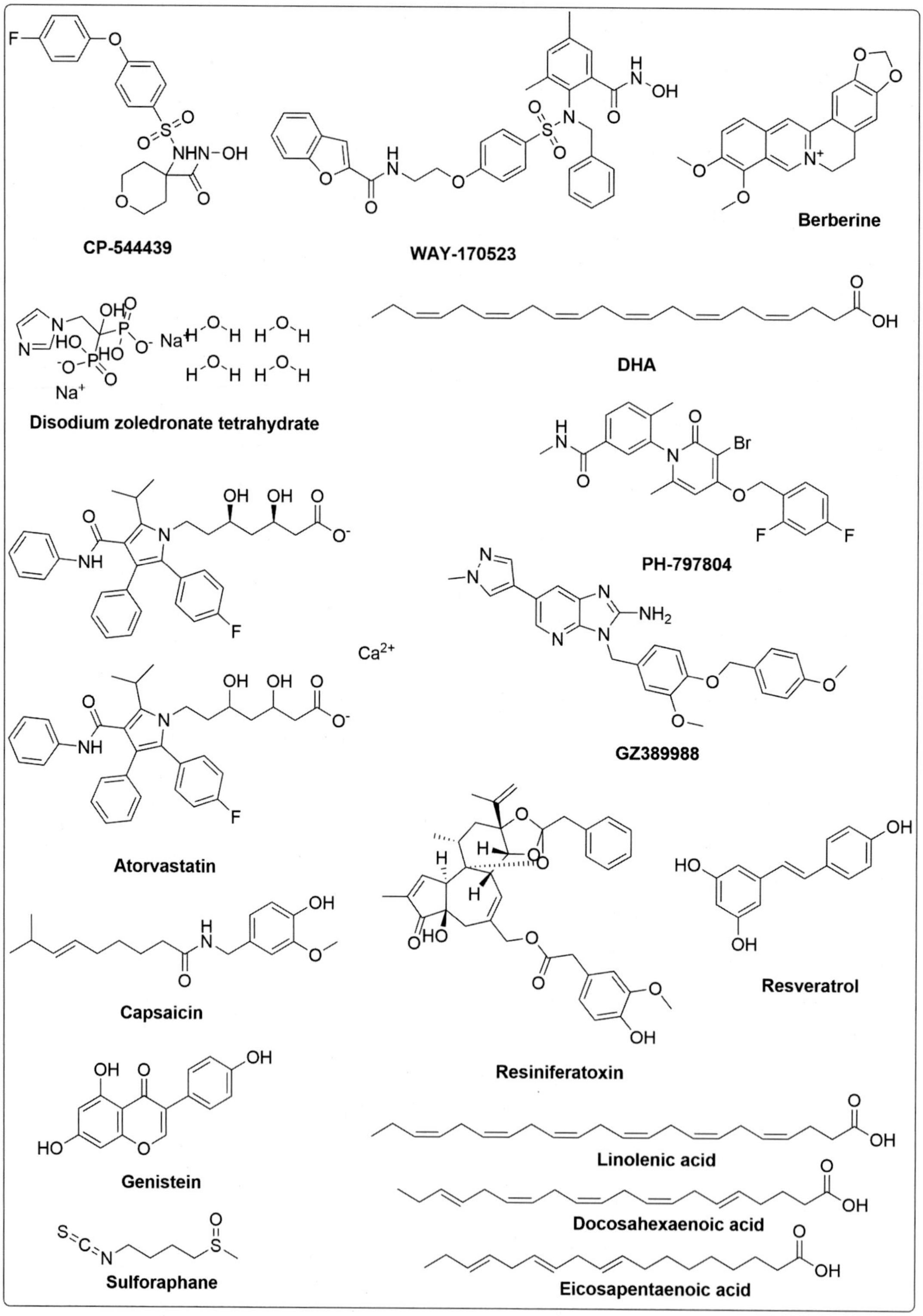

FIG. 5 Structure of compounds used in the treatment therapy of osteoarthritis.

chondrocyte proliferation. Its phase 2 trial in individuals with primary osteoarthritis of the knee was recently finished (clinicaltrials.gov: NCT01919164). In participants with radiographic knee osteoarthritis (symptomatic), intra-articular injections of sprifermin (100 g) every 6/12 months versus placebo improved total femorotibial joint cartilage thickness, but the therapeutic significance remained unclear after 2 years. Another sprifermin study in patients with acute or isolated cartilage injury of the knee was halted due to a lack of participants [53,54].

BMP-7 has been shown to improve articular cartilage repair and has a pro-anabolic impact. It has completed phase 1 (ClinicalTrials.gov Identifier: NCT01133613) and phase 2 (ClinicalTrials.gov Identifier: NCT01111045) trials in subjects with knee osteoarthritis to evaluate two different formulations of BMP-7 in a double-blind randomized trial and to determine the safety and efficacy of the intra-articular injected drug [55].

MMP inhibitors have been shown to have an anticatabolic effect, which inhibits the enzyme that causes cartilage deterioration. Such agents include CP-544439, AZD-8955, and WAY-170523, which are still in clinical trials [56].

7.2 Stem cell therapies inducing regeneration

Many studies on the therapeutic potential of stem cell therapy for osteoarthritis have been published on clinicaltrials.gov, but academics remain skeptical that it is the best instrument for regeneration. The essential issue here is that stem cell therapeutic activities are paracrine and unaffected by engrafted cells. They tend to fade away after stem cell induction, but the immunomodulatory and stem cell effects remain for a long time. Stem cell therapy, specifically mesenchymal cell therapy, is now being used to treat knee osteoarthritis. Transplantation of mesenchymal cell therapy, for example, is an intrusive procedure, whereas intra-articular injection of mesenchymal stem cells is a less invasive and safer alternative to transplantation [79,80]. Exosome, an extracellular vesicle that has been demonstrated to ameliorate the aberrant pattern in an arthritic mice model, is now a more improved strategy than stem cells. These pleiotropic exosomes have a beneficial effect on cartilage pathologies while being less invasive [81–83].

7.3 Bisphosphonate therapies

Bisphosphonates work by blocking osteoclasts and slowing bone turnover; however, their efficiency is debatable. Treatments with zoledronic acid for 6 months (randomized controlled study) significantly enhance visual analog scale pain score and lower BML, but the second multicenter trial could not confirm it, and Vaysbrot and group [84–86] found the same results. The safety and efficacy of disodium zoledronate tetrahydrate (AXS-02) is being studied in a phase 3 trial (ClinicalTrials.gov Identifier: NCT02746068, recruitment status: unclear) in participants with knee osteoarthritis, but the results have not been updated, according to clinicaltrials.gov. Clinically available medications can slow bone turnover and be helpful in subjects with BML, as well as relieve pain, but their usefulness as a whole is still in dispute [57]. In a murine osteoarthritis model, researchers discovered that osteoclasts and their related activities can cause osteoarthritis pain by causing sensory intervention in osteoarthritis [87].

7.4 Agents targeting bone cells

Cathepsin K (protease released by osteoclasts) suppression, such as MIV-711, was shown to be particularly effective in the rabbit osteoarthritis model [58]. MIV-711 (ClinicalTrials.gov Identifier: NCT03037489) recently completed a phase 2 trial to assess its safety, effectiveness, and tolerability in osteoarthritis patients. Another drug, Denosumab, has completed a phase 2 trial in participants with hand osteoarthritis (ClinicalTrials.gov Identifier: NCT02771860); however, the data have not been published as reported by clinicaltrials.gov. Parathyroid hormones, such as teriparatide, which are currently undergoing a phase II trial (ClinicalTrials.gov Identifier: NCT03072147, Recruitment Status: Active, not recruiting), have been used in chondroregenerative therapy, and the same agent was found to be effective in slowing the progression of osteoarthritis in rats [59].

7.5 Role of statins and metabolic targets in osteoarthritis

Recent research has shown that the mTOR signaling pathway can promote autophagy, which could be beneficial in the treatment of osteoarthritis [88]. According to the studies, removing AMP kinase, especially in arthritic chondrocytes, can lead to enhanced catabolic activity and biochemical damage. Agents like metformin activate AMPK, which counteracts the effects, indicating the importance of AMPK activation in cartilage deterioration [89,90]. In a mouse model of osteoarthritis, Farnahgi and colleagues investigated the effects of hypercholesterolemia on the course of the disease. The administration of a statin (atorvastatin) improved the symptoms of osteoarthritis, indicating that hypercholesterolemia plays a role in osteoarthritis [60]. Clinical trials on the role of a combination containing statin and metformin in osteoarthritis in terms of metabolic syndrome have yielded mixed results. More research is needed to link metabolic syndrome to osteoarthritis.

7.6 Role of inflammatory mediators and associated pathways

Various preclinical and experimental models have shown the production of proinflammatory mediators such as cytokines, prostaglandins, and chemokines [91]. Synovitis is a common symptom of osteoarthritis that can be detected with MRI or ultrasound [92,93]. The use of NSAIDs and glucocorticoids to treat osteoarthritis is common, but they can have substantial side effects [94,95]. In a mouse osteoarthritis model, granulocyte/macrophage colony-stimulating factors have been linked to inflammatory pain [96,97]. GSK3196165 (ClinicalTrials.gov Identifier: NCT02683785), an antigranulocyte/macrophage colony-stimulating factor, has completed a phase 2 trial to investigate the safety and efficacy of inflammatory hand osteoarthritis [61]. The identification of a single candidate chemical that targets proinflammatory signaling pathways in osteoarthritis seems to be a significant challenge. Although the complement system may be an essential target, there is no single therapeutic treatment that can be utilized to treat osteoarthritis [98–100]. The upstream initiator of the proinflammatory signaling cascade is currently being studied. A few clinical agents are available, such as PH-797804 (ClinicalTrials.gov Identifier: NCT01102660), which has completed a phase 2 trial in knee osteoarthritis patients alongside naproxen.

7.7 Treatment targeting pain

The only reason the subjects arrive at the patient is because of pain, which is a hallmark of osteoarthritis. Osteoarthritis has a complicated etiology, and the pain's underlying mechanism is still unknown [101,102]. During the course of osteoarthritis, pain is not uniform in participants, and synovitis and joint effusion are closely connected to pain [99,103,104]. Some of the medications, such as NSAIDs and opioids, have substantial side effects. Some new treatments for osteoarthritis include antinerve growth factor antibodies and receptor strategies. In human and preclinical osteoarthritis models, several clinical findings have revealed that nerve growth factors are generated by a different inflammatory mediator from multiple cells including osteocytes, chondrocytes, and synovial fibroblasts [105,106]. Although the first results and use of these agents were unsatisfactory, dose adjustments and the good effects outweighing the negative effects helped these agents gain market acceptance [62,63]. Only a few of these medicines, such as tanezumab, are in the race and are effective in terms of pain relief, but their safety remains a concern. Inhibiting nerve growth factor-induced pain by antagonizing tropomyosin-related kinase A and p75NTR was found to effectively diminish pain in preclinical animals [64,65]. GZ389988, AR786, ASP7962, ONO-4474, and VM902A are some of the drugs that block the TrkA receptor. LEVI-04 (Clinicaltrials.gov identifier: NCT03227796) is a p75NTR that is currently in phase 1 testing. Ion channels, including voltage-gated sodium channels like Nav1.7/Nav1.8 and transient receptor potential, have recently become a hot topic in osteoarthritis research. TRP vanilloid 1 (TRPV1) channel agonists, such as capsaicin or resiniferatoxin, can be employed as a target in the treatment of osteoarthritis pain since they are highly expressed by sensory neurons. Although these drugs are effective at reducing pain, the outcomes are mixed [66,67]. One of these drugs is trans-capsaicin (CNTX-4975), which is presently being studied for its osteoarthritic action [68]. A-803467, a specific Nav1.8 inhibiting drug, was found to be effective in monoiodoacetate-induced OA by interrupting pain signal transmission. Other drugs used to treat osteoarthritis include kappa-specific opioid receptor agonists like Difelikefalin, which has completed a phase 2 trial (clinicaltrials.gov: NCT02944448) and is being tested for pain reduction in people with hip and knee osteoarthritis [69].

7.8 Role of nutraceuticals in the management of osteoarthritis

The biochemical route implicated in osteoarthritis is influenced or modulated by nutrient components, which are responsible for executing structural activities. Antiinflammatory, antioxidant, and anticatabolic effects were found in the dietary supplements [107]. At present, there are a variety of nutritional supplements that can help slow down the growth of osteoarthritis. In this part, we will look at a couple of them.

MMP-3/13, aggrecanase-1/2, and JNK are all activated by IL-1 expression, and glucosamine and chondroitin can help. They are employed in the management of symptoms as a combination or monotherapy, and they help to improve tissue anatomy [108–110]. Extracellular matrix breakdown is inhibited by hyaluronic acid (an important component of synovial fluid). NF-B and ERK1/2 pathways are inhibited by hyaluronic acid, and ADAMTS-4 expression is reduced [111,112]. The chondroprotective action of avocado/soybean unsaponifiables has been linked to transforming growth factor expression. The induction of plasminogen activator inhibitors also inhibited metalloproteinase and the plasmin cascade [113]. Soy includes the isoflavone genistein, which has estrogenic properties. COX-2, NO, iNOS, and MMP are all inhibited by genistein [70,71]. An anticatabolic effect was found in fatty acids such as DHA and omega-3 fatty acids, which inhibited matrix degradation and regulated gene expression involved in inflammation and proteolysis. The researchers also discovered that eicosapentaenoic acid (intra-articular) protects chondrocytes from oxidative stress-induced apoptosis and lowers MMP-13 expression in rats [72,73]. Chondrocytes can be protected against oxidative stress caused by inflammatory cytokines by sulforaphane. It also reduced the expression of COX-2, MMP-2, and ADAMTS-5, all of which are involved in joint degradation [74,75]. The antiinflammatory properties of polyphenol molecules such as oleocanthal, hydroxytyrosoltyrosol, and oleuropein are well established in degenerative illnesses [114].

Resveratrol, for example, is widely known for its antiinflammatory, immunomodulatory, and antiapoptotic properties. Resveratrol has a chondroprotective effect and lowers cartilage loss in the early stages of osteoarthritis, according to a study [76]. Resveratrol contributed to the prevention of IL-1-mediated apoptosis by inhibiting NF-B and its related gene [115]. Wogonin is a flavone found in the *Scutellaria baicalensis* plant. It may help to promote joint health and reduce pathology such as cyst-like lesions [116]. Berberine, an isoquinoline alkaloid, is well known for its antioxidant and antiinflammatory properties. MMP-1/5/13, COX-2, and ADMATS-5, among other osteoarthritic indicators, have been demonstrated to be downregulated by berberine [117,118]. The antiinflammatory and anticatabolic actions were attributed to the IL-1-induced inflammation and the inhibition of the MAPK signaling pathway [119]. Berberine has a limited bioavailability; nonetheless, berberine nanoparticles containing chitosan have been shown to improve OA in rats [120]. Spermidine has been found to protect cartilage from damage by inhibiting the NF-B pathway and reducing DNA damage [77,78]. By inhibiting the NF-B signal, naringin-treated animals showed a protective effect against cartilage injury [121,122].

8 Conclusions

Osteoarthritis is a complex and varied illness that affects the entire joint. Understanding the underlying mechanisms, such as temporal changes throughout disease development, such as increased bone turnover to decreased bone turnover, is a priority. Current osteoarthritis trends have given information on the disease's pathology and found a new target for treatment. A single-tissue monotherapy may not be beneficial, and there are currently no single medications that can address all of the clinical criteria in the treatment of osteoarthritis or reverse the pathology. The correct drug, as well as targeted suppression of the target, can help to alleviate symptoms. When combined with other treatments, such as disease-modifying osteoarthritic medications, patient compliance improves. There has been a lot of study done on the safety and efficacy of medicines that target bone and cartilage while reducing or inhibiting inflammation and pain. TRPV1/TrkA inhibitors aid in alleviating pain, while sprifermin inhibitors help to rebuild joint structure. In the treatment of osteoarthritis, the current goal is to repair the anatomy and biochemical mechanism. Many novel medicines, such as regenerative approaches and stem cell therapy, have been proposed to address these issues, although there is still worry about their safety. The identification of targets, as well as the restoration of anatomy and biological pathways, aids in the discovery and development of new medicines, as well as the reprofile of potential compounds.

References

[1] https://www.mayoclinic.org/diseases-conditions/osteoarthritis/symptoms-causes/syc-20351925. (Accessed 10 August 2021).
[2] I. Schwarz, B. Hills, Surface-active phospholipid as the lubricating component of lubricin, Br. J. Rheumatol. 37 (1998) 21–26.
[3] https://www.arthritis.org/health-wellness/about-arthritis/understanding-arthritis/what-is-arthritis. (Accessed 10 August 2021).
[4] D. Qi-ping, Q. Min-lei, S. Ping, Clinical observation on treatment of 60 cases of osteoarthritis of knee joint by electroacupuncture, J. Acupunct. Tuina Sci. 1 (2003) 38–40.
[5] B. Hills, K.J. Thomas, Joint stiffness and 'articular gelling': inhibition of the fusion of articular surfaces by surfactant, Br. J. Rheumatol. 37 (1998) 532–538.
[6] N.A. Segal, N.A. Glass, J. Torner, M. Yang, D.T. Felson, L. Sharma, et al., Quadriceps weakness predicts risk for knee joint space narrowing in women in the MOST cohort, Osteoarthr. Cartil. 18 (2010) 769–775.
[7] N. Smidt, H.C. de Vet, L.M. Bouter, J. Dekker, Effectiveness of exercise therapy: a best-evidence summary of systematic reviews, J. Physiother. 51 (2005) 71–85.
[8] https://www.medicinenet.com/types_of_osteoarthritis_medications/drug-class.htm. (Accessed 10 August 2021).
[9] Z. Ashkavand, H. Malekinejad, B.S. Vishwanath, The pathophysiology of osteoarthritis, J. Pharm. Res. 7 (2013) 132–138.
[10] E. Losina, A.D. Paltiel, A.M. Weinstein, E. Yelin, D.J. Hunter, S.P. Chen, et al., Lifetime medical costs of knee osteoarthritis management in the United States: impact of extending indications for total knee arthroplasty, Arthritis Care Res. 67 (2015) 203–215.
[11] F.M. Cicuttini, T.D. Spector, Osteoarthritis in the aged, Drugs Aging 6 (1995) 409–420.
[12] T.D. Spector, A. MacGregor, Risk factors for osteoarthritis: genetics, Osteoarthr. Cartil. 12 (2004) 39–44.
[13] Arthritis Research UK, Osteoarthritis in General Practice: Data and Perspectives, 2013. https://www.arthritisresearchuk.org/~/media/Files/Policy%20files/Policy%20pages%20files/Osteoarthritis%20in%20general%20practice%20%20July%202013%20%20Arthritis%20Research%20UK%20PDF%20421%20MB.ashx. (Accessed 10 August 2021).
[14] T. Neogi, The epidemiology and impact of pain in osteoarthritis, Osteoarthr. Cartil. 21 (2013) 1145–1153.
[15] D. Bobinac, J. Spanjol, S. Zoricic, I. Maric, Changes in articular cartilage and subchondral bone histomorphometry in osteoarthritic knee joints in humans, Bone 32 (2003) 284–290.
[16] E.L. Radin, I.L. Paul, Does cartilage compliance reduce skeletal impact loads? the relative force-attenuating properties of articular cartilage, synovial fluid, periarticular soft tissues and bone, Arthritis Rheumatol. 13 (1970) 139–144.
[17] Y. Nagaosa, P. Lanyon, M. Doherty, Characterisation of size and direction of osteophyte in knee osteoarthritis: a radiographic study, Ann. Rheum. Dis. 61 (2002) 319–324.
[18] B. Li, R.M. Aspden, Composition and mechanical properties of cancellous bone from the femoral head of patients with osteoporosis or osteoarthritis, J. Bone Miner. Res. 12 (1997) 641–651.
[19] G. Bentley, The surgical treatment of chondromalacia patellae, J. Bone Jt. Surg 60 (1978) 74–81.
[20] B.W. Penninx, H. Abbas, W. Ambrosius, B.J. Nicklas, C. Davis, S.P. Messier, et al., Inflammatory markers and physical function among older adults with knee osteoarthritis, J. Rheumatol. 31 (2004) 2027–2031.
[21] M.B. Goldring, Osteoarthritis and cartilage: the role of cytokines, Curr. Rheumatol. Rep. 2 (2002) 459–465.
[22] W. Van den Berg, The role of cytokines and growth factors in cartilage destruction in osteoarthritis and rheumatoid arthritis, Z. Rheumatol. 58 (1999) 136–141.
[23] G. Janossy, O. Duke, L. Poulter, G. Panayi, M. Bofill, G. Goldstein, Rheumatoid arthritis: a disease of T-lymphocyte/macrophage immunoregulation, Lancet 318 (1981) 839–842.

[24] C.A. Dinarello, Biologic basis for interleukin-1 in disease, Blood (1996) 2095–2147.

[25] D. Taskiran, M. Stefanovicracic, H. Georgescu, C. Evans, Nitricoxide mediates suppression of cartilage proteoglycan synthesis by interleukin-1, Biochem. Biophys. Res. Commun. 200 (1994) 142–148.

[26] J. Bondeson, K.A. Browne, F.M. Brennan, B.M. Foxwell, M. Feldmann, Selective regulation of cytokine induction by adenoviral gene transfer of IκBα into human macrophages: lipopolysaccharide-induced, but not zymosan-induced, proinflammatory cytokines are inhibited, but IL-10 is nuclear factor-κB independent, J. Immunol. 162 (1999) 2939–2945.

[27] W.-W. Lin, M. Karin, A cytokine-mediated link between innate immunity, inflammation, and cancer, J. Clin. Investig. 117 (2007) 1175–1183.

[28] T. Niki, S. Tsutsui, S. Hirose, S. Aradono, Y. Sugimoto, K. Takeshita, et al., Galectin-9 is a high affinity IgE-binding lectin with anti-allergic effect by blocking IgE-antigen complex formation, J. Biol. Chem. 284 (2009) 32344–32352.

[29] K. Kühn, A.R. Shikhman, M. Lotz, Role of nitric oxide, reactive oxygen species, and p38 MAP kinase in the regulation of human chondrocyte apoptosis, J. Cell. Physiol. 197 (2003) 379–387.

[30] T. Tamura, T. Nakanishi, Y. Kimura, T. Hattori, K. Sasaki, H. Norimatsu, et al., Nitric oxide mediates interleukin-1-induced matrix degradation and basic fibroblast growth factor release in cultured rabbit articular chondrocytes: a possible mechanism of pathological neovascularization in arthritis, Endocrinology 137 (1996) 3729–3737.

[31] S.R. Goldring, M.B. Goldring, The role of cytokines in cartilage matrix degeneration in osteoarthritis, Clin. Orthop. Relat. Res. 427 (2004) S27–S36.

[32] H.-M. Shen, S. Pervaiz, TNF receptor superfamily-induced cell death: redox-dependent execution, FASEB J. 20 (2006) 1589–1598.

[33] J. Zhang, Yin and yang interplay of IFN-γ in inflammation and autoimmune disease, J. Clin. Investig. 117 (2007) 871–873.

[34] B. Beutler, A. Cerami, Cachectin (tumor necrosis factor): a macrophage hormone governing cellular metabolism and inflammatory response, Endocr. Rev. 9 (1988) 57–66.

[35] P.M. van der Kraan, M.-J. Goumans, E.B. Davidson, P. Ten Dijke, Age-dependent alteration of TGF-β signalling in osteoarthritis, Cell Tissue Res. 347 (2012) 257–265.

[36] T.N. Wight, M.G. Kinsella, E.E. Qwarnström, The role of proteoglycans in cell adhesion, migration and proliferation, Curr. Opin. Cell Biol. 4 (1992) 793–801.

[37] C. Kiani, C. Liwen, Y.J. Wu, J.Y. Albert, B.Y. Burton, Structure and function of aggrecan, Cell Res. 12 (2002) 19–32.

[38] B.M. Vertel, The ins and outs of aggrecan, Trends Cell Biol. 5 (1995) 458–464.

[39] B. Bau, P.M. Gebhard, J. Haag, T. Knorr, E. Bartnik, T.J.A. Aigner, et al., Relative messenger RNA expression profiling of collagenases and aggrecanases in human articular chondrocytes in vivo and in vitro, Arthritis Rheum. 46 (2002) 2648–2657.

[40] G. Murphy, H. Nagase, Reappraising metalloproteinases in rheumatoid arthritis and osteoarthritis: destruction or repair? Nat. Clin. Pract. Rheumatol. 4 (2008) 128–135.

[41] J. Bondeson, S.D. Wainwright, S. Lauder, N. Amos, C.E. Hughes, The role of synovial macrophages and macrophage-produced cytokines in driving aggrecanases, matrix metalloproteinases, and other destructive and inflammatory responses in osteoarthritis, Arthritis Res. Ther. 8 (2006) 1–12.

[42] H. Nagase, M. Kashiwagi, Aggrecanases and cartilage matrix degradation, Arthritis Res. Ther. 5 (2003) 1–10.

[43] J.L. Greene, G.M. Leytze, J. Emswiler, R. Peach, J. Bajorath, W. Cosand, et al., Covalent dimerization of CD28/CTLA-4 and oligomerization of CD80/CD86 regulate T cell costimulatory interactions, J. Biol. Chem. 271 (1996) 26762–26771.

[44] J.A. Uría, A.A. Ferrando, G. Velasco, J.M. Freije, C. López-Otín, Structure and expression in breast tumors of human TIMP-3, a new member of the metalloproteinase inhibitor family, Cancer Res. 54 (1994) 2091–2094.

[45] P. Reboul, J.-P. Pelletier, G. Tardif, J.-M. Cloutier, J.J.T. Martel-Pelletier, The new collagenase, collagenase-3, is expressed and synthesized by human chondrocytes but not by synoviocytes: A role in osteoarthritis, J. Clin. Invest. 97 (1996) 2011–2019.

[46] E.J. Bates, D.A. Lowther, C.C. Johnson, Hyaluronic acid synthesis in articular cartilage: an inhibition by hydrogen peroxide, Biochem. Biophys. Res. Commun. 132 (1985) 714–720.

[47] C.K. Mukhopadhyay, I.B. Chatterjee, Free metal ion-independent oxidative damage of collagen. Protection by ascorbic acid, J. Biol. Chem. 269 (1994) 30200–30205.

[48] M.D. Carlo Jr., R.F. Loeser, Increased oxidative stress with aging reduces chondrocyte survival: correlation with intracellular glutathione levels, Arthritis Rheum. 48 (2003) 3419–3430.

[49] R. Stanescu, V. Stanescu, P. Maroteaux, J. Peyron, Constitutional articular cartilage dysplasia with accumulation of complex lipids in chondrocytes and precocious arthrosis, Arthritis Rheum. 24 (1981) 965–968.

[50] P.M. Arnstein, Evolution of topical NSAIDs in the guidelines for treatment of osteoarthritis in elderly patients, Drugs Aging 29 (2012) 523–531.

[51] B.R. da Costa, E. Nüesch, R. Kasteler, E. Husni, V. Welch, A.W. Rutjes, et al., Oral or transdermal opioids for osteoarthritis of the knee or hip, Cochrane Database Syst. Rev. 9 (2014).

[52] B.R. da Costa, R. Hari, P. Jüni, Intra-articular corticosteroids for osteoarthritis of the knee, JAMA 316 (2016) 2671–2672.

[53] M.C. Hochberg, A. Guermazi, H. Guehring, A. Aydemir, S. Wax, P. Fleuranceau-Morel, et al., Effect of intra-articular sprifermin vs placebo on femorotibial joint cartilage thickness in patients with osteoarthritis: the FORWARD randomized clinical trial, JAMA 322 (2019) 1360–1370.

[54] M. Karsdal, M. Michaelis, C. Ladel, A. Siebuhr, A. Bihlet, J. Andersen, et al., Disease-modifying treatments for osteoarthritis (DMOADs) of the knee and hip: lessons learned from failures and opportunities for the future, Osteoarthr. Cartil. 24 (2016) 2013–2021.

[55] C.H. Evans, V.B. Kraus, L.A. Setton, Progress in intra-articular therapy, Nat. Rev. Rheumatol. 10 (2014) 11–22.

[56] P.S. Burrage, K.S. Mix, C.E. Brinckerhoff, Matrix metalloproteinases: role in arthritis, Front. Biosci. 11 (2006) 529–543.

[57] L.A. Deveza, S.M. Bierma-Zeinstra, W.E. Van Spil, W.M. Oo, B.T. Saragiotto, T. Neogi, et al., Efficacy of bisphosphonates in specific knee osteoarthritis subpopulations: protocol for an OA Trial Bank systematic review and individual patient data meta-analysis, BMJ Open 8 (2018), e023889.

[58] P.G. Conaghan, M.A. Bowes, S.R. Kingsbury, A. Brett, G. Guillard, B. Rizoska, et al., Disease-modifying effects of a novel cathepsin K

inhibitor in osteoarthritis: a randomized controlled trial, Ann. Intern. Med. 172 (2020) 86–95.

[59] C.-H. Chen, M.-L. Ho, L.-H. Chang, L. Kang, Y.-S. Lin, S.-Y. Lin, et al., Parathyroid hormone-(1–34) ameliorated knee osteoarthritis in rats via autophagy, J. Appl. Physiol. 124 (2018) 1177–1185.

[60] S. Farnaghi, I. Prasadam, G. Cai, T. Friis, Z. Du, R. Crawford, et al., Protective effects of mitochondria-targeted antioxidants and statins on cholesterol-induced osteoarthritis, FASEB J. 31 (2017) 356–367.

[61] S. Grässel, D. Muschter, Recent advances in the treatment of osteoarthritis, F100 Research 9 (2020) 325.

[62] M. Schmelz, P. Mantyh, A.-M. Malfait, J. Farrar, T. Yaksh, L. Tive, et al., Nerve growth factor antibody for the treatment of osteoarthritis pain and chronic low-back pain: mechanism of action in the context of efficacy and safety, Pain 160 (2019) 2210.

[63] R.E. Miller, A.-M. Malfait, J.A. Block, Current status of nerve growth factor antibodies for the treatment of osteoarthritis pain, Clin. Exp. Rheumatol. 35 (Suppl. 107) (2017) 85.

[64] S. Ashraf, K.S. Bouhana, J. Pheneger, S.W. Andrews, D.A. Walsh, Selective inhibition of tropomyosin-receptor-kinase A (TrkA) reduces pain and joint damage in two rat models of inflammatory arthritis, Arthritis Res. Ther. 18 (2016) 1–11.

[65] L.N. Nwosu, P.I. Mapp, V. Chapman, D.A. Walsh, Blocking the tropomyosin receptor kinase A (TrkA) receptor inhibits pain behaviour in two rat models of osteoarthritis, Ann. Rheum. Dis. 75 (2016) 1246–1254.

[66] W. Rahman, A.J.N. Dickenson, Osteoarthritis-dependent changes in antinociceptive action of Nav1. 7 and Nav1. 8 sodium channel blockers: An in vivo electrophysiological study in the rat, Neuroscience 295 (2015) 103–116.

[67] T. Galindo, J. Reyna, A.J.P. Weyer, Evidence for transient receptor potential (TRP) channel contribution to arthritis pain and pathogenesis, Pharmaceuticals 11 (2018) 105.

[68] N. Schuelert, J.J. McDougall, Involvement of Nav 1.8 sodium ion channels in the transduction of mechanical pain in a rodent model of osteoarthritis, Arthritis Res. Ther. 14 (2012) 1–9.

[69] J.M.K. Hesselink, CR845 (Difelikefalin), a kappa receptors agonist in phase III by CARA therapeutics: a case of 'Spin'In scientific writing? J. Pharmacol. Clin. Res. Int. J. Mol. Sci. 2 (2017), 555588.

[70] F.-C. Liu, C.-C. Wang, J.-W. Lu, C.-H. Lee, S.-C. Chen, Y.-J. Ho, et al., Chondroprotective effects of genistein against osteoarthritis induced joint inflammation, Nutrients 11 (2019) 1180.

[71] S. Hooshmand, D.Y. Soung, E.A. Lucas, S.V. Madihally, C.W. Levenson, B.H. Arjmandi, Genistein reduces the production of proinflammatory molecules in human chondrocytes, J. Nutr. Biochem. 18 (2007) 609–614.

[72] S. Sakata, S. Hayashi, T. Fujishiro, K. Kawakita, N. Kanzaki, S. Hashimoto, et al., Oxidative stress-induced apoptosis and matrix loss of chondrocytes is inhibited by eicosapentaenoic acid, J. Orthop. Res. 33 (2015) 359–365.

[73] Z. Zainal, A.J. Longman, S. Hurst, K. Duggan, B. Caterson, C.E. Hughes, et al., Relative efficacies of omega-3 polyunsaturated fatty acids in reducing expression of key proteins in a model system for studying osteoarthritis, Osteoarthr. Cartil. 17 (2009) 896–905.

[74] J.-Y. Ko, Y.-J. Choi, G.-J. Jeong, G.-I. Im, Sulforaphane–PLGA microspheres for the intra-articular treatment of osteoarthritis, Biomaterials 34 (2013) 5359–5368.

[75] A. Facchini, I. Stanic, S. Cetrullo, R.M. Borzì, G. Filardo, F. Flamigni, Sulforaphane protects human chondrocytes against cell death induced by various stimuli, J. Cell. Physiol. 226 (2011) 1771–1779.

[76] N. Elmali, I. Esenkaya, A. Harma, K. Ertem, Y. Turkoz, B. Mizrak, Effect of resveratrol in experimental osteoarthritis in rabbits, Inflamm. Res. 54 (2005) 158–162.

[77] S. D'Adamo, S. Cetrullo, S. Guidotti, Y. Silvestri, M. Minguzzi, S. Santi, et al., Spermidine rescues the deregulated autophagic response to oxidative stress of osteoarthritic chondrocytes, Free Radic. Biol. Med. 153 (2020) 159–172.

[78] P.K. Sacitharan, S. Lwin, G.B. Gharios, J.R. Edwards, Spermidine restores dysregulated autophagy and polyamine synthesis in aged and osteoarthritic chondrocytes via EP300, Exp. Mol. Med. 50 (2018) 1–10.

[79] P. Mancuso, S. Raman, A. Glynn, F. Barry, J.M. Murphy, Mesenchymal stem cell therapy for osteoarthritis: the critical role of the cell secretome, Front. Bioeng. Biotechnol. 7 (2019) 9.

[80] C. Roubille, J.-P. Pelletier, J. Martel-Pelletier, New and emerging treatments for osteoarthritis management: will the dream come true with personalized medicine? Expert Opin. Pharmacother. 14 (2013) 2059–2077.

[81] J. Wu, L. Kuang, C. Chen, J. Yang, W.-N. Zeng, T. Li, et al., miR-100-5p-abundant exosomes derived from infrapatellar fat pad MSCs protect articular cartilage and ameliorate gait abnormalities via inhibition of mTOR in osteoarthritis, Biomaterials 206 (2019) 87–100.

[82] J. Malda, J. Boere, C.H. Van De Lest, P.R. Van Weeren, M.H. Wauben, Extracellular vesicles—new tool for joint repair and regeneration, Nat. Rev. Rheumatol. 12 (2016) 243–249.

[83] D. D'Arrigo, A. Roffi, M. Cucchiarini, M. Moretti, C. Candrian, G. Filardo, Secretome and extracellular vesicles as new biological therapies for knee osteoarthritis: a systematic review, J. Clin. Med. 8 (2019) 1867.

[84] L.L. Laslett, D.A. Doré, S.J. Quinn, P. Boon, E. Ryan, T.M. Winzenberg, et al., Zoledronic acid reduces knee pain and bone marrow lesions over 1 year: a randomised controlled trial, Ann. Rheum. Dis. 71 (2012) 1322–1328.

[85] W.E. Van Spil, O. Kubassova, M. Boesen, A.-C. Bay-Jensen, A. Mobasheri, Osteoarthritis phenotypes and novel therapeutic targets, Biochem. Pharmacol. 165 (2019) 41–48.

[86] E. Vaysbrot, M. Osani, M.-C. Musetti, T. McAlindon, R. Bannuru, Are bisphosphonates efficacious in knee osteoarthritis? A meta-analysis of randomized controlled trials, Osteoarthr. Cartil. 26 (2018) 154–164.

[87] S. Zhu, J. Zhu, G. Zhen, Y. Hu, S. An, Y. Li, et al., Subchondral bone osteoclasts induce sensory innervation and osteoarthritis pain, J. Clin. Investig. 129 (2019) 1076–1093.

[88] M. Lotz, B. Caramés, Autophagy: a new therapeutic target in cartilage injury and osteoarthritis, J. Am. Acad. Orthop. Surg. 20 (2012) 261–262.

[89] A. Mobasheri, M.P. Rayman, O. Gualillo, J. Sellam, P. Van Der Kraan, U. Fearon, The role of metabolism in the pathogenesis of osteoarthritis, Nat. Rev. Rheumatol. 13 (2017) 302–311.

[90] M. Husa, F. Petursson, M. Lotz, R. Terkeltaub, R. Liu-Bryan, C/EBP homologous protein drives pro-catabolic responses in chondrocytes, Arthritis Res. Ther. 15 (2013) 1–10.

[91] F. Berenbaum, Osteoarthritis as an inflammatory disease (osteoarthritis is not osteoarthrosis!), Osteoarthr. Cartil. 21 (2013) 16–21.

[92] A. Mathiessen, P.G. Conaghan, Synovitis in osteoarthritis: current understanding with therapeutic implications, Arthritis Res. Ther. 19 (2017) 1–9.

[93] D. Hayashi, F.W. Roemer, A. Katur, D.T. Felson, S.-O. Yang, F. Alomran, et al., Imaging of synovitis in osteoarthritis: current status and outlook, Semin. Arthritis Rheum. 41 (2) (2011) 116–130.

[94] J.-P. Pelletier, J. Martel-Pelletier, F. Rannou, C. Cooper, Efficacy and safety of oral NSAIDs and analgesics in the management of osteoarthritis: evidence from real-life setting trials and surveys, Semin. Arthritis Rheum. 45 (4) (2016) S22–S27.

[95] O. Savvidou, M. Milonaki, S. Goumenos, D. Flevas, P. Papagelopoulos, P.J.M. Moutsatsou, et al., Glucocorticoid signaling and osteoarthritis, Mol. Cell. Endocrinol. 480 (2019) 153–166.

[96] A.D. Cook, S. Pobjoy, S. Steidl, M. Dürr, E.L. Braine, A.L. Turner, et al., Granulocyte-macrophage colony-stimulating factor is a key mediator in experimental osteoarthritis pain and disease development, Arthritis Res. Ther. 14 (2012) 1–9.

[97] R. Grieshaber-Bouyer, T. Kämmerer, N. Rosshirt, T.A. Nees, P. Koniezke, E. Tripel, et al., Divergent mononuclear cell participation and cytokine release profiles define hip and knee osteoarthritis, J. Clin. Med. 8 (2019) 1631.

[98] D. Ricklin, D.C. Mastellos, J.D. Lambris, Therapeutic targeting of the complement system, Nat. Rev. Drug Discov. (2019).

[99] N. Rosshirt, S. Hagmann, E. Tripel, T. Gotterbarm, J. Kirsch, F. Zeifang, et al., A predominant Th1 polarization is present in synovial fluid of end-stage osteoarthritic knee joints: analysis of peripheral blood, synovial fluid and synovial membrane, Clin. Exp. Immunol. 195 (3) (2019) 395–406.

[100] W. Zhu, X. Zhang, Y. Jiang, X. Liu, L. Huang, Q. Wei, et al., Alterations in peripheral T cell and B cell subsets in patients with osteoarthritis, Clin. Rheumatol. 39 (2020) 523–532.

[101] A.-P. Trouvin, S. Perrot, Pain in osteoarthritis. Implications for optimal management, Joint Bone Spine 85 (2018) 429–434.

[102] K. Fu, S.R. Robbins, J.J. McDougall, Osteoarthritis: the genesis of pain, Rheumatology (Oxford) 57 (Suppl_4) (2018). iv43-iv50.

[103] T. Alliston, C.J. Hernandez, D.M. Findlay, D.T. Felson, O.D. Kennedy, Bone marrow lesions in osteoarthritis: what lies beneath, J. Orthop. Res. 36 (2018) 1818–1825.

[104] N. Mesci, E. Mesci, D.G. Külcü, Association of neuropathic pain with ultrasonographic measurements of femoral cartilage thickness and clinical parameters in patients with knee osteoarthritis, J. Phys. Ther. Sci. 28 (2016) 2190–2195.

[105] Y. Sakurai, M. Fujita, S. Kawasaki, T. Sanaki, T. Yoshioka, K. Higashino, et al., Contribution of synovial macrophages to rat advanced osteoarthritis pain resistant to cyclooxygenase inhibitors, Pain 160 (2019) 895–907.

[106] E. Pecchi, S. Priam, M. Gosset, A. Pigenet, L. Sudre, M.-C. Laiguillon, et al., Induction of nerve growth factor expression and release by mechanical and inflammatory stimuli in chondrocytes: possible involvement in osteoarthritis pain, Arthritis Res. Ther. 16 (2014) 1–11.

[107] D.J. Leong, M. Choudhury, D.M. Hirsh, J.A. Hardin, N.J. Cobelli, H.B. Sun, Nutraceuticals: potential for chondroprotection and molecular targeting of osteoarthritis, Int. J. Mol. Sci. 14 (2013) 23063–23085.

[108] J. Jerosch, Effects of glucosamine and chondroitin sulfate on cartilage metabolism in OA: outlook on other nutrient partners especially omega-3 fatty acids, Int. J. Rheumatol. 2011 (2011).

[109] K.M. Neil, M.W. Orth, P.M. Coussens, P.-S. Chan, J.P. Caron, Effects of glucosamine and chondroitin sulfate on mediators of osteoarthritis in cultured equine chondrocytes stimulated by use of recombinant equine interleukin-1β, Am. J. Vet. Res. 66 (2005) 1861–1869.

[110] P.-S. Chan, J.P. Caron, M.W. Orth, Effect of glucosamine and chondroitin sulfate on regulation of gene expression of proteolytic enzymes and their inhibitors in interleukin-1–challenged bovine articular cartilage explants, Am. J. Vet. Res. 66 (2005) 1870–1876.

[111] T. Yatabe, S. Mochizuki, M. Takizawa, M. Chijiiwa, A. Okada, T. Kimura, et al., Hyaluronan inhibits expression of ADAMTS4 (aggrecanase-1) in human osteoarthritic chondrocytes, Ann. Rheum. Dis. 68 (2009) 1051–1058.

[112] R.C. Gupta, R. Lall, A. Srivastava, A. Sinha, Hyaluronic acid: molecular mechanisms and therapeutic trajectory, Front. Vet. Sci. 6 (2019) 192.

[113] K. Boumediene, N. Felisaz, P. Bogdanowicz, P. Galera, J.P. Pujol, Avocado/soya unsaponifiables enhance the expression of transforming growth factor β1 and β2 in cultured articular chondrocytes, Arthritis Rheum. 42 (1999) 148–156.

[114] M.A. Karković, J. Torić, M. Barbarić, C. Jakobušić Brala, Hydroxytyrosol, tyrosol and derivatives and their potential effects on human health, Molecules 24 (2019) 2001.

[115] M. Dave, M. Attur, G. Palmer, H.E. Al-Mussawir, L. Kennish, J. Patel, et al., The antioxidant resveratrol protects against chondrocyte apoptosis via effects on mitochondrial polarization and ATP production, Arthritis Rheum. 58 (2008) 2786–2797.

[116] J.F. Smith, E.G. Starr, M.A. Goodman, R.B. Hanson, T.A. Palmer, J.B. Woolstenhulme, et al., Topical application of wogonin provides a novel treatment of knee osteoarthritis, Front. Physiol. 11 (2020) 80.

[117] P.-f. Hu, W.-p. Chen, J.-l. Tang, J.-p. Bao, L.-d. Wu, Protective effects of berberine in an experimental rat osteoarthritis model, Phytother. Res. 25 (2011) 878–885.

[118] P.D. Moon, H.S. Jeong, C.S. Chun, H.M. Kim, Baekjeolyusin-tang and its active component berberine block the release of collagen and proteoglycan from IL-1β-stimulated rabbit cartilage and down-regulate matrix metalloproteinases in rabbit chondrocytes, Phytother. Res. 25 (2011) 844–850.

[119] X. Li, P. He, Y. Hou, S. Chen, Z. Xiao, J. Zhan, et al., Berberine inhibits the interleukin-1 beta-induced inflammatory response via MAPK downregulation in rat articular chondrocytes, Drug Dev. Res. 80 (2019) 637–645.

[120] Y. Zhou, S.-q. Liu, H. Peng, L. Yu, B. He, Q. Zhao, In vivo antiapoptosis activity of novel berberine-loaded chitosan nanoparticles effectively ameliorates osteoarthritis, Int. Immunopharmacol. 28 (2015) 34–43.

[121] Q. Xu, Z.-f. Zhang, W.-x. Sun, Effect of naringin on monosodium iodoacetate-induced osteoarthritis pain in rats, Med. Sci. Monit. 23 (2017) 3746.

[122] Y. Zhao, Z. Li, W. Wang, H. Zhang, J. Chen, P. Su, et al., Naringin protects against cartilage destruction in osteoarthritis through repression of NF-κB signaling pathway, Inflammation 39 (2016) 385–392.

Chapter 8

Advanced therapeutics for targeting atherosclerosis

Shome Sankar Bhunia[a] and Utsab Debnath[b]

[a]School of Pharmacy, The Assam Kaziranga University, Jorhat, Assam, India, [b]School of Health Sciences and Technology, University of Petroleum and Energy Studies, Dehradun, Uttarakhand, India

1 Introduction

Cardiovascular disorders (CVD) caused by atherosclerosis are one of the most serious health problems in recent times causing millions of deaths worldwide [1]. The earlier understanding behind the development of atherosclerosis and its related cardiovascular complications was linked exclusively with an increase in the plasma low-density lipoproteins (LDL) resulting in lipid deposition in the arterial wall (Fig. 1) [2]. This may further worsen with the endothelium disruption and blood clot formation, impairing flow of blood that may require antithrombotic therapy [3,4]. This concept has gradually changed over time to include both dyslipidemia and inflammation as crucial factors in the development of atherosclerosis. The elevated levels of chylomicrons (CM), low-density lipoprotein (LDL), and very low-density lipoprotein (VLDL) or decreased levels of high-density lipoprotein (HDL) distinguish dyslipidemia, which includes hypercholesterolemia and hypertriglyceridemia (HDL) [5]. Statins are acknowledged to be the most effective therapeutic medications for lowering atherogenic lipoprotein levels and preventing major cardiovascular events [6–8]. In addition, statins have antiinflammatory actions that are independent of LDL reduction and may help to prevent atherogenesis and other cardiovascular illnesses [6]. In this context, the new proprotein convertase subtilisin/kexin type 9 (PCSK9) inhibitors have also shown significant LDL lowering activity [9–12]. Despite statins and new inhibitors of proprotein convertase subtilisin/kexin type 9 (PCSK9) decreasing low-density lipoprotein (LDL) levels and cardiovascular events, residual cardiovascular burden remains substantial even in the subset of patients taking statin treatment [13,14]. The relevance of epigenetic processes as a new layer of biological control in CVD has been highlighted by emerging data over the last two decades. The role of epigenetics in the formation and vulnerability of atherosclerotic plaques is crucial and may lead to new therapies in atherosclerosis [15].

The primary therapeutic agents, such as bile acid sequestrants, statins, ezetimibe, and recently discovered PCSK9 inhibitors, all operate exclusively or by either increasing LDLR activity and/or LDL-C clearance [16]. Further LDL-C reduction can be accomplished by inhibiting the formation of LDL-C or its precursors with either lomitapide [17], a microsomal triglyceride transfer protein (MTP) inhibitor, or mipomersen [18], an antisense oligonucleotide that inhibits apoB synthesis. Despite the promising results obtained in decreasing LDL-C by 50%–60% by statins and ezetimibe, a substantial proportion of patients fail to meet the required LDL-C targets due to extreme LDL-C levels [19–22].

Therefore, alternative therapeutic agents in combination with current drugs alone or as a single entity should be considered to reduce the atherosclerotic complications in patients.

2 LDL-C-lowering therapy and TG-lowering therapy

2.1 HMG-CoA reductase inhibitors (statins)

HMG-CoA reductase inhibitors used in the treatment of hypercholesterolemia act by lowering total cholesterol (TC), low-density lipoprotein cholesterol (LDL-C), and triglycerides (TG) while increasing high-density lipoprotein cholesterol (HDL-C) [23]. Statins, beside maintaining a healthy lifestyle beneficial for heart, are recommended in clinically significant cardiovascular disease patients to lower the risk of myocardial infarction, stroke, or revascularization procedures [23,24]. A major amount of cholesterol production occurs at night when the body is in fasting condition; statins having a shorter half-life [such as simvastatin, pravastatin, or fluvastatin (Fig. 1)] are recommended orally before sleep to enhance their effectiveness. The outcome of meta-analysis study on statins in the prevention of major coronary events and in mortality showed that atorvastatin

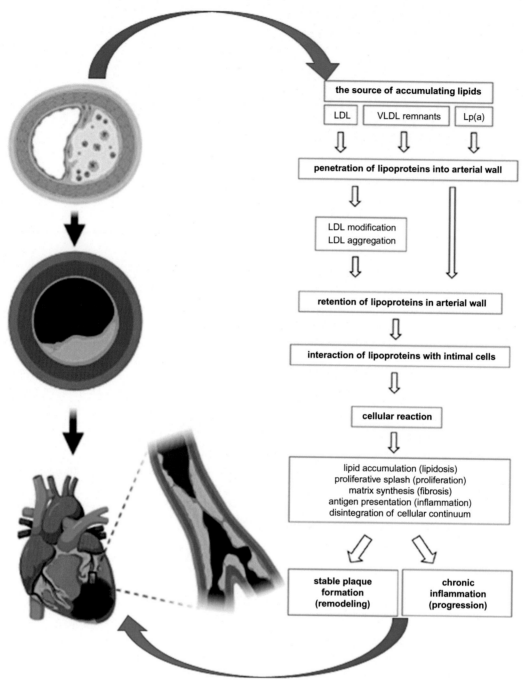

FIG. 1 Different stages of atherosclerosis.

and fluvastatin were more efficient in reducing major coronary events as compared to rosuvastatin. For secondary prevention of major coronary events, atorvastatin was substantially more efficacious than pravastatin (OR 0.65, 95% CI: 0.43–0.99) and simvastatin (OR 0.68, 95% CI: 0.38–0.98). Overall, atorvastatin (80%), fluvastatin (79%), and simvastatin (62%) had the highest overall chance of being the optimal treatment in terms of both outcomes across all age groups [25]. All statins reduced LDL and total cholesterol levels in the blood, at higher doses resulting in greater pretreatment LDL and total cholesterol reductions. In terms of decreasing LDL cholesterol, the statins such as atorvastatin, rosuvastatin, and simvastatin showed similar effectiveness [26]. In meta-analysis studies, statin therapy was found to reduce the incidence of stroke, myocardial infarction, unstable angina, and coronary revascularization to levels comparable to those reported in coronary artery disease studies. Statins also lowered the relative risk of mortality from any cause by 10% in persons with low cardio-vascular risk [27]. There are safety variations among individual statins when evaluated in network meta-analyses, with simvastatin and pravastatin having a better safety profile as compared to other statins; however, simvastatin at high dose increase creatinine kinase levels. Elevation of transaminase levels was observed with greater doses of atorvasatin, fluvastatin, lovastatin, and simvastatin [28].

3 LDL-C-lowering therapy

3.1 Cholesterol absorption inhibitors

Cholesterol absorption inhibitors decrease the cholesterol transported to the liver by preventing the intestinal absorption of dietary and biliary cholesterol. Reduced cholesterol delivery to the liver causes increased hepatic LDL (low-density lipoprotein) receptor activity, resulting in higher LDL cholesterol clearance. Cholesterol O-acyl transferases (ACAT) catalyze the esterification and absorption of cholesterol in intestinal mucosal cells and maintain cholesterol levels in the blood. One of the most attractive options for treating hyperlipidemia is inhibiting the ACAT enzymes. According to a literature review, ACAT inhibitory effects can be found in a wide range of structurally varied substances. Ezetimibe is the first drug in a new class of selective cholesterol absorption inhibitors recently licensed for treatment in the United States by the Food and Drug Administration. The biliary and dietary cholesterol absorption from the small intestine is blocked by Ezetimibe

without altering fat-soluble vitamins, triglycerides, or bile acids absorption. Ezetimibe binds to the small intestine's brush barrier and inhibits cholesterol uptake by enterocytes. Ezetimibe is a cholesterol absorption inhibitor that inhibits the Niemann-Pick C1 Like 1 (NPC1L1) transporter in the small intestine [29]. Ezetimibe has been shown in preclinical tests to have lipid-lowering characteristics as a monotherapy and to have a synergistic impact when combined with inhibitors of 3-hydroxy-3-methylglutaryl coenzyme A reductase (statins). Ezetimibe reduces low-density lipoprotein cholesterol (LDL) by 15%–20% when used alone or in combination with statins or fenofibrate, while boosting high-density lipoprotein cholesterol by 2.5%–5%. Ezetimibe, unlike other intestinally acting lipid-lowering medications, has no deleterious effects on triglyceride levels and has few drug interactions due to its poor systemic absorption [30,31]. Avasimibe is a new ACAT inhibitor that has been studied in human phase III trials. Avasimibe inhibits foam cell production in human macrophages in vitro not only by increasing free cholesterol efflux but also by reducing the uptake of modified LDL.

Avasimibe was the first ACAT inhibitor to achieve clinical proof of concept; however, it was discontinued in phases for the treatment of atherosclerosis (Fig. 2). In a recent study, Avasimibe (7.5, 15, and 30 M) reduced tumor cell colony growth by decreasing the synthesis of DNA [32]. The dual ACAT1 and ACAT2 inhibitor pactimibe slowed the progression of atherosclerosis in animal models by inhibiting the formation of cholesteryl ester in macrophages [33]. Pactimibe failed to diminish the carotid intima-media

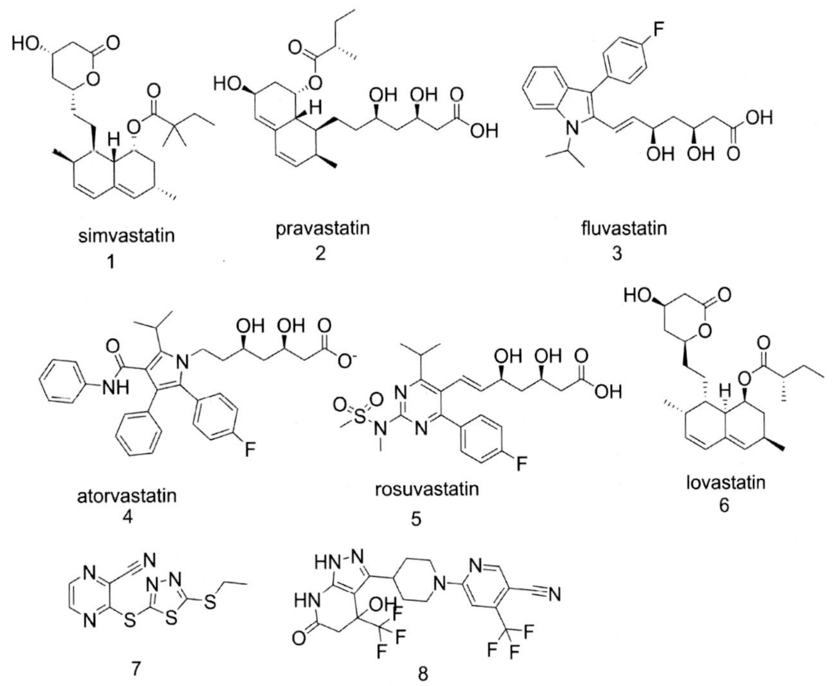

FIG. 2 Representative class of antiatherosclerotic agents.

thickness (CIMT) in patients with familial hypercholesterolemia and carotid atherosclerosis and it was observed that CIMT progressed faster with pactimibe as compared to placebo in the CAPTIVATE trial. In the parallel ACTIVATE trial, the effect of pactimibe on coronary artery disease progression also showed no promising results, and hence it was discontinued [34].

3.2 Bile acid sequestrants

Bile acid sequestrants are positively charged molecules that prevent cholesterol absorption by attaching to negatively charged bile acids in the gut and prevent lipid solubilizing. They reduce the bile acid pool by inhibiting the reabsorption of bile acids that leads to increased bile acid synthesis, and competes with cholesterol synthesis in the liver, that leads to low serum cholesterol levels. The bile acid sequestrants colesevelam, colestipol, and cholestyramine have been authorized by the Food and Drug Administration (FDA) for patients with hypercholesterolemia without hypertriglyceridemia. In statin-intolerant individuals, bile acid sequestrants are an effective treatment option (myalgia and myopathy). They can be used with niacin and ezetimibe, a cholesterol absorption inhibitor, to help patients accomplish their primary and secondary preventive goals. The major benefit of bile acid sequestrants is their safety profile when used in combination with other antidiabetic medicines and statins. Cholestyramine (24 g/d) as compared to placebo decreased the coronary heart disease (CHD) and nonfatal myocardial infarction (MI) by 19% in individuals with primary hypercholesterolemia as observed in the Coronary Primary Prevention Trial (LRC-CPPT) [35]. The reduction of LDL-C and hemoglobin (Hb)A1c by colesevelam HCL (COL) was observed in individuals with Type II diabetes mellitus (T2D) in three double-blind, placebo-controlled studies. The FDA approved COL as an adjunct to exercise and food restriction for improving glucose control in T2D patients based on these findings [36]. For colestipol, over the course of 7 years, a significant lowering of LDL-C levels was observed in participants by the use of bile acid sequestrant in Type IIA hyperproteinemia, randomized to a reduced cholesterol diet with either placebo or colestipol (30 mg) [37,38].

3.3 ATP-citrate lyase inhibitors

Bempedoic acid has been discovered to be a strong inhibitor of ATP-citrate lyase (ACLY), a target for LDL cholesterol lowering (LDL-C). ACLY, a crucial enzyme connecting glucose catabolism to lipogenesis, is inhibited by the liver-specific activation of bempedoic acid, which catalyzes the production of acetyl-CoA from mitochondrial-derived citrate for de novo synthesis of fatty acids and cholesterol [39].

In the assessment of the Long-Term Safety and Efficacy of Bempedoic Acid (BA) (CLEAR Harmony OLE). The 78 weeks of BA treatment resulted in long-term cholesterol reduction, and patient adherence to BA medication was strong (86.2%). With no additional adverse findings, overall safety throughout the OLE was identical to outcomes reported in the 52-week-long CLEAR Harmony trial in the entire BA phase 3 clinical program (Table 1). In the CLEAR Wisdom in patients with hyperlipidemia and at high cardiovascular risk, the evaluation of long-term efficacy of bempedoic acid (ETC-1002) is safe and effective in lowering the LDL-C compared with placebo in patients with ASCVD or heterogeneous FH on maximum-tolerated statin therapy (Table 1). The add-on of Bempedoic Acid (ETC-1002) to ezetimibe therapy in patients with elevated LDL-C (CLEAR Tranquility) BA was safe and effective in the oral therapeutic option complementary to ezetimibe in statin-intolerant patients who require additional LDL-C lowering. [43] The evaluation of long-term safety and tolerability of ETC-1002 in high-risk patients with hyperlipidemia and high cv risk (CLEAR Harmony) that provided significant evidence that bempedoic acid treatment as an addition to statin regimens based on guidelines had an acceptable safety profile [45]. Bempedoic acid successfully reduces LDL-C as monotherapy, coupled with ezetimibe, added to statin treatment, and in statin-intolerant hypercholesterolemic patients, according to phase 2 and 3 clinical studies [39].

3.4 Proprotein convertase subtilisin/kexin type-9 inhibitors

Injectable monoclonal antibodies, known as PCSK9 inhibitors, increase the availability of low-density lipoprotein (LDL) receptors, lowering serum LDL cholesterol levels (LDL-C). When taken as monotherapy or in combination with other lipid-lowering treatments, the PCSK9 inhibitors alirocumab and evolocumab significantly reduced (55%–60%) LDL-C values as compared to placebo [13,48]. The effect of statins on the risk of cardiovascular events over an average of 5 years of treatment has been estimated by the use of the CTT regression line and it was observed that the PCSK9 inhibitors and statins used for the same length of time have strikingly comparable effects on the risk of cardiovascular events [48]. The total duration of the therapy as observed from the results of the FOURIER, SPIRE 2 trials and the CTT meta-analysis statin trials indicates that both PCSK9 inhibitors and statins have similar effects on the risk of cardiovascular events per unit change in LDL-C. This suggests that both PCSK9 inhibitors and statins reduce the risk of cardiovascular events due to the reduction in LDL-C, without any pleiotropic consequences.

TABLE 1 Recent clinical trials for the treatment of aaherosclerosis.

Sl. No	Name of the therapeutic	Description of the study	NCT number	Phase	End date	Outcome
1.	Rosuvastatin	A phase 3 study measuring the effect of rosuvastatin 20mg on carotid intima-media thickness in Chinese subjects with subclinical atherosclerosis	NCT02546323	Phase 3	December 11, 2019	Measuring effects on intima-media thickness: an evaluation of rosuvastatin in Chinese subjects with subclinical atherosclerosis-design, rationale, and methodology of the METEOR-China study
2.	Canakinumab (ACZ885)	Cardiovascular risk reduction study (reduction in recurrent major cv disease events) (CANTOS)	NCT01327846	Phase 3	January 22, 2020	Study showed a significant 15% reduction of major adverse cardiovascular events (MACE) in people with a prior heart attack and inflammatory atherosclerosis who were treated with 150mg of ACZ885, in addition to standard of care including lipid-lowering therapy. Effect driven by 24% relative reduction in risk of heart attack; a nonsignificant 10% reduction in risk of cardiovascular death was observed [https://www.acc.org/latest-in-cardiology/clinical-trials/2017/08/26/08/35/cantos]
3.	Darapladib	The stabilization of atherosclerotic plaque by initiation of darapladib therapy trial (STABILITY)	NCT00799903	Phase 3	August 10, 2017	The results of the STABILITY trial indicate that inhibition of Lp-PLA$_2$ and sustained lowering of its levels with darapladib was not associated with an improvement in the primary endpoint of cardiovascular death/MI/stroke at a median of 3.7 years in patients with established CAD, as compared with placebo. However, some of the secondary endpoints that included a need for coronary revascularization were significantly lower. It is possible that this drug might have potential benefit in specific subsets (such as smokers), and will need to be further prospectively explored in future studies.[https://www.acc.org/Latest-in-Cardiology/Clinical-Trials/2014/09/01/16/30/STABILITY?w_nav=RI]
4.	Rosuvastatin	Does rosuvastatin delay progression of atherosclerosis in HIV	NCT01813357	Phase 4	August 28, 2020	Rosuvastatin effectively lowers LDL and appears to substantially slow progression of CCA-IMT in patients with treated HIV infection. In conclusion, 10mg of daily rosuvastatin lowers LDL by 20–25% and appears to slow progression of caroid IMT in patients with treated HIV infection [40].

Continued

TABLE 1 Recent clinical trials for the treatment of aaherosclerosis—cont'd

Sl. No	Name of the therapeutic	Description of the study	NCT number	Phase	End date	Outcome
5.	Alirocumab	ODYSSEY outcomes: evaluation of cardiovascular outcomes after an acute coronary syndrome during treatment with alirocumab	NCT01663402	Phase 3	March 18, 2019	The ODYSSEY OUTCOMES trial showed that use of alirocumab, taken every other week, significantly reduces ischemic events, including all-cause mortality and MI, compared with placebo among patients with an ACS event within the preceding 1–12 months.[https://www.acc.org/latest-in-cardiology/clinical-trials/2018/03/09/08/02/odyssey-outcomes]
6.	Anacetrapib	REVEAL: randomized evaluation of the effects of anacetrapib through lipid-modification (REVEAL)	NCT01252953	Phase 3	June 17, 2020	The HPS3/TIMI55-REVEAL trial showed that anacetrapib was superior to placebo at preventing adverse cardiac events [41].
7.	Inclisiran Sodium	Inclisiran for participants with atherosclerotic cardiovascular disease and elevated low-density lipoprotein cholesterol (ORION-10)	NCT03399370 NCT03400800	Phase 3	October 5, 2020	Reductions in LDL cholesterol levels of approximately 50% were obtained with inclisiran, administered subcutaneously every 6 months. More injection-site adverse events occurred with inclisiran than with placebo [42].
8.	Bempedoic Acid	Evaluation of the efficacy and safety of bempedoic acid (ETC-1002) as add-on to ezetimibe therapy in patients with elevated LDL-C (CLEAR Tranquility)	NCT03001076	Phase 3	May 11, 2020	Bempedoic acid may provide an oral therapeutic option complementary to ezetimibe in statin intolerant patients who require additional LDL-C lowering [43].
9.	EpaNova	Outcomes study to assess statin residual risk reduction with EpaNova in high CV risk patients with hypertriglyceridemia (STRENGTH)	NCT02104817	Phase 3	July 28, 2021	The STRENGTH trial failed to show that omega-3 CA was superior to placebo at reducing adverse cardiovascular outcomes.[https://www.acc.org/latest-in-cardiology/clinical-trials/2020/11/21/29/strength]
10.	Bempedoic Acid	Assessment of the long-term safety and efficacy of bempedoic acid (CLEAR Harmony OLE)	NCT03067441	Phase 3	March 1, 2021	Durable lipid lowering was observed through 78 weeks of BA treatment and patient adherence to BA therapy was high (86.2%). Overall safety during the OLE was similar to results reported in the 52-week-long CLEAR Harmony study and the overall BA phase 3 clinical program, with no new safety findings [44].

#	Drug	Title	NCT Number	Phase	Date	Description
11.	Bempedoic Acid	Evaluation of long-term efficacy of bempedoic acid (ETC-1002) in patients with hyperlipidemia at high cardiovascular risk (CLEAR Wisdom)	NCT02991118	Phase 3	April 27, 2020	The CLEAR Wisdom trial showed that bempedoic acid is safe and effective in reducing LDL-C compared with placebo among patients with ASCVD or heterogeneous FH on maximum-tolerated statin therapy. [https://www.acc.org/latest-in-cardiology/clinical-trials/2019/03/16/23/43/clear-wisdom]
12.	Bempedoic Acid	Evaluation of long-term safety and tolerability of ETC-1002 in high-risk patients with hyperlipidemia and high CV risk (CLEAR Harmony)	NCT02666664	Phase 3	May 11, 2020	Safety and efficacy of bempedoic acid to reduce LDL cholesterol [45].
13.	Inclisiran	Inclisiran for subjects with ASCVD or ASCVD-risk equivalents and elevated low-density lipoprotein cholesterol (ORION-11)	NCT03399370NCT03400800	Phase 3	August 21, 2020	Reductions in LDL cholesterol levels of approximately 50% were obtained with inclisiran, administered subcutaneously every 6 months. More injection-site adverse events occurred with inclisiran than with placebo [42].
14.	EzetimibeNiaspan	Effectiveness of intensive lipid modification medication in preventing the progression of peripheral arterial disease (The ELIMIT Study)	NCT00687076	Phase 4	February 6, 2020	The effect of lipid modification on peripheral artery disease after endovascular intervention trial (ELIMIT) [46].
15.	Darapladib	The stabilization of plaques using darapladib-thrombolysis in myocardial infarction 52 trial (SOLID-TIMI 52)	NCT01000727	Phase 3	August 10, 2017	Study design and rationale for the stabilization of plaques using darapladib-thrombolysis in myocardial infarction (SOLID-TIMI 52) trial in patients after an acute coronary syndrome [https://www.acc.org/latest-in-cardiology/articles/2014/08/31/03/00/solid-timi-52-the-stabilization-of-plaques-using-darapladib-thrombolysis-in-mi-52].
16.	Bempedoic Acid + Ezetimibe	A Study evaluating the safety and efficacy of bempedoic acid plus ezetimibe fixed-dose combination compared to bempedoic acid, ezetimibe, and placebo in patients treated with maximally tolerated statin therapy	NCT03337308	Phase 3	April 8, 2020	Bempedoic acid plus ezetimibe fixed-dose combination in patients with hypercholesterolemia and high CVD risk treated with maximally tolerated statin therapy [47].

The SPIRE-2 trial reduced the risk of major vascular events (CVD, MI, stroke, or urgent revascularization) by 1 year of bococizumab treatment by 14.5% per mmol/L reduction in LDL-C (HR: 0.85, 95% CI: 0.75–0.98), which is very similar to the CTT meta-analysis's that showed 12% reduction in major vascular events after 1 year of statin treatment. Similarly, the FOURIER trial found that 2.2 years of evolocumab treatment reduced the risk of major vascular events by 16% per mmol/L reduction in LDL-C (HR: 0.84, 95% CI: 0.80–0.88), which is nearly identical to the CTT meta-analysis's of 17% reduction in major vascular events after 2 years of statin treatment. The effectiveness of PCSK9 inhibitors in lowering LDL-C was enhanced in the FOURIER and ODYSSER OUTCOME studies [48–50].

4 HDL-C increasing therapy

4.1 Cholesteryl ester transfer protein (CETP) inhibitors

High-density lipoprotein (HDL) and apolipoprotein B100-containing lipoproteins can interchange triglycerides and cholesteryl ester through the Cholesteryl Ester Transfer Protein (CETP). CETP has the overall effect of transporting CE from HDL to both VLDL and LDL, while TG is transported in the other way [51]. The fact that common gene variations and hereditary CETP impairment have been discovered to be related to hyperalphaproteinemia, lower LDL-C levels, and a lower risk of CHD that encouraged the identification of CETP inhibition as a pharmacological target. However, the results observed for the CETP inhibitors in the clinical trials are not promising due to their associated side effects that resulted in their discontinuation. The CETP inhibitors dalcetrapib and evacetrapib lack clinically meaningful efficacy and were discontinued from further development [52], while toracetib was withdrawn due to the increased risk of death [53]. Another CETP inhibitor anacetrapib in the REVEAL (randomized evaluation of the effects of anacetrapib through lipid modification) trial doubled HDL cholesterol, reduced non-HDL cholesterol, and reduced major vascular events by 9% over 4 years; however, anacetrapib was found to accumulate in adipose tissue, so despite its early promise, CETP inhibition does not give enough cardiovascular benefit for therapeutic usage [51].

4.2 LCAT inhibitors

HDL combines cholesterol from cholesterol-rich macrophages, which is subsequently esterified by the lecithin:cholesterol acyltransferase (LCAT) attached to HDL in the process of reverse cholesterol transport (RCT). ApoA-I, the most abundant structural apolipoprotein in HDL, promotes LCAT esterification of cholesterol in HDL. In a phase I research, recombinant human LCAT (rhLCAT:

MEDI6012), which elevates HDL-C and enhances cholesterol efflux, was shown to be safe and tested for CHD in phase II studies. In this phase 2a double-blind study, 48 subjects with stable coronary heart disease on a statin were randomly assigned to receive a single dose of MEDI6012 or placebo (6:2) (NCT02601560), with ascending doses administered intravenously (24, 80, 240, and 800 mg) and subcutaneously (24, 80, 240, and 800 mg) (80 and 600 mg). MEDI6012 with an area under the concentration-time curves from 0 to 96 h, showed dose-dependent increases in high-density lipoprotein cholesterol. MEDI6012 had a good safety profile and improved the efflux capacity of high-density lipoprotein cholesterol, endogenous apoA1, and non-ATP-binding cassette transporter A1 cholesterol while decreasing the amount of atherogenic low-density lipoprotein particles [54].

Several small molecule inhibitors targeting LCAT have been discovered, such as (3-(5-(ethylthio)-1,3,4-thiadiazol-2-ylthio)pyrazine-2-carbonitrile)), which binds covalently to Cys31 in the active site of LCAT, monocyclic β-lactams, piperidinylpyrazolopyridine activator, and isopropyl dodecyl fluorophosphonate (IDFP), a covalent inhibitors with (3-(5-(ethylthio)-1,3,4-thiadiazol-2-ylthio)pyrazine-2-carbonitrile)), and monocyclic β-lactams showing off target effects. However, such side effects were less observed for the piperidinylpyrazolopyridine activator [55].

5 Angiopoietin-like 3 (ANGPTL3) inhibition

Hypertriglyceridemia is linked to an elevated risk of cardiovascular disease and is thought to be caused by a reduction in lipoprotein clearance. Angiopoietin-like protein 3 (ANGPTL3) increases triglycerides and other lipids via inhibiting lipoprotein lipase function. Two approaches have been considered in the targeting ANGPTL3 (1) monoclonal antibody that neutralizes serum levels of ANGPTL3 such as evinacumab [56] and (2) an antisense oligonucleotide that inhibits hepatocyte synthesis of ANGPTL3 such as vupanorsen [57]. In two Phase 1 trials, Evinacumab, an ANGPTL3 inhibitor, decreased triglycerides in healthy adult volunteers and was well tolerated. Lipid alterations in hypertriglyceridemia were comparable to those seen in ANGPTL3 loss-of-function mutants. ANGPTL3 inhibition may enhance the clinical result, since it is linked to a lower risk of cardiovascular disease.

Vupanorsen is an antisense oligonucleotide that prevents ANGPTL3 from being produced upstream. Patients with hypertriglyceridemia, type 2 diabetes, and hepatic steatosis were treated with subcutaneous vupanorsen or placebo in a phase 2 double-blind, placebo-controlled study to see if their triglyceride levels changed. Vupanorsen treatment was linked to a 53% decrease in triglycerides after 6 months (CI −43% to −60%; p-value 0.0001). Secondary endpoints revealed Apo-C III (58%) reductions, remnant cholesterol (38%) reductions, total cholesterol (19%) reductions, and HDL-C (24%) reductions [all p 0.0001], but no significant change in LDL-C.

6 Immunotherapy for atherosclerosis and cardiovascular disease

A recent review of the relationship between lipids, lipid-lowering treatment, and inflammation concluded that inflammation is a key regulator of atherosclerosis, both reliant and independent of lipids. The Canakinumab Antiinflammatory Thrombosis Outcome Study (CANTOS) has demonstrated that targeting a proinflammatory mediator, interleukin (IL)-1β, is effective in lowering the risk of CVD deaths in patients with residual inflammation without affecting the LDL levels [58]. Despite the limitations of immunotherapy in CVD Anti IL-1β medication, according to a substudy from the CANTOS trial, decreased the number of post-MI patients with hsCRP levels who were hospitalized for HF, as well as HF-related mortality in this patient group, suggesting that immunotherapy may be helpful for a specific population of HF patients [59]. Recent research has demonstrated that, in addition to the innate immune system, adaptive immunity plays an important role in HF. Effector T cells are harmful to normal cardiac remodeling after MI, and regulatory T cells have been shown to inhibit effector T-cell responses in experimental HF [60]. The activation of a network of immune cells and inflammatory pathways occurs during the inflammatory phase in atherosclerosis. Apart from the IL1b-IL6-CRP axis, research over the last three decades has revealed that four other inflammatory pathways are important in atherosclerosis and may 1 day become a therapeutic medication target for the treatment of CVD. Chemokines and their receptors, immunological checkpoints, immune-metabolism pathways, and hormones and lipid mediators are all examples of these pathways [61].

7 Epigenetics in atherosclerosis

Several vascular cells in atherosclerosis (primarily endothelial cells, VSMCs, and monocytes/macrophages) have global epigenetic changes that complement genetic abnormalities. Many comparable processes exist in the development of cardiovascular illnesses and malignancies, such as oxidative stress, inflammation, and sensitivity to shared risk factors. There have been several published studies on the role of epigenetics in CVD. In this context, several epigenetic drugs are used in the treatment of atherosclerosis. In numerous well-established animal models of atherosclerosis, including diet-induced atherosclerosis, the 5-Aza-2′-deoxycytidine are FDA-approved nucleoside-based DNMTi that block DNA methylation efficiently suppresses atherosclerosis progression. By pharmacologically activating KLF2, a prospective target for treating atherosclerosis, the pan-HDAC inhibitor SAHA (suberoylanilide hydroxamic acid), a clinically utilized medication for treating T cell cutaneous lymphoma, reduces vascular inflammation and atherosclerotic lesion. Furthermore, the pan-HDAC inhibitors phenylbutyrate and valproic acid, which have also shown therapeutic benefits in mice models of experimental atherosclerosis. By selectively binding to the BD2 domain (second bromodomain) of BRD4, the BET inhibitor (bromodomain and extra-terminal domain) RVX-208 (also known as apabetalone) raises ApoAI and HDL levels, therefore enhancing HDL functioning (such as cholesterol efflux and antiinflammatory properties). RVX-208 patients exhibit lower levels of circulating inflammatory cytokines and a decreased risk of severe adverse cardiac events.

MiRNA is a viable therapeutic target for treating atherosclerosis because of its complex regulatory network. MiRNA mimics or inhibitors can be delivered locally or systemically [15].

8 MicroRNAs in atherosclerosis

The most prevalent hereditary type of dyslipidemia, familial hypercholesterolemia (FH), is a leading cause of early cardiovascular disease. The effectiveness of therapies that lower plasma low-density lipoprotein (LDL) cholesterol (LDL-C) concentrations is crucial in the management of FH. RNA-based methods have shown promise as new treatments for human diseases during the last decade. Endogenously produced noncoding short hairpin RNAs, called miRs and siRNAs, limit gene expression via RNA interference (RNAi) pathways. The introduction of a synthetic siRNA into target cells is used in siRNA-based therapeutic methods to inhibit the production of a specific mRNA and produce a gene silencing effect. Inclisiran (previously ALN-PCS), an siRNA-based cholesterol-lowering drug, has completed a phase II study in 497 patients with a baseline LDL-C of less than 130 mg/dL. Inclisiran was generally well tolerated, with 54% of patients experiencing treatment-emergent adverse events, regardless of whether they were given placebo or inclisiran, and no differences in inclisiran dosages. Inclisiran caused injection site responses in 3.2% of patients, which were mild to severe and usually transitory. With modest and occasional subcutaneous injections, Inclisiran appears to produce a long-lasting decrease in PCSK9 and LDL-C levels [19].

9 New therapeutic opportunities for atherosclerosis

TET2 is a methylcytosine dioxygenase that converts 5-methylcytosine (5mC) to 5-hydroxymethylcytosine (5hmC). TET2 deficiency is linked to progressive atherosclerotic lesions. TET2 has been linked to phenotypic change of vascular smooth muscle cells, endothelial dysfunction, and macrophage inflammation, all of which are important contributors in atherosclerosis. As a result, TET2 might be a therapeutic target for atherosclerosis [62].

Interferon-activated macrophages generate neopterin, a guanosine triphosphate metabolite that is expressed at high levels in atheromatous plaques in the human carotid and coronary arteries, as well as the aorta. The amount of neopterin in the blood is linked to the degree of coronary artery disease. In individuals with atherosclerosis, however, a prospective cohort study found that neopterin helps to prevent plaque development in the carotid arteries. Furthermore, neopterin's atheroprotective properties have been demonstrated in a recent study employing both in vitro and in vivo studies. Tetrahydroneopterin (BH4), a neopterin derivative that acts as a cofactor for nitric oxide (NO) synthases, inhibits atherosclerosis and vascular injury-induced neointimal hyperplasia suggesting neopterin derivatives are a novel therapeutic target for atherosclerosis [63,64].

Long noncoding RNAs (lncRNAs) are expressed differently at various stages of atherosclerosis. In advanced atherosclerotic lesions and macrophages, the key lncRNA involved in the development and intervention of atherosclerosis (RAPIA) is substantially expressed. By competitively binding to microRNA-183-5p, which represses the production of ITGB1 (integrin 1), RAPIA partly stimulates macrophage proliferation and prevents apoptosis.

Inhibition of RAPIA in vivo slows the development of atherosclerosis and has atheroprotective effects on advanced atherosclerotic plaques comparable to atorvastatin.

Inhibition of RAPIA/MIR222HG might be a viable alternative therapy for advanced atherosclerotic plaques, particularly in individuals who are statin resistant or intolerant [65].

In patients with acute MI, inhibiting the terminal complement component with pexelizumab, for example, had no effect on outcomes [66]. The preliminary phase of a large-scale clinical study with the MAPK inhibitor losmapimod (LATITUDE) also failed to show therapeutic advantages, necessitating the target's removal [67]. Treatment of CVD with methotrexate, a broad-spectrum antiinflammatory drug, on the other hand, had no effect in lowering CVD risk or death [68].

Caveolin-1 is a key pathophysiological component in the progression of atherosclerosis. Caveolin-1 has been shown in previous research to have a pathogenic role in atherosclerosis through regulating membrane trafficking, cholesterol metabolism, and cellular signal transduction. Endothelial caveolin-1 is important in the early stages of atherosclerosis because it promotes ox-LDL absorption by endocytosis and perhaps transcytosis across endothelial cells, as well as endothelial permeability disruption. Despite caveolin-1's

inhibitory impact on eNOS, a noninhibitory caveolin-1 (Cav1 F92A), created by replacing alanine with phenylalanine, was found to enhance eNOS expression and NO production [69].

The main receptor for oxidized low-density lipoprotein (Ox-LDL) in the aorta of elderly rats is lectin-like oxidized low-density lipoprotein receptor-1 (LOX-1). Both animal and human individuals with hypercholesterolemia activate LOX-1 in the endothelium of lipid-accumulating sites. Targeting LOX-1 for hypercholesterolemia and vascular disorders might be a potential diagnostic approach. Atorvastatin was found to interact with LOX1, and aegeline at a dosage of 20 mg/kg body weight is beneficial in lowering lipid abnormalities in elderly hypercholesterolemic rats [70].

10 Conclusions

Atherosclerosis is a chronic inflammatory reaction of the vascular wall including the inflammatory influx of leukocytes and the activation of resident vascular cells in response to dyslipidemia and endothelial distress. In order to regulate atherosclerosis, lipid-lowering medication is a fundamental cornerstone of medical treatment for cardiovascular disease. The most effective way to reduce cardiovascular risk is through primary prevention. Obesity is the most pressing issue, and it has pleiotropic effects on blood pressure, lipid profiles, glucose metabolism, inflammation, and the advancement of atherothrombotic illness. The effectiveness of primary prevention is questionable, given the present constraints. Simultaneously, the repercussions of inaction and delay will undoubtedly be terrible, heightening the sense of urgency. Current recommendations already prescribe statins, ezetimibe, and new PCSK9-inhibitors, which have been demonstrated to enhance lipid profiles and reduce the risk of ischemic events and cardiovascular death. LDL, bempedoic acid, and the siRNA inclisiran have all shown encouraging outcomes. Furthermore, a monoclonal antibody named evinacumab as well as an antisense oligonucleotide targeting ANGPTL3 were found to be beneficial in reducing TG. The CANTOS study has produced compelling proof-of-concept for the inflammatory theory of atherosclerosis in humans, paving the path for the development of CVD immunotherapy. Canakinumab therapy significantly reduced the risk of main (MI, stroke, and CV mortality) and secondary endpoints. The discovery of new therapeutics and the recent advances may further open newer avenues for the treatment of atherosclerosis.

References

[1] E.J. Benjamin, S.S. Virani, C.W. Callaway, A.M. Chamberlain, A.-R. Chang, S. Cheng, S.E. Chiuve, M. Cushman, F.N. Delling, R. Deo, S.D. de Ferranti, J.F. Ferguson, M. Fornage, C. Gillespie,

C.R. Isasi, M.C. Jiménez, L.C. Jordan, S.E. Judd, D. Lackland, J.H. Lichtman, L. Lisabeth, S. Liu, C.T. Longenecker, P.L. Lutsey, J.S. Mackey, D.B. Matchar, K. Matsushita, M.E. Mussolino, K. Nasir, M. O'Flaherty, L.P. Palaniappan, A. Pandey, D.K. Pandey, M.J. Reeves, M.D. Ritchey, C.J. Rodriguez, G.A. Roth, W.D. Rosamond, U.K.A. Sampson, G.M. Satou, S.H. Shah, N.L. Spartano, D.L. Tirschwell, C.W. Tsao, J.H. Voeks, J.Z. Willey, J.T. Wilkins, J.H. Wu, H.M. Alger, S.S. Wong, P. Muntner, Heart disease and stroke Statistics-2018 update: a report from the American Heart Association, Circulation 137 (2018) e67–e492.

[2] M. Rafieian-Kopaei, M. Setorki, M. Doudi, A. Baradaran, H. Nasri, Atherosclerosis: process, indicators, risk factors and new hopes, Int. J. Prev. Med. 5 (2014) 927–946.

[3] S.S. Bhunia, K.K. Roy, A.K. Saxena, Profiling the structural determinants for the selectivity of representative factor-Xa and thrombin inhibitors using combined ligand-based and structure-based approaches, J. Chem. Inf. Model. 51 (2011) 1966–1985.

[4] S.S. Bhunia, A. Misra, I.A. Khan, S. Gaur, M. Jain, S. Singh, A. Saxena, T. Hohlfield, M. Dikshit, A.K. Saxena, Novel glycoprotein VI antagonists as Antithrombotics: synthesis, biological evaluation, and molecular modeling studies on 2,3-disubstituted Tetrahydropyrido(3,4-b)indoles, J. Med. Chem. 60 (2017) 322–337.

[5] J. Borén, M.J. Chapman, R.M. Krauss, C.J. Packard, J.F. Bentzon, C.J. Binder, M.J. Daemen, L.L. Demer, R.A. Hegele, S.J. Nicholls, B.G. Nordestgaard, G.F. Watts, E. Bruckert, S. Fazio, B.A. Ference, I. Graham, J.D. Horton, U. Landmesser, U. Laufs, L. Masana, G. Pasterkamp, F.J. Raal, K.K. Ray, H. Schunkert, M.-R. Taskinen, B. van de Sluis, O. Wiklund, L. Tokgozoglu, A.L. Catapano, H.N. Ginsberg, Low-density lipoproteins cause atherosclerotic cardiovascular disease: pathophysiological, genetic, and therapeutic insights: a consensus statement from the European atherosclerosis society consensus panel, Eur. Heart J. 41 (2020) 2313–2330.

[6] G.R. Geovanini, P. Libby, Atherosclerosis and inflammation: overview and updates, Clin. Sci. (Lond.) 132 (2018) 1243–1252.

[7] C.C. Low Wang, C.N. Hess, W.R. Hiatt, A.B. Goldfine, Clinical update: cardiovascular disease in diabetes mellitus: atherosclerotic cardiovascular disease and heart failure in type 2 diabetes mellitus - mechanisms, management, and clinical considerations, Circulation 133 (2016) 2459–2502.

[8] V. Lahera, M. Goicoechea, S.G. de Vinuesa, M. Miana, N. de las Heras, V. Cachofeiro, J. Luño, Endothelial dysfunction, oxidative stress and inflammation in atherosclerosis: beneficial effects of statins, Curr. Med. Chem. 14 (2007) 243–248.

[9] M. Shahreyar, S.A. Salem, M. Nayyar, L.K. George, N. Garg, S.K.G. Koshy, Hyperlipidemia: management with Proprotein convertase Subtilisin/Kexin type 9 (PCSK9) inhibitors, J. Am. Board Fam. Med. 31 (2018) 628–634.

[10] D. Leong, P.E. Wu, Proprotein convertase subtilisin-kexin type 9 (PCSK9) inhibitors, CMAJ 191 (2019) E894.

[11] M. Alkhalil, Proprotein convertase Subtilisin/Kexin type 9 (PCSK9) inhibitors, reality or dream in managing patients with cardiovascular disease, Curr. Drug Metab. 20 (2019) 72–82.

[12] R.S. Rosenson, R.A. Hegele, S. Fazio, C.P. Cannon, The evolving future of PCSK9 inhibitors, J. Am. Coll. Cardiol. 72 (2018) 314–329.

[13] K.H. Cho, Y.J. Hong, Proprotein convertase subtilisin/kexin type 9 inhibition in cardiovascular disease: current status and future perspectives, Korean J. Intern. Med. 35 (2020) 1045–1058.

[14] N. Bergeron, B.A.P. Phan, Y. Ding, A. Fong, R.M. Krauss, Proprotein convertase subtilisin/Kexin Type 9 inhibition, Circulation 132 (2015) 1648–1666.

[15] S. Xu, D. Kamato, P.J. Little, S. Nakagawa, J. Pelisek, Z.G. Jin, Targeting epigenetics and non-coding RNAs in atherosclerosis: from mechanisms to therapeutics, Pharmacol. Ther. 196 (2019) 15–43.

[16] C.T. Lambert, P. Sandesara, I. Isiadinso, M.C. Gongora, D. Eapen, N. Bhatia, J.T. Baer, L. Sperling, Current treatment of familial Hypercholesterolaemia, Eur. Cardiol. 9 (2014) 76–81.

[17] R. Alonso, A. Cuevas, P. Mata, Lomitapide: a review of its clinical use, efficacy, and tolerability, Core Evid. 14 (2019) 19–30.

[18] R.S. Geary, B.F. Baker, S.T. Crooke, Clinical and preclinical pharmacokinetics and pharmacodynamics of mipomersen (kynamro(®)): a second-generation antisense oligonucleotide inhibitor of apolipoprotein B, Clin. Pharmacokinet. 54 (2015) 133–146.

[19] A.A. Momtazi, M. Banach, M. Pirro, E.A. Stein, A. Sahebkar, MicroRNAs: new therapeutic targets for familial hypercholesterolemia? Clin Rev Allergy Immunol 54 (2018) 224–233.

[20] C.P. Cannon, M.A. Blazing, R.P. Giugliano, A. McCagg, J.A. White, P. Theroux, H. Darius, B.S. Lewis, T.O. Ophuis, J.W. Jukema, G.M. De Ferrari, W. Ruzyllo, P. De Lucca, K. Im, E.A. Bohula, C. Reist, S.D. Wiviott, A.M. Tershakovec, T.A. Musliner, E. Braunwald, R.M. Califf, Ezetimibe added to statin therapy after acute coronary syndromes, N. Engl. J. Med. 372 (2015) 2387–2397.

[21] A.L. Catapano, I. Graham, G. De Backer, O. Wiklund, M.J. Chapman, H. Drexel, A.W. Hoes, C.S. Jennings, U. Landmesser, T.R. Pedersen, Ž. Reiner, G. Riccardi, M.R. Taskinen, L. Tokgozoglu, W.M.M. Verschuren, C. Vlachopoulos, D.A. Wood, J.L. Zamorano, M.T. Cooney, 2016 ESC/EAS guidelines for the Management of Dyslipidaemias, Eur. Heart J. 37 (2016) 2999–3058.

[22] M. Banach, P. Jankowski, J. Jóźwiak, B. Cybulska, A. Windak, T. Guzik, A. Mamcarz, M. Broncel, T. Tomasik, J. Rysz, A. Jankowska-Zduńczyk, P. Hoffman, A. Mastalerz-Migas, PoLA/ CFPiP/PCS guidelines for the Management of Dyslipidaemias for family physicians 2016, Arch. Med. Sci. 13 (2017) 1–45.

[23] A. Endo, The discovery and development of HMG-CoA reductase inhibitors, J. Lipid Res. 33 (1992) 1569–1582.

[24] D.S. Gesto, C.M.S. Pereira, N.M.F.S. Cerqueira, S.F. Sousa, An atomic-level perspective of HMG-CoA-reductase: the target enzyme to treat hypercholesterolemia, Molecules (Basel, Switzerland) 25 (2020) 3891.

[25] H. Naci, J.J. Brugts, R. Fleurence, B. Tsoi, H. Toor, A.E. Ades, Comparative benefits of statins in the primary and secondary prevention of major coronary events and all-cause mortality: a network metaanalysis of placebo-controlled and active-comparator trials, Eur. J. Prev. Cardiol. 20 (2013) 641–657.

[26] H. Naci, J.J. Brugts, R. Fleurence, A.E. Ades, Dose-comparative effects of different statins on serum lipid levels: a network metaanalysis of 256,827 individuals in 181 randomized controlled trials, Eur. J. Prev. Cardiol. 20 (2013) 658–670.

[27] M. Tonelli, A. Lloyd, F. Clement, J. Conly, D. Husereau, B. Hemmelgarn, S. Klarenbach, F.A. McAlister, N. Wiebe, B. Manns, Efficacy of statins for primary prevention in people at low cardiovascular risk: a meta-analysis, CMAJ 183 (2011) E1189–E1202.

[28] H. Naci, J. Brugts, T. Ades, Comparative tolerability and harms of individual statins: a study-level network meta-analysis of 246 955

participants from 135 randomized, controlled trials, Circ. Cardiovasc. Qual. Outcomes 6 (2013) 390–399.

[29] J.W. Clader, The discovery of ezetimibe: a view from outside the receptor, J. Med. Chem. 47 (2004) 1–9.

[30] E.A. Nutescu, N.L. Shapiro, Ezetimibe: a selective cholesterol absorption inhibitor, Pharmacotherapy 23 (2003) 1463–1474.

[31] M.L.A.D. Lestari, F. Ardiana, G. Indrayanto, Chapter 3—Ezetimibe, in: H.G. Brittain (Ed.), Profiles of Drug Substances, Excipients and Related Methodology, Academic Press, 2011, pp. 103–149.

[32] J.-y. Liu, W.-q. Fu, X.-j. Zheng, W. Li, L.-w. Ren, J.-h. Wang, C. Yang, G.-h. Du, Avasimibe exerts anticancer effects on human glioblastoma cells via inducing cell apoptosis and cell cycle arrest, Acta Pharmacol. Sin. 42 (2021) 97–107.

[33] J.A. Sikorski, 6.20 - Atherosclerosis/lipoprotein/cholesterol metabolism, in: J.B. Taylor, D.J. Triggle (Eds.), Comprehensive Medicinal Chemistry II, Elsevier, Oxford, 2007, pp. 459–494.

[34] Clinical Trial, Atherosclerosis drug fails to meet Phase III trial end point, Nat. Rev. Drug Discov. 8 (2009) 348.

[35] Clinical Trial, The Lipid Research Clinics Coronary Primary Prevention Trial results. I. Reduction in incidence of coronary heart disease, JAMA 251 (1984) 351–364.

[36] I. Jialal, S.L. Abby, S. Misir, S. Nagendran, Concomitant reduction in low-density lipoprotein cholesterol and glycated hemoglobin with colesevelam hydrochloride in patients with type 2 diabetes: a pooled analysis, Metab. Syndr. Relat. Disord. 7 (2009) 255–258.

[37] J.F. Brensike, R.I. Levy, S.F. Kelsey, E.R. Passamani, J.M. Richardson, I.K. Loh, N.J. Stone, R.F. Aldrich, J.W. Battaglini, D.J. Moriarty, et al., Effects of therapy with cholestyramine on progression of coronary arteriosclerosis: results of the NHLBI type II coronary intervention study, Circulation 69 (1984) 313–324.

[38] C.F. Semenkovich, A.C. Goldberg, I.J. Goldberg, CHAPTER 37—Disorders of lipid metabolism, in: S. Melmed, K.S. Polonsky, P.R. Larsen, H.M. Kronenberg (Eds.), Williams Textbook of Endocrinology, twelfth ed., W.B. Saunders, Philadelphia, 2011, pp. 1633–1674.

[39] A.C. Burke, D.E. Telford, M.W. Huff, Bempedoic acid: effects on lipoprotein metabolism and atherosclerosis, Curr. Opin. Lipidol. 30 (2019) 1–9.

[40] C.T. Longenecker, A. Sattar, R. Gilkeson, G.A. McComsey, Rosuvastatin slows progression of subclinical atherosclerosis in patients with treated HIV infection, AIDS 30 (2016) 2195–2203.

[41] L. Bowman, F. Chen, E. Sammons, J.C. Hopewell, K. Wallendszus, W. Stevens, E. Valdes-Marquez, S. Wiviott, C.P. Cannon, E. Braunwald, R. Collins, M.J. Landray, Randomized evaluation of the effects of Anacetrapib through lipid-modification (REVEAL)-a large-scale, randomized, placebo-controlled trial of the clinical effects of anacetrapib among people with established vascular disease: trial design, recruitment, and baseline characteristics, Am. Heart J. 187 (2017) 182–190.

[42] K.K. Ray, R.S. Wright, D. Kallend, W. Koenig, L.A. Leiter, F.J. Raal, J.A. Bisch, T. Richardson, M. Jaros, P.L.J. Wijngaard, J.J.P. Kastelein, Two phase 3 trials of Inclisiran in patients with elevated LDL cholesterol, N. Engl. J. Med. 382 (2020) 1507–1519.

[43] C.M. Ballantyne, M. Banach, G.B.J. Mancini, N.E. Lepor, J.C. Hanselman, X. Zhao, L.A. Leiter, Efficacy and safety of bempedoic acid added to ezetimibe in statin-intolerant patients with hypercholesterolemia: a randomized, placebo-controlled study, Atherosclerosis 277 (2018) 195–203.

[44] C.M. Ballantyne, M. Banach, H.E. Bays, A.L. Catapano, U. Laufs, E.S.G. Stroes, L. Bloedon, A. Feng, P. Robinson, K.K. Ray, Long-term safety and efficacy of bempedoic acid in patients at high risk of atherosclerotic cardiovascular disease: results from the CLEAR harmony open-label extension study, Eur. Heart J. 41 (2020).

[45] K.K. Ray, H.E. Bays, A.L. Catapano, N.D. Lalwani, L.T. Bloedon, L.R. Sterling, P.L. Robinson, C.M. Ballantyne, Safety and efficacy of bempedoic acid to reduce LDL cholesterol, N. Engl. J. Med. 380 (2019) 1022–1032.

[46] G. Brunner, E.Y. Yang, A. Kumar, W. Sun, S.S. Virani, S.I. Negi, T. Murray, P.H. Lin, R.C. Hoogeveen, C. Chen, J.F. Dong, P. Kougias, A. Taylor, A.B. Lumsden, V. Nambi, C.M. Ballantyne, J.D. Morrisett, The effect of lipid modification on peripheral artery disease after endovascular intervention trial (ELIMIT), Atherosclerosis 231 (2013) 371–377.

[47] C.M. Ballantyne, U. Laufs, K.K. Ray, L.A. Leiter, H.E. Bays, A.C. Goldberg, E.S. Stroes, D. MacDougall, X. Zhao, A.L. Catapano, Bempedoic acid plus ezetimibe fixed-dose combination in patients with hypercholesterolemia and high CVD risk treated with maximally tolerated statin therapy, Eur. J. Prev. Cardiol. 27 (2020) 593–603.

[48] B.A. Ference, C.P. Cannon, U. Landmesser, T.F. Lüscher, A.L. Catapano, K.K. Ray, Reduction of low density lipoprotein-cholesterol and cardiovascular events with proprotein convertase subtilisin-kexin type 9 (PCSK9) inhibitors and statins: an analysis of FOURIER, SPIRE, and the cholesterol treatment Trialists collaboration, Eur. Heart J. 39 (2018) 2540–2545.

[49] R.A. Alali, A short review of proprotein convertase subtilisin/kexin type 9 inhibitors, Rev. Cardiovasc. Med. 20 (2019) 1–8.

[50] C. Singh, D.J. Valero, J. Nisar, J.I. Trujillo Ramirez, K.K. Kothari, S. Isola, A.M. San Hernandez, D.K. Gordon, Statins versus Proprotein convertase Subtilisin/Kexin type 9 inhibitors- are we doing better? A systematic review on treatment disparity, Cureus 12 (2020). e10965.

[51] J.A. Hunt, Z. Lu, Cholesteryl ester transfer protein (CETP) inhibitors, Curr. Top. Med. Chem. 9 (2009) 419–427.

[52] H. Taheri, K.B. Filion, S.B. Windle, P. Reynier, M.J. Eisenberg, Cholesteryl ester transfer protein inhibitors and cardiovascular outcomes: a systematic review and meta-analysis of randomized controlled trials, Cardiology 145 (2020) 236–250.

[53] A. Ali, J. Duffy, 8.11—case histories: Anacetrapib, in: S. Chackalamannil, D. Rotella, S.E. Ward (Eds.), Comprehensive Medicinal Chemistry III, Elsevier, Oxford, 2017, pp. 284–307.

[54] R.T. George, L. Abuhatzira, S.M. Stoughton, S.K. Karathanasis, D. She, C. Jin, N. Buss, R. Bakker-Arkema, E.L. Ongstad, M. Koren, B. Hirshberg, MEDI6012: recombinant human lecithin cholesterol acyltransferase, high-density lipoprotein, and Low-density lipoprotein receptor-mediated reverse cholesterol transport, J. Am. Heart Assoc. 10 (2021), e014572.

[55] K.A. Manthei, S.-M. Yang, B. Baljinnyam, L. Chang, A. Glukhova, W. Yuan, L.A. Freeman, D.J. Maloney, A. Schwendeman, A.T. Remaley, A. Jadhav, J.J.G. Tesmer, Molecular basis for activation of lecithin:cholesterol acyltransferase by a compound that increases HDL cholesterol, Elife 7 (2018), e41604.

[56] F.E. Dewey, V. Gusarova, R.L. Dunbar, C. O'Dushlaine, C. Schurmann, O. Gottesman, S. McCarthy, C.V. Van Hout, S. Bruse, H.M. Dansky, J.B. Leader, M.F. Murray, M.D. Ritchie, H.L. Kirchner, L. Habegger, A. Lopez, J. Penn, A. Zhao, W. Shao, N. Stahl, A.J. Murphy, S. Hamon, A. Bouzelmat, R. Zhang, B. Shumel, R. Pordy, D. Gipe, G.A. Herman, W.H.H. Sheu, I.T. Lee,

K.-W. Liang, X. Guo, J.I. Rotter, Y.-D.I. Chen, W.E. Kraus, S.H. Shah, S. Damrauer, A. Small, D.J. Rader, A.B. Wulff, B.G. Nordestgaard, A. Tybjærg-Hansen, A.M. van den Hoek, H.M.G. Princen, D.H. Ledbetter, D.J. Carey, J.D. Overton, J.G. Reid, W.J. Sasiela, P. Banerjee, A.R. Shuldiner, I.B. Borecki, T.M. Teslovich, G.D. Yancopoulos, S.J. Mellis, J. Gromada, A. Baras, Genetic and pharmacologic inactivation of ANGPTL3 and cardiovascular disease, N. Engl. J. Med. 377 (2017) 211–221.

[57] M.J. Graham, R.G. Lee, T.A. Brandt, L.-J. Tai, W. Fu, R. Peralta, R. Yu, E. Hurh, E. Paz, B.W. McEvoy, B.F. Baker, N.C. Pham, A. Digenio, S.G. Hughes, R.S. Geary, J.L. Witztum, R.M. Crooke, S. Tsimikas, Cardiovascular and metabolic effects of ANGPTL3 antisense oligonucleotides, N. Engl. J. Med. 377 (2017) 222–232.

[58] P.M. Ridker, B.M. Everett, T. Thuren, J.G. MacFadyen, W.H. Chang, C. Ballantyne, F. Fonseca, J. Nicolau, W. Koenig, S.D. Anker, J.J.P. Kastelein, J.H. Cornel, P. Pais, D. Pella, J. Genest, R. Cifkova, A. Lorenzatti, T. Forster, Z. Kobalava, L. Vida-Simiti, M. Flather, H. Shimokawa, H. Ogawa, M. Dellborg, P.R.F. Rossi, R.P.T. Troquay, P. Libby, R.J. Glynn, Antiinflammatory therapy with Canakinumab for atherosclerotic disease, N. Engl. J. Med. 377 (2017) 1119–1131.

[59] B.M. Everett, J.H. Cornel, M. Lainscak, S.D. Anker, A. Abbate, T. Thuren, P. Libby, R.J. Glynn, P.M. Ridker, Anti-inflammatory therapy with Canakinumab for the prevention of hospitalization for heart failure, Circulation 139 (2019) 1289–1299.

[60] S.S. Bansal, M.A. Ismahil, M. Goel, G. Zhou, G. Rokosh, T. Hamid, S.D. Prabhu, Dysfunctional and Proinflammatory regulatory T-lymphocytes are essential for adverse cardiac remodeling in ischemic cardiomyopathy, Circulation 139 (2019) 206–221.

[61] E. Lutgens, D. Atzler, Y. Döring, J. Duchene, S. Steffens, C. Weber, Immunotherapy for cardiovascular disease, Eur. Heart J. 40 (2019) 3937–3946.

[62] Y. Liu, W. Peng, K. Qu, X. Lin, Z. Zeng, J. Chen, D. Wei, Z. Wang, TET2: a novel epigenetic regulator and potential intervention target for atherosclerosis, DNA Cell Biol. 37 (2018) 517–523.

[63] T. Watanabe, Neopterin derivatives - a novel therapeutic target rather than biomarker for atherosclerosis and related diseases, Vasa 50 (2021) 165–173.

[64] J.B. Pierce, M.W. Feinberg, Long noncoding RNAs in atherosclerosis and vascular injury: pathobiology, biomarkers, and targets for therapy, Arterioscler. Thromb. Vasc. Biol. 40 (2020) 2002–2017.

[65] C. Sun, Y. Fu, X. Gu, X. Xi, X. Peng, C. Wang, Q. Sun, X. Wang, F. Qian, Z. Qin, W. Qu, M. Piao, S. Zhong, S. Liu, M. Zhang, S. Fang, J. Tian, C. Li, L. Maegdefessel, J. Tian, B. Yu, Macrophage-enriched lncRNA RAPIA, Arterioscler. Thromb. Vasc. Biol. 40 (2020) 1464–1478.

[66] P.W. Armstrong, C.B. Granger, P.X. Adams, C. Hamm, D. Holmes Jr., W.W. O'Neill, T.G. Todaro, A. Vahanian, F. Van de Werf, Pexelizumab for acute ST-elevation myocardial infarction in patients undergoing primary percutaneous coronary intervention: a randomized controlled trial, JAMA 297 (2007) 43–51.

[67] M.L. O'Donoghue, R. Glaser, M.A. Cavender, P.E. Aylward, M.P. Bonaca, A. Budaj, R.Y. Davies, M. Dellborg, K.A. Fox, J.A. Gutierrez, C. Hamm, R.G. Kiss, F. Kovar, J.F. Kuder, K.A. Im, J.J. Lepore, J.L. Lopez-Sendon, T.O. Ophuis, A. Parkhomenko, J.B. Shannon, J. Spinar, J.F. Tanguay, M. Ruda, P.G. Steg, P. Theroux, S.D. Wiviott, I. Laws, M.S. Sabatine, D.A. Morrow, Effect of Losmapimod on cardiovascular outcomes in patients hospitalized with acute myocardial infarction: a randomized clinical trial, JAMA 315 (2016) 1591–1599.

[68] P.M. Ridker, B.M. Everett, A. Pradhan, J.G. MacFadyen, D.H. Solomon, E. Zaharris, V. Mam, A. Hasan, Y. Rosenberg, E. Iturriaga, M. Gupta, M. Tsigoulis, S. Verma, M. Clearfield, P. Libby, S.Z. Goldhaber, R. Seagle, C. Ofori, M. Saklayen, S. Butman, N. Singh, M. Le May, O. Bertrand, J. Johnston, N.P. Paynter, R.J. Glynn, Low-dose methotrexate for the prevention of atherosclerotic events, N. Engl. J. Med. 380 (2018) 752–762.

[69] J. Tian, M.S. Popal, R. Huang, M. Zhang, X. Zhao, M. Zhang, X. Song, Caveolin as a novel potential therapeutic target in cardiac and vascular diseases: a Mini review, Aging Dis. 11 (2020) 378–389.

[70] A. Singh, A.K. Srinivasan, L.N. Chakrapani, P. Kalaiselvi, LOX-1, the common therapeutic target in hypercholesterolemia: a new perspective of Antiatherosclerotic action of Aegeline, Oxid. Med. Cell. Longev. 2019 (2019) 8285730.

Chapter 9

Targeting vascular inflammation in atherosclerosis with plant extracts, phytochemicals, and their advanced drug formulations

Kushal Sharma[a,*], Keshav Raj Paudel[b,*], Nisha Pantha[a], Saurav Kumar Jha[c], and Hari Prasad Devkota[d]

[a]College of Pharmacy and Natural Medicine Research Institute, Mokpo National University, Muan-gun, Jeonnam, Republic of Korea, [b]Department of Oriental Medicine Resources, Mokpo National University, Muan-gun, Jeonnam, Republic of Korea, [c]Department of Biomedicine, Health & Life Convergence Sciences, BK21, Mokpo National University, Muan-gun, Jeonnam, Republic of Korea, [d]Graduate School of Pharmaceutical Sciences, Kumamoto University, Kumamoto, Japan

1 Introduction

Atherosclerosis is an inflammatory disorder of blood vessels characterized by narrowing of vessel lumen that results in restricted blood flow and further cardiovascular complications [1]. The factors involved in the narrowing of vessels include the accumulation of modified lipids in the lumen, migration, and the proliferation of vascular smooth muscle cells (VSMCs) from tunica media to tunica intima (at the site of the atherogenic lesion) [2,3]. Various cells such as endothelial cells, macrophages, and VSMCs are involved in vascular inflammation [4,5]. The first event that triggers vascular inflammation initiation is endothelial dysfunction that attracts circulating cells and facilitates their adhesion to the endothelial layer mediated by the overexpression of adhesion molecules such as intercellular adhesion molecule (ICAM) and vascular cell adhesion molecule (VCAM) [6,7]. Then, circulating monocyte are recruited at the site of inflammation by monocyte chemoattractant protein-1 (MCP-1) followed by a change in phenotype from monocyte to tissue macrophage [8]. These macrophages are activated by various factors such as interferon (IFN)-γ, tumor necrosis factor (TNF)-α, and interleukin (IL)-4 followed by the release of reactive oxygen species, various inflammatory cytokines (IL-6, IL-1β, IL-8), and nitric oxide, and overexpression of cyclooxygenase (COX)-2 and inducible nitric oxide synthase (iNOS) protein [9–11]. Similarly, VSMCs are stimulated by mitogens such as TNF-α, VSMC-derived microparticles, and growth factors such as insulin and platelet-derived growth factor (PDGF) to undergo proliferation mediated by mitogen-activated protein kinase (MAPK) cell signaling pathway, and migration facilitates by overexpression of matrix metalloproteinase (MMP)-9 and MAPK [12–15]. Increasing number of studies are being conducted to explore a potential therapeutic agent that can target these inflammatory events to prevent or delay the progression of vascular inflammation [16]. Plant extracts and phytochemicals (plant-derived bioactive compounds) are also being investigated for their potential role in targeting vascular inflammation [17]. Meanwhile, to overcome the problems associated with the solubility and bioavailability of these phytochemicals, various novel drug delivery systems are also being investigated [18–21]. In this chapter, the role of plant extracts, phytochemicals, and their advanced drug formulation strategies for the management of atherosclerosis by controlling key hallmark features of vascular inflammation are discussed.

2 Plant extracts

Medicinal plants are one of the important sources of therapeutic agents for the management of multiple diseases such as cardiovascular disease [22], respiratory disease [23,24], cancer [25], diabetes [26,27], and hepatic disease [28]. Among these medicinal plants, few herbal extracts with promising beneficial activity against vascular inflammation/atherosclerosis are described below.

---

*Equal contribution.

Recent Developments in Anti-Inflammatory Therapy. https://doi.org/10.1016/B978-0-323-99988-5.00004-8

2.1 *Camellia japonica*

A high-fat diet (HDF)-fed rats as a model of atherosclerosis was developed by Lee et al. by feeding Wistar rats with 60% HFD for 1 month. To reveal the antiatherogenic activity of *C. japonica* fruit extracts, rats were orally administered 100, 400, and 800 mg/kg body weight of extract for 1 month along with HFD. The endpoint results showed dose-dependent decrease in serum total cholesterol, triglyceride, and low-density lipoprotein, and inhibition of the formation of oxidized low-density lipoprotein (LDL) as revealed by lipid peroxidation assay. This suggests that *C. japonica* fruits may act as a potent herbal therapeutic option for the management of atherosclerosis and hypercholesterolemia [29].

2.2 *Camellia sinensis*

Chungtaejeon (CTJ) is a Korean fermented tea prepared from tea leaves of *C. sinensis* which prevents the risk of atherosclerosis. Oral administration of 100, 200, and 400 mg/kg of CTJ for 20 days along with 60% HFD showed that CTJ dose dependently decreased the HFD and increased total (serum) cholesterol and hepatic cholesterol, LDL, while no significant change was observed in high-density lipoprotein. Similarly, there was an inhibition of PDGF-induced VSMC proliferation, MMP-9 enzymatic activity, and VSMC migration in both wound healing and transwell cell migration assay. Thus, consumption of green tea (*C. sinensis*) would be beneficial to prevent vascular inflammation/atherosclerosis [30].

2.3 *Morus alba*

The ethanol extract of *M. alba* root bark possess vascular protection activity by promoting endothelium-depending vasorelaxation in rat thoracic aorta in a dose-dependent manner. Mechanistically, it was revealed that the extract stimulates NO-mediated endothelium-dependent relaxation via nitric oxide-soluble guanylate cyclase pathway [31].

2.4 *Terminalia chebula*

An in vitro model of vascular inflammation established with human VSMC and mice macrophage (RAW264.7) was used to test the efficacy of *T. chebula* fruit aqueous extract. The results show that 24-h treatment of aqueous extract in VSMC stimulated with PDGF-BB inhibited proliferation by targeting MAPK expression (ERK, JNK, p38) and migration by targeting both MMP-9 protein expression and enzyme level. Furthermore, there was a dose-dependent decrease in cell adhesion molecules pFAK, Cdc42, and RhoA in VSMC. In RAW264,7 aqueous extract inhibited LPS and induced nitric oxide production and expression of iNOS and COX-2 protein [32].

2.5 Mixture of plant extracts

Kim et al. investigated the beneficial activity of seven different traditional Korean formulations (made from a mixture of medicinal plants) on rat model of atherosclerosis induced by balloon catheter injury of carotid artery. Among seven formulation, 4 weeks of oral administration of Samhwang-sasim-tang (a mixture of *Scutellaria baicalensis* radix, *Coptis japonica* rhizome and *Rheum palmatum* rhizome) at 400 mg/kg body weight significantly inhibited the intimal narrowing of carotid artery 28 days after balloon injury. Moreover, there was inhibition of VSMC proliferation and MMP-2 enzymatic activity in vitro suggesting potent efficacy of mixture of traditional Korean formulation against animal model of experimental atherosclerosis [33].

3 Phytochemicals

3.1 Terpenoids

Various phytochemicals isolated from plants not only have served as one of the main sources for modern drugs discovery, but are also widely used as functional foods, nutraceuticals, and supplements. Many compounds belonging to different chemical classes such as alkaloids, polyphenols, saponins, terpenoids, etc., are studied for their role in the prevention and management of vascular inflammation. Some of these compounds are explained in detail below.

3.2 Alkaloids

Nelumbo nucifera (lotus) is a good source of alkaloids such as neferine, liensinine, isoliensinine with potent in vitro and in vivo activity against vascular inflammation [34]. Jun et al. investigated the beneficial activity of alkaloid-rich fraction (ARF) from lotus in rat model of atherosclerosis induced by balloon injury of carotid artery. It was observed from the histological staining that ARF remarkably inhibited the narrowing of rat's carotid artery lumen [35]. Similarly, in vitro study carried in VSMC showed that liensinine (an alkaloid from lotus, Fig. 1) attenuate vascular inflammation by inhibiting PDGF-induced proliferation, TNF-a-induced migration by targeting MMP-9 enzymatic activity and IL-6 release [36]. Likewise, cepharanthine (a bisbenzylisoquinoline alkaloid, Fig. 1) from *Stephania cepharantha* was found to inhibit VSMC proliferation by inhibiting MAPK and NF-kB pathway and reduce the release of inflammation markers (nitric oxide, iNOS protein, COX-2 protein, and prostaglandin E_2 enzyme) from mice macrophage cell line RAW264.7 [11].

3.3 Polyphenols

Paudel et al. investigated the mechanism of attenuation of vascular inflammation by baicalin (a potent flavonoid

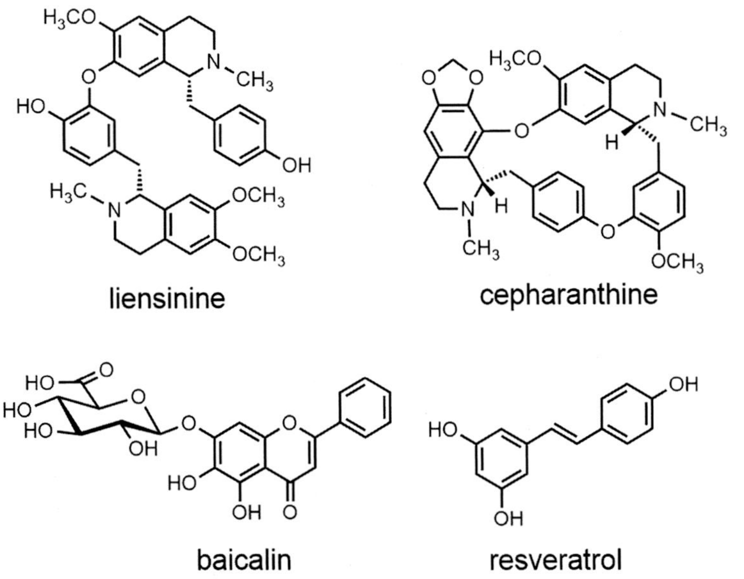

FIG. 1 Chemical structure of liensinine, cepharanthine, baicalin, and resveratrol. *(No permission required.)*

present in *Scutellaria baicalensis*, Fig. 1) using in vitro model in VSMC, macrophage, and endothelial cell line. Microparticles were isolated from these cells after stimulation (TNF-α for VSMC, LPS for macrophage and endothelial cells) and treated to healthy/unstimulated cells showed the hallmark features of vascular inflammation. This was revealed by endothelial dysfunction (ROS production, upregulation of ICAM, and downregulation of pENOS and pAkt), markers of inflammation from macrophage (iNOS, COX-2), VSMC proliferation, and migration. In contrast, treatment of baicalin at various dose ranging from 1 to 25 μM inhibited marker of endothelial dysfunction, release of inflammatory mediators from macrophage, VSMC proliferation, and migration [37].

Resveratrol (Fig. 1), a natural polyphenol, is abundantly present in grapes, red wines, peanut grapes, mulberries, and other plants [38]. Several animal and human studies have shown that resveratrol prevents atherosclerosis progression. Oxidation of low-density lipoprotein (LDL) is an early and critical event in the advancement of atherosclerosis [39]. The study showed that resveratrol ameliorates ROS production and enhances antioxidant enzymes (superoxide dismutase, catalase, glutathione peroxidase) [40]. Resveratrol inhibits LDL oxidation through its antioxidant activity and prevents the progression of atherosclerosis [41]. Similarly, resveratrol inhibits the production of inflammatory mediators, critical molecules in the genesis of atherosclerosis. A study showed that it inhibits interleukin-1, -2, -8, and -12, interferon-γ, and TNF-α [42]. In addition, it inhibits MCP1-induced monocyte migration, which is one mechanism to cause atherosclerosis [43]. Resveratrol decreases the expression of cell adhesion molecules such as ELAM, VCAM-1, and ICAM-1 [44]. Resveratrol suppresses VSMC proliferation,

a key mechanism to induce atherosclerosis [45]. It also inhibits platelet aggregation, an agent involved in the genesis of atherosclerosis [41].

Carotenoids, belonging to a class of terpenoids, are present in dark green, red, and dark orange fruits and vegetables [46]. Various in vitro studies have indicated that carotenoids can reduce the plasma level of cholesterol by inhibiting HMG-CoA reductase, which is the rate-limiting enzyme in cholesterol synthesis [47]. It may protect against atherosclerosis by reducing the oxidative damage of proteins, lipids, and lipoproteins. They are effective in lowering LDL peroxidation and preventing the development of atherosclerotic lesion. It has been shown to reduce numerous inflammatory biomarkers such as C-reactive proteins and interleukin related to atherosclerosis development [48]. Few studies have stated that carotenoid could also reduce cytokine level, which helps control diseases like atherosclerosis [49].

3.4 Saponins

Saponins, such as *Panax notoginseng* saponins (PNS), exert beneficial effects on atherosclerosis [50]. It was reported that notoginsenoside R1 significantly alleviated atherosclerotic lesions in ApoE$^{-/-}$ mice [51]. This attenuation was marked by a reduction in lipid deposition and inhibition of the production of inflammatory cytokines such as IL-2, IL-6, TNF-α, and γ-IFN [51]. Similarly, saponins from sea cucumber (SSC) might inhibit the progression of atherosclerotic lesions via their antiinflammatory and lipid-lowering biological properties. SSC could promote the cholesterol reverse transport in the liver and inhibit the expression of inflammatory cytokines in aortic lesions and peritoneal macrophages [52].

4   Vitamins

Vitamins are considered as promising nutraceuticals for the prevention of diverse pathologies, including atherosclerosis. Vitamin E has received the most attention since it considered potent antioxidants. Vitamin E is present in various foods and oils such as sunflowers, almonds, peanut butter, spinach, and corn. Several pieces of evidence have indicated that vitamin E is a protective agent against the progression of atherosclerosis. It ameliorates LDL oxidation and proliferation of smooth muscle cells. Similarly, it inhibits cholesterol synthesis by inhibiting HMG-CoA reductase and reduces synthesis of ICAM-1 and VCAM-1 [53,54]. It inhibits platelet adhesion and aggregation, adhesion molecules, leukotrienes synthesis, and monocyte adhesion [55]. It can lower circulating C reactive protein levels, an inflammatory marker associated with atherosclerosis [56].

5   Advanced drug delivery technology in targeting atherosclerosis

Currently, nanotechnology and nanomedicine as an advanced drug delivery system in cardiovascular diseases (CVDs) deal with four main aspects that either control or aids in the management of CVDs. These areas of nanotechnology are molecular imaging, diagnostics, targeted drug delivery, and tissue engineering [57]. In addition, there are various types of nanoparticulate drug delivery carriers or devices that are being used in CVDs and atherosclerosis. Moreover, atherosclerotic molecular markers could be the major targets, which can be exploited effectively to develop and deliver abovementioned potent herbal extract via targeted nanoparticles conjugated with specific ligands. Cellular components at atherosclerotic plaques are exposed to the circulation by the high expression of certain molecules and therefore could be efficiently targeted by nanoparticles. Nevertheless, the upregulated cellular receptors such as VCAM-I, ICAM-I, P-selectin, E-selectin, and avb3-integrin that are highly expressed on the endothelia of the luminal wall of microvasculature could be a promising target [58]. Interestingly, high-density lipoprotein (HDL) is responsible for the modulation of systemic inflammation. When there is no inflammation, HDL has a complement of antioxidant enzymes that function to maintain an anti-inflammatory state. While, in the case of systemic inflammation, these antioxidant enzymes can be inactivated and HDL can accumulate oxidized lipoproteins that make it proinflammatory. Thus, HDL is a vital factors in the targeted therapy of atherosclerosis. Therefore, increasing the half-life of HDL by PEGylating HDL could further favor its antiatherogenic functions [59].

Kulandaivelu et al. found that tea polyphenol (TPP) nanoparticles possess prolonged antioxidant activity (measured by in vitro free radical scavenging activity) compared with free TPP. Furthermore, in mice model, oral administration of TPP resulted in a significant decrease in cholesterol and triglyceride (a risk factor of atherosclerosis) [60]. Similarly, marrubiin (a widely known diterpenoid lactone)-loaded solid lipid nanoparticles were found to be protective against TNF-a-induced oxidative stress in human umbilical vein endothelial cells and this activity was higher compared to intact molecule (unloaded marrubiin) [61]. Tanshinone IIA was formulated into two different forms; discoidal and spherical recombinant high-density lipoprotein loaded (TA-d-rHDL and TA-s-rHDL) to study the pharmacokinetics and efficacy against atherosclerosis lesion. It was observed that both TA-d-rHDL and TA-s-rHDL improve the pharmacokinetics profile in rabbits and ex vivo imaging revealed that both formulations (s- and d-HDL) bound with strong affinity to atherosclerotic lesions than normal vascular walls. Comparatively, s-rHDL showed more precise targeting effect than d-HDL. On top of that, both formulations (d- and s-rHDL) showed better anti-atherogenic efficacy than traditional TA-nanostructured lipid carrier, TA liposomes, and commercial drug sulfotanshinone sodium injection [62].

Different types of nanocarriers like liposomes, metallic nanoparticles, dendrimers, micelles, and polymeric carriers are being used to effectively treat atherosclerosis. However, polymeric nanoparticles are considered as ideal nanodevice for targeting, because their small size not only facilitates the drug absorption into the wall of artery but also sustains release property. Furthermore, chelators like ethylenediaminetetraacetic acid (EDTA) can reabsorb the calcium mineral deposit, and therefore could be highly effective in treating atherosclerosis. However, its systemic use could have significant side effects. Hence, oral nanoparticulate delivery of chelating agent could be efficacious treatment modality for atherosclerosis. Although various cardiovascular nanocarriers are being widely investigated both in vitro and in vivo in preclinical and clinical trials, their commercialization is still under development. The stability and biological efficacy of tea polyphenol (TPP) in cardiovascular disease can be improved by formulating into solid lipid nanoparticles. Some of the common obstacles are lack of institutional and industrial interest, absence of proper infrastructure, poor monitoring of patient outcomes, and affordability [63].

6   Conclusions

Vascular inflammation in atherosclerosis involves various cellular mechanisms, and these inflammatory processes are being studied as targets for therapeutic agents in the management of atherosclerosis and other related disorders. Extracts of medicinal plants, isolated single phytochemicals such as liensenins, cepharanthine, resveratrol, baicalin, etc., have also shown promising activities in controlling vascular inflammation through different mechanisms. However, there is still a need for research related to the identification of active compounds in plant extracts. Similarly, many phytochemicals have low solubility and poor oral bioavailability, which could be improved using various advanced drug delivery systems.

References

[1] K.R. Paudel, N. Panth, D.W. Kim, Circulating endothelial microparticles: a key Hallmark of atherosclerosis progression, Scientifica (Cairo) 2016 (2016) 8514056.

[2] A.J. Lusis, Atherosclerosis, Nature 407 (6801) (2000) 233–241.

[3] P. Libby, J.E. Buring, L. Badimon, G.K. Hansson, J. Deanfield, M.S. Bittencourt, L. Tokgozoglu, E.F. Lewis, Atherosclerosis, Nat. Rev. Dis. Primers. 5 (1) (2019) 56.

[4] M. Li, M. Qian, K. Kyler, J. Xu, Endothelial-vascular smooth muscle cells interactions in atherosclerosis, Front Cardiovasc. Med. 5 (2018) 151.

[5] Y.V. Bobryshev, E.A. Ivanova, D.A. Chistiakov, N.G. Nikiforov, A. N. Orekhov, Macrophages and their role in atherosclerosis: pathophysiology and transcriptome analysis, Biomed. Res. Int. 2016 (2016) 9582430.

[6] J. Davignon, P. Ganz, Role of endothelial dysfunction in atherosclerosis, Circulation 109 (23 Suppl 1) (2004) III27-32.

[7] Y. Nakashima, E.W. Raines, A.S. Plump, J.L. Breslow, R. Ross, Upregulation of VCAM-1 and ICAM-1 at atherosclerosis-prone sites on the endothelium in the ApoE-deficient mouse, Arterioscler. Thromb. Vasc. Biol. 18 (5) (1998) 842–851.

[8] R.J. Aiello, P.A. Bourassa, S. Lindsey, W. Weng, E. Natoli, B.J. Rollins, P.M. Milos, Monocyte chemoattractant protein-1 accelerates atherosclerosis in apolipoprotein E-deficient mice, Arterioscler. Thromb. Vasc. Biol. 19 (6) (1999) 1518–1525.

[9] D.M. Mosser, J.P. Edwards, Exploring the full spectrum of macrophage activation, Nat. Rev. Immunol. 8 (12) (2008) 958–969.

[10] N. Panth, K.R. Paudel, K. Parajuli, Reactive oxygen species: a key Hallmark of cardiovascular disease, Adv. Med. 2016 (2016) 9152732.

[11] K.R. Paudel, R. Karki, D.W. Kim, Cepharanthine inhibits in vitro VSMC proliferation and migration and vascular inflammatory responses mediated by RAW264.7, Toxicol. In Vitro 34 (2016) 16–25.

[12] S. Goetze, X.P. Xi, Y. Kawano, H. Kawano, E. Fleck, W.A. Hsueh, R. E. Law, TNF-alpha-induced migration of vascular smooth muscle cells is MAPK dependent, Hypertension 33 (1 Pt 2) (1999) 183–189.

[13] C.C. Wang, I. Gurevich, B. Draznin, Insulin affects vascular smooth muscle cell phenotype and migration via distinct signaling pathways, Diabetes 52 (10) (2003) 2562–2569.

[14] J. Li, S.L. Huang, Z.G. Guo, Platelet-derived growth factor stimulated vascular smooth muscle cell proliferation and its molecular mechanism, Acta Pharmacol. Sin. 21 (4) (2000) 340–344.

[15] K.R. Paudel, M.H. Oak, D.W. Kim, Smooth muscle cell derived microparticles acts as autocrine activation of smooth muscle cell proliferation by mitogen associated protein kinase upregulation, J. Nanosci. Nanotechnol. 20 (9) (2020) 5746–5750.

[16] O. Soehnlein, P. Libby, Targeting inflammation in atherosclerosis—from experimental insights to the clinic, Nat. Rev. Drug Discov. 20 (8) (2021) 589–610.

[17] M. Sedighi, M. Bahmani, S. Asgary, F. Beyranvand, M. Rafieian-Kopaei, A review of plant-based compounds and medicinal plants effective on atherosclerosis, J. Res. Med. Sci. 22 (2017) 30.

[18] K.R. Paudel, R. Wadhwa, X.N. Tew, N.J.X. Lau, T. Madheswaran, J. Panneerselvam, F. Zeeshan, P. Kumar, G. Gupta, K. Anand, S.K. Singh, N.K. Jha, R. MacLoughlin, N.G. Hansbro, G. Liu, S.D. Shukla, M. Mehta, P.M. Hansbro, D.K. Chellappan, K. Dua, Rutin loaded liquid crystalline nanoparticles inhibit non-small cell lung cancer proliferation and migration in vitro, Life Sci. 276 (2021), 119436.

[19] M. Mehta, K.R. Paudel, S.D. Shukla, M.D. Shastri, S. Satija, S.K. Singh, M. Gulati, H. Dureja, F.C. Zacconi, P.M. Hansbro, D.K. Chellappan, K. Dua, Rutin-loaded liquid crystalline nanoparticles attenuate oxidative stress in bronchial epithelial cells: a PCR validation, Future Med. Chem. 13 (6) (2021) 543–549.

[20] R. Wadhwa, K.R. Paudel, L.H. Chin, C.M. Hon, T. Madheswaran, G. Gupta, J. Panneerselvam, T. Lakshmi, S.K. Singh, M. Gulati, H. Dureja, A. Hsu, M. Mehta, K. Anand, H.P. Devkota, J. Chellian, D.K. Chellappan, P.M. Hansbro, K. Dua, Anti-inflammatory and anti-cancer activities of Naringenin-loaded liquid crystalline nanoparticles in vitro, J. Food Biochem. 45 (1) (2021), e13572.

[21] N. Solanki, M. Mehta, D.K. Chellappan, G. Gupta, N.G. Hansbro, M. M. Tambuwala, A. Aa Aljabali, K.R. Paudel, G. Liu, S. Satija, P.M. Hansbro, K. Dua, H. Dureja, Antiproliferative effects of boswellic acid-loaded chitosan nanoparticles on human lung cancer cell line A549, Future Med. Chem. 12 (22) (2020) 2019–2034.

[22] B. Manandhar, K.R. Paudel, B. Sharma, R. Karki, Phytochemical profile and pharmacological activity of *Aegle marmelos* Linn, J. Integr. Med. 16 (3) (2018) 153–163.

[23] P. Prasher, M. Sharma, M. Mehta, K.R. Paudel, S. Satija, D.K. Chellappan, H. Dureja, G. Gupta, M.M. Tambuwala, P. Negi, P.R. Wich, N.G. Hansbro, P.M. Hansbro, K. Dua, Plants derived therapeutic strategies targeting chronic respiratory diseases: chemical and immunological perspective, Chem. Biol. Interact. 325 (2020), 109125.

[24] T.M. Kim, K.R. Paudel, D.W. Kim, Eriobotrya japonica leaf extract attenuates airway inflammation in ovalbumin-induced mice model of asthma, J. Ethnopharmacol. 253 (2020), 112082.

[25] N. Panth, B. Manandhar, K.R. Paudel, Anticancer activity of *Punica granatum* (pomegranate): a review, Phytother. Res. 31 (4) (2017) 568–578.

[26] A.I. Dirar, A. Adhikari-Devkota, R.M. Kunwar, K.R. Paudel, T. Belwal, G. Gupta, D.K. Chellappan, P.M. Hansbro, K. Dua, H.P. Devkota, Genus Blepharis (Acanthaceae): a review of ethnomedicinally used species, and their phytochemistry and pharmacological activities, J. Ethnopharmacol. 265 (2021), 113255.

[27] A.K. Jugran, S. Rawat, H.P. Devkota, I.D. Bhatt, R.S. Rawal, Diabetes and plant-derived natural products: from ethnopharmacological approaches to their potential for modern drug discovery and development, Phytother. Res. 35 (1) (2021) 223–245.

[28] N. Panth, K.R. Paudel, R. Karki, Phytochemical profile and biological activity of *Juglans regia*, J. Integr. Med. 14 (5) (2016) 359–373.

[29] H.H. Lee, K.R. Paudel, J. Jeong, A.J. Wi, W.S. Park, D.W. Kim, M.H. Oak, Antiatherogenic effect of *Camellia japonica* fruit extract in high fat diet-fed rats, Evid. Based Complement. Alternat. Med. 2016 (2016) 9679867.

[30] K.R. Paudel, U.W. Lee, D.W. Kim, Chungtaejeon, a Korean fermented tea, prevents the risk of atherosclerosis in rats fed a high-fat atherogenic diet, J. Integr. Med. 14 (2) (2016) 134–142.

[31] N. Panth, K.R. Paudel, D.S. Gong, M.H. Oak, Vascular protection by ethanol extract of Morus alba root bark: endothelium-dependent relaxation of rat aorta and decrease of smooth muscle cell migration and proliferation, Evid. Based Complement. Alternat. Med. 2018 (2018) 7905763.

[32] H.H. Lee, K.R. Paudel, D.W. Kim, Terminalia chebula Fructus inhibits migration and proliferation of vascular smooth muscle cells and production of inflammatory mediators in RAW 264.7, Evid. Based Complement. Alternat. Med. 2015 (2015), 502182.

[33] S.B. Kim, K.R. Paudel, D.W.J.K. Kim, Preventive Effect of traditional Korean formulations on intimal thickening of rat carotid artery injured by balloon catheter, Korean J. Plant Res. 26 (6) (2013) 678–685.

[34] K.R. Paudel, N. Panth, Phytochemical profile and biological activity of *Nelumbo nucifera*, Evid. Based Complement. Alternat. Med. 2015 (2015), 789124.

[35] M.Y. Jun, R. Karki, K.R. Paudel, B.R. Sharma, D. Adhikari, D.W. Kim, Alkaloid rich fraction from *Nelumbo nucifera* targets VSMC proliferation and migration to suppress restenosis in balloon-injured rat carotid artery, Atherosclerosis 248 (2016) 179–189.

[36] M.Y. Jun, R. Karki, K.R. Paudel, N. Panth, H.P. Devkota, D.-W.J.A.S. Kim, Liensinine prevents vascular inflammation by attenuating inflammatory mediators and modulating VSMC function, Appl. Sci. 11 (1) (2021) 386.

[37] K.R. Paudel, D.W. Kim, Microparticles-mediated vascular inflammation and its amelioration by antioxidant activity of Baicalin, Antioxidants (Basel) 9 (9) (2020) 1–23.

[38] D. Perrone, M.P. Fuggetta, F. Ardito, A. Cottarelli, A. De Filippis, G. Ravagnan, S. De Maria, L. Lo Muzio, Resveratrol (3,5,4′-trihydroxystilbene) and its properties in oral diseases, Exp. Ther. Med. 14 (1) (2017) 3–9.

[39] M.F. Linton, P.G. Yancey, S.S. Davies, W.G. Jerome, E.F. Linton, W.L. Song, A.C. Doran, K.C. Vickers, The role of lipids and lipoproteins in atherosclerosis, in: K.R. Feingold, B. Anawalt, A. Boyce, G. Chrousos, W.W. de Herder, K. Dhatariya, et al. (Eds.), Endotext [Internet], MDText.com, Inc., South Dartmouth, MA, 2019.

[40] E.B. Kurutas, The importance of antioxidants which play the role in cellular response against oxidative/nitrosative stress: current state, Nutr. J. 15 (1) (2016) 71.

[41] K. Prasad, Resveratrol, wine, and atherosclerosis, Int. J. Angiol. 21 (1) (2012) 7–18.

[42] S. Kany, J.T. Vollrath, B. Relja, Cytokines in inflammatory disease, Int. J. Mol. Sci. 20 (23) (2019) 1–31.

[43] I. Cicha, M. Regler, K. Urschel, M. Goppelt-Struebe, W.G. Daniel, C.D. Garlichs, Resveratrol inhibits monocytic cell chemotaxis to MCP-1 and prevents spontaneous endothelial cell migration through rho kinase-dependent mechanism, J. Atheroscler. Thromb. 18 (12) (2011) 1031–1042.

[44] Y. Zhang, H. Liu, W. Tang, Q. Qiu, J. Peng, Resveratrol prevents TNF-alpha-induced VCAM-1 and ICAM-1 upregulation in endothelial progenitor cells via reduction of NF-kappaB activation, J. Int. Med. Res. 48 (9) (2020), https://doi.org/10.1177/0300060520945131.

[45] A.M. Thompson, K.A. Martin, E.M. Rzucidlo, Resveratrol induces vascular smooth muscle cell differentiation through stimulation of SirT1 and AMPK, PLoS One 9 (1) (2014), e85495.

[46] Mezzomo, N.; Ferreira, S.R.S., Carotenoids functionality, sources, and processing by supercritical technology: a review. J. Chem. 2016, *2016*.

[47] P. Palozza, A. Catalano, R.E. Simone, M.C. Mele, A. Cittadini, Effect of lycopene and tomato products on cholesterol metabolism, Ann. Nutr. Metab. 61 (2) (2012) 126–134.

[48] R.W.S. Chung, P. Leanderson, A.K. Lundberg, L. Jonasson, Lutein exerts anti-inflammatory effects in patients with coronary artery disease, Atherosclerosis 262 (2017) 87–93.

[49] X.R. Xu, Z.Y. Zou, Y.M. Huang, X. Xiao, L. Ma, X.M. Lin, Serum carotenoids in relation to risk factors for development of atherosclerosis, Clin. Biochem. 45 (16–17) (2012) 1357–1361.

[50] L. Duan, X. Xiong, J. Hu, Y. Liu, J. Li, J. Wang, Panax notoginseng Saponins for treating coronary artery disease: a functional and mechanistic overview, Front. Pharmacol. 8 (2017) 702.

[51] C. Jia, M. Xiong, P. Wang, J. Cui, X. Du, Q. Yang, W. Wang, Y. Chen, T. Zhang, Notoginsenoside R1 attenuates atherosclerotic lesions in ApoE deficient mouse model, PLoS One 9 (6) (2014), e99849.

[52] L. Ding, T.-T. Zhang, H.-X. Che, L.-Y. Zhang, C.-H. Xue, Y.-G. Chang, Y.-M. Wang, Saponins of sea cucumber attenuate atherosclerosis in ApoE−/− mice via lipid-lowering and anti-inflammatory properties, J. Funct. Foods 48 (2018) 490–497.

[53] B. Rashidi, Z. Hoseini, A. Sahebkar, H. Mirzaei, Anti-atherosclerotic effects of vitamins D and E in suppression of Atherogenesis, J. Cell. Physiol. 232 (11) (2017) 2968–2976.

[54] H.N. Siti, Y. Kamisah, J. Kamsiah, The role of oxidative stress, antioxidants and vascular inflammation in cardiovascular disease (a review), Vascul. Pharmacol. 71 (2015) 40–56.

[55] D. Kirmizis, D. Chatzidimitriou, Antiatherogenic effects of vitamin E: the search for the holy grail, Vasc. Health Risk Manag. 5 (2009) 767–774.

[56] S. Saboori, S. Shab-Bidar, J.R. Speakman, E. Yousefi Rad, K. Djafarian, Effect of vitamin E supplementation on serum C-reactive protein level: a meta-analysis of randomized controlled trials, Eur. J. Clin. Nutr. 69 (8) (2015) 867–873.

[57] A. Nakhlband, M. Eskandani, Y. Omidi, N. Saeedi, S. Ghaffari, J. Barar, A. Garjani, Combating atherosclerosis with targeted nanomedicines: recent advances and future prospective, Bioimpacts 8 (1) (2018) 59–75.

[58] E. Westein, U. Flierl, C.E. Hagemeyer, K. Peter, Destination known: targeted drug delivery in atherosclerosis and thrombosis, Drug Dev. Res. 74 (7) (2013) 460–471.

[59] M. Navab, G.M. Anantharamaiah, S.T. Reddy, B.J. Van Lenten, B.J. Ansell, A.M. Fogelman, Mechanisms of disease: proatherogenic HDL—an evolving field, Nat. Clin. Pract. Endocrinol. Metab. 2 (9) (2006) 504–511.

[60] K. Kulandaivelu, A.K. Mandal, Positive regulation of biochemical parameters by tea polyphenol encapsulated solid lipid nanoparticles at in vitro and in vivo conditions, IET Nanobiotechnol. 10 (6) (2016) 419–424.

[61] A. Nakhlband, M. Eskandani, N. Saeedi, S. Ghafari, Y. Omidi, J. Barar, A. Garjani, Marrubiin-loaded solid lipid nanoparticles' impact on TNF-alpha treated umbilical vein endothelial cells: a study for cardioprotective effect, Colloids Surf. B Biointerfaces 164 (2018) 299–307.

[62] W. Zhang, H. He, J. Liu, J. Wang, S. Zhang, S. Zhang, Z. Wu, Pharmacokinetics and atherosclerotic lesions targeting effects of tanshinone IIA discoidal and spherical biomimetic high density lipoproteins, Biomaterials 34 (1) (2013) 306–319.

[63] T. Matoba, K. Egashira, Nanoparticle-mediated drug delivery system for cardiovascular disease, Int. Heart J. 55 (4) (2014) 281–286.

Chapter 10

Targeting cancer-inducing inflammation: Current advancements and future prospects

Yinghan Chan[a], Hui Shan Liew[b,c], Lesley Jia Wei Pua[b,c], Laura Soon[a], Sin Wi Ng[a], Joycelin Zhu Xin Tan[a], Dinesh Kumar Chellappan[d], and Kamal Dua[e]

[a]School of Pharmacy, International Medical University (IMU), Kuala Lumpur, Malaysia, [b]School of Postgraduate Studies, International Medical University (IMU), Kuala Lumpur, Malaysia, [c]Center for Cancer and Stem Cell Research, Institute for Research, Development and Innovation (IRDI), International Medical University (IMU), Kuala Lumpur, Malaysia, [d]Department of Life Sciences, School of Pharmacy, International Medical University (IMU), Kuala Lumpur, Malaysia, [e]Discipline of Pharmacy, Graduate School of Health, University of Technology Sydney, Sydney, NSW, Australia

1 Introduction

Cancer is a complex disease that is characterized by uncontrolled cell proliferation and acquisition of metastatic properties, in which normal cells transform into a conglomeration of abnormal cells, thereby forming a mass of tumor tissues that can either be malignant or benign. The major risk factors of cancer are prior family history and genetic mutations, exposure to ultraviolet radiation, and unhealthy diet, as well as alcohol consumption and use of tobacco [1,2]. Cancer can affect multiple types of cells or tissues within the human body, whereby the most common types of cancer include cancers of the lungs, breast, colon, pancreas, blood, skin, and nasopharyngeal. These cancers can generally be diagnosed through screenings, imaging, and laboratory testing [1]. Despite advancements in medical research, cancer remains as one of the leading causes of worldwide deaths with new cases projected to increase by 70% in the coming years. The high mortality rate of cancer has also been reported by the World Health Organization (WHO), as 9.6 million people worldwide are estimated to have succumbed to cancer in 2018 alone [3,4]. The growing cancer burden throughout the world has prompted medical researchers to urgently address the tremendous physical, emotional, and financial strains brought upon by the disease on individuals, communities, and public health systems. As such, a thorough understanding of the mechanisms underlying cancer initiation, development, and progression is essential to develop therapeutic agents that can effectively target the pathogenesis of the disease.

The presence of leukocytes within tumor tissues, which was observed in 1863 by Rudolf Virchow, the father of modern pathology, has provided the first indication that there may be a possible link between cancer and inflammation [5,6]. Inflammation is a robust defense system of the human body that involves the activation, recruitment, and actions of cells of both innate and adaptive immune systems. Initially emphasized for its crucial role in host defense fighting against pathogens, inflammation is also equally important in the repair, regeneration, and remodeling of damaged tissue from physical injury, ischemic injury, toxin exposure, infection, or other types of traumas. Therefore, subtle forms of inflammation are highly essential for an optimal regulation of tissue homeostasis [7,8]. Nevertheless, if the cause of inflammation persists or when certain mechanisms that regulate such a process fail, chronic inflammation can occur. It is now a generally accepted paradigm that chronic inflammation often creates an environment that facilitates the development of cancer through the secretion of multiple growth factors, cytokines, and chemokines by inflammatory cells, which then further modulates various processes during tumorigenesis, such as cellular transformation, promotion, proliferation, survival, angiogenesis, invasion, and metastasis [5,6,8]. Research and studies have also found that the underlying chronic inflammatory reactions are associated with approximately 15%–20% of all cancer-related deaths [5]. Thus, the events and molecules involved in the cross talk between the inflammatory processes and tumor microenvironment have attracted great interest as potential targets in the development of anticancer therapeutics.

Advancements in medical research have led to the discovery of potent compounds and development of various anticancer therapeutics to combat different types of cancer with respect to their underlying inflammatory mechanisms. These include nonsteroidal antiinflammatory drugs

Recent Developments in Anti-Inflammatory Therapy. https://doi.org/10.1016/B978-0-323-99988-5.00001-2

(NSAIDs), glucocorticoids, small interfering ribonucleic acids (siRNAs), and certain natural products [9,10]. Despite that, the full pharmacological success of these agents is limited by several drawbacks. For example, the systemic circulation of naked siRNAs may be challenged by rapid enzymatic degradation in biological and physiological media, recognition by the immune system, poor tissue penetration, entrapment by phagocytes, as well as off-target effects, thereby reducing their therapeutic efficacy in cancer [11,12]. Besides, although certain compounds demonstrated remarkable antiinflammatory activity, these compounds have poor water solubility and poor biodistribution, thereby necessitating higher doses to achieve a therapeutically effective concentration, resulting in higher occurrence of adverse drug reactions [12–14]. Collectively, these limitations have hindered therapeutic success due to low drug accumulation within the tumor tissues and possible incidences of off-target side effects [12]. For this instance, nanomedicine-based strategies offer a feasible tool to enhance the physicochemical properties of these agents, which can subsequently improve their therapeutic index in the management of cancer. Typically, nanoencapsulation of therapeutic agents within drug delivery systems can promote drug stability and prevent premature drug degradation, thereby improving drug solubilization and prolonging its biodistribution. At the same time, the versatility of drug delivery systems allows for surface modification to facilitate selective targeting of therapeutic agents to specific tumor tissues, thereby improving drug accumulation while reducing off-target side effects and avoiding multidrug resistance [1,12,13,15–17]. In this chapter, we discuss the relationship between inflammation and cancer, and provide an insight into the currently available anticancer therapeutics that exploit the inflammatory pathways underlying cancer development. We also discuss the perspectives for the use of novel nanomedicine-based strategies in the management of cancer, justified by various recent studies that are conducted in this field of research thus far.

2 Inflammation and cancer

Inflammation is a physiologic process of the immune system in response to harmful stimuli, such as pathogens, toxic compounds, damaged cells and tissues, or irradiation. As it acts to remove injurious stimuli and facilitates the healing process of damaged tissues, inflammation is a part of the body's defense mechanism that is essential in the maintenance of health [8,18]. As the primary effectors of an inflammatory response, the recruitment of neutrophils at the site of infection or injury is influenced by the release of pathogen-associated molecular patterns (PAMP) from the invading pathogens or damage-associated molecular patterns (DAMP) from damaged cells [10,19]. These signals

can be recognized locally by tissue-resident innate immune cells, such as dendritic cells, resident macrophages, endothelial cells, and fibroblasts that express pattern recognition receptors (PRR), which include C-type lectin receptors, Toll-like receptors, nucleotide-binding and oligomerization domain (NOD)-like receptors, and retinoic acid-inducible gene I (RIG-I)-like receptors [10,19,20]. Activation of these PRRs can lead to the production and secretion of cytokines such as interleukins (IL)-6, −1β, and tumor necrosis factor (TNF), chemokines such as C-X-C motif chemokine ligand 1 (CXCL1) and 2 (CXCL2), as well as other neutrophil chemoattractants such as a platelet-activating factor and leukotriene B4 (LTB4), which collectively promote the migration of leukocytes and the inflammatory response [10,20]. Generally, the neutrophil recruitment cascade involves a four-step mechanism, namely, of P-, E-, and L-selectin-mediated tethering of free-flowing neutrophils to the surface of the endothelium, rolling of neutrophils along the luminal side of the endothelium adjacent to the infection or injury site in the direction of blood flow, chemokine-induced integrin-mediated adhesion of neutrophils, and lastly, intraluminal crawling and transmigration of neutrophils to the inflammatory sites [19–21].

In most cases, an inflammatory response is self-limiting, and its duration is influenced by several molecules with dual proinflammatory and antiinflammatory activities. Resolution of inflammation is a highly regulated process that involves spatially and temporally controlled secretion of mediators, during which chemokine gradients are diluted over time [18]. Despite the crucial roles of neutrophils in the proper elimination of inflammogenic substances, the exaggerated influx of neutrophils is often highly deleterious as compared to the injury or infection itself; therefore, they have been regarded as a negative marker of tissue homeostasis. As such, the depletion of neutrophils from the local inflamed sites is the primary histological feature during the resolution of acute inflammation [22]. Generally, the processes involved in the resolution of inflammation to restore tissue homeostasis include reduction or cessation of neutrophil infiltration in tissues, apoptosis of spent neutrophils, counter-regulation of cytokines and chemokines, transformation of macrophages from classically to alternatively activated cells, as well as initiation of healing. An effective resolution can ultimately prevent the progression from acute inflammation to chronic inflammation, thereby avoiding excessive tissue damage and giving little opportunity for the development of chronic inflammatory diseases [18,23]. However, if the acute inflammatory mechanisms fail to resolve tissue injury, or if dysregulation of one or more steps of the inflammatory resolution processes occurs, it can result in nonresolving, persistent chronic inflammation that is characterized by the presence of macrophages and lymphocytes with abnormal morphology that consistently produce growth factors and cytokines [10,18,22].

In terms of cancer, such persistent secretion of inflammatory mediators can result in DNA and tissue damage through the generation of a microenvironment which promotes cell proliferation and predisposes to the development of the disease [10]. In the following sections, we provide a general overview on several key mediators involved in cancer-associated inflammation and describe the roles of inflammation in driving tumorigenesis, from initiation through tumor promotion, all the way to metastatic progression of tumor tissues.

2.1 Molecular basis and mediators of cancer-related inflammation

The traditional dogma of tumor infiltrating leukocytes is that they are the manifestations of an intrinsic defense mechanism against developing tumor cells. Subsequently, it was identified that the presence of leukocytes in tumors is an aborted attempt of the immune system to reject the tumor [5]. There is also increasing evidence that indicates that the infiltration of leukocytes can induce tumor phenotypes. This can be attributed to the inflammatory cells that modulate cancer promotion via the secretion of cytokines, chemokines, growth factors, and proteases that promote the proliferation and invasiveness of tumor cells [5,6].

Inflammation and cancer can be linked by two different pathways, namely the extrinsic and intrinsic pathways (Fig. 1). The extrinsic pathway refers to the activation by inflammatory stimuli, such as tissue injury, infection, carcinogen exposure, and dietary habits that contribute to the risk of cancer, whereas the intrinsic pathway refers to genetic alterations that contribute to the induction of inflammatory pathways in both premalignant and malignant cells; therefore, not only inflammation contributes to cancer, but cancer can also contribute to inflammation [24]. Generally, both extrinsic and intrinsic factors can lead to the expression of several proinflammatory transcription factors within the tumor cells, such as nuclear factor kappa B (NF-κB), signal transducer and activator of transcription (STAT) 3, and hypoxia inducible factor 1 subunit alpha (HIF1α). These transcription factors modulate the expressions of major cytokines and chemokines, such as TNF-α and IL-6, as well as other inflammatory enzymes such as cyclooxygenase (COX)-2 to form a complex and rich network of inflammatory responses within the tumor microenvironment when activated. Immune response is then mediated by host leukocytes including dendritic cells, macrophages, T cells, and mast cells which are recruited by chemokines and function within the tumor stroma. Within the tumor microenvironment, the activities of these cells are further sustained by autocrine and paracrine effects of cytokine release.

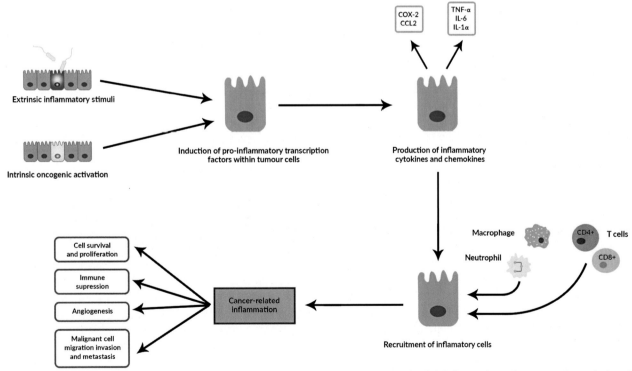

FIG. 1 Overview of the molecular basis of cancer-associated inflammation. The two pathways that link inflammation and cancer are the extrinsic and intrinsic pathways, in which the activation of specific transcription factors by these pathways influences the secretion of cytokines and chemokines, as well as other inflammatory mediators, thereby resulting in the development of an inflammatory tumor microenvironment.

Finally, inflammatory enzymes catalyze the key steps in the synthesis of prostaglandins, which then regulate multiple physiological processes involved in cancer-associated inflammation, thereby driving the process of tumorigenesis [24,25].

2.1.1 Cytokines

Cytokines are low molecular weight proteins that play a role in the modulation of cell-to-cell communication. They are synthesized by immune and stromal cells such as fibroblasts and endothelial cells and they play a role in the regulation of cell proliferation, survival, differentiation, migration, and death [26]. Cytokines can generally be classified into two different classes, namely proinflammatory cytokines such as IL-1β, IL-6, and TNF-κ, as well as antiinflammatory cytokines such as IL-10, interferon (IFN)-α, and TGF-β. Depending on the tumor and its microenvironment, cytokines can either induce an antitumoral activity or trigger cell transformation and malignancy for the development of cancer [26,27].

TNF-α is a key multifunctional cytokine that has pleiotropic actions in the regulation of immune responses associated with inflammation. It is primarily synthesized by macrophages, as well as by natural killer (NK) cells, CD4 + T lymphocytes, mast cells, neutrophils, eosinophils, and neurons [24,26]. There have been controversies regarding the roles of TNF-α in cancer. Initially, this cytokine was named for its antitumor properties as it can induce hemorrhagic necrosis of tumors, in which studies have shown that about 28% of cancers are susceptible to direct cell killing by soluble TNF-α, in part through its action on tumor vasculature to disrupt blood supply [28,29]. Since this discovery, however, accumulating evidence suggested that TNF-α also exhibits paradoxical effects on tumor cells, either through the induction of carcinogenesis or the promotion of establish tumors progression. The tumor promotion mechanism of TNF-α is based on the activation of the NF-κB pathway, as well as the production of reactive oxygen species (ROS) and reactive nitrogen species (RNS) that lead to DNA damage. Besides, TNF-α can also contribute to the escape of tumor cells from immunosurveillance and promote tumor metastasis by upregulating the immunosuppressive property of myeloid-derived suppressor cells and regulatory T (Treg) cells [26,29]. Therefore, as the primary cytokine within the tumor microenvironment that is capable of modulating other cytokines and chemokines to influence several hallmarks of cancer, agents that modify TNF-α signaling can be exploited for the potential treatment of various malignancies.

Initially identified as a B cell growth factor, IL-6 is another example of a proinflammatory cytokine, and it has since been demonstrated to provide important survival and proliferative signals to various populations of leukocytes, thereby orchestrating immune response [30]. The close association between IL-6 and the development of human cancer can be reflected by the high levels of IL-6 present within the tumor microenvironment, and its overexpression has been shown in almost all types of tumors. As such, the high serum concentration of IL-6 is regarded as a prognostic indicator of poor outcomes especially in patients with diverse histological tumor types, including lung cancer, breast cancer, pancreatic cancer, gastric cancer, colorectal cancer, as well as multiple myeloma and lymphomas [30,31]. Classically, IL-6 signaling is mediated through its binding to the IL-6 receptor α (IL-6Rα) subunit, followed by the binding of the IL-6/IL-6Rα complex to the signal transducing subunit glycoprotein 130 (gp130), thereby leading to the activation of Janus kinases (JAK) and the STAT-3 signaling pathway [30,32]. The activation of the IL-6/JAK/STAT-3 signaling axis is an important event in cancer as it promotes tumorigenesis by modulating all hallmarks of cancer, which include survival, proliferation, angiogenesis, invasiveness, metastasis, and apoptosis. Besides, IL-6 can also shield tumor cells from therapy-induced DNA damage, oxidative stress, and apoptosis by facilitating their repair and inducing pro-survival, antiapoptotic, and antioxidative counter-signaling pathways [31]. Hence, agents that block the activity of IL-6 or its associated signaling, as well as the activity of JAK and STAT-3, can be a potential therapeutic strategy for the management of multiple human cancers.

TGF-β is another superfamily of antiinflammatory cytokines that encompasses widespread and evolutionary conserved polypeptide growth factors which play a role in the regulation and orchestration of growth and differentiation in various cells and tissues [26,33]. Apart from regulating asymmetric cell division and determining cell fate during embryogenesis and early development, TGF-β has a well-documented role in modulating immune and hormonal responses, cell growth, death, and immortalization, tissue remodeling and repair, bone formation, as well as erythropoiesis throughout adult life [33]. Upon binding of TGF-β to its receptor on the cell membrane, a signaling cascade is induced via the phosphorylation of Smad2/3, in which phosphorylated Smad2/3 binds to Smad4 to form a complex that translocates to the nucleus from the cytoplasm for the activation of end effectors transcription, such as p15, p21, and parathyroid hormone-related protein (PTHrP) [34]. The role of TGF-β in cancer is complex and paradoxical depending on the cell type and stage of tumorigenesis. Primarily, it is a tumor suppressor which inhibits proliferation and triggers apoptosis of premalignant epithelial cells. However, TGF-β functions as the promoter of metastasis during the later stages of cancer progression through the induction of epithelial-mesenchymal transition, thereby resulting in enhanced invasion of cancer cells, as well as by the induction of genes associated with metastatic colonization of secondary organ sites [34,35]. Although the mechanism of the role switch in TGF-β is not clearly understood, there have been much effort to develop cancer therapeutics by targeting TGF-β in both the tumor and its microenvironment due to the key role of its signaling pathway in the development of cancer. Nonetheless, due to their potent tumor suppressive properties in early-stage disease, targeting TGF-β too early during disease progression may be detrimental, and the timing of TGF-β-targeting therapies must be carefully considered for an effective anticancer response [35].

Apart from that, IL-10 is widely known as a potent anti-inflammatory cytokine, and it is produced by almost every immune cell, including B cells, T cells, macrophages, monocytes, granulocytes, mast cells, and dendritic cells [36]. It is also regarded as an immunosuppressive cytokine as it can reduce the antigen-presenting activity of dendritic cells, as well as suppress the cytotoxic and cytokine-release functions performed by T and NK lymphocytes [37]. Nevertheless, the role of IL-10 in tumorigenesis and cancer development remains controversial at this point, there are certain studies that suggest that IL-10 positively contributes to the growth and promotion of tumor, whereas other studies indicate that IL-10 contributes to the suppression and eradication of angiogenesis and metastasis, thereby improving long-term patient survival [38–40]. In terms of tumor promotion, IL-10 has been considered to promote escape from tumor immune surveillance due to its immunosuppressive behavior, which subsequently diminishes antitumor immune response within the tumor microenvironment. Multiple studies have demonstrated a positive correlation between IL-10 and poor patient prognosis, whereby the presence of the mRNA and protein of IL-10 has been reported in various freshly excised human tumors, including lung, breast, ovarian, renal cell, and metastatic melanoma [39,40]. On the other hand, there is also a large amount of evidence which suggests the potent antitumor effects of IL-10. In several studies, it has been found that established tumors displayed retarded growth rates upon IL-10 injection and inhibited metastasis in an immune-dependent manner. Notably, there was reduced mRNA expression of vascular endothelial growth factor (VEGF), which is a crucial angiogenic factor, as well as matrix metalloproteinase (MMP)-9, which is essential for both angiogenic and metastatic processes [40,41]. In short, IL-10 may play a dual role in tumorigenesis, in which IL-10 may predominantly act in the stimulation of NK and cytotoxic T lymphocytes (CTL) through the downregulation of a major histocompatibility complex (MHC) for killing tumor cells as cancer begins to form. If tumor cells managed to survive, the production of IL-10 within the tumor microenvironment may primarily act as a potent cancer promoter [26,39,40].

2.1.2 Chemokines

Chemokines are soluble, low molecular weight chemoattractants that bind to their cognate G-protein coupled receptors (GPCR) to produce a cellular response. The chemokine family is generally classified into four major subfamilies, namely CC, CXC, CX3C, and XC, depending on the number and location of the highly conserved cysteine residues on the N-terminus, as well as the presence or absence of the intervening amino acids [42]. Apart from their pivotal role in coordinating the chemotaxis of immune cells to inflammatory sites, chemokines are also essential in various biological events including the development of lymphoid tissues, maturation of immune cells, as well as the generation and delivery of adaptive immune responses. Therefore, dysregulation in the expression of chemokines and/or their receptors can result in various human diseases, such as autoimmune and inflammatory diseases, as well as cancer [43]. In cancer, chemokines are involved in tumor angiogenesis and in homing of tumor cells to the sentinel lymph nodes, metastasis to other organs, as well as metastasis of the metastatic lesions in addition to their roles in inducing chronic inflammation linked with tumor progression. Besides, chemokines can also directly impact tumor cells and endothelial cells within the tumor microenvironment to regulate the growth and proliferation of tumor cells, thereby influencing tumor immunity and cancer progression [42,44]. Thus, chemokines and chemokine receptors can act as promising targets in cancer immunotherapy due to their paramount role in disease progression.

2.1.3 Nuclear factor kappa B

NF-κB is a family of transcription factors that regulates the expression of genes responsible for various crucial physiological responses, including inflammatory responses and cell adhesion, proliferation, differentiation, and apoptosis [45]. In its inactivated form, NF-κB can be found in the cytosol bound to an inhibitor protein, IκBα. Various inflammatory stimuli can lead to the activation of the IκB kinase (IKK) enzyme via the involvement of membrane receptors, leading to the phosphorylation of IκBα and its subsequent ubiquitination and proteasomal degradation. Ultimately, NF-κB is activated, followed by its translocation into the nucleus for the induction of inflammatory processes [46]. Therefore, a well-regulated NF-κB signaling is essential for the maintenance of human health, as aberrant NF-κB signaling can result in the development of various autoimmune, inflammatory, and malignant diseases.

In terms of cancer, various types of tumors presented constitutively active NF-κB, in which activated NF-κB upregulates genes expression that maintains cell proliferation and shields the cells from conditions that would otherwise result in apoptosis. Thus, constitutively activated NF-κB is closely associated with multiple aspects of tumorigenesis, which include promotion of cancer cell proliferation, suppression of apoptosis, as well as the promotion of the angiogenic and metastatic potential of tumor cells [45,47]. Apart from that, continuous NF-κB activity can also induce the generation of ROS, thereby resulting in DNA damage of the surrounding epithelial cells [45,48]. Continuously elevated NF-κB activity in tumor cells can generally be established by both intrinsic and extrinsic factors. Specifically, mutations of NF-κB genes and/or oncogenes that upregulate the NF-κB signaling pathway can directly induce the activity of NF-κB in tumor cells. On the other hand, a tumor can achieve increased NF-κB activity via the elevated release of proinflammatory cytokines from the tumor microenvironment [47]. In short, NF-κB strictly links inflammation and cancer since it generates cytokines, growth factors, and adhesion molecules that possess pro-tumorigenic effects. Hence, inhibition of NF-κB as a means of cancer treatment has been prioritized. These inhibitors are primarily designed to target the key elements essential to the activation of the NF-κB signaling pathway, such as IKK, NF-κB subunit dimers, proteasome 26S, and the Ub-ligase complex [49].

2.1.4   Prostaglandins and leukotrienes

Prostaglandins (PGs) are members of prostanoids, which are a subclass of eicosanoids, and they are classified depending on the structures of the cyclopentane ring as well as the number of double bonds within their hydrocarbon structures. These are crucial lipid mediators that are responsible for the modulation of body immune responses and homeostasis, in which their biosynthesis is found to be remarkably elevated in inflamed tissues, thereby contributing to the development of the cardinal signs of inflammation [50,51]. The synthesis of PGs takes place in a series of steps, in which it is initiated when phospholipase A2 (PLA2) acts on membrane phospholipids to produce arachidonic acid (AA). The process is then followed by the conversion of AA into PGH2 via reduction of the intermediate PGG2 by PG G/H synthases, or colloquially known as cyclooxygenases (COXs) [51,52]. COX is a bifunctional enzyme that plays an important role in the arachidonic acid pathway for the synthesis of PGs, which exists in two isoforms, namely the constitutively expressed COX-1, which is constantly expressed in a wide range of cells and tissues under most pathological or physiological conditions, and the inducible COX-2, which is normally absent in most cells and tissues, but its expression is greatly induced during inflammatory responses [53,54]. Mainly, COX-1 is the major source of prostanoids that plays a role in housekeeping activities, such as maintenance of homeostasis and gastric epithelial cytoprotection, whereas COX-2 is the source of prostanoid synthesis during inflammation and in proliferative diseases,

including cancer [50]. Finally, diverse PGs are synthesized from PGH2, which include thromboxane A2 (TXA2), PGE2, PGD2, PGI2, and PGF2α, depending on the type of synthase involved during the process [51,52].

PGE2 is the major product of COXs that plays a pivotal role in the induction of cancer progression. There are many biological activities that have been associated with PGE2 in both physiological and pathological conditions. For instance, in physiological processes, PGE2 facilitates the regulation of fever, pain, kidney function, mucosal integrity, inflammation, and blood vessel homeostasis, whereas in pathological conditions such as cancer, production of PGE2 by cancer stromal cells can induce the proliferation and survival of tumor cells, enhance angiogenesis, and promote metastasis [55,56]. These effects of PGE2 are believed to be mediated through mechanisms, including (i) activation of VEGF; (ii) upregulation of protooncogenes, BCL2, and epidermal growth factor receptor (EGFR) via the mitogen-activated protein kinase (MAPK) and phosphoinositide 3-kinase (PI3K)/protein kinase B (AKT) signaling pathways; (iii) promotion of invasion and metastasis via induction of MMP-2 and MMP-9; (iv) increased expression of the NF-κB signaling pathway; and (v) immunosuppression by decreasing the production of IL-12 [57]. Typically, an increase in the concentration of PGE2 is often an indication of altered expression of COXs, particularly COX-2, as it has been found to be overexpressed in multiple tumor cells and is positively correlated with progressive tumor growth, as well as the emergence of tumor cells resistance to radiotherapy and conventional chemotherapy. Furthermore, evidence has also demonstrated that elevated COX-2 expression and the subsequent increase in PGE2 release can contribute to the repopulation of tumors and inefficient therapy in cancer [58,59]. Such an increase in COX-2-dependent PGE$_2$ synthesis can contribute to tumorigenesis via suppression of natural killer (NK) cells, T-cells, and dendritic cells, as well as promotion of type-1 or even type-2 immunity which further induces tumor immune evasion [58]. Another COX-2 derived prostanoid that is increasingly implicated in the progression of cancer is TXA2, and it has been demonstrated to modulate inflammatory processes and is also involved in the regulation of acquired immunity, allergic reactions, angiogenesis, as well as cancer cell metastasis [59,60].

On top of PGs, leukotrienes (LTs) are also potent eicosanoid lipid mediators that are derived from AA. In contrast to PGs that are formed by most cells in the body, LTs are mainly synthesized by inflammatory cells such as mast cells, macrophages, neutrophils, eosinophils, and polymorphonuclear leukocytes [61,62]. 5-Lipoxygenase (5-LO) is the key enzyme involved in the production of LTs, in which LTs can be converted from AA in a concerted three-step reaction (Fig. 2): (i) deoxygenation of AA into 5-

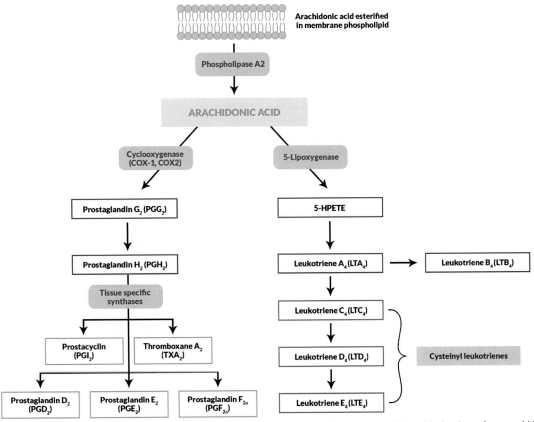

FIG. 2   General overview of the cyclooxygenase and lipoxygenase pathways in the synthesis of prostanoids and leukotrienes from arachidonic acid.

hydroperoxy-6-trans-8,11,14-cis-eicosatetraenoic acid (5-HPETE), (ii) dehydration of 5-HPETE forming the transient epoxide intermediate LTA4, and (iii) depending on the presence of 5-LO and its functional coupling to its downstream enzymes, LTA4 is converted to LTC4 by LTC4 synthase, or LTB4 by LTA4 hydrolase [62,63]. LTB4 is a potent chemoattractant for eosinophils, neutrophils, and monocytes, which stimulates their adhesion and extravasation through vascular endothelial barriers, their migration to inflammatory sites, as well as their subsequent activation [64]. LTC4 can also be further converted into LTD4 by γ-glutamyl transferase and subsequently LTD4 to LTE4 by membrane-bound dipeptidase. Collectively, LTC4, LTD4, and LTE4 are known as cysteinyl leukotrienes and they are responsible for the recruitment of inflammatory cells, contraction of smooth muscles, vasodilation, and vessel permeability [65]. Elevated levels of 5-LO and LTs, as well as their receptors, have been reported in different types of cancer, in which there has been evidence that suggests the involvement of 5-LO and LTs as proinflammatory mediators that influence tumorigenesis by the modulation of tumor cells proliferation, apoptosis, migration, and invasion [62]. Besides, 5-LO and LTs can promote the shaping of the tumor microenvironment via the induction of immune cells recruitment, migration and activation, growth factors production, as well as the synthesis of

proinflammatory and angiogenic factors. The migration of tumor cells can also be influenced by 5-LO and LTs by their interaction with the blood and lymphatic endothelium. As such, the inhibition of 5-LO may be beneficial in suppressing tumor growth and development by reducing inflammation and exerting a direct action on the modulation of tumor cells [62,66].

Hence, due to their paramount roles in the cross talk between inflammation and cancer, both the 5-LO and COX pathways provide an interesting avenue for the development of a targeted therapeutic strategy for the modulation of a tumor microenvironment and the subsequent prevention or inhibition of tumorigenesis.

2.1.5   Signal transducer and activator of transcription and Janus kinases

The signal transducer and activator of transcription (STAT) proteins belong to a class of transcription factors that can be activated by various peptide ligands, growth factors, and cytokines. Multiple physiological processes are regulated by STAT proteins, including cell proliferation, apoptosis, division, and differentiation, whereby in healthy cells the activation of STATs is regulated tightly to avoid uncontrolled gene expression. As such, the prolonged activation of STATs as observed in tumor cells may lead to remarkable adverse effects, including poor disease prognosis and resistance to therapies [67,68]. In particular, STAT3 and STAT5 have been implicated in the progression of cancer, in which dysregulated activation of STAT3 and/or STAT5 is known to induce the development of chronic inflammation that increases the susceptibility of healthy cells to carcinogenesis [68]. On the other hand, Janus kinases (JAKs) are a family of inactive receptor protein tyrosine kinases that are highly essential for the growth, survival, development, and differentiation of immune and hematopoietic cells [69]. Upon engagement with specific ligands such as cytokines, receptor-associated JAKs become activated, leading to the phosphorylation of each other and the intracellular tail of their receptors, as well as the creation of docking sites for STAT proteins. This is followed by JAK-mediated phosphorylation of STAT on its retained tyrosine residues, which is then released from the receptor and forms a dimer by binding with another phosphorylated STAT molecule.

Lastly, the STAT complex translocates into the nucleus and binds DNA to act as transcription factors for the genes that are involved in cell survival and proliferation (Fig. 3) [70,71].

Abnormal activation of the JAK/STAT signaling pathway occurs when a ligand constitutively binds to its receptor, or when there is an inappropriate stimulation of tyrosine kinase [72]. In the context of cancer, an aberrant activation of the JAK/STAT signaling pathway can result in enhanced tumorigenic and metastatic abilities, transition of cancer stem cells, as well as chemoresistance through the induction of epithelial-mesenchymal transition (EMT). EMT is the key regulator in cancer progression to control the invasion, spread, and survival of tumor cells [72,73]. Besides, an activated JAK/STAT pathway can initiate the transcription of genes that are involved in tumorigenesis, such as cyclin D1 that acts as cell cycle regulators, VEGF that acts as an angiogenic inducer, as well as Bcl-2, Bcl-xL, and survivin that act as apoptosis inhibitors. The

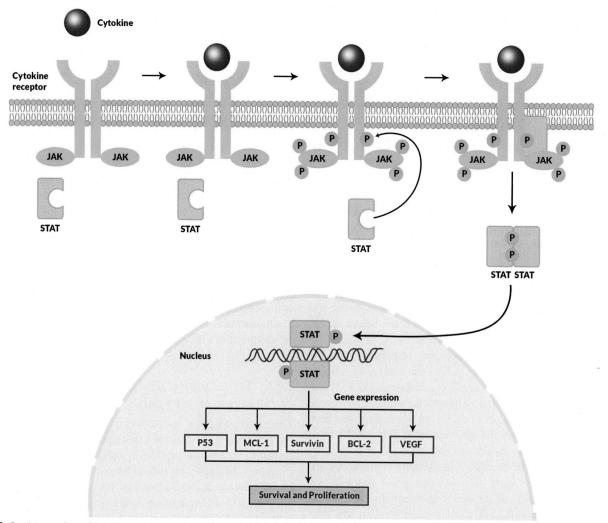

FIG. 3 An overview of the JAK/STAT signaling pathway that is involved in upregulating the genes responsible for the proliferation and survival of tumor cells.

activation of NF-κB can also be further triggered, thereby resulting in the promotion of inflammatory cascades involved in tumorigenesis [72]. As such, the blockade of JAK/STAT signaling in tumor cells can potentially inhibit the expression of target genes that regulate essential cell functions, thus preventing tumor cells from the evasion of the normal growth regulation mechanism, such as apoptosis and invasion.

2.1.6 Mitogen-activated protein kinases

Mitogen-activated protein kinase (MAPK) is a complex interconnected signaling pathway that is frequently involved in the regulation of cell proliferation, differentiation, migration, and apoptosis, immune and stress responses, as well as gene expressions [74]. The activation of MAPKs occurs via consecutive phosphorylations, where the most upstream kinase directly phosphorylates the middle kinase upon responding to various intracellular and extracellular signals, followed by the middle kinase-mediated phosphorylation and activation of an MAPK that often has various substrates that exert a specific cell fate decision corresponding to the input signal [75]. There are three major pathways mediated by MAPKs, namely the extracellular-regulated kinases (ERK) 1/2, the c-Jun-N-terminal kinases (JNKs) 1/2/3, and the p38 MAPKs α, β, γ, and δ. Generally, ERK1/2 are activated by cytokines and growth factors, and they are involved in upregulating transcription factors, such as cAMP response element-binding protein (CREB) and NF-κB; the JNK pathway is activated by growth factors, radiation, and environmental stresses, and it is responsible for regulating responses to inflammation, stress, and apoptosis; and lastly, p38 APKs mediates autoimmunity and are activated by hormones, chemical stresses, and cytokines such as TNF and ILs, and they target several transcription factors, including NF-κB [74–76]. In short, the MAPK cascade represents a crucial signaling pathway for the survival and dissemination of tumor cells, as well as its resistance to therapies. Thus, MAPK pathways are viable targets in the management of cancer, with the ERK pathway being the most prominent and frequently utilized target. Despite that, the JNK and p38 MAPK pathways are equally important as they also play crucial immunomodulatory roles that can alter tumor cells' response to therapies, as well as metabolic and epigenetic modulators [75,77].

2.1.7 Phosphoinositide 3-kinase

Phosphoinositide-3-kinases (PI3Ks) are a large family of lipid enzymes that phosphorylate the 3′-OH group of phosphatidylinositols on the plasma membrane. PI3Ks signaling is essential in the regulation of a plethora of cellular processes, including inflammation, metabolism, cell survival and motility, as well as cancer progression [78]. Under physiological conditions, the activation of PI3K is usually induced by multiple extracellular stimuli, including hormones, cytokines, and growth factors. Once activated, PI3K catalyzes the phosphorylation of phosphatidylinositol-4,5-biphosphate (PIP2) into phosphatidylinositol-3,4,5-triphosphate (PIP3), which is a process that can be reversed by phosphatase and the tensin homolog deleted on chromosome 10 (PTEN). PIP3 is a second messenger that binds and recruits pleckstrin homology (pH)-containing proteins such as 3-phosphoinositide-dependent kinase 1 (PDK1) and AKT, thereby leading to their localization to the cell membrane for the activation of cell growth and cell survival pathways [78,79]. AKT, on its own, can also modulate several cell processes involved in cell survival and cell cycle progression. Moreover, AKT can induce the stimulation of the mammalian target of rapamycin (mTOR), which is a key protein evolutionary conserved from yeast to man and is crucial for life. The activity of mTOR in normal cells is controlled by positive regulators such as growth factors and their receptors, which transmit signals to mTOR via the PI3K/AKT pathway, and negative regulators such as PTEN that suppress signaling via the PI3K/AKT pathway [78,80]. The activation of mTOR can lead to the elevation of multiple proteins, including those that are implicated in the development of various tumors, such as the hypoxia-inducible factor (HIF) that induces proangiogenic growth factors, and cyclin D1 that allows cell progression through the cell cycle [80]. As such, the dysregulation of the PI3K/AKT/mTOR pathway has been identified in almost all types of human cancer, which signifies the great value of targeting this pathway as a potential strategy in the management of cancer [79].

2.2 Inflammation and inflammatory mediators in tumorigenesis

2.2.1 Tumor initiation

Tumor initiation requires an accumulation of genetic mutations and/or epigenetic alterations in the genes for tumor suppression in normal cells. In this respect, the involvement of chronic inflammatory responses has contributed to the initiation of signaling cascades that are involved in tumorigenic processes. Specifically, activated inflammatory cells, such as neutrophils and macrophages, produce large amounts of ROS and RNS which are known to induce genomic instability and DNA damage in cells. Inflammatory cells can also utilize cytokines to further induce the accumulation of ROS in neighboring epithelial cells. These mutations change cells by removing their control in proliferation and apoptosis [8,81]. This was supported by the findings from Canli et al. which showed that myeloid cell-derived hydrogen peroxide triggered genome-wide DNA mutations to induce invasive growth in intestinal epithelial cells. At the same time, increased ROS production in myeloid cells initiated tumor growth in multiple organs without the presence of a carcinogen challenge [82]. Another example is colitis-associated cancer, whereby chronic inflammation was found to induce DNA oxidative damage, leading to early p53 mutations. Signaling by cytokines produced by inflammatory cells also upregulated DNA methyltransferases, including DNMT1 and DNMT3, which mediate the silencing of numerous target genes in mouse and human colon cancers. Such epigenetic silencing can reduce the expression of several proteins which function as tumor suppressors. Collectively, these contributed to the initiation of carcinogenesis and development of colon cancer [83,84]. Also, in prostate cancer, environmental and mutagenic exposure and genetic variations were found to predispose the prostate gland to inflammation, leading to an elevated level of critical inflammatory mediators such as TGF-β, IL-1β, IL-6, and IL-8, and ultimately drives the initiation of prostate cancer [85].

Another mechanism linking chronic inflammation to tumor initiation is that inflammation-induced mutagenesis can lead to the repression or inactivation of mismatch response genes, while ROS can directly induce oxidative inactivation of mismatch repair enzymes. As such, this leads to the dysregulation of the mismatch repair system, thereby enhancing mutagenesis and inactivating several crucial tumor suppressors, such as Bax and TGF-β receptor 2 (TGFBR2) [86]. Chronic inflammation can also promote the initiation of tumor by conferring stem cell-like phenotype on premalignant cells and forming niches which support the survival and maintenance of tumor-initiating cells, which eventually expands the cell pool for mutagenesis [81]. Moreover, chronic inflammation increases the exposure toward mutagens and carcinogenic agents. One explanation is that chronic inflammation weakens the barrier function, thereby exposing the stem cell compartment to cancer-inducing agents or bringing stem cells to the active inflammatory cells producing genotoxic compounds in a close proximity [8].

2.2.2 Tumor promotion

In the second stage of tumorigenesis, the survival and proliferation of a single initiated cell is promoted by various growth stimuli and growth factors to form a fully developed primary tumor [81,86]. Specifically, the production of tumor-promoting cytokines by inflammatory cells which then activates various transcription factors that upregulate genes responsible for stimulating cell proliferation and survival, including STAT3, NF-κB, and AP-1 in premalignant cells, is the primary tumor-promoting mechanism [86]. Apart from tumor cells, inflammatory signals can also impact the components of the tumor stroma, including fibroblasts, endothelial cells, and immune cells, thereby shaping

the tumor microenvironment that supports tumor promotion and progression [81]. These correlated to the findings in a study which reported that myeloid cell-specific inactivation of NF-κB resulted in suppression of tumor growth in various cancer models. Several experiments utilizing mice with knocked-out genes that are involved in encoding cytokines and/or their receptors have also demonstrated significant suppression of tumor growth, indicating the contribution of inflammatory pathways to tumor promotion [81,87]. In one study, mice deficient in IL-1β or wild-type mice treated with anti-IL-1β antibodies had demonstrated regression of implanted breast cancer tumors. Such regression can be attributed to elevated dendritic cell function and activated CD8 lymphocytes, which increase antitumoral immunity, and decrease tumor-related immunosuppression that are primarily mediated by macrophages [88].

2.2.3 Tumor angiogenesis

Tumor angiogenesis is defined as the growth of blood vessels that supply tumor with oxygen and nutrients to survive and grow. Angiogenesis is often triggered by tumor hypoxia and is dependent on the recruitment of tumor-associated macrophages, which can detect hypoxic signals to produce various chemokines and proangiogenic factors [86,89]. Generally, the process of angiogenesis in tumors can be classified into three different phases, namely inflammatory, proliferative, and remodeling. In the inflammatory phase, inflammatory cells such as leukocytes and monocytes would accumulate at the site of the tumor and produce proangiogenic chemokines and cytokines [90]. The inflammatory mediators NF-κB, STAT3, and AP-1 in tumor-associated macrophages, myeloid-derived suppressor cells, and other inflammatory cells can also directly regulate multiple proangiogenic factors, such as IL-8, CXCL-1, CXCL-8, VEGF, and HIF1α [86]. Besides, the production of ROS by the activation of inflammatory cells also plays a role in angiogenic signaling via VEGF-dependent pathways [91]. On the other hand, during the proliferative phase, which is the most essential for successful tumor angiogenesis, fibroblasts would proliferate along with endothelial cells, thereby producing components of the extracellular matrix that increase the hyperpermeability and degradation of the basement membrane. Growth factors, platelet factors, proteases, and heparin are also released to promote the formation of new blood vessels at this stage [90]. Lastly, during the remodeling phase, blood vessels are remodeled, pruned, and allowed to mature, where the newly formed vascular supply can contribute to the further exacerbation of inflammation by inducing the inflammatory cell migration to sites of inflammation [90,92].

There have been several studies that demonstrated the role of inflammatory mediators in the promotion of tumor angiogenesis. For example, Protopsaltis et al. have reported that IL-22, a major cytokine expressed by Th17 cells, acts directly on endothelial cells to promote tumor angiogenesis by inducing endothelial cell proliferation, survival, and chemotaxis in vitro, as well as neovascularization in an ex vivo mouse choroid explant model. This can be attributed to the ability of Th17 cells to induce recruitment of proangiogenic myeloid cells to the tumor microenvironment [93]. Apart from that, in a model of experimental angiogenesis utilizing mouse corneas, it was found that inflammatory cytokines induced tissue infiltration of macrophages, which led to the production of chemokines and proangiogenic factors, including VEGF, IL-8, MMPs, and ROS. IL-1β, a key inflammatory cytokine, was also found to induce tumor growth and angiogenesis along with macrophage infiltration and activation. As COX-2 is one of the key inflammatory mediators that is involved in tumor angiogenesis by catalyzing the production of prostanoids, its knockdown or suppression of its activity has led to almost complete attenuation of IL-1β-induced mouse corneal angiogenesis [94].

2.2.4   Tumor metastasis

Metastasis is defined as the spread of neoplastic cells to neighboring or distant sites where these cells would continue to proliferate into tumor cells. It is regarded as the most critical aspect of tumorigenesis from a clinical perspective, as over 90% of cancer-related mortality is the result of metastasis [86]. Generally, the process of metastasis can be divided into four different steps. The first step is EMT; it is one of the major events during metastasis, where epithelial tumor cells acquire mesenchymal characteristics that enhance cell motility and migratory properties which allow them to invade epithelial linings and basal membrane, and to reach efferent blood vessels and lymphatics. As such, EMT can be regarded as a leading process that regulates cancer invasion, cell phenotypic heterogeneity, stemness, immune escape, and therapeutic resistance [95,96]. Various inflammatory mediators including IL-1β, IL-6, IL-8, IL-11, and TNF-α are known as the potent inducers of EMT [97]. For instance, Ershaid et al. reported that cancer-associated fibroblasts (CAFs) activated the NLRP3 inflammasome pathway and upregulated proinflammatory signaling and production of IL-1β. Such CAF-derived inflammasome signaling facilitated the metastasis of breast carcinomas to the lungs, which was attenuated upon ablation of NLRP3 or IL-1β due to modulation on the mesenchymal transition and invasive properties of tumor cells [98]. The process is followed by the intravasation of tumor cells into blood vessels and lymphatics, which is induced by chronic inflammation thorough the production of mediators and remodeling of the tumor stroma that increase vascular permeability. For instance, tumor-associated macrophages produce MMPs that destroy cell-to-cell adhesions and the extracellular matrix, which can

eventually lead to an effective migration and invasion of tumor cells [86,99]. The third step is the maintenance of metastasis-initiated cells survival and travel throughout the circulation, followed by the extravasation of circulating tumor cells via integrin-mediated arrest. Typically, an inflamed environment with an abundance of proinflammatory cytokines can impact the formation of metastases due to the induction of ligands overexpression, which are specific to cancer cell integrins on endothelial cells. As such, these ligands increase the likelihood of metastatic cells' adherence to the endothelium of secondary organs [12]. Within the circulation, the survival of metastatic tumor cells is supported by various inflammatory mediators that are released by immune cells, which later support their colonization in the target organ. The migration of tumor cells can also be guided by the generation of chemokine gradients within the tumor microenvironment, which can be detected by chemokine receptors in a manner similar to the trafficking of leukocytes [81,86,100]. Lastly, metastatic progenitors interact with inflammatory, immune, and stromal cells for their proliferation [86].

3   Current antiinflammatory therapies against cancer

As discussed above, it has long been established that inflammation plays a key role in promoting tumorigenesis by encouraging proliferation, metastasis, angiogenesis and by decreasing the feedback toward the immune system and chemotherapeutics. Besides, an inflamed microenvironment can contribute to genomic damage as well as the enhancement of cell proliferation and survival, thus inducing neoplastic risk. As such, given its myriad of pro-tumorigenic effects, inflammation has become a great target for the prevention and therapeutics of cancer. Various antiinflammatory agents including nonsteroidal antiinflammatory drugs (NSAIDs) have been investigated for their potential in cancer therapeutics. These agents can modify the tumor itself or might impede tumor microenvironment by decreasing cell migration, enhancing cell apoptosis, and increasing chemosensitivity [101]. Hence, the use of antiinflammatory agents either alone or in combination with chemotherapeutic agents can potentially produce beneficial effects in the prevention and treatment of cancer, which ultimately improves disease prognosis and patients' quality of life.

3.1   Nonsteroidal antiinflammatory drugs

The use of NSAIDs in cancer prevention and treatment has been intensively studied in the past decades since the discovery of the correlation between cancer and chronic inflammation [102]. NSAIDs are a group of medications that are commonly prescribed for their analgesic, antipyretic, and antiinflammatory properties. NSAIDs such as mefenamic acid, aspirin, celecoxib, ibuprofen, and diclofenac sodium work by inhibiting the COX enzyme or PGH synthase to exert pain-relieving effects in several conditions ranging from arthritis, menstrual pain to postoperative pain [103]. In terms of cancer, several clinical studies have demonstrated that NSAIDs had notable anticancer activity and their long-term usage can possibly reduce the occurrence of esophageal, colorectal, lung, and breast cancers, with a lowered incidence rate of primary or recurrent tumors [104,105]. Besides, the mortality rate is found to be significantly decreased in cancer individuals after including NSAIDs in their therapeutic regimen [106]. Some published studies have also reported that antiinflammatory drugs may enhance cell apoptosis and sensitivity toward conventional treatment and thus reduce tumor cell invasion and metastasis which in turn deemed them as suitable agents in the treatment of cancer [107–110]. Moreover, NSAIDS were proved to arrest tumor progression by interrupting the inflammatory tumor microenvironment and had lower toxicity or reduced side effects as compared to conventional chemotherapeutics [107].

Nonaspirin NSAIDs have been proven to possess cancer-protective effects. For instance, in a rat mammary model, celecoxib demonstrated a 90% tumor suppression and 25% decrease in palpable tumor growth [111]. Yao et al. also revealed that ibuprofen can lead to a 41%–81% reduction in tumor growth and decrease in liver metastases in mice with colorectal cancer [112]. Moreover, loxoprofen was shown to halt the maturation of implanted Lewis lung cancer in mice. The loxoprofen-treated mice with a dose of 120 mg daily for a week displayed a prominent reduction in intratumoral vessel density and plasma levels of VEGF which effectively suppressed angiogenesis [113]. On top of that, aspirin was also reported to exert antitumor effects. In a study by Xiang et al., aspirin was found to exert antiproliferative and antiapoptotic effects on cervical cancer (HeLa) cells [114]. The reason underlying aspirin's antiapoptotic effects was attributed to the inhibition of Bcl-2 expression and suppression of the activation of AKT as well as ERK [114]. Besides, aspirin was shown to exert both in vitro and in vivo synergism with doxorubicin on HepG2 human hepatocellular carcinoma [115].

Surprisingly, most of the antitumor effects displayed by NSAIDs are not dependent on COX enzyme inhibition. Regardless of the level of COX enzyme expression in tumor cells, NSAIDs still exert great apoptotic and antiproliferative effects [116,117]. This mechanism is further exemplified with a study which demonstrated that the growth-suppressing effects of NSAIDs are irreversible despite supplementation with PGs [118]. Besides, indomethacin was found to induce cell apoptosis in esophageal adenocarcinoma cells by a COX-2-independent upregulation of Bax, a central cell death regulator, and the translocation of cytochrome C in mitochondria [117]. This was also affirmed by Vogt et al. who also suggested that cell apoptosis induced by NSAIDs was not related to the COX-2 enzyme [116]. Previous reviews have shown that the COX-independent activities by NSAIDS in cancer treatment include the suppression of NF-κB, adenosine monophosphate-activated protein kinase (AMPK) and AKT signaling pathways, modulation of cyclic guanosine monophosphate (cGMP)-specific phosphodiesterase signaling, induction of PPAR-γ promoter activity, as well as inhibition of metastasis and angiogenesis [119].

Nonetheless, there are several drawbacks and limitations regarding the current evidence on the use of NSAIDs in cancer therapy. Although epidemiological data demonstrated that the mortality and incidence rates of cancer patients who are prescribed NSAIDs were lower than those who are not given NSAIDs, these findings are only well studied and documented for colorectal and lung cancer [120,121]. For instance, among the various studies which evaluated the connection between NSAIDs and the risk of developing breast cancer, only half of the studies demonstrated a potential reduction of breast cancer risk with the use of NSAIDs [10]. Specifically, one randomized clinical trial has shown that breast cancer risk is not decreased with the long-term use of aspirin, whereas in terms of its prevention, no promising data were documented [122].

3.2 Glucocorticoids

Glucocorticoids are the first-line agents for the treatment of inflammation and chronic inflammation diseases. Traditionally, glucocorticoids were first known as a strong, potent antiinflammatory drug for treating rheumatoid arthritis [123]. Since then, natural and/or synthetic glucocorticoids have been commonly prescribed as immunosuppressive agents [124]. Generally, glucocorticoids exhibit their antiinflammatory effects through almost all cell types within the immune system [125]. Commonly, dexamethasone, an example of a synthetic glucocorticoid, is widely utilized in chemotherapy protocols to enhance tumor cell apoptosis in malignant lymphoid cancers such as Hodgkin's lymphoma, non-Hodgkin's lymphoma, multiple myeloma, as well as acute and chronic lymphocytic leukemia [126].

Glucocorticoids reduce leukocyte recruitment by inhibiting vascular permeability that occurs after inflammation and activate immune cells by inducing cell apoptosis, alteration of cell differentiation, as well as inhibition of cell migration and cytokine release [127]. The antiinflammatory and immunosuppressive effects of glucocorticoids are mostly attributed to trans-repression control of glucocorticoid receptors via their attachment to different DNA-bound transcription factors such as NF-κB, activating protein-1 (AP-1), interferon regulatory factor 3 (IRF3), CREB, nuclear factor of activated T cells (NFAT), T-box expressed in T cells (T-Bet), STAT, and GATA-3

[128,129]. This further leads to downregulation of the genes that produce proinflammatory molecules including COX-2, IFN-γ, IL-1β, IL-2, IL-4, IL-5, IL-6, IL-8, IL-12, IL-18, inducible NO synthase (iNOS), E-selectin, intercellular adhesion molecule (ICAM), TNF-α, vascular cell adhesion molecule (VCAM), and monocyte chemoattractant protein (MCP)-1 [129]. In addition, the antiinflammatory activities brought upon by glucocorticoid receptors can be associated with the induction of glucocorticoid response elements (GRE)-dependent genes such as dual-specificity phosphatase 1 (DUSP1) [130]. One study has proven that DUSP1 causes dephosphorylation of JNK and p38 MAPK in both cell lines and animal models, which ultimately led to the reduction of proinflammatory gene expression [131,132].

One may argue that glucocorticoids have the benefits of counteracting the side effects caused by chemotherapy and radiotherapy, but in some studies, glucocorticoids were found to exert prominent antitumor effects with or without treatment combination. Despite an inconclusive understanding of its mechanism, glucocorticoids have been proven to be beneficial in increasing the survival rate of cancer patients. For example, preclinical studies have shown the remarkable efficacy of dexamethasone in treating breast and renal cancer by inhibiting cell growth and progression [133]. In another study, the incidence rate of lung cancer was decreased after treatment with dexamethasone in tobacco smoke-exposed mice [134]. Besides, the antitumor effects of conventional medications were also found to be induced by the administration of dexamethasone in several in vivo studies [135,136]. Not only dexamethasone, but also other glucocorticoids such as hydrocortisone and prednisone demonstrated significant anticancer effects both in vitro and in vivo [137].

To date, the role of glucocorticoids in cancer metastasis has not been fully studied. They have been shown to suppress cell invasion and migration via different mechanisms including the induction of e-cadherin, as well as the downregulation of MMP2/9, IL-6, and the ras homolog gene family member A (RhoA) [138–140]. Treatment with glucocorticoids has also been correlated to the modulation of angiogenesis, as they can suppress the development of new blood vessels through the downregulation of proangiogenic factors such as VEGF and IL-8 [137]. Lin et al. have reported that miR-708, one of the metastasis suppressor micro-RNA, was believed to be the regulatory mechanism of glucocorticoids in inhibiting cancer metastasis in an in vivo orthotopic xenograft mouse model. It was found that synthetic glucocorticoids can promote miR-708 transcription followed by the suppression of Rap1B, which resulted in reduced tumor cell adhesion, migration, and abdominal metastasis [141]. The recognition of micro-RNAs as a downstream target for glucocorticoids might be helpful for the elucidation of glucocorticoid-associated gene regulation in cancer cell progression and metastasis, which may contribute to additional targets in the treatment of cancer.

Nevertheless, induction of resistance is observed in several in vitro and in vivo studies that utilized corticosteroids in combination with other chemotherapeutics or radiotherapeutics. Such occurrence was observed in kidney, bladder, prostate, testis, breast, ovary, brain, colon, lung, cervix, liver, and pancreatic cancers. This has raised the concern of physicians with regard to the feasibility of utilizing corticosteroids as a combination with the cancer therapeutic regimen [142–148]. The induction of glucocorticoid-mediated resistance was mostly due to the upregulation of threonine/serine survival kinase 1 (SGK1), IκBα, and mitogen-activated protein kinase phosphatase (MKP1/DUSP1) [149,150]. However, no clinical studies have been conducted to support these findings despite the emerging in vitro evidence of the suppression of cell apoptosis by glucocorticoids in different cancer cells. For instance, there was no significant difference observed on the occurrence of adverse events between ovarian cancer patients who received chemotherapy concurrently with glucocorticoids or not [151]. Nevertheless, the action of glucocorticoids in promoting or inhibiting cancer cell progression remains controversial in nonhematologic cancer [133]. Thus, a firm conclusion can only be drawn once more investigations from animal model experiments or retrospective clinical studies have been carried out.

3.3 Small interfering RNA

Advancements in scientific research have led to the development of multiple innovative tools for the treatment of various abnormalities, from inflammation to a vast range of human cancers. RNA interference is one of the technologies that has attracted great attention as a novel therapeutic tool among the research community. Small interfering RNA (siRNA) is a long 20–25 base pairs oligonucleotide that is commonly used to reduce mRNA target expressions through annealing via RNAi to its complementary sequences (Fig. 4) [152,153]. Many recent research works have utilized high-throughput RNAi screenings to identify new therapeutic targets for cancer treatment and to characterize key genes that are involved in certain malignancies. As such, siRNAs have gained importance as potentially effective agents against specific genes involved in the pathogenesis of different cancers [154–162].

In the recent years, siRNA has been poised as an agent for cancer therapeutics due to its extensive ability to target mRNA sequencing [163–165]. However, due to its highly unstable behavior and chances to destroy the human body's immune system, siRNA is not recommended to be administered directly into living organisms [166]. Besides, the negative charge of siRNA, which is attributed to the existence

FIG. 4 The mechanism of RNAi in gene silencing. RNAi begins with the cutting of dsRNA into siRNA by Dicer, followed by the formation of an RISC complex which unwinds the siRNA. The unwound siRNA pairs with complementary mRNA which guides the RNAi machinery to target the mRNA. Finally, the mRNA is cleaved and degraded, thus silencing the gene.

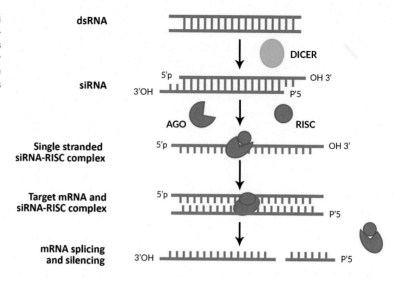

of an anionic phosphate backbone, may further induce toxicity in living organisms. In a study by Niu et al., siRNA-only drug was injected subcutaneously in a model of murine cervical cancer, but it was only successful after multiple trials. This is mostly due to the negative charges surrounding siRNA which prevent its penetration through the lipophilic plasma membrane, thereby resulting in low intracellular delivery [167]. Thus, siRNA is highly not recommended to be injected nakedly. Instead, a delivery vehicle is necessary for the delivery of siRNA into the human body to allow effective delivery to the targeted site while protecting the siRNA from immune surveillance.

Recently, research on the tumor-targeted siRNA delivery system as an antimetastatic biotherapy has been well studied. For example, poly(ethyleneimine) complexed to siRNA-epidermal growth factor receptor (siRNA-EGFR) was injected into mice with lung cancer xenograft had successfully suppressed tumor growth [168,169]. Besides, the introduction of 2-o-methyl residues into the selected sugar structure of the nucleotides in siRNA strands can halt the activation of immune response toward siRNA, where such an approach has been patented. The incorporation of siRNA with cholesterol might also prevent siRNA from exposing its endonuclease activity prematurely [170]. siRNA-loaded 1,2-dioleoyl-3-trimethylammonium-propane (DOTAP) lipoplex nanoparticles have successfully achieved remarkable TNF-α inhibition which attenuated inflammation [171]. Polyethylene glycol (PEG)-arginine-glycine-aspartate (RGD)-siRNAs conjugated to gold nanoparticles have also been shown to reduce tumor growth by downregulating the expression of the c-Myc oncogene via αvβ integrin interactions in alveolar epithelial type-2 adenocarcinoma cells [172]. Lipid/calcium/phosphate (LCP)-based nanoparticles have also been developed to deliver siRNA to inactivate the c-Myc pathway to induce antimetastatic and

antiinflammatory effects [173]. Taken together, these findings from multiple studies indicate that it is feasible to administer siRNA with/without chemotherapeutics by the utilization of a delivery system which might greatly augment the quality and effects of cancer treatment.

3.4 Natural products

The relation of medicinal plants and their role in the management of various health conditions has been conceptualized since ancient times, in which there have been a vast cornucopia of herbs and plants as an integral part of culture and history, serving as the backbone of traditional healing systems in multiple countries. To date, various plants and foods, such as garlic, red wine, grapes, and curry powder, have been proven to possess antiinflammatory effects that are beneficial for the management and/or prevention of cancer [174–178].

Owing to their ability to induce cell cycle arrest or cell apoptosis, these natural products can exhibit inhibitory effects on tumor cells. It has been proven that multiple natural bioactive compounds derived from plants and herbs exert their anticancer effects by either targeting the proinflammatory MAPK, NF-κB, and JNK signaling pathways, or by inhibiting COX and VEGF enzymes [174–176]. One clinical study has reported that the usage of natural compounds as an adjuvant presented convincing results as cancer therapy. It was shown that the combination of 5-fluorouracil and vinorelbine with curcumin led to a synergistic effect in preventing colon cancer cells from proliferation [179]. Besides, ginseng saponins sensitized tumor cells toward conventional chemotherapeutic agents and minimized hematologic toxicity after radiotherapy [176]. Garlic compounds were also found to promote cytotoxicity exhibited by fludarabine and cytarabine in myeloid leukemia cells [177]. At the same time, garlic compounds can reduce the side effects and increase the response of prostate cancer cells toward docetaxel [178]. In addition, S-allylmercaptocysteine, another garlic compound, had augmented the inhibitory efficacy of sulindac toward cellular growth and activated cellular apoptosis [180]. Apart from that, berberine, found in plants of the genera *Coptis*, too presented inhibitory effects on the transcription factor NF-κB and downregulated COX-2 to act as an anticarcinogenic, antiinflammatory, and pro-apoptotic agent toward colon cancer cells [181].

Chemoresistance has become a major concern in recent years as it is the topmost challenging aspect in terms of effective cancer treatment, especially in prostate cancer and nonsmall cell lung cancer (NSCLC) [182,183]. The burden of drug resistance further increases the expenditures incurred during treatment and higher toxicity associated with chemotherapy [184,185]. Among the cancer-related deaths, approximately 80%–90% of them are attributed to drug resistance, whereas around 90% of therapeutic failure occurs during recurrent cancer therapy [186,187]. Interestingly, herbal compounds had shown promising affect to decrease resistance against cancer therapeutics in addition to their antiinflammatory and anticancer effects. Several recent published data on the efficacy of natural products against chemoresistance demonstrated that they can halt the activity of multidrug resistance proteins (MRP) or decrease their protein expressions [188]. For example, silybin, a natural lignan found in *Silybum marianum*, enabled doxorubicin to conquer drug resistance through inhibition of MRP expression in colorectal cancer [189]. Eleven polyoxypregnanes from *Marsdenia tenacissima* have also been proven to overcome doxorubicin resistance by inhibiting ATP-binding cassette (ABC) transporters in multidrug resistance cancer cells [190]. The transporter P-glycoprotein (P-gp) is inhibited by bisbenzylisoquinoline alkaloids, resulting in substantial doxorubicin accumulation in MCF7/ADR breast cancer cells which significantly enhanced cytotoxicity [191]. Several ergot alkaloids isolated from *Claviceps purpurea* had been reported that may overcome chemoresistance in various cancers, although their exact mechanisms of action are yet to be identified [192]. In addition, ellagic acid can overcome chemoresistance toward cisplatin in ovarian cancer cells [193]. Moreover, (Z)-3,4,3′,5′-tetramethoxystilbene, or stilbenoid, enhanced anticancer effectiveness of cisplatin in vitro and in vivo in cisplatin-resistant osteosarcoma cells [194]. Resveratrol, another known stilbenoid, improved the uptake and efficacy of cisplatin in colorectal cancer cells [195]. β-phenylethyl isothiocyanate and 6-gingerol reduced the cellular level of glutathione, which simultaneously reversed drug resistance toward cisplatin and doxorubicin in resistant-uterine sarcoma cells [196,197]. Taken together, all these findings suggested that natural herbs and plants may bring upon advantageous effects in overcoming

chemoresistance and improve the treatment outcomes of recurrent cancers when used in combination with conventional drugs or therapies.

4 Nanomedicine-based approach for the management of cancer

Despite the standard therapies and antiinflammatory intervention currently available, the overall prognosis of patients, especially those with high risk or recurring cancer, remained poor. Besides, most patients are still suffering from adverse effects brought upon by aggressive cancer therapy, while some develop multidrug resistance that leads to drug inactivation and/or drug efflux from tumor cells, which can ultimately result in therapeutic failure. Therefore, these limitations of conventional cancer therapeutics have prompted researchers to elucidate next-generation strategies to achieve more effective and safer cancer therapy while minimizing the occurrence of undesirable adverse reactions. Although the discovery of novel drug compounds that target various signaling pathways underlying the disease can be a straightforward strategy to improve therapeutic outcomes in cancer patients, we believe that a more convincing strategy is by enhancing the therapeutic profiles of existing agents which have already been known to produce anticancer activities to a certain extent.

Nanotechnology is a field of scientific research which involves the know-how of the manufacturing, as well as the study of the structure, property, and behavior of nanomaterials. On the other hand, the field where nanomaterials and nanotechnology are employed for the design and engineering of novel drug delivery systems to enhance the efficacy of the loaded therapeutic agents is known as nanomedicine. These can be engineered using lipids, polymers, metals, or other nanomaterials that enable the encapsulation of various chemical moieties [198–200]. Over the years, nanomedicine-based strategies have been employed as an alternative to conventional therapeutics in various diseases and have presented promising outcomes in multiple studies, which include increased solubility of poorly water-soluble drug moieties leading to the improved biodistribution and bioavailability of therapeutic agents, reduced drug clearance, as well as minimal premature degradation of unstable compounds [198,199,201–205]. Thus, in terms of cancer research, nanomedicine can offer great opportunities in overcoming the drawbacks of conventional therapeutics, along with their uniquely appealing properties such as their nanoscale size, high surface-to-volume ratio, tunable drug release profile, and ability to differentiate and target malignant cells with selectivity. Nanomedicine has gained considerable interest among cancer researchers [205,206]. Furthermore, the convergence of nanomedicine has allowed the development of more advanced and innovative nanocarriers that allow the targeted delivery of chemotherapeutic agents and monitoring of therapeutic effectiveness at the same time [207]. Undoubtedly, the nanomedicine-based approach may be useful in the management of cancer with respect to their beneficial properties, in particular, their ability to achieve safety through specific targeting of malignant tumor cells.

4.1 Enhanced permeability and retention effect

The basis of the tumor-targeted delivery system is the ability of drug-loaded nanocarriers to accumulate in targeted tumor cells and tissues. As such, a passive targeting strategy based on the enhanced permeability and retention (EPR) effect can facilitate tumor targeting where molecules of 10–1000 nm preferentially accumulate within tumor tissues instead of normal tissues [208,209]. Since tumor cells are generally not responsive to cell signaling processes involved in regulating vasculogenesis, the endothelial gap of angiogenic tumor vasculature is often larger than that of normal vasculature. Therefore, it allows the entry of macromolecules into the tumor through its leaky vasculature and its abnormally wide pores. The lack of a lymphatic drainage system in the tumor tissues can also result in higher retention due to the reduced molecule clearance [208–210]. Thus, nanocarriers can be engineered to carry therapeutic agents to target tumor tissues via the EPR effect, whereby a high concentration of these agents can be retained within specific sites while minimizing any off-target side effects, leading to more effective cancer therapy.

4.2 Active tumor targeting

Active targeting refers to the strategy where nanocarriers are designed to demonstrate favorable binding toward complementary molecules presented by malignant cells via the functionalization of surface-bound ligands. Typically, such attachment can contribute to the specific localization of drug-loaded nanocarriers to malignant cells instead of nonmalignant cells, while reducing nonspecific interactions of the nanocarrier with the cell plasma membrane at the same time [210,211]. As such, an active targeting strategy can be employed as a complementary strategy to EPR-based passive targeting to enhance the accumulation of therapeutic agents within tumor tissues. Advancements in the field of nanotechnology have allowed the surface of nanocarriers to be functionalized with one or more ligands, such as the epidermal growth factor receptor, death receptor complexes, folic acid, transferrin, monoclonal antibodies, as well as macromolecules including carbohydrates and proteins, thereby facilitating their binding and receptor-mediated endocytosis by malignant cells [212,213]. Moreover, hydrophilic molecules such as poly(ethylene glycol) can also be functionalized onto the surface of nanocarriers as an attempt to maximize their bio-circulation time by avoiding recognition and clearance by the reticulo-endothelial system (RES) [214]. Nonetheless, the targeting efficiency of ligands may differ depending on their molecular weight, valency, targeting affinity, density, and their biocompatibility with the nanocarrier. Thus, to ensure an effective targeting of nanocarriers to tumor cells and optimization of their intended therapeutic effects, it is of the utmost importance that targeting ligands are designed based on the specificity of overexpressed antigen on the surface of tumor cells, while considering their biocompatibility with the nanomaterials [210,213,215].

4.3 Targeting the tumor microenvironment

As discussed earlier, the physiological state of the tumor microenvironment can greatly influence the pathogenesis and disease outcome of cancer. Therefore, the profile of the tumor microenvironment has a significant impact on the efficacy of anticancer therapeutics and patient prognosis. It has been well established that the tumor microenvironment, which consists of the extracellular matrix, fibroblasts, myofibroblasts, inflammatory cells, and mesenchymal stromal cells, can modulate aberrant tissues and lead to the resulting evolution of cell malignancies [216,217]. As such, researchers have invested their attention in the development of novel therapeutics that exclusively target the tumor microenvironment for the effective management of cancer. Unlike conventional passive and active targeting mechanisms, the tumor microenvironment targeted nanocarriers can respond to various physiological features of the tumor, including hypoxia, redox environment, ROS, and pH abnormality [218–220]. Hence, the nanomedicine-based strategy represents a feasible tool in providing a universal approach for the effective management of cancer.

For instance, in terms of pH-responsiveness, the pKa value of nanomaterials can be optimized to be of similar value as the interstitial pH of the tumor. The slightly acidic condition of the tumor microenvironment can facilitate a pH-dependent structural transformation of the drug-loaded nanocarriers where the protonation or dissociation of pH-sensitive moieties can be triggered when the nanocarriers arrive at the tumor site, thereby resulting in the targeted release of loaded therapeutic agents in the tumor tissues with specificity [205,221]. Besides that, the upregulation of MMP, an enzyme involved in the proliferation of tumor cells that is commonly observed in the tumor microenvironment, can be exploited for the functionalization of nanocarriers with specific substrates that induce binding with MMP in the tumor tissues. This can produce enhanced therapeutic efficacy as the loaded drugs can be directly delivered and retained in the tumor tissues at a relatively high concentration [219,222]. Another unique feature of the tumor microenvironment is hypoxia, which has a crucial role in the induction of tumor angiogenesis and tumor metastasis, as well as the suppression of immune reactivity. Therefore, nanocarriers can be incorporated with a hypoxia-sensitive electron receptor, such as nitroimidazole, to target the hypoxic regions of the tumor [220]. A study has shown that the hypoxic environment of tumor tissues mediated the conversion of hydrophobic nitroimidazole into hydrophilic 2-amino-nitroimidazole, thereby disrupting the hydrophilic-hydrophobic balance to achieve specific release of loaded drugs from the nanocarriers into the tumor tissues [223]. Apart from that, the higher temperature of tumor tissues can also be exploited for the engineering of temperature-sensitive nanocarriers, where the temperature difference between tumor tissues and normal tissues can trigger the targeted release of loaded drugs from the nanocarriers [219].

4.4 Cancer theranostics

Theranostics refers to the simultaneous integration of diagnostics and therapy in a single pharmaceutical formulation [224]. Generally, theranostics approaches enable disease therapy and diagnosis via imaging methods such as optical and ultrasound imaging, magnetic resonance imaging, and computed tomography, as well as real-time monitoring of therapeutic progress and efficacy, all with one therapeutic agent [225]. In recent years, the application of multifunctional nanocarriers for cancer theranostics has emerged as a novel strategy for the safe and effective management of cancers, as it offers the advantage of improved diagnosis on top of the advanced capabilities of nanocarriers, including tumor-specific delivery, sustained and controlled release profile, enhanced transport efficiency, stimuli-responsive release, as well as reduced toxicity to normal tissues [226,227]. As cancer is a highly heterogeneous disease, one type of treatment may only be effective for a subset of the patient population and may not be effective in another. As such, the capability of theranostic nanomedicine to monitor drug accumulation in targeted tissues and therapeutic responses allows for an individualized feedback where researchers and medical practitioners can fine-tune treatment strategies such as drug dosage to meet the personal needs of each patient [225,228]. In principle, nanomaterials are highly useful for this purpose due to their high surface area to volume ratio and their versatility for chemical modifications to augment imaging sensitivity, while allowing a high amount of therapeutic and imaging agents to be loaded into a single nanocarrier [229,230]. Hence, biocompatible multifunctional nanocarriers with appropriate intrinsic physicochemical properties can be engineered to provide a platform for the simultaneous incorporation of therapeutic agents and imaging probes, which enables an accurate diagnosis and efficient monitoring of therapeutic efficacy for a personalized approach in cancer management.

5 Antiinflammatory applications of novel drug delivery systems in cancer

5.1 Lipid-based nanocarriers

Liposomes are sphere-shaped lipid vesicles that are composed of cholesterol and other natural nontoxic phospholipids. They are the most common and well-studied nanocarriers utilized for targeted drug delivery, attributed to their amphiphilicity and their unique ability to entrap both hydrophilic and hydrophobic agents, thereby allowing a wide range of therapeutic agents to be encapsulated by liposomes [231,232]. There have been multiple studies utilizing liposomes as nanocarriers of antiinflammatory agents for the treatment of various cancers. One study by Quagliariello et al. has developed chitosan-coated and uncoated liposomes loaded with butyric acid and evaluated their anticancer effects in the hepatoblastoma HepG2 cell line. Butyric acid is a short-chain fatty acid with antiinflammatory effects, but its clinical applications are limited due to its unpleasant taste and low intestinal absorption. The results showed that both the coated and uncoated nanoformulations had a remarkably higher cytotoxicity as compared with free butyric acid, with a great reduction in IC50 values at 72 h of more than 65% and significantly lowered expressions of proinflammatory cytokines IL-8, IL-6, TNF-α, and TGF-β. A more pronounced effect was observed for the coated liposomes as compared to the uncoated liposomes due to greater internalization by the HepG2 cells. This indicates that liposomes can be employed as a nanocarrier to improve the pharmacokinetic profile of free butyric acid leading to enhanced antiinflammatory effects and improved liver cell survival [233]. Similarly, Kroon et al. evaluated the anticancer efficacy of dexamethasone-loaded liposomes in a mouse model of prostate cancer bone metastases. Although dexamethasone is a highly effective antiinflammatory drug, it is believed that a high tumor concentration of dexamethasone is required for the modulation of tumor-associated inflammation, which is only achieved by high and frequent dosing that can lead to detrimental glucocorticoid-related adverse effects. It was reported that the liposomal formulation was localized efficiently to bone metastases and remarkably inhibited tumor growth, with great inhibition on osteoclast differentiation and osteoclastic bone resorption. In terms of prostate carcinogenesis, liposomal dexamethasone downregulated the expression of IL-6 in macrophages and monocyte-like cells, thereby modulating the proliferation, apoptosis, migration, invasion, angiogenesis, and survival of prostate cancer stem cells. Notably, the antitumor effects of liposomal dexamethasone were significantly greater as compared to free dexamethasone, and it was found to be well tolerated at a clinically relevant dosage that elicits potent antitumor activities. Taken together, the liposomal encapsulation of dexamethasone may present as a promising novel strategy for advanced metastatic prostate cancer [234]. In another work, Sakpakdeejaroen et al. employed transferrin-functionalized liposomes for the targeted delivery of plumbagin to tumor cells. Plumbagin, a naphthoquinone derived from the roots of *Plumbaginaceae* plants, exerts anticancer effects by modulating various signaling pathways including NF-κB, STAT3, JNK, p35, p38, MAPK, and MMP2/9. However, plumbagin suffers from poor water solubility, low stability, and low oral bioavailability which hampered its clinical application. This study demonstrated that the liposomal formulation of plumbagin had improved antiproliferative and apoptotic activities in vitro as compared with free plumbagin solution, whereas in vivo, liposomal plumbagin led to tumor suppression and tumor regression, in contrast tumors treated free plumbagin solution which were progressive. The uptake of plumbagin-loaded liposomes was further enhanced by the functionalization of transferrin, whose receptors are overexpressed on multiple tumor cells, thereby resulting in selective delivery of plumbagin to tumor tissues [235].

Solid-lipid nanoparticles (SLNs) are newer types of lipid-based nanocarriers based on solid lipid matrix, therefore that they remain in a solid state at both storage and body temperature. As such, they are considered as an improvement to liposomes due to their ability to achieve sustained drug release due to their solid matrix [236]. SLNs also offer the feasibility of carrying both hydrophilic and lipophilic drugs, with a higher entrapment efficiency for hydrophobic drugs as they do not contain an aqueous core like liposomes [237,238]. In one study, Rahman et al. encapsulated resveratrol, a phytoalexin with poor oral bioavailability, in cationic SLNs for the treatment of hepatocellular carcinoma. It was found that the SLN nanoformulation had a sustained drug release profile with a remarkably higher cytotoxicity on HepG2 cells in contrast to free resveratrol solution. There were also a notable reduction in tumor volume and increased retention of resveratrol in the tumor tissues in vivo as compared to the free drug solution. The antitumor effects were most likely attributed to the downregulation of proinflammatory cytokines, including TNF-α, IL-1β, and IL-6, as well as NF-κB, while balancing antioxidative enzymes [239]. Apart from that, Thakkar et al. formulated a chitosan-coated SLN drug delivery system encapsulating ferulic acid, an antioxidant, and aspirin, an NSAID, and evaluated its potential as a chemopreventive agent for pancreatic cancer. The researchers demonstrated that there were 5- and 40-fold decrease in the required dose of ferulic acid and aspirin to produce a reduction in the viability of pancreatic cancer cells when encapsulated within chitosan-coated SLNs. The nanoformulation also produced increases in the apoptosis of pancreatic cancer cells in vitro, whereas in vivo, drug-loaded SLNs significantly suppressed tumor growth in contrast to free drugs [240]. Hence, these studies suggest that SLNs can potentially be utilized as a drug nanocarrier to enhance therapeutic efficacy on cancer.

On the other hand, nanostructured lipid carriers (NLCs) are referred to as the second generation of SLNs, as they are mainly developed to overcome the shortcomings of SLNs. While SLNs are composed of solid lipids, NLCs consist of an unstructured lipid matrix that results from a blend of solid and liquid lipids [231,241]. Therefore, NLCs offer an increased drug loading capacity while preventing drug expulsion for long-term drug stability, due to their highly unordered structures that offer a firmer inclusion of the drug molecules within the matrix [241,242]. Thymoquinone is a bioactive compound extracted from *Nigella sativa* that exhibits antiinflammatory, antioxidative, and antitumor effects; however, it cannot be orally administered due to its poor hydrophilicity. As an attempt to overcome this drawback, Haron et al. loaded thymoquinone into NLC and evaluated its therapeutic potential on liver cancer cells Hep3B. The results showed that the nanoformulation induced nonphase-specific cell cycle arrest and inhibited the growth and proliferation of Hep3B cells in a time- and dose-dependent manner, which accompanied the upregulation of caspase-3 and -7. Unlike free thymoquinone, thymoquinone-loaded NLCs acted as an antioxidant which reduced the level of ROS [243]. Besides, Nordin et al. studied the antitumor and antimetastatic effects of citral-loaded NLC in a 4T1-induced breast cancer mouse model. Citral-loaded NLC was found to produce higher efficacy than free citral, signified by the greater inhibition of metastasis via the downregulation of metastatic genes, including MMP-8 and NF-κB, as well as angiogenesis-associated proteins including VEGF, eotaxin, and IL-1α. These findings indicated that NLC is an effective delivery system in the targeting of tumor cells, thereby resulting in enhanced antitumor and antimetastatic effects [244].

5.2 Polymer-based nanocarriers

Polymer-based nanocarriers have received considerable attention in drug delivery research and have been widely regarded as a promising tool for improving therapeutic outcomes in the treatment of diseases [245]. Naturally occurring polymeric nanomaterials are commonly utilized in the design of drug delivery systems due to their abundance, biocompatibility, biodegradability, as well as low toxicity. With respect to that, chitosan is the most widely used natural polymeric nanomaterial for drug delivery due to its capability to blend with other polymers and ease of surface modification, along with lower toxicity and its non-immunogenic property. Besides, the cationic property of chitosan enables it to interact with negatively charged components, such as nucleic acids and cell surface macromolecules [246]. In terms of cancer therapeutics, one study by Wang et al., which utilized chitosan nanoparticles for the co-delivery of 5-fluorouracil and aspirin, has shown promising antitumor activity on hepatocellular carcinoma cells. The results showed that when compared with free aspirin and free 5-fluoruracil, the application of 5-fluoruracil and aspirin-loaded chitosan nanoparticles led to a notable decrease in cell viability and strongly induced cell apoptosis. Aspirin also downregulated the NF-κB pathway and inhibited the expressions of COX-2 and PGE2, which promoted 5-fluoruracil-mediated apoptosis. Thus, it can be deduced that chitosan nanoparticles enhanced the intracellular concentration of both drugs to exert synergistic antitumor effects [247]. Likewise, chitosan encapsulation was also found to promote the efficacy of curcumin in the management of lung carcinogenesis. Like most natural products, the chemopreventive potential of curcumin is limited by its poor aqueous solubility and bioavailability. The study reported that chitosan nanocurcumin drastically enhanced lung localization in vivo as compared with free curcumin. Notably, the nanoformulation exhibited higher efficacy in reducing tumor incidence at a significantly lower dosage, namely, at a dose equivalent to one-fourth of free curcumin. The sustained drug release profile of chitosan nanoparticles also allowed prolonged retention of curcumin in tumor tissues [248].

Nevertheless, natural polymeric nanomaterials suffer from a few disadvantages, such as a high degree of variability, complex structures, as well as a complicated and expensive extraction process. This has led to the advent of synthetic polymeric nanomaterials which offer several advantages over natural polymeric nanomaterials in drug delivery applications. Typically, synthetic polymeric nanomaterials can be easily fabricated using reproducible protocols, thereby producing the near-exact polymers with negligible batch-to-batch variation [249]. One example of a synthetic polymeric nanomaterial that is commonly utilized in cancer therapeutics is poly(lactic-glycolic acid) (PLGA), which is a copolymer synthesized from poly(lactic acid) (PLA) and poly(glycolic acid) (PGA) [250]. Over the years, PLGA nanoparticles have been employed as a potential tool to enhance the therapeutic outcomes of cancer in various studies. For instance, Acharya and Guru reported that prednisolone-loaded PLGA nanoparticles enhanced the antiinflammatory and antiproliferative activities of free prednisolone in C6 glial cell lines. The researchers showed that the PLGA nanoformulation shielded the drug from premature degradation and achieved a biphasic drug release profile; therefore, it can remarkably control the release of proinflammatory cytokines such as TNF-α and nitric oxide for an extended period as compared to free prednisolone. Besides, C6 glial cells also exhibited a significantly lowered cell proliferation upon treatment with the nanoformulation, indicating that the therapeutic efficacy of prednisolone was more pronounced when encapsulated within PLGA nanoparticles

[251]. In another work, the anticancer effects of crocetin-loaded PLGA nanoparticles on the MCF-7 breast cancer cell line were investigated. Crocetin is a carotenoid extracted from the dried stigma of the *Crocus sativus* flower which has demonstrated excellent antiinflammatory, antioxidative, and anticancer activities. However, its poor hydrophilicity has limited its clinical application as a potential chemotherapeutic agent. The encapsulation of crocetin into PLGA nanoparticles had resulted in augmented antiproliferative effects which significantly decreased the IC50 value of MCF-7 cells in a dose-dependent manner, in contrast to that of free crocetin. Such findings may be attributed to the enhanced cellular uptake and improved aqueous solubility that further increased the ability of crocetin to induce apoptosis in cancer cells. This study reaffirmed that PLGA nanoparticles can enhance the efficacy of therapeutic agents for the management of cancer [252].

Another example of a synthetic polymeric nanomaterial that has been widely used for various drug delivery applications is poly(ethylene glycol) (PEG). It is commonly known for its 'stealth' behavior, where therapeutic agents can be directly conjugated with PEG, or it can be functionalized to the surface of various drug delivery systems, which is a technique known as PEGylation, to improve drug bioavailability and cellular uptake. This is one typical approach to achieve greater site-specific targeting, as the high level of hydration of the polyether backbone of PEG prevents nonspecific protein adsorption through steric repulsion. At the same time, it also helps to avoid rapid recognition of the nanocarriers by the immune system, thereby increasing their bio-circulation time in the body [214,253,254]. Chen et al. in a study developed PEG–PLA nanoparticles for the co-delivery of erlotinib and fedratinib to NSCLC cells. As both erlotinib and fedratinib have been linked with poor aqueous solubility and various adverse effects, an effective delivery system is in high demand to enhance the therapeutic efficacy of the drugs. Besides, the upregulation of the JAK2/STAT3 signaling pathway has been shown to induce acquired erlotinib resistance in NSCLC cells with EGFR mutation, whereas fedratinib, a highly selective JAK2 inhibitor, has been shown to sensitize resistant EGFR-mutant NSCLC cells to erlotinib. As such, the combined application of erlotinib and fedratinib may enhance the cytotoxicity of erlotinib and suppress the growth of NSCLC cells. Indeed, the results showed that the nanoformulation exhibited good stability with an efficient release of erlotinib and fedratinib in the acidic microenvironment of the tumor cells. The JAK2/STAT3 signaling pathway was downregulated, thereby reversing erlotinib resistance to induce antitumor activity both in vitro and in vivo. The PEG–PLA nanoparticles also produced remarkably less systemic toxicity as compared to free drugs, indicating the potential of this nanoformulation in treating NSCLC [255]. In another research, EGFR-targeting GE11 peptide-conjugated PLGA-PEG nanoparticles were developed as a nanocarrier to deliver curcumin into EGFR-expressing MCF-7 cells. Indeed, the conjugation of GE11 peptides to curcumin-loaded PLGA-PEG nanoparticles enhanced the delivery of curcumin to EGFR-expressing tumor cells which subsequently improved the inhibition of PI3K signaling and augmented apoptotic tumor cell death. The rapid accumulation of curcumin in tumor cells can be attributed to active receptor-mediated endocytosis as well as passive uptake through the cell membrane. In contrast to free curcumin, the nanoformulation greatly decreased tumor cell viability, systemic drug clearance, and tumor burden, indicating that the therapeutic efficacy of antitumor agents can be enhanced via their delivery in the form of surface-modified nanocarriers to effectively target specific malignant tumor cells [256].

5.3 Inorganic nanocarriers

Inorganic nanocarriers are another group of drug delivery systems that are commonly evaluated for their potential in therapeutic and imaging applications due to their multitude of benefits, including high loading capacity, large surface area, controlled release profile, improved bioavailability, and good tolerance toward various organic solvents [257]. In a work, anti-p65 antibody-loaded TAT peptide-conjugated mesoporous silica nanoparticles (MSNP) have been employed to inhibit the function of NF-κB and induce antitumor effects. It was found that TAT peptide facilitated nonendocytosis cell membrane transduction of MSNP and its convergence toward the perinuclear region, where the nanoparticles were successful in their attack on NF-κB p65 and inhibition of p65 nuclear translocation. As the blockade of NF-κB activation can overcome tumor resistance to chemotherapeutic agents, cotreatment of the nanoformulation with doxorubicin led to a significant suppression of tumor growth in 4T1 tumor-bearing mice. The nanoformulation itself also demonstrated a remarkable inhibition of tumor growth; however, it is incomplete, thereby signifying that this strategy can potentially be useful in the management of cancer by combining with another antitumor agent to maximize its therapeutic efficacy [258]. Gold nanoparticles are another example of an inorganic nanocarrier that is widely employed in imaging, theranostics, and drug delivery applications. This can be attributed to their unique biochemical, optical, sensing, and electronic properties, as well as other advantages such as high functionality, stability, and biocompatibility [259]. Sulaiman et al. encapsulated hesperidin, a flavanone glycoside extracted from citrus fruits, into gold nanoparticles and evaluated their cytotoxic effect on the human breast cancer cell line. It was revealed that the nanoformulation significantly decreased the proliferation and growth of the treated cells in vitro. The nanoformulation also presented antioxidative activities and exerted protective effects against hydrogen peroxide-induced DNA damage. Besides, in vivo studies showed that hesperidin-loaded gold nanoparticles ameliorated the functional activity of macrophages against Ehrlich ascites tumor cells bearing mice. The production of proinflammatory cytokines including TNF-α, IL-1β, and IL-6 was also remarkably suppressed. Collectively, these findings suggested that gold nanoparticles is a suitable carrier and may be applicable as a novel anticancer therapy without inducing excessive adverse effects [260].

6 Conclusions

Inflammation has a great impact on the composition of the tumor microenvironment as well as the plasticity of both tumor and stromal cells. As such, inflammation can predispose to the development of cancer and promotes all stages of tumorigenesis, from the initiation of cancer to the metastatic spread of tumor cells. Therefore, targeting inflammation represents a plausible strategy for the prevention and treatment of cancer. Despite various antiinflammatory agents currently utilized in cancer therapeutics, the therapeutic success of these agents is limited by several drawbacks, such as poor biodistribution and poor bioavailability that necessitate higher dosage to achieve an optimal therapeutic concentration, poor site-specific targeting, adverse effects, as well as drug resistance. In recent years, efforts have been made by researchers to develop novel strategies to replace or complement existing therapeutic agents in the management of cancer. The emerging field of nanomedicine has great potential in addressing these shortcomings of conventional therapeutics, as drug delivery nanocarriers typically possess unique physicochemical characteristics that enable them to exploit the biological and physical features of the tumor microenvironment, thereby increasing targeting specificity and drug retention within the tumor tissues, resulting in enhanced therapeutic efficacy. Various types of drug delivery nanocarriers have been developed and studied for their benefits over conventional therapeutics in the management of cancer, with promising outcomes presented in many preclinical studies conducted thus far, offering an opportunity for the successful application of cancer nanomedicine in improving the quality of life of cancer patients throughout the world. Despite that, the complex pathogenesis of cancer remained as an obstacle for this novel strategy, as certain aspects including their biodistribution, elimination, safety profile, and underlying molecular mechanisms are yet to be fully elucidated. Hence, further research must be performed with emphasis on clinical studies, as the findings obtained from cell lines and animal models may differ drastically in human subjects due to the presence of a complex biological environment within the human body. Interdisciplinary collaboration between medical researchers, scientists, medical practitioners, and oncologists is crucial to ensure research success and the eventual clinical translation of this novel approach as the future therapeutics in the management of cancer.

Declaration of competing interest

The authors declare that they have no known competing financial interests or personal relationships that could have appeared to influence the work reported in this paper.

References

[1] Y.Y. Tan, P.K. Yap, G.L. Xin Lim, M. Mehta, Y. Chan, S.W. Ng, D.N. Kapoor, P. Negi, K. Anand, S.K. Singh, N.K. Jha, L.C. Lim, T. Madheswaran, S. Satija, G. Gupta, K. Dua, D.K. Chellappan, Perspectives and advancements in the design of nanomaterials for targeted cancer theranostics, Chem. Biol. Interact. 329 (2020) 109221, https://doi.org/10.1016/J.CBI.2020.109221.

[2] S. Sarkar, G. Horn, K. Moulton, A. Oza, S. Byler, S. Kokolus, M. Longacre, Cancer development, progression, and therapy: an epigenetic overview, Int. J. Mol. Sci. 14 (2013) 21087, https://doi.org/10.3390/IJMS141021087.

[3] Cancer, World Health Organization. (n.d.). https://www.who.int/health-topics/cancer#tab=tab_1 (Accessed 16 July 2021).

[4] S. Tran, P.-J. DeGiovanni, B. Piel, P. Rai, Cancer nanomedicine: a review of recent success in drug delivery, Clin. Transl. Med. 6 (2017) 44, https://doi.org/10.1186/S40169-017-0175-0.

[5] N. Eiró, F.J. Vizoso, Inflammation and cancer, World J. Gastrointest. Surg. 4 (2012) 62, https://doi.org/10.4240/WJGS.V4.I3.62.

[6] N. Singh, D. Baby, J.P. Rajguru, P.B. Patil, S.S. Thakkannavar, V.B. Pujari, Inflammation and cancer, Ann. Afr. Med. 18 (2019) 121, https://doi.org/10.4103/AAM.AAM_56_18.

[7] L. Munn, Cancer and inflammation, Wiley Interdiscip. Rev. Syst. Biol. Med. 9 (2017), https://doi.org/10.1002/WSBM.1370.

[8] F.R. Greten, S.I. Grivennikov, Inflammation and cancer: triggers, mechanisms and consequences, Immunity 51 (2019) 27, https://doi.org/10.1016/J.IMMUNI.2019.06.025.

[9] E.R. Rayburn, S.J. Ezell, R. Zhang, Anti-inflammatory agents for cancer therapy, Mol. Cell. Pharmacol. 1 (2009) 29, https://doi.org/10.4255/MCPHARMACOL.09.05.

[10] S. Zappavigna, A.M. Cossu, A. Grimaldi, M. Bocchetti, G.A. Ferraro, G.F. Nicoletti, R. Filosa, M. Caraglia, Anti-inflammatory drugs as anticancer agents, Int. J. Mol. Sci. 21 (2020) 2605, https://doi.org/10.3390/ijms21072605.

[11] N. Gupta, D.B. Rai, A.K. Jangid, D. Pooja, H. Kulhari, Nanomaterials-based siRNA delivery: routes of administration, hurdles and role of nanocarriers, Nanotechnol. Mod. Anim. Biotechnol. 67 (2019), https://doi.org/10.1007/978-981-13-6004-6_3.

[12] R. Molinaro, C. Corbo, M. Livingston, M. Evangelopoulos, A. Parodi, C. Boada, M. Agostini, E. Tasciotti, Inflammation and cancer: in medio Stat Nano, Curr. Med. Chem. 25 (2018) 4208, https://doi.org/10.2174/09298673246661709 20160030.

[13] Y. Chan, M. Mehta, K.R. Paudel, T. Madheswaran, J. Panneerselvam, G. Gupta, Q.P. Su, P.M. Hansbro, R. MacLoughlin, K. Dua, D.K. Chellappan, Versatility of liquid crystalline

[14] Y. Chan, S.W. Ng, K. Dua, D.K. Chellappan, Plant-based chemical moieties for targeting chronic respiratory diseases, Target. Cell. Signall. Pathways Lung Dis. (2021) 741–781, https://doi.org/10.1007/978-981-33-6827-9_34.

[15] M.Z. El-Readi, M.A. Althubiti, Cancer nanomedicine: a new era of successful targeted therapy, J. Nanomater. 2019 (2019), https://doi.org/10.1155/2019/4927312.

[16] J. Shi, P.W. Kantoff, R. Wooster, O.C. Farokhzad, Cancer nanomedicine: progress, challenges and opportunities, Nat. Rev. Cancer 17 (1) (2016) 20–37, https://doi.org/10.1038/nrc.2016.108.

[17] S.W. Ng, Y. Chan, X.Y. Ng, K. Dua, D.K. Chellappan, Neuroblastoma: current advancements and future therapeutics, Adv. Drug Deliv. Syst. Manage. Cancer (2021) 281–297, https://doi.org/10.1016/B978-0-323-85503-7.00001-8.

[18] L. Chen, H. Deng, H. Cui, J. Fang, Z. Zuo, J. Deng, Y. Li, X. Wang, L. Zhao, Inflammatory responses and inflammation-associated diseases in organs, Oncotarget 9 (2018) 7204, https://doi.org/10.18632/ONCOTARGET.23208.

[19] E. Kolaczkowska, P. Kubes, Neutrophil recruitment and function in health and inflammation, Nat. Rev. Immunol. 13 (3) (2013) 159–175, https://doi.org/10.1038/nri3399.

[20] M.-B. Voisin, S. Nourshargh, Neutrophil transmigration: emergence of an adhesive Cascade within venular walls, J. Innate Immun. 5 (2013) 336–347, https://doi.org/10.1159/000346659.

[21] P.X. Liew, P. Kubes, The Neutrophil's role during health and disease, Physiol. Rev. 99 (2019) 1223–1248, https://doi.org/10.1152/PHYSREV.00012.2018.

[22] M.A. Sugimoto, L.P. Sousa, V. Pinho, M. Perretti, M.M. Teixeira, Resolution of inflammation: what controls its onset? Front. Immunol. 7 (2016) 160, https://doi.org/10.3389/FIMMU.2016.00160.

[23] M.F. Neurath, Resolution of inflammation: from basic concepts to clinical application, Semin. Immunopathol. 41 (6) (2019) 627–631, https://doi.org/10.1007/S00281-019-00771-2.

[24] S.M. Crusz, F.R. Balkwill, Inflammation and cancer: advances and new agents, Nat. Rev. Clin. Oncol. 12 (2015) 584–596, https://doi.org/10.1038/NRCLINONC.2015.105.

[25] E.A. Comen, R.L. Bowman, M. Kleppe, Underlying causes and therapeutic targeting of the inflammatory tumor microenvironment, Front. Cell Dev. Biol. 6 (2018) 56, https://doi.org/10.3389/FCELL.2018.00056.

[26] G. Landskron, M.D. la Fuente, P. Thuwajit, C. Thuwajit, M.A. Hermoso, Chronic inflammation and cytokines in the tumor microenvironment, J. Immunol. Res. 2014 (2014), https://doi.org/10.1155/2014/149185.

[27] B.F. Zamarron, W. Chen, Dual roles of immune cells and their factors in cancer development and progression, Int. J. Biol. Sci. 7 (2011) 651, https://doi.org/10.7150/IJBS.7.651.

[28] S.F. Josephs, T.E. Ichim, S.M. Prince, S. Kesari, F.M. Marincola, A.R. Escobedo, A. Jafri, Unleashing endogenous TNF-alpha as a cancer immunotherapeutic, J. Transl. Med. 16 (2018) 242, https://doi.org/10.1186/S12967-018-1611-7.

[29] G.D. Kalliolias, L.B. Ivashkiv, TNF biology, pathogenic mechanisms and emerging therapeutic strategies, Nat. Rev. Rheumatol. 12 (2016) 49, https://doi.org/10.1038/NRRHEUM.2015.169.

[30] D.T. Fisher, M.M. Appenheimer, S.S. Evans, The two faces of IL-6 in the tumor microenvironment, Semin. Immunol. 26 (2014) 38, https://doi.org/10.1016/J.SMIM.2014.01.008.

[31] N. Kumari, B.S. Dwarakanath, A. Das, A.N. Bhatt, Role of interleukin-6 in cancer progression and therapeutic resistance, Tumor Biol. 37 (2016) 11553–11572, https://doi.org/10.1007/S13277-016-5098-7.

[32] P. Zarogoulidis, L. Yarmus, K. Darwiche, R. Walter, H. Huang, Z. Li, B. Zaric, K. Tsakiridis, K. Zarogoulidis, Interleukin-6 cytokine: a multifunctional glycoprotein for cancer, Immun. Res. 9 (2013) 16535, https://doi.org/10.1186/2090-5009-9-1.

[33] J.-C. Neel, L. Humbert, J.-J. Lebrun, The dual role of TGFβ in human cancer: from tumor suppression to cancer metastasis, ISRN Mol. Biol. 2012 (2012) 1–28, https://doi.org/10.5402/2012/381428.

[34] N. Sun, A. Taguchi, S. Hanash, Switching roles of TGF-β in cancer development: implications for therapeutic target and biomarker studies, J. Clin. Med. 5 (2016) 109, https://doi.org/10.3390/JCM5120109.

[35] D.R. Principe, J.A. Doll, J. Bauer, B. Jung, H.G. Munshi, L. Bartholin, B. Pasche, C. Lee, P.J. Grippo, TGF-β: Duality of Function Between Tumor Prevention and Carcinogenesis, JNCI J. Natl. Cancer Inst. 106 (2014), https://doi.org/10.1093/JNCI/DJT369.

[36] R. Sabat, G. Grütz, K. Warszawska, S. Kirsch, E. Witte, K. Wolk, J. Geginat, Biology of interleukin-10, Cytokine Growth Factor Rev. 21 (2010) 331–344, https://doi.org/10.1016/J.CYTOGFR.2010.09.002.

[37] P. Berraondo, M.F. Sanmamed, M.C. Ochoa, I. Etxeberria, M.A. Aznar, J.L. Pérez-Gracia, M.E. Rodríguez-Ruiz, M. Ponz-Sarvise, E. Castañón, I. Melero, Cytokines in clinical cancer immunotherapy, Br. J. Cancer 120 (1) (2018) 6–15, https://doi.org/10.1038/s41416-018-0328-y.

[38] M. Oft, IL-10: master switch from tumor-promoting inflammation to antitumor immunity, Cancer Immunol. Res. 2 (2014) 194–199, https://doi.org/10.1158/2326-6066.CIR-13-0214.

[39] T. Sato, M. Terai, Y. Tamura, V. Alexeev, M.J. Mastrangelo, S.R. Selvan, Interleukin 10 in the tumor microenvironment: a target for anticancer immunotherapy, Immunol. Res. 51 (2) (2011) 170–182, https://doi.org/10.1007/S12026-011-8262-6.

[40] M.H. Mannino, Z. Zhu, H. Xiao, Q. Bai, M.R. Wakefield, Y. Fang, The paradoxical role of IL-10 in immunity and cancer, Cancer Lett. 367 (2015) 103–107, https://doi.org/10.1016/J.CANLET.2015.07.009.

[41] K.L. Dennis, N.R. Blatner, F. Gounari, K. Khazaie, Current status of IL-10 and regulatory T-cells in cancer, Curr. Opin. Oncol. 25 (2013) 637, https://doi.org/10.1097/CCO.0000000000000006.

[42] H.T.T. Do, C.H. Lee, J. Cho, Chemokines and their receptors: multifaceted roles in cancer progression and potential value as cancer prognostic markers, Cancers 12 (2020), https://doi.org/10.3390/CANCERS12020287.

[43] M.T. Chow, A.D. Luster, Chemokines in cancer, Cancer Immunol. Res. 2 (2014) 1125, https://doi.org/10.1158/2326-6066.CIR-14-0160.

[44] D. Raman, P.J. Baugher, Y.M. Thu, A. Richmond, Role of chemokines in tumor growth, Cancer Lett. 256 (2007) 137, https://doi.org/10.1016/J.CANLET.2007.05.013.

[45] M.H. Park, J.T. Hong, Roles of NF-κB in cancer and inflammatory diseases and their therapeutic approaches, Cells 5 (2016) 15, https://doi.org/10.3390/CELLS5020015.

[46] V. Tergaonkar, V. Bottero, M. Ikawa, Q. Li, I.M. Verma, IκB kinase-independent IκBα degradation pathway: functional NF-κB activity and implications for cancer therapy, Mol. Cell. Biol. 23 (2003) 8070–8083, https://doi.org/10.1128/MCB.23.22.8070-8083.2003.

[47] B. Hoesel, J.A. Schmid, The complexity of NF-κB signaling in inflammation and cancer, Mol. Cancer 12 (2013) 86, https://doi.org/10.1186/1476-4598-12-86.

[48] K. Lingappan, NF-κB in oxidative stress, Curr. Opin. Toxicol. 7 (2018) 81, https://doi.org/10.1016/J.COTOX.2017.11.002.

[49] L. Xia, S. Tan, Y. Zhou, J. Lin, H. Wang, L. Oyang, Y. Tian, L. Liu, M. Su, H. Wang, D. Cao, Q. Liao, Role of the NFκB-signaling pathway in cancer, Onco. Targets. Ther. 11 (2018) 2063, https://doi.org/10.2147/OTT.S161109.

[50] E. Ricciotti, G.A. FitzGerald, Prostaglandins and inflammation, Arterioscler. Thromb. Vasc. Biol. 31 (2011) 986, https://doi.org/10.1161/ATVBAHA.110.207449.

[51] M.J. Seo, D.K. Oh, Prostaglandin synthases: molecular characterization and involvement in prostaglandin biosynthesis, Prog. Lipid Res. 66 (2017) 50–68, https://doi.org/10.1016/J.PLIPRES.2017.04.003.

[52] M. Hofer, Z. Hoferová, M. Falk, Brief story on prostaglandins, inhibitors of their synthesis, hematopoiesis, and acute radiation syndrome, Molecules 24 (2019), https://doi.org/10.3390/MOLECULES24224019.

[53] D. Wang, R.N. Dubois, Prostaglandins and cancer, Gut 55 (2006) 115–122, https://doi.org/10.1136/gut.2004.047100.

[54] K. Kobayashi, K. Omori, T. Murata, Role of prostaglandins in tumor microenvironment, Cancer Metastasis Rev. 37 (2) (2018) 347–354, https://doi.org/10.1007/S10555-018-9740-2.

[55] F. Finetti, C. Travelli, J. Ercoli, G. Colombo, E. Buoso, L. Trabalzini, Prostaglandin E2 and cancer: insight into tumor progression and immunity, Biology 9 (2020) 1–26, https://doi.org/10.3390/BIOLOGY9120434.

[56] S. Donnini, F. Finetti, E. Terzuoli, M. Bazzani, M. Ziche, Targeting PGE2 signaling in tumor progression and angiogenesis, Onco Therapeut. 5 (2014) 223–232, https://doi.org/10.1615/FORUMIMMUNDISTHER.2015014095.

[57] L.Y. Pang, E.A. Hurst, D.J. Argyle, Cyclooxygenase-2: a role in cancer stem cell survival and repopulation of cancer cells during therapy, Stem Cells Int. 2016 (2016), https://doi.org/10.1155/2016/2048731.

[58] B. Liu, L. Qu, S. Yan, Cyclooxygenase-2 promotes tumor growth and suppresses tumor immunity, Cancer Cell Int. 15 (2015) 106, https://doi.org/10.1186/S12935-015-0260-7.

[59] R.N. Gomes, S.F. da Costa, A. Colquhoun, Eicosanoids and cancer, Clinics 73 (2018), https://doi.org/10.6061/CLINICS/2018/E530S.

[60] N. Nakahata, Thromboxane A2: physiology/pathophysiology, cellular signal transduction and pharmacology, Pharmacol. Ther. 118 (2008) 18–35, https://doi.org/10.1016/J.PHARMTHERA.2008.01.001.

[61] C.D. Funk, Prostaglandins and leukotrienes: advances in eicosanoid biology, Science 294 (2001) 1871–1875, https://doi.org/10.1126/SCIENCE.294.5548.1871.

[62] W. Tian, X. Jiang, D. Kim, T. Guan, M.R. Nicolls, S.G. Rockson, Leukotrienes in tumor-associated inflammation, Front. Pharmacol. 11 (2020), https://doi.org/10.3389/FPHAR.2020.01289.

[63] D. Wang, R.N. DuBois, Eicosanoids and cancer, Nat. Rev. Cancer 10 (2010) 181, https://doi.org/10.1038/NRC2809.

[64] L.M. Knab, P.J. Grippo, D.J. Bentrem, Involvement of eicosanoids in the pathogenesis of pancreatic cancer: the roles of cyclooxygenase-2 and 5-lipoxygenase, World J Gastroenterol: WJG 20 (2014) 10729, https://doi.org/10.3748/WJG.V20.I31.10729.

[65] G.Y. Moore, G.P. Pidgeon, Cross-talk between cancer cells and the tumour microenvironment: the role of the 5-lipoxygenase pathway, Int. J. Mol. Sci. 18 (2017), https://doi.org/10.3390/IJMS18020236.

[66] C. Schneider, A. Pozzi, Cyclooxygenases and lipoxygenases in cancer, Cancer Metastasis Rev. 30 (2011) 277, https://doi.org/10.1007/S10555-011-9310-3.

[67] Y. Gu, I.S. Mohammad, Z. Liu, Overview of the STAT-3 signaling pathway in cancer and the development of specific inhibitors, Oncol. Lett. 19 (2020) 2585, https://doi.org/10.3892/OL.2020.11394.

[68] C.-Y. Loh, A. Arya, A.F. Naema, W.F. Wong, G. Sethi, C.Y. Looi, Signal transducer and activator of transcription (STATs) proteins in cancer and inflammation: functions and therapeutic implication, Front. Oncol. 9 (2019) 48, https://doi.org/10.3389/FONC.2019.00048.

[69] K. Ghoreschi, A. Laurence, J.J. O'Shea, Janus kinases in immune cell signaling, Immunol. Rev. 228 (2009) 273, https://doi.org/10.1111/J.1600-065X.2008.00754.X.

[70] S.J. Thomas, J.A. Snowden, M.P. Zeidler, S.J. Danson, The role of JAK/STAT signalling in the pathogenesis, prognosis and treatment of solid tumours, Br. J. Cancer 113 (2015) 365, https://doi.org/10.1038/BJC.2015.233.

[71] J.J. O'Shea, D.M. Schwartz, A.V. Villarino, M. Gadina, I.B. McInnes, A. Laurence, The JAK-STAT pathway: impact on human disease and therapeutic intervention, Annu. Rev. Med. 66 (2015) 311, https://doi.org/10.1146/ANNUREV-MED-051113-024537.

[72] S. Bose, S. Banerjee, A. Mondal, U. Chakraborty, J. Pumarol, C.R. Croley, A. Bishayee, Targeting the JAK/STAT signaling pathway using phytocompounds for cancer prevention and therapy, Cell 9 (2020), https://doi.org/10.3390/CELLS9061451.

[73] W. Jin, Role of JAK/STAT3 signaling in the regulation of metastasis, the transition of cancer stem cells, and chemoresistance of cancer by epithelial–mesenchymal transition, Cell 9 (2020), https://doi.org/10.3390/CELLS9010217.

[74] M.L. Slattery, L.E. Mullany, L.C. Sakoda, R.K. Wolff, W.S. Samowitz, J.S. Herrick, The MAPK-signaling pathway in colorectal cancer: dysregulated genes and their association with micro RNAs, Cancer Inform. 17 (2018), https://doi.org/10.1177/11769351 18766522.

[75] S. Lee, J. Rauch, W. Kolch, Targeting MAPK signaling in cancer: mechanisms of drug resistance and sensitivity, Int. J. Mol. Sci. 21 (2020), https://doi.org/10.3390/IJMS21031102.

[76] C. Braicu, M. Buse, C. Busuioc, R. Drula, D. Gulei, L. Raduly, A. Rusu, A. Irimie, A.G. Atanasov, O. Slaby, C. Ionescu, I.-Berindan-Neagoe, A comprehensive review on MAPK: a promising therapeutic target in cancer, Cancers 11 (2019) 1618, https://doi.org/10.3390/CANCERS11101618.

[77] M. Burotto, V.L. Chiou, J.-M. Lee, E.C. Kohn, The MAPK pathway across different malignancies: a new perspective, Cancer 120 (2014) 3446–3456, https://doi.org/10.1002/CNCR.28864.

[78] E. Hirsch, M. Martini, M. Chiara, D. Santis, L. Braccini, F. Gulluni, PI3K/AKT signaling pathway and cancer: an updated review, Ann. Med. (2014), https://doi.org/10.3109/07853890.2014.912836.

[79] J. Yang, J. Nie, X. Ma, Y. Wei, Y. Peng, X. Wei, Targeting PI3K in cancer: mechanisms and advances in clinical trials, Mol. Cancer 18 (2019), https://doi.org/10.1186/S12943-019-0954-X.

[80] C. Porta, C. Paglino, A. Mosca, Targeting PI3K/Akt/mTOR signaling in cancer, Front. Oncol. 4 (2014), https://doi.org/10.3389/FONC.2014.00064.

[81] S. Hibino, T. Kawazoe, H. Kasahara, S. Itoh, T. Ishimoto, M. Sakata-Yanagimoto, K. Taniguchi, Inflammation-induced tumorigenesis and metastasis, Int. J. Mol. Sci. 22 (2021) 5421, https://doi.org/10.3390/IJMS22115421.

[82] Ö. Canli, A.M. Nicolas, J. Gupta, F. Finkelmeier, O. Goncharova, M. Pesic, T. Neumann, D. Horst, M. Löwer, U. Sahin, F.R. Greten, Myeloid cell-derived reactive oxygen species induce epithelial mutagenesis, Cancer Cell 32 (2017) 869–883.e5, https://doi.org/10.1016/J.CCELL.2017.11.004.

[83] R. Pathania, S. Ramachandran, S. Elangovan, R. Padia, P. Yang, S. Cinghu, R. Veeranan-Karmegam, P. Arjunan, J.P. Gnana-Prakasam, F. Sadanand, L. Pei, C.-S. Chang, J.-H. Choi, H. Shi, S. Manicassamy, P.D. Prasad, S. Sharma, V. Ganapathy, R. Jothi, M. Thangaraju, DNMT1 is essential for mammary and cancer stem cell maintenance and tumorigenesis, Nat. Commun. 6 (1) (2015) 1–11, https://doi.org/10.1038/ncomms7910.

[84] J.E. Axelrad, S. Lichtiger, V. Yajnik, Inflammatory bowel disease and cancer: the role of inflammation, immunosuppression, and cancer treatment, World J. Gastroenterol. 22 (2016) 4794, https://doi.org/10.3748/WJG.V22.I20.4794.

[85] M. Archer, N. Dogra, N. Kyprianou, Inflammation as a driver of prostate cancer metastasis and therapeutic resistance, Cancers 12 (2020) 2984, https://doi.org/10.3390/CANCERS12102984.

[86] S.I. Grivennikov, F.R. Greten, M. Karin, Immunity, inflammation, and cancer, Cell 140 (2010) 883, https://doi.org/10.1016/J.CELL.2010.01.025.

[87] H. Oshima, T. Ishikawa, G.J. Yoshida, K. Naoi, Y. Maeda, K. Naka, X. Ju, Y. Yamada, T. Minamoto, N. Mukaida, H. Saya, M. Oshima, TNF-α/TNFR1 signaling promotes gastric tumorigenesis through induction of Noxo1 and Gna14 in tumor cells, Oncogene 33 (2013) 3820–3829, https://doi.org/10.1038/onc.2013.356.

[88] I. Kaplanov, Y. Carmi, R. Kornetsky, A. Shemesh, G.V. Shurin, M.R. Shurin, C.A. Dinarello, E. Voronov, R.N. Apte, Blocking IL-1β reverses the immunosuppression in mouse breast cancer and synergizes with anti–PD-1 for tumor abrogation, Proc. Natl. Acad. Sci. 116 (2019) 1361–1369, https://doi.org/10.1073/PNAS.1812266115.

[89] D. Aguilar-Cazares, R. Chavez-Dominguez, A. Carlos-Reyes, C.-Lopez-Camarillo, O.N. Hernadez de la Cruz, J.S. Lopez-Gonzalez, Contribution of angiogenesis to inflammation and cancer, Front. Oncol. (2019) 1399, https://doi.org/10.3389/FONC.2019.01399.

[90] C.A. Whipple, M. Korc, Angiogenesis signaling pathways as targets in cancer therapy, Handbook Cell Signal. 2 (3) (2010) 2895–2905, https://doi.org/10.1016/B978-0-12-374145-5.00333-8.

[91] Y.-W. Kim, X.Z. West, T.V. Byzova, Inflammation and oxidative stress in angiogenesis and vascular disease, J. Mol. Med. 91 (2013) 323–328, https://doi.org/10.1007/S00109-013-1007-3.

[92] D. Ribatti, Inflammation and angiogenesis, Inflamm. Angiogen. (2017) 25–26, https://doi.org/10.1007/978-3-319-68448-2_6.

[93] N.J. Protopsaltis, W. Liang, E. Nudleman, N. Ferrara, Interleukin-22 promotes tumor angiogenesis, Angiogenesis 22 (2018) 311–323, https://doi.org/10.1007/S10456-018-9658-X.

[94] M. Ono, Molecular links between tumor angiogenesis and inflammation: inflammatory stimuli of macrophages and cancer cells as targets for therapeutic strategy, Cancer Sci. 99 (2008) 1501–1506, https://doi.org/10.1111/J.1349-7006.2008.00853.X.

[95] I. Pastushenko, A. Brisebarre, A. Sifrim, M. Fioramonti, T. Revenco, S. Boumahdi, A. van Keymeulen, D. Brown, V. Moers, S. Lemaire, S. de Clercq, E. Minguijón, C. Balsat, Y. Sokolow, C. Dubois, F. de Cock, S. Scozzaro, F. Sopena, A. Lanas, N. D'Haene, I. Salmon, J.-C. Marine, T. Voet, P.A. Sotiropoulou, C. Blanpain, Identification of the tumour transition states occurring during EMT, Nature 556 (2018) 463–468, https://doi.org/10.1038/s41586-018-0040-3.

[96] R. Derynck, R.A. Weinberg, EMT and cancer: more than meets the eye, Dev. Cell 49 (2019) 313–316, https://doi.org/10.1016/J.DEVCEL.2019.04.026.

[97] A. Sistigu, F. di Modugno, G. Manic, P. Nisticò, Deciphering the loop of epithelial-mesenchymal transition, inflammatory cytokines and cancer immunoediting, Cytokine Growth Factor Rev. 36 (2017) 67–77, https://doi.org/10.1016/J.CYTOGFR.2017.05.008.

[98] N. Ershaid, Y. Sharon, H. Doron, Y. Raz, O. Shani, N. Cohen, L. Monteran, L. Leider-Trejo, A. Ben-Shmuel, M. Yassin, M. Gerlic, A. Ben-Baruch, M. Pasmanik-Chor, R. Apte, N. Erez, NLRP3 inflammasome in fibroblasts links tissue damage with inflammation in breast cancer progression and metastasis, Nat. Commun. 10 (1) (2019) 1–15, https://doi.org/10.1038/s41467-019-12370-8.

[99] S. Shang, X. Ji, L. Zhang, J. Chen, C. Li, R. Shi, W. Xiang, X. Kang, D. Zhang, F. Yang, R. Dai, P. Chen, S. Chen, Y. Chen, Y. Li, H. Miao, Macrophage ABHD5 suppresses NFκB-dependent matrix metalloproteinase expression and cancer metastasis, Cancer Res. 79 (2019) 5513–5526, https://doi.org/10.1158/0008-5472.CAN-19-1059.

[100] Z. Zhou, G. Xia, Z. Xiang, M. Liu, Z. Wei, J. Yan, W. Chen, J. Zhu, N. Awasthi, X. Sun, K.-M. Fung, Y. He, M. Li, C. Zhang, A C-X-C chemokine receptor type 2–dominated cross-talk between tumor cells and macrophages drives gastric cancer metastasis, Clin. Cancer Res. 25 (2019) 3317–3328, https://doi.org/10.1158/1078-0432.CCR-18-3567.

[101] J. Todoric, L. Antonucci, M. Karin, Targeting inflammation in cancer prevention and therapy, Cancer Prev. Res. 9 (2016) 895–905, https://doi.org/10.1158/1940-6207.CAPR-16-0209.

[102] R. Virchow, As based upon physiological and pathological histology, Nutr. Rev. 47 (1989) 23–25, https://doi.org/10.1111/J.1753-4887.1989.TB02747.X.

[103] W.L. Smith, D.L. DeWitt, R.M. Garavito, Cyclooxygenases: structural, cellular, and molecular biology, Annu. Rev. Biochem. 69 (2003) 145–182, https://doi.org/10.1146/ANNUREV.BIOCHEM.69.1.145.

[104] G.A. Kune, S. Kune, L.F. Watson, Colorectal cancer risk, chronic illnesses, operations and medications: case–control results from the Melbourne colorectal cancer study, Int. J. Epidemiol. 36 (2007) 951–957, https://doi.org/10.1093/IJE/DYM193.

[105] W.R. Waddell, R.W. Loughry, Sulindac for polyposis of the colon, J. Surg. Oncol. 24 (1983) 83–87, https://doi.org/10.1002/JSO.2930240119.

[106] K. Kashfi, Anti-inflammatory agents as cancer therapeutics, Adv. Pharmacol. (San Diego, CA) 57 (2009) 31–89, https://doi.org/10.1016/s1054-3589(08)57002-5.

[107] D.J.A. de Groot, E.G.E. de Vries, H.J.M. Groen, S. de Jong, Nonsteroidal anti-inflammatory drugs to potentiate chemotherapy effects: from lab to clinic, Crit. Rev. Oncol. Hematol. 61 (2007) 52–69, https://doi.org/10.1016/j.critrevonc.2006.07.001.

[108] A. Zlotnik, Involvement of chemokine receptors in organ-specific metastasis, Contrib. Microbiol. 13 (2006) 191–199, https://doi.org/10.1159/000092973.

[109] N.R. Jana, NSAIDs and apoptosis, Cell. Mol. Life Sci. 65 (2008) 1295–1301, https://doi.org/10.1007/s00018-008-7511-x.

[110] B. Arun, P. Goss, The role of COX-2 inhibition in breast cancer treatment and prevention, Semin. Oncol. 31 (2004) 22–29, https://doi.org/10.1053/j.seminoncol.2004.03.042.

[111] G.A. Alshafie, H.M. Abou-Issa, K. Seibert, R.E. Harris, Chemotherapeutic evaluation of celecoxib, a cyclooxygenase-2 inhibitor, in a rat mammary tumor model, Oncol. Rep. 7 (2000) 1377–1381, https://doi.org/10.3892/or.7.6.1377.

[112] M. Yao, W. Zhou, S. Sangha, A. Albert, A.J. Chang, T.C. Liu, M.M. Wolfe, Effects of nonselective cyclooxygenase inhibition with low-dose ibuprofen on tumor growth, angiogenesis, metastasis, and survival in a mouse model of colorectal cancer, Clin. Cancer Res. 11 (2005) 1618–1628, https://doi.org/10.1158/1078-0432.CCR-04-1696.

[113] A. Kanda, S. Ebihara, H. Takahashi, H. Sasaki, Loxoprofen sodium suppresses mouse tumor growth by inhibiting vascular endothelial growth factor, Acta Oncol. 42 (2003) 62–70, https://doi.org/10.1080/08910603100022258.

[114] S. Xiang, Z. Sun, Q. He, F. Yan, Y. Wang, J. Zhang, Aspirin inhibits ErbB2 to induce apoptosis in cervical cancer cells, Med. Oncol. 27 (2010) 379–387, https://doi.org/10.1007/s12032-009-9221-0.

[115] M.A. Hossain, D.H. Kim, J.Y. Jang, Y.J. Kang, J.H. Yoon, J.O. Moon, H.Y. Chung, G.Y. Kim, Y.H. Choi, B.L. Copple, N.D. Kim, Aspirin enhances doxorubicin-induced apoptosis and reduces tumor growth in human hepatocellular carcinoma cells in vitro and in vivo, Int. J. Oncol. 40 (2012) 1636–1642, https://doi.org/10.3892/ijo.2012.1359.

[116] T. Vogt, M. McClelland, B. Jung, S. Popova, T. Bogenrieder, B. Becker, G. Rumpler, M. Landthaler, W. Stolz, Progression and NSAID-induced apoptosis in malignant melanomas are independent of cyclooxygenase II, Melanoma Res. 11 (2001) 587–599, https://doi.org/10.1097/00008390-200112000-00005.

[117] S. Aggarwal, N. Taneja, L. Lin, M.B. Orringer, A. Rehemtulla, D.G. Beer, Indomethacin-induced apoptosis in esophageal adenocarcinoma cells involves upregulation of bax and translocation of mitochondrial cytochrome C independent of COX-2 expression, Neoplasia 2 (2000) 346–356, https://doi.org/10.1038/sj.neo.7900097.

[118] T.A. Chan, P.J. Morin, B. Vogelstein, K.W. Kinzler, Mechanisms underlying nonsteroidal antiinflammatory drug-mediated apoptosis, Proc. Natl. Acad. Sci. U. S. A. 95 (1998) 681–686, https://doi.org/10.1073/pnas.95.2.681.

[119] E. Gurpinar, W.E. Grizzle, G.A. Piazza, NSAIDs inhibit tumorigenesis, but how? Clin. Cancer Res. 20 (2014) 1104–1113, https://doi.org/10.1158/1078-0432.CCR-13-1573.

[120] C. Gridelli, C. Gallo, A. Ceribelli, V. Gebbia, T. Gamucci, F. Ciardiello, F. Carozza, A. Favaretto, B. Daniele, D. Galetta, S. Barbera, F. Rosetti, A. Rossi, P. Maione, F. Cognetti, A. Testa, M. di Maio, A. Morabito, F. Perrone, Factorial phase III randomised trial of rofecoxib and prolonged constant infusion of gemcitabine in advanced non-small-cell lung cancer: the GEmcitabine-COxib in NSCLC (GECO) study, Lancet Oncol. 8 (2007) 500–512, https://doi.org/10.1016/S1470-2045(07)70146-8.

[121] W.E. Smalley, R.N. DuBois, Colorectal cancer and nonsteroidal anti-inflammatory drugs, Adv. Pharmacol. 39 (1997) 1–20, https://doi.org/10.1016/S1054-3589(08)60067-8.

[122] S.M. Zhang, N.R. Cook, J.E. Manson, I.M. Lee, J.E. Buring, Low-dose aspirin and breast cancer risk: results by tumour characteristics from a randomised trial, Br. J. Cancer 98 (2008) 989–991, https://doi.org/10.1038/sj.bjc.6604240.

[123] P.S. Hench, E.C. Kendall, The effect of a hormone of the adrenal cortex (17-hydroxy-11-dehydrocorticosterone; compound E) and of pituitary adrenocorticotropic hormone on rheumatoid arthritis, Proc. Staff Meet. Mayo Clin. 24 (1949) 181–197.

[124] A.R. Clark, M.G. Belvisi, Maps and legends: the quest for dissociated ligands of the glucocorticoid receptor, Pharmacol. Ther. 134 (2012) 54–67, https://doi.org/10.1016/j.pharmthera.2011.12.004.

[125] U. Baschant, J. Tuckermann, The role of the glucocorticoid receptor in inflammation and immunity, J. Steroid Biochem. Mol. Biol. 120 (2010) 69–75, https://doi.org/10.1016/j.jsbmb.2010.03.058.

[126] D.W. Kufe, R.E. Pollock, R.R. Weichselbaum, R.C. Bast, T.S. Gansler, J.F. Holland, E. Frei (Eds.), Holland-Frei Cancer Medicine, 6th ed., n.d. https://www.ncbi.nlm.nih.gov/books/NBK12354/ (Accessed 23 June 2021).

[127] M. Perretti, A. Ahluwalia, The microcirculation and inflammation: site of action for glucocorticoids, Microcirculation 7 (2000) 147–161, https://doi.org/10.1111/j.1549-8719.2000.tb00117.x.

[128] K. de Bosscher, W. van den Berghe, G. Haegeman, The interplay between the glucocorticoid receptor and nuclear factor-κB or activator protein-1: molecular mechanisms for gene repression, Endocr. Rev. 24 (2003) 488–522, https://doi.org/10.1210/er.2002-0006.

[129] A.C. Liberman, J. Druker, M.J. Perone, E. Arzt, Glucocorticoids in the regulation of transcription factors that control cytokine synthesis, Cytokine Growth Factor Rev. 18 (2007) 45–56, https://doi.org/10.1016/j.cytogfr.2007.01.005.

[130] S.M. Abraham, A.R. Clark, Dual-specificity phosphatase 1: a critical regulator of innate immune responses, Biochem. Soc. Trans. 34 (2006) 1018–1023, https://doi.org/10.1042/BST0341018.

[131] S.M. Abraham, T. Lawrence, A. Kleiman, P. Warden, M. Medghalchi, J. Tuckermann, J. Saklatvala, A.R. Clark, Antiinflammatory effects of dexamethasone are partly dependent on induction of dual specificity phosphatase 1, J. Exp. Med. 203 (2006) 1883–1889, https://doi.org/10.1084/jem.20060336.

[132] S. Bhattacharyya, D.E. Brown, J.A. Brewer, S.K. Vogt, L.J. Muglia, Macrophage glucocorticoid receptors regulate toll-like receptor 4-mediated inflammatory responses by selective inhibition of p38 MAP kinase, Blood 109 (2007) 4313–4319, https://doi.org/10.1182/blood-2006-10-048215.

[133] B.D. Keith, Systematic review of the clinical effect of glucocorticoids on nonhematologic malignancy, BMC Cancer 8 (2008), https://doi.org/10.1186/1471-2407-8-84.

[134] H. Witschi, I. Espiritu, M. Ly, D. Uyeminami, The chemopreventive effects of orally administered dexamethasone in strain A/J mice following cessation of smoke exposure, Inhal. Toxicol. 17 (2005) 119–122, https://doi.org/10.1080/08958370590899712.

[135] H. Wang, Y. Wang, E.R. Rayburn, D.L. Hill, J.J. Rinehart, R. Zhang, Dexamethasone as a chemosensitizer for breast cancer chemotherapy: potentiation of the antitumor activity of adriamycin, modulation of cytokine expression, and pharmacokinetics, Int. J. Oncol. 30 (2007) 947–953, https://doi.org/10.3892/ijo.30.4.947.

[136] H. Wang, M. Li, J.J. Rinehart, R. Zhang, Pretreatment with dexamethasone increases antitumor activity of carboplatin and gemcitabine in mice bearing human cancer xenografts: in vivo activity, pharmacokinetics, and clinical implications for cancer chemotherapy, Clin. Cancer Res. 10 (2004) 1633–1644, https://doi.org/10.1158/1078-0432.CCR-0829-3.

[137] A. Yano, Y. Fujii, A. Iwai, Y. Kageyama, K. Kihara, Glucocorticoids suppress tumor angiogenesis and in vivo growth of prostate cancer cells, Clin. Cancer Res. 12 (2006) 3003–3009, https://doi.org/10.1158/1078-0432.CCR-05-2085.

[138] N.M. Rubenstein, Y. Guan, P.L. Woo, G.L. Firestone, Glucocorticoid down-regulation of RhoA is required for the steroid-induced organization of the junctional complex and tight junction formation in rat mammary epithelial tumor cells, J. Biol. Chem. 278 (2003) 10353–10360, https://doi.org/10.1074/jbc.M213121200.

[139] Y. Zheng, K. Izumi, Y. Li, H. Ishiguro, H. Miyamoto, Contrary regulation of bladder cancer cell proliferation and invasion by dexamethasone-mediated glucocorticoid receptor signals, Mol. Cancer Ther. 11 (2012) 2621–2632, https://doi.org/10.1158/1535-7163.MCT-12-0621.

[140] M.E. Law, P.E. Corsino, S.C. Jahn, B.J. Davis, S. Chen, B. Patel, K. Pham, J. Lu, B. Sheppard, P. Nørgaard, J. Hong, P. Higgins, J.S. Kim, H. Luesch, B.K. Law, Glucocorticoids and histone deacetylase inhibitors cooperate to block the invasiveness of basal-like breast cancer cells through novel mechanisms, Oncogene 32 (2013) 1316–1329, https://doi.org/10.1038/onc.2012.138.

[141] K.T. Lin, Y.M. Yeh, C.M. Chuang, S.Y. Yang, J.W. Chang, S.P. Sun, Y.S. Wang, K.C. Chao, L.H. Wang, Glucocorticoids mediate induction of microRNA-708 to suppress ovarian cancer metastasis through targeting Rap1B, Nat. Commun. 6 (2015) 1–13, https://doi.org/10.1038/ncomms6917.

[142] C. Zhang, J. Mattern, A. Haferkamp, J. Pfitzenmaier, M. Hohenfellner, W. Rittgen, L. Edler, K.M. Debatin, E. Groene, I. Herr, Corticosteroid-induced chemotherapy resistance in urological cancers, Cancer Biol. Ther. 5 (2006) 59–64, https://doi.org/10.4161/cbt.5.1.2272.

[143] S. Benedetti, B. Pirola, P.L. Poliani, L. Cajola, B. Pollo, R. Bagnati, L. Magrassi, P. Tunici, G. Finocchiaro, Dexamethasone inhibits the anti-tumor effect of interleukin 4 on rat experimental gliomas, Gene Ther. 10 (2003) 188–192, https://doi.org/10.1038/sj.gt.3301863.

[144] M. Sui, F. Chen, Z. Chen, W. Fan, Glucocorticoids interfere with therapeutic efficacy of paclitaxel against human breast and ovarian xenograft tumors, Int. J. Cancer 119 (2006) 712–717, https://doi.org/10.1002/ijc.21743.

[145] M.C. Kamradt, N. Mohideen, E. Krueger, S. Walter, A.T.M. Vaughan, Inhibition of radiation-induced apoptosis lay dexamethasone in cervical carcinoma cell lines depends upon increased HPV E6/E7, Br. J. Cancer 82 (2000) 1709–1716, https://doi.org/10.1054/bjoc.2000.1114.

[146] C. Zhang, A. Kolb, J. Mattern, N. Gassler, T. Wenger, K. Herzer, K.M. Debatin, M. Büchler, H. Friess, W. Rittgen, L. Edler, I. Herr, Dexamethasone desensitizes hepatocellular and colorectal tumours toward cytotoxic therapy, Cancer Lett. 242 (2006) 104–111, https://doi.org/10.1016/j.canlet.2005.10.037.

[147] N. Gassler, C. Zhang, T. Wenger, P.A. Schnabel, H. Dienemann, K.M. Debatin, J. Mattern, I. Herr, Dexamethasone-induced cisplatin and gemcitabine resistance in lung carcinoma samples treated ex vivo, Br. J. Cancer 92 (2005) 1084–1088, https://doi.org/10.1038/sj.bjc.6602453.

[148] C. Zhang, A. Kolb, P. Büchler, A.C.B. Cato, J. Mattern, W. Rittgen, L. Edler, K.M. Debatin, M.W. Büchler, H. Friess, I. Herr, Corticosteroid co-treatment induces resistance to chemotherapy in surgical resections, xenografts and established cell lines of pancreatic cancer, BMC Cancer 6 (2006), https://doi.org/10.1186/1471-2407-6-61.

[149] C.A. Mikosz, D.R. Brickley, M.S. Sharkey, T.W. Moran, S.D. Conzen, Glucocorticoid receptor-mediated protection from apoptosis is associated with induction of the serine/threonine survival kinase gene, sgk-1, J. Biol. Chem. 276 (2001) 16649–16654, https://doi.org/10.1074/jbc.M010842200.

[150] W. Wu, S. Chaudhuri, D.R. Brickley, D. Pang, T. Karrison, S.D. Conzen, Microarray analysis reveals glucocorticoid-regulated survival genes that are associated with inhibition of apoptosis in breast

epithelial cells, Cancer Res. 64 (2004) 1757–1764, https://doi.org/10.1158/0008-5472.CAN-03-2546.

[151] K. Münstedt, D. Borces, M.K. Bohlmann, M. Zygmunt, R. von Georgi, Glucocorticoid administration in antiemetic therapy: is it safe? Cancer 101 (2004) 1696–1702, https://doi.org/10.1002/cncr.20534.

[152] D.M. Dykxhoorn, C.D. Novina, P.A. Sharp, Killing the messenger: short RNAs that silence gene expression, Nat. Rev. Mol. Cell Biol. 4 (2003) 457–467, https://doi.org/10.1038/nrm1129.

[153] D.H. Kim, J.J. Rossi, Strategies for silencing human disease using RNA interference, Nat. Rev. Genet. 8 (2007) 173–184, https://doi.org/10.1038/nrg2006.

[154] K. Liew, G.Q.S. Yu, L.J. Wei Pua, L.Z. Wong, S.Y. Tham, L.W. Hii, W.M. Lim, B.M. OuYong, C.K. Looi, C.W. Mai, F. Fei-Lei Chung, L.P. Tan, M. Ahmad, A. Soo-Beng Khoo, C.O. Leong, Parallel genome-wide RNAi screens identify lymphocyte-specific protein tyrosine kinase (LCK) as a targetable vulnerability of cell proliferation and chemoresistance in nasopharyngeal carcinoma, Cancer Lett. 504 (2021) 81–90, https://doi.org/10.1016/j.canlet.2021.02.006.

[155] L.W. Hii, F.F.L. Chung, C.W. Mai, Z.Y. Yee, H.H. Chan, V.J. Raja, N.E. Dephoure, N.J. Pyne, S. Pyne, C.O. Leong, Sphingosine kinase 1 regulates the survival of breast cancer stem cells and non-stem breast cancer cells by suppression of STAT1, Cell 9 (2020), https://doi.org/10.3390/cells9040886.

[156] F.F.L. Chung, P.F.T.M. Tan, V.J. Raja, B.S. Tan, K.H. Lim, T.S. Kam, L.W. Hii, S.H. Tan, S.J. See, Y.F. Tan, L.Z. Wong, W.K. Yam, C.W. Mai, T.D. Bradshaw, C.O. Leong, Jerantinine A induces tumor-specific cell death through modulation of splicing factor 3b subunit 1 (SF3B1), Sci. Rep. 7 (2017), https://doi.org/10.1038/srep42504.

[157] J.L. Er, P.N. Goh, C.Y. Lee, Y.J. Tan, L.W. Hii, C.W. Mai, F.F.L. Chung, C.O. Leong, Identification of inhibitors synergizing gemcitabine sensitivity in the squamous subtype of pancreatic ductal adenocarcinoma (PDAC), Apoptosis 23 (2018) 343–355, https://doi.org/10.1007/s10495-018-1459-6.

[158] K.H. Tiong, B.S. Tan, H.L. Choo, F.F.L. Chung, L.W. Hii, S.H. Tan, N.T. Woei Khor, S.F. Wong, S.J. See, Y.F. Tan, R. Rosli, S.K. Cheong, C.O. Leong, Fibroblast growth factor receptor 4 (FGFR4) and fibroblast growth factor 19 (FGF19) autocrine enhance breast cancer cells survival, Oncotarget 7 (2016) 57633–57650, https://doi.org/10.18632/oncotarget.9328.

[159] J. Campbell, C.J. Ryan, R. Brough, I. Bajrami, H.N. Pemberton, I.Y. Chong, S. Costa-Cabral, J. Frankum, A. Gulati, H. Holme, R. Miller, S. Postel-Vinay, R. Rafiq, W. Wei, C.T. Williamson, D.A. Quigley, J. Tym, B. Al-Lazikani, T. Fenton, R. Natrajan, S.J. Strauss, A. Ashworth, C.J. Lord, Large-scale profiling of kinase dependencies in cancer cell lines, Cell Rep. 14 (2016) 2490–2501, https://doi.org/10.1016/j.celrep.2016.02.023.

[160] T. He, D. Surdez, J.K. Rantala, S. Haapa-Paananen, J. Ban, M. Kauer, E. Tomazou, V. Fey, J. Alonso, H. Kovar, O. Delattre, K. Iljin, High-throughput RNAi screen in Ewing sarcoma cells identifies leucine rich repeats and WD repeat domain containing 1 (LRWD1) as a regulator of EWS-FLI1 driven cell viability, Gene 596 (2017) 137–146, https://doi.org/10.1016/j.gene.2016.10.021.

[161] E. Siebring-van Olst, M. Blijlevens, R.X. de Menezes, I.H. van der Meulen-Muileman, E.F. Smit, V.W. van Beusechem, A genome-wide siRNA screen for regulators of tumor suppressor p53 activity in human non-small cell lung cancer cells identifies components of the RNA splicing machinery as targets for anticancer treatment,

Mol. Oncol. 11 (2017) 534–551, https://doi.org/10.1002/1878-0261.12052.

[162] T. Davoli, K.E. Mengwasser, J. Duan, T. Chen, C. Christensen, E.C. Wooten, A.N. Anselmo, M.Z. Li, K.K. Wong, K.T. Kahle, S.J. Elledge, Functional genomics reveals that tumors with activating phosphoinositide 3-kinase mutations are dependent on accelerated protein turnover, Genes Dev. 30 (2016) 2684–2695, https://doi.org/10.1101/gad.290122.116.

[163] M.H. Darvishi, A. Nomani, M. Amini, M.A. Shokrgozar, R. Dinarvand, Novel biotinylated chitosan-graft-polyethyleneimine copolymer as a targeted non-viral vector for anti-EGF receptor siRNA delivery in cancer cells, Int. J. Pharm. 456 (2013) 408–416, https://doi.org/10.1016/j.ijpharm.2013.08.069.

[164] J. Das, S. Das, A. Paul, A. Samadder, S.S. Bhattacharyya, A.R. Khuda-Bukhsh, Assessment of drug delivery and anticancer potentials of nanoparticles-loaded siRNA targeting STAT3 in lung cancer, in vitro and in vivo, Toxicol. Lett. 225 (2014) 454–466, https://doi.org/10.1016/j.toxlet.2014.01.009.

[165] T.S.C. Li, T. Yawata, K. Honke, Efficient siRNA delivery and tumor accumulation mediated by ionically cross-linked folic acid-poly (ethylene glycol)-chitosan oligosaccharide lactate nanoparticles: for the potential targeted ovarian cancer gene therapy, Eur. J. Pharm. Sci. 52 (2014) 48–61, https://doi.org/10.1016/j.ejps.2013.10.011.

[166] A. Sharma, N.K. Jha, K. Dahiya, V.K. Singh, K. Chaurasiya, A.N. Jha, S.K. Jha, P.C. Mishra, S. Dholpuria, R. Astya, P. Nand, A. Kumar, J. Ruokolainen, K.K. Kesari, Nanoparticulate RNA delivery systems in cancer, Cancer Reports 3 (2020), https://doi.org/10.1002/cnr2.1271.

[167] X.Y. Niu, Z.L. Peng, W.Q. Duan, H. Wang, P. Wang, Inhibition of HPV 16 E6 oncogene expression by RNA interference in vitro and in vivo, Int. J. Gynecol. Cancer 16 (2006) 743–751, https://doi.org/10.1111/j.1525-1438.2006.00384.x.

[168] T. Sasaki, K. Hiroki, Y. Yamashita, The role of epidermal growth factor receptor in cancer metastasis and microenvironment, Biomed. Res. Int. (2013), https://doi.org/10.1155/2013/546318.

[169] P. Zhang, N. Xu, L. Zhou, X. Xu, Y. Wang, K. Li, Z. Zeng, X. Wang, X. Zhang, C. Bai, A linear polyethylenimine mediated siRNA-based therapy targeting human epidermal growth factor receptor in SPC-A1 xenograft mice, Transl. Respirat. Med. 1 (2013) 2, https://doi.org/10.1186/2213-0802-1-2.

[170] Google Patents, (n.d.), US8334373B2 - Nuclease resistant double-stranded ribonucleic acid. https://patents.google.com/patent/US8334373B2/en (Accessed 25 June 2021).

[171] M. Khoury, P. Louis-Plence, V. Escriou, D. Noel, C. Largeau, C. Cantos, D. Scherman, C. Jorgensen, F. Apparailly, Efficient new cationic liposome formulation for systemic delivery of small interfering RNA silencing tumor necrosis factor α in experimental arthritis, Arthritis Rheum. 54 (2006) 1867–1877, https://doi.org/10.1002/art.21876.

[172] J. Conde, F. Tian, Y. Hernández, C. Bao, D. Cui, K.P. Janssen, M.R. Ibarra, P.V. Baptista, T. Stoeger, J.M. de la Fuente, In vivo tumor targeting via nanoparticle-mediated therapeutic siRNA coupled to inflammatory response in lung cancer mouse models, Biomaterials 34 (2013) 7744–7753, https://doi.org/10.1016/j.biomaterials.2013.06.041.

[173] Y. Zhang, L. Peng, R.J. Mumper, L. Huang, Combinational delivery of c-myc siRNA and nucleoside analogs in a single, synthetic nanocarrier for targeted cancer therapy, Biomaterials 34 (2013) 8459–8468, https://doi.org/10.1016/j.biomaterials.2013.07.050.

[174] S. Das, D.K. Das, Anti-inflammatory responses of resveratrol, Inflamm. Allergy Drug Targets 6 (2007) 168–173, https://doi.org/10.2174/187152807781696464.

[175] P. Anand, C. Sundaram, S. Jhurani, A.B. Kunnumakkara, B.B. Aggarwal, Curcumin and cancer: an "old-age" disease with an "age-old" solution, Cancer Lett. 267 (2008) 133–164, https://doi.org/10.1016/j.canlet.2008.03.025.

[176] L.J. Hofseth, M.J. Wargovich, Inflammation, cancer, and targets of ginseng, J. Nutr. (2007) 183S–185S, https://doi.org/10.1093/jn/137.1.183s. American Institute of Nutrition.

[177] H.T. Hassan, Ajoene (natural garlic compound): a new anti-leukaemia agent for AML therapy, Leuk. Res. 28 (2004) 667–671, https://doi.org/10.1016/j.leukres.2003.10.008.

[178] E.W. Howard, D.T. Lee, T.C. Yung, W.C. Chee, X. Wang, C.W. Yong, Evidence of a novel docetaxel sensitizer, garlic-derived S-allylmercaptocysteine, as a treatment option for hormone refractory prostate cancer, Int. J. Cancer 122 (2008) 1941–1948, https://doi.org/10.1002/ijc.23355.

[179] B. Du, L. Jiang, Q. Xia, L. Zhong, Synergistic inhibitory effects of curcumin and 5-fluorouracil on the growth of the human colon cancer cell line HT-29, Chemotherapy 52 (2005) 23–28, https://doi.org/10.1159/000090238.

[180] H. Shirin, J.T. Pinto, Y. Kawabata, J. Soh, T. Delohery, S.F. Moss, V. Murty, R.S. Rivlin, P.R. Holt, I.B. Weinstein, Antiproliferative effects of S-allylmercaptocysteine on colon cancer cells when tested alone or in combination with sulindac sulfide, Cancer Res. 61 (2001) 725–731.

[181] K. Fukuda, Y. Hibiya, M. Mutoh, M. Koshiji, S. Akao, H. Fujiwara, Inhibition by berberine of cyclooxygenase-2 transcriptional activity in human colon cancer cells, J. Ethnopharmacol. 66 (1999) 227–233, https://doi.org/10.1016/S0378-8741(98)00162-7.

[182] A. Chang, Chemotherapy, chemoresistance and the changing treatment landscape for NSCLC, Lung Cancer 71 (2011) 3–10, https://doi.org/10.1016/j.lungcan.2010.08.022.

[183] C.A. Wade, N. Kyprianou, Profiling prostate cancer therapeutic resistance, Int. J. Mol. Sci. 19 (2018), https://doi.org/10.3390/ijms19030904.

[184] G. Housman, S. Byler, S. Heerboth, K. Lapinska, M. Longacre, N. Snyder, S. Sarkar, Drug resistance in cancer: an overview, Cancers 6 (2014) 1769–1792, https://doi.org/10.3390/cancers6031769.

[185] H.C. Zheng, The molecular mechanisms of chemoresistance in cancers, Oncotarget 8 (2017) 59950–59964, https://doi.org/10.18632/oncotarget.19048.

[186] B. Mansoori, A. Mohammadi, S. Davudian, S. Shirjang, B. Baradaran, The different mechanisms of cancer drug resistance: a brief review, Adv. Pharmaceut. Bull. 7 (2017) 339–348, https://doi.org/10.15171/apb.2017.041.

[187] R. Yuan, Y. Hou, W. Sun, J. Yu, X. Liu, Y. Niu, J.J. Lu, X. Chen, Natural products to prevent drug resistance in cancer chemotherapy: a review, Ann. N. Y. Acad. Sci. 1401 (2017) 19–27, https://doi.org/10.1111/nyas.13387.

[188] E. Turrini, L. Ferruzzi, C. Fimognari, Natural compounds to overcome cancer chemoresistance: toxicological and clinical issues, Expert Opin. Drug Metab. Toxicol. 10 (2014) 1677–1690, https://doi.org/10.1517/17425255.2014.972933.

[189] D. Catanzaro, D. Gabbia, V. Cocetta, M. Biagi, E. Ragazzi, M. Montopoli, M. Carrara, Silybin counteracts doxorubicin resistance by inhibiting GLUT1 expression, Fitoterapia 124 (2018) 42–48, https://doi.org/10.1016/j.fitote.2017.10.007.

[190] K.K.W. To, X. Wu, C. Yin, S. Chai, S. Yao, O. Kadioglu, T. Efferth, Y. Ye, G. Lin, Reversal of multidrug resistance by Marsdenia tenacissima and its main active ingredients polyoxypregnanes, J. Ethnopharmacol. 203 (2017) 110–119, https://doi.org/10.1016/j.jep.2017.03.051.

[191] Y.F. Sun, M. Wink, Tetrandrine and fangchinoline, bisbenzylisoquinoline alkaloids from Stephania tetrandra can reverse multidrug resistance by inhibiting P-glycoprotein activity in multidrug resistant human cancer cells, Phytomedicine 21 (2014) 1110–1119, https://doi.org/10.1016/j.phymed.2014.04.029.

[192] M. Mrusek, E.J. Seo, H.J. Greten, M. Simon, T. Efferth, Identification of cellular and molecular factors determining the response of cancer cells to six ergot alkaloids, Invest. New Drugs 33 (2015) 32–44, https://doi.org/10.1007/s10637-014-0168-4.

[193] L.H. Engelke, A. Hamacher, P. Proksch, M.U. Kassack, Ellagic acid and resveratrol prevent the development of cisplatin resistance in the epithelial ovarian cancer cell line A2780, J. Cancer 7 (2016) 353–363, https://doi.org/10.7150/jca.13754.

[194] H. Xu, (Z)-3,4,3′,5′-Tetramethoxystilbene, a natural product, induces apoptosis and reduces viability of paclitaxel-And cisplatin-resistant osteosarcoma cells, J. Cancer Res. Ther. 12 (2016) 1261–1265, https://doi.org/10.4103/0973-1482.158035.

[195] A.M.M. Osman, H.S. Al-Malki, S.E. Al-Harthi, A.A. El-Hanafy, H.M. Elashmaoui, M.F. Elshal, Modulatory role of resveratrol on cytotoxic activity of cisplatin, sensitization and modification of cisplatin resistance in colorectal cancer cells, Mol. Med. Rep. 12 (2015) 1368–1374, https://doi.org/10.3892/mmr.2015.3513.

[196] W.J. Wu, Y. Zhang, Z.L. Zeng, X.B. Li, K.S. Hu, H.Y. Luo, J. Yang, P. Huang, R.H. Xu, β-Phenylethyl isothiocyanate reverses platinum resistance by a GSH-dependent mechanism in cancer cells with epithelial-mesenchymal transition phenotype, Biochem. Pharmacol. 85 (2013) 486–496, https://doi.org/10.1016/j.bcp.2012.11.017.

[197] A. Angelini, C. di Ilio, M.L. Castellani, P. Conti, F. Cuccurullo, Modulation of multidrug resistance p-glycoprotein activity by flavonoids and honokiol in human doxorubicin- resistant sarcoma cells (MES-SA/Dx-5): implications for natural sedatives as chemosensitizing agents in cancer therapy, J. Biol. Regul. Homeost. Agents 24 (2010) 197–205.

[198] Y. Chan, S.W. Ng, H.S. Liew, L.J.W. Pua, L. Soon, J.S. Lim, K. Dua, D.K. Chellappan, Introduction to chronic respiratory diseases: a pressing need for novel therapeutic approaches, Med. Plants Lung Dis. (2021) 47–84, https://doi.org/10.1007/978-981-33-6850-7_2.

[199] Y. Xin, M. Yin, L. Zhao, F. Meng, L. Luo, Recent progress on nanoparticle-based drug delivery systems for cancer therapy, Cancer Biol. Med. 14 (2017) 228–241. http://www.cancerbiomed.org/index.php/cocr/article/view/1045/1171. (Accessed 12 August 2021).

[200] Y. Chan, X.H. Wu, B.W. Chieng, N.A. Ibrahim, Y.Y. Then, Superhydrophobic Nanocoatings as intervention against biofilm-associated bacterial infections, Nano 11 (2021) 1046, https://doi.org/10.3390/NANO11041046.

[201] P. Pandey, S. Satija, R. Wadhwa, M. Mehta, D. Purohit, G. Gupta, P. Prasher, D.K. Chellappan, R. Awasthi, H. Dureja, K. Dua, Emerging trends in nanomedicine for topical delivery in skin disorders: current and translational approaches, Dermatol. Ther. 33 (2020), e13292, https://doi.org/10.1111/DTH.13292.

[202] A.K. Thakur, D.K. Chellappan, K. Dua, M. Mehta, S. Satija, I. Singh, Patented therapeutic drug delivery strategies for targeting pulmonary diseases, Expert Opin. Ther. Pat. 30 (2020), https://doi.org/10.1080/13543776.2020.1741547.

[203] Y. Chan, P. Prasher, R. Löbenberg, G. Gupta, S.K. Singh, B.G. Oliver, D.K. Chellappan, K. Dua, Applications and practice of advanced drug delivery systems for targeting toll-like receptors in pulmonary diseases, Nanomedicine 16 (2021) 783–786, https://doi.org/10.2217/NNM-2021-0056.

[204] Y. Chan, R. MacLoughlin, F.C. Zacconi, M.M. Tambuwala, R.M. Pabari, S.K. Singh, T.J.A. de Pinto, G. Gupta, D.K. Chellappan, K. Dua, Advances in nanotechnology-based drug delivery in targeting PI3K signaling in respiratory diseases, Nanomedicine 16 (2021) 1351–1355, https://doi.org/10.2217/NNM-2021-0087.

[205] J. Wang, Y. Li, G. Nie, Y. Zhao, Precise design of nanomedicines: perspectives for cancer treatment, Natl. Sci. Rev. 6 (2019) 1107–1110, https://doi.org/10.1093/NSR/NWZ012.

[206] M. Arruebo, N. Vilaboa, B. Sáez-Gutierrez, J. Lambea, A. Tres, M. Valladares, Á. González-Fernández, Assessment of the evolution of cancer treatment therapies, Cancers 3 (2011) 3279–3330, https://doi.org/10.3390/CANCERS3033279.

[207] R.G. Bai, K. Muthoosamy, S. Manickam, Nanomedicine in theranostics, Nanotechnol. Appl. Tissue Eng. (2015) 195–213, https://doi.org/10.1016/B978-0-323-32889-0.00012-1.

[208] Y. Shi, R. van der Meel, X. Chen, T. Lammers, The EPR effect and beyond: strategies to improve tumor targeting and cancer nanomedicine treatment efficacy, Theranostics 10 (2020) 7921–7924, https://doi.org/10.7150/THNO.49577.

[209] S.K. Golombek, J.N. May, B. Theek, L. Appold, N. Drude, F. Kiessling, T. Lammers, Tumor targeting via EPR: strategies to enhance patient responses, Adv. Drug Deliv. Rev. 130 (2018) 17–38, https://doi.org/10.1016/J.ADDR.2018.07.007.

[210] D. Rosenblum, N. Joshi, W. Tao, J.M. Karp, D. Peer, Progress and challenges towards targeted delivery of cancer therapeutics, Nat. Commun. 9 (1) (2018) 1–12, https://doi.org/10.1038/s41467-018-03705-y.

[211] Y. Zhang, J. Cao, Z. Yuan, Strategies and challenges to improve the performance of tumor-associated active targeting, J. Mater. Chem. B 8 (2020) 3959–3971, https://doi.org/10.1039/D0TB00289E.

[212] A. Gonda, N. Zhao, J.V. Shah, H.R. Calvelli, H. Kantamneni, N.L. Francis, V. Ganapathy, Engineering tumor-targeting nanoparticles as vehicles for precision nanomedicine, Med One 4 (2019), https://doi.org/10.20900/MO.20190021.

[213] U. Chitgupi, Y. Qin, J.F. Lovell, Targeted nanomaterials for phototherapy, Nanotheranostics 1 (2017) 38–58, https://doi.org/10.7150/NTNO.17694.

[214] J.S. Suk, Q. Xu, N. Kim, J. Hanes, L.M. Ensign, PEGylation as a strategy for improving nanoparticle-based drug and gene delivery, Adv. Drug Deliv. Rev. 99 (2016) 28–51, https://doi.org/10.1016/J.ADDR.2015.09.012.

[215] A.G. Arranja, V. Pathak, T. Lammers, Y. Shi, Tumor-targeted nanomedicines for cancer theranostics, Pharmacol. Res. 115 (2017) 87–95, https://doi.org/10.1016/J.PHRS.2016.11.014.

[216] J. Liu, Q. Chen, L. Feng, Z. Liu, Nanomedicine for tumor microenvironment modulation and cancer treatment enhancement, Nano Today 21 (2018) 55–73, https://doi.org/10.1016/J.NANTOD.2018.06.008.

[217] B. Zhang, Y. Hu, Z. Pang, Modulating the tumor microenvironment to enhance tumor nanomedicine delivery, Front. Pharmacol. 8 (2017) 952, https://doi.org/10.3389/FPHAR.2017.00952.

[218] C. Roma-Rodrigues, R. Mendes, P.V. Baptista, A.R. Fernandes, Targeting tumor microenvironment for cancer therapy, Int. J. Mol. Sci. 20 (2019) 840, https://doi.org/10.3390/IJMS20040840.

[219] S. Uthaman, K.M. Huh, I.-K. Park, Tumor microenvironment-responsive nanoparticles for cancer theragnostic applications, Biomater. Res. 22 (2018) 1–11, https://doi.org/10.1186/S40824-018-0132-Z.

[220] C. Fernandes, D. Suares, M.C. Yergeri, Tumor microenvironment targeted Nanotherapy, Front. Pharmacol. 0 (2018) 1230. doi:https://doi.org/10.3389/FPHAR.2018.01230.

[221] L. Feng, Z. Dong, D. Tao, Y. Zhang, Z. Liu, The acidic tumor microenvironment: a target for smart cancer nano-theranostics, Natl. Sci. Rev. 5 (2018) 269–286, https://doi.org/10.1093/NSR/NWX062.

[222] Y. Lyu, Q. Xiao, Y. Li, Y. Wu, W. He, L. Yin, "Locked" cancer cells are more sensitive to chemotherapy, Bioeng. Transl. Med. 4 (2019), https://doi.org/10.1002/BTM2.10130.

[223] L. Sun, S. Xie, J. Qi, E. Liu, D. Liu, Q. Liu, S. Chen, H. He, V.C. Yang, Cell-permeable, MMP-2 activatable, nickel ferrite and his-tagged fusion protein self-assembled fluorescent nanoprobe for tumor magnetic-targeting and imaging, ACS Appl. Mater. Interfaces 9 (2017) 39209–39222, https://doi.org/10.1021/ACSAMI.7B12918.

[224] Z. Fan, P.P. Fu, H. Yu, P.C. Ray, Theranostic nanomedicine for cancer detection and treatment, J. Food Drug Anal. 22 (2014) 3–17, https://doi.org/10.1016/J.JFDA.2014.01.001.

[225] S.D. Jo, S.H. Ku, Y.Y. Won, S.H. Kim, I.C. Kwon, Targeted nanotheranostics for future personalized medicine: recent progress in cancer therapy, Theranostics 6 (2016) 1362–1377, https://doi.org/10.7150/THNO.15335.

[226] P.P. Shanbhag, S.V. Jog, M.M. Chogale, S.S. Gaikwad, Theranostics for cancer therapy, Curr. Drug Deliv. 10 (2013) 357–362, https://doi.org/10.2174/1567201811310030013.

[227] V.S. Madamsetty, A. Mukherjee, S. Mukherjee, Recent trends of the bio-inspired nanoparticles in cancer theranostics, Front. Pharmacol. 0 (2019) 1264. doi:https://doi.org/10.3389/FPHAR.2019.01264.

[228] S.M. Janib, A.S. Moses, J.A. MacKay, Imaging and drug delivery using theranostic nanoparticles, Adv. Drug Deliv. Rev. 62 (2010) 1052–1063, https://doi.org/10.1016/J.ADDR.2010.08.004.

[229] M.S. Muthu, D.T. Leong, L. Mei, S.S. Feng, Nanotheranostics—application and further development of nanomedicine strategies for advanced theranostics, Theranostics 4 (2014) 660–677, https://doi.org/10.7150/THNO.8698.

[230] H. Chen, Z. Zhen, T. Todd, P.K. Chu, J. Xie, Nanoparticles for improving cancer diagnosis, Mater. Sci. Eng.: R: Rep. 74 (2013) 35–69, https://doi.org/10.1016/J.MSER.2013.03.001.

[231] B. García-Pinel, C. Porras-Alcalá, A. Ortega-Rodríguez, F. Sarabia, J. Prados, C. Melguizo, J.M. López-Romero, Lipid-based nanoparticles: Application and recent advances in cancer treatment, Nanomaterials 9 (2019), https://doi.org/10.3390/nano9040638.

[232] A. Akbarzadeh, R. Rezaei-Sadabady, S. Davaran, S.W. Joo, N. Zarghami, Y. Hanifehpour, M. Samiei, M. Kouhi, K. Nejati-Koshki, Liposome: classification, preparation, and applications, Nanoscale Res. Lett. 8 (2013) 102, https://doi.org/10.1186/1556-276X-8-102.

[233] V. Quagliariello, M. Masarone, E. Armenia, A. Giudice, M. Barbarisi, A. Caraglia, M. Barbarisi, M. Persico, Chitosan-coated liposomes loaded with butyric acid demonstrate anticancer and anti-

inflammatory activity in human hepatoma HepG2 cells, Oncol. Rep. 41 (2019) 1476–1486, https://doi.org/10.3892/OR.2018.6932.

[234] J. Kroon, J.T. Buijs, G. van der Horst, H. Cheung, M. van der Mark, L. van Bloois, L.Y. Rizzo, T. Lammers, R.C. Pelger, G. Storm, G. van der Pluijm, J.M. Metselaar, Liposomal delivery of dexamethasone attenuates prostate cancer bone metastatic tumor growth in vivo, Prostate 75 (2015) 815–824, https://doi.org/10.1002/PROS.22963.

[235] I. Sakpakdeejaroen, S. Somani, P. Laskar, M. Mullin, C. Dufès, Transferrin-bearing liposomes entrapping plumbagin for targeted cancer therapy, J. Interdiscip. Nanomed. 4 (2019) 54, https://doi.org/10.1002/JIN2.56.

[236] M. Harms, C.C. Müller-Goymann, Solid lipid nanoparticles for drug delivery, J. Drug Deliv. Sci. Technol. 21 (2011) 89–99, https://doi.org/10.1016/S1773-2247(11)50008-5.

[237] R.K. Shirodkar, L. Kumar, S. Mutalik, S. Lewis, Solid lipid nanoparticles and nanostructured lipid carriers: emerging lipid based drug delivery systems, Pharm. Chem. J. 53 (2019) 440–453, https://doi.org/10.1007/s11094-019-02017-9.

[238] Y. Duan, A. Dhar, C. Patel, M. Khimani, S. Neogi, P. Sharma, N. Siva Kumar, R.L. Vekariya, A brief review on solid lipid nanoparticles: part and parcel of contemporary drug delivery systems, RSC Adv. 10 (2020) 26777–26791, https://doi.org/10.1039/d0ra03491f.

[239] M. Rahman, W.H. Almalki, O. Afzal, A.S.A. Altamimi, I. Kazmi, F. A. Al-Abbasi, H. Choudhry, S.K. Alenezi, M.A. Barkat, S. Beg, V. Kumar, A. Alhalmi, Cationic solid lipid nanoparticles of resveratrol for hepatocellular carcinoma treatment: systematic optimization, in vitro characterization and preclinical investigation, Int. J. Nanomedicine 15 (2020) 9283–9299, https://doi.org/10.2147/IJN.S277545.

[240] A. Thakkar, S. Chenreddy, J. Wang, S. Prabhu, Ferulic acid combined with aspirin demonstrates chemopreventive potential towards pancreatic cancer when delivered using chitosan-coated solid-lipid nanoparticles, Cell Biosci. 5 (2015) 1–14, https://doi.org/10.1186/S13578-015-0041-Y.

[241] A. Beloqui, M.Á. Solinís, A. Rodríguez-Gascón, A.J. Almeida, V. Préat, Nanostructured lipid carriers: promising drug delivery systems for future clinics, Nanomed. Nanotechnol. Biol. Med. 12 (2016) 143–161, https://doi.org/10.1016/j.nano.2015.09.004.

[242] F.Q. Hu, S.P. Jiang, Y.Z. Du, H. Yuan, Y.Q. Ye, S. Zeng, Preparation and characterization of stearic acid nanostructured lipid carriers by solvent diffusion method in an aqueous system, Colloids Surf. B Biointerfaces 45 (2005) 167–173, https://doi.org/10.1016/j.colsurfb.2005.08.005.

[243] A.S. Haron, S.S. Syed Alwi, L. Saiful Yazan, R. Abd Razak, Y.S. Ong, F.H. Zakarial Ansar, H. Roshini Alexander, Cytotoxic effect of thymoquinone-loaded nanostructured lipid carrier (TQ-NLC) on liver cancer cell integrated with hepatitis B genome, Hep3B, Evid. Based Complement. Alternat. Med. (2018), https://doi.org/10.1155/2018/1549805.

[244] N. Nordin, S.K. Yeap, H.S. Rahman, N.R. Zamberi, N.E. Mohamad, N. Abu, M.J. Masarudin, R. Abdullah, N.B. Alitheen, Antitumor and anti-metastatic effects of Citral-loaded nanostructured lipid carrier in 4T1-induced breast cancer mouse model, Molecules 25 (2020) 2670, https://doi.org/10.3390/MOLECULES25112670.

[245] A. Zielinska, F. Carreiró, A.M. Oliveira, A. Neves, B. Pires, D. Nagasamy Venkatesh, A. Durazzo, M. Lucarini, P. Eder, A.M. Silva, A. Santini, E.B. Souto, Polymeric nanoparticles: production, characterization, toxicology and ecotoxicology, Molecules 25 (2020), https://doi.org/10.3390/molecules25163731.

[246] A. George, P.A. Shah, P.S. Shrivastav, Natural biodegradable polymers based nano-formulations for drug delivery: a review, Int. J. Pharm. 561 (2019) 244–264, https://doi.org/10.1016/j.ijpharm.2019.03.011.

[247] P. Wang, Y. Shen, L. Zhao, Chitosan nanoparticles loaded with aspirin and 5-fluorouracil enable synergistic antitumour activity through the modulation of NF-κB/COX-2 signalling pathway, IET Nanobiotechnol. 14 (2020) 479–484, https://doi.org/10.1049/IET-NBT.2020.0002.

[248] V. Vijayakurup, A.T. Thulasidasan, M. Shankar G, A.P. Retnakumari, C.D. Nandan, J. Somaraj, J. Antony, V.V. Alex, B.S. Vinod, V.B. Liju, S. Sundaram, G.S.V. Kumar, R.J. Anto, Chitosan encapsulation enhances the bioavailability and tissue retention of curcumin and improves its efficacy in preventing B[a]P-induced lung carcinogenesis, Cancer Prev. Res. 12 (2019) 225–236, https://doi.org/10.1158/1940-6207.CAPR-18-0437.

[249] K.K. Bansal, J.M. Rosenholm, Synthetic polymers from renewable feedstocks: an alternative to fossil-based materials in biomedical applications, Ther. Deliv. 11 (2020) 297–300, https://doi.org/10.4155/tde-2020-0033.

[250] S. Rezvantalab, N.I. Drude, M.K. Moraveji, N. Güvener, E.K. Koons, Y. Shi, T. Lammers, F. Kiessling, PLGA-based nanoparticles in cancer treatment, Front. Pharmacol. 9 (2018) 1260, https://doi.org/10.3389/fphar.2018.01260.

[251] S. Acharya, B.R. Guru, Prednisolone encapsulated PLGA nanoparticles: characterization, cytotoxicity, and anti-inflammatory activity on C6 glial cells, J. Appl. Pharmaceut. Sci. 10 (2020) 14–21, https://doi.org/10.7324/JAPS.2020.104003.

[252] Z.H. Ghahestani, F.A. Langroodi, A. Mokhtarzadeh, M. Ramezani, M. Hashemi, Evaluation of anti-cancer activity of PLGA nanoparticles containing crocetin, Artif. Cells Nanomed. Biotechnol. 45 (2016) 955–960, https://doi.org/10.1080/21691401.2016.1198359.

[253] Z. Hussain, S. Khan, M. Imran, M. Sohail, S.W.A. Shah, M. de Matas, PEGylation: a promising strategy to overcome challenges to cancer-targeted nanomedicines: a review of challenges to clinical transition and promising resolution, Drug Deliv. Transl. Res. 9 (3) (2019) 721–734, https://doi.org/10.1007/S13346-019-00631-4.

[254] M.S.H. Akash, K. Rehman, S. Chen, Natural and synthetic polymers as drug carriers for delivery of therapeutic proteins, Polym. Rev. 55 (2015) 371–406, https://doi.org/10.1080/15583724.2014.995806.

[255] D. Chen, F. Zhang, J. Wang, H. He, S. Duan, R. Zhu, C. Chen, L. Yin, Y. Chen, Biodegradable nanoparticles mediated co-delivery of erlotinib (ELTN) and Fedratinib (FDTN) toward the treatment of ELTN-resistant non-small cell lung cancer (NSCLC) via suppression of the JAK2/STAT3 Signaling pathway, Front. Pharmacol. 0 (2018) 1214. doi:https://doi.org/10.3389/FPHAR.2018.01214.

[256] H. Jin, J. Pi, Y. Zhao, J. Jiang, T. Li, X. Zeng, P. Yang, C.E. Evans, J. Cai, EGFR-targeting PLGA-PEG nanoparticles as a curcumin delivery system for breast cancer therapy, Nanoscale 9 (2017) 16365–16374, https://doi.org/10.1039/C7NR06898K.

[257] S. Senapati, A.K. Mahanta, S. Kumar, P. Maiti, Controlled drug delivery vehicles for cancer treatment and their performance, Signal Transduct. Target. Ther. 3 (1) (2018) 1–19, https://doi.org/10.1038/s41392-017-0004-3.

[258] Y.P. Chen, C.T. Chen, T.P. Liu, F.C. Chien, S.H. Wu, P. Chen, C.Y. Mou, Catcher in the rel: nanoparticles-antibody conjugate as NF-κB nuclear translocation blocker, Biomaterials 246 (2020) 119997, https://doi.org/10.1016/J.BIOMATERIALS.2020.119997.

[259] X. Bai, Y. Wang, Z. Song, Y. Feng, Y. Chen, D. Zhang, L. Feng, The basic properties of gold nanoparticles and their applications in tumor diagnosis and treatment, Int. J. Mol. Sci. 21 (2020), https://doi.org/10.3390/IJMS21072480.

[260] G.M. Sulaiman, H.M. Waheeb, M.S. Jabir, S.H. Khazaal, Y.H. Dewir, Y. Naidoo, Hesperidin loaded on gold nanoparticles as a drug delivery system for a successful biocompatible, Anti-Cancer, Anti-Inflamm. Phagocyt. Inducer Model Scient. Rep. 10 (1) (2020) 1–16, https://doi.org/10.1038/s41598-020-66419-6.

Chapter 11

Interplay between gut microbiota in immune homeostasis and inflammatory diseases

Nidhi Tiwari[a], Manvi Suri[b], Jyoti Upadhyay[b], Mohd Nazam Ansari[c], and Abdul Samad[d]

[a]Institute of Nuclear Medicine and Allied Sciences, Defence Research and Development Organization, New Delhi, Delhi, India, [b]School of Health Sciences and Technology, University of Petroleum and Energy Studies, Dehradun, Uttarakhand, India, [c]Department of Pharmacology & Toxicology, College of Pharmacy, Prince Sattam Bin Abdulaziz University, Al-Kharj, Saudi Arabia, [d]Faculty of Pharmacy, Tishk International University, Erbil, Kurdistan Region, Iraq

1 Introduction

Human body organs like skin, gut, and mucosal surroundings host a tremendous number of microbes that are collectively known as the microbiome. Over the past few decades, the interesting interrelationship between microorganism in this environment and human beings has greatly enhanced. The microbial community living inside the digestive tract is called "gut microbiota." Many researchers are working to interpret the microbial and bacterial genomes in the gut environment, facilitated by advanced culture-independent genomic procedures. Gut microbiota play an essential role in immunity development, nutrition, and growth of the body [1]. Recent advancement in this field revealed that the gut microbiota are not only an inactive component but has also play an active role in several host functions such as immunity, metabolism, nutritional responses, and circadian rhythmicity [2,3]. The human immune system comprises an intricate framework of adaptive and innate immune components present in all types of tissues, performs a major function against pathogens and external toxic agents, and regulates the homeostatic imbalance caused by these pathogens. From the environmental viewpoint, it was observed that mammals and their gut microbiota coevolved toward homeostasis and mutualism and require proper host immune functioning to prevent overexploitation of the host machinery in regulating immune tolerance to noxious stimuli [4,5]. Disturbances in the gut microbial environment by factors such as diet, antibiotics, or demographic changes may impair host immune interfaces and can cause pathogenic invasion of microbes and abnormal immune responses. However, this pathogenic invasion and interaction of microbe-immune responses are found to be involved in

gastrointestinal noncommunicable disorders such as celiac diseases [6], inflammatory bowel disease (IBD) [7], and other extra-intestinal diseases such as neurodegenerative diseases [8], metabolic syndrome [9], rheumatoid arthritis [10], and cancer [11]. The gut microbiota, host immune system, and homeostasis interrelationship is a complex, context-dependent, and dynamic process. In this chapter, we have reviewed the current knowledge about the interrelationship between gut microbiota and highlighted the key concepts that link gut microbes and host immune system development and functions. We have also discussed the important role of microbiome-targeted approaches in understanding the pathogenesis of diseases and in the development of microbiome-associated therapeutic interventions.

2 Gut microbiota and immune system development

Microbial colonization in the host mucosal membrane during the early phase of life plays a significant role in the development and maturation of host body immune organization [12]. Many of the critical events related to immune response occur in the first year of life where gut microbes demonstrate greater inter- and intraindividual inconsistency before gaining a more stable configuration attained during adult age [13]. In newborns and infants, it was observed that their immature immune system has an increased susceptibility toward pathogenic infectious agents [14]. This renders infectious diseases in children and is considered as the leading cause of mortality among them [15]. In contrast to this, increased susceptibility toward severe inflammation is also encountered in premature babies as demonstrated by a more distressing disorder, i.e., necrotizing enterocolitis [16]. It was analyzed in some studies that microbial colonization to a major extent mainly originates from the maternal microbial environment [17]. There are several factors that modulate microbial colonization including mode of delivery that has a considerable impact on the arrangement of microbiota across several body system habitats [18]. In addition, breastmilk feeding provides maternal antibodies that offer protection against several pathogenic infections [19]. One study in mice model showed that breastfeeding provides an antibody-generated protective immune response in rat neonates [20]. In one study, a germ-free (GF) animal model determined the mechanistic role of gut microbes and host immune system. Previously, a GF animal study established the association between absence of gut microbes and intense impairment in the lymphoid tissue structure of the intestines and immune response [21]. It was observed in GF mice that the level of intraepithelial lymphocytes (IELs-$\alpha\beta$ and $\gamma\delta$) was significantly declined as compared to normal gut-microbe-colonized mice [22]. Substantial decline in the level of IgA antibodies, which are the backbone of humoral immune responses identified in germ-free mice, was also observed and was restored after microbial colonization [23]. Maternal gestational colonization shows increased level of ILC3s (innate lymphoid cells) and mononuclear cells (F4/80$^+$CD11c$^+$) in neonates [17]. High number of inflammatory mediators such as IL-$^{17+}$ CD^{4+} T (Th17) cells were found in the thin layer of the small intestine (lamina propria) representing potent immunomodulatory endogenous proteins [24]. In GF mice, Th17 cells were found to be absent but are inducible during colonization of microbes, especially with SFB (segmented filamentous bacteria) [25] and with other commensal microbes. SFB causes the adhesion of Th17 cells to the epithelial cells, which causes their activation [26]. Gut bacteria, *Bacteroides fragilis*, causes maturation of immune cell development in mice with the help of this bacteria-derived polysaccharide. It also corrected the deficiency of T cells and lymphoid tissue Th1/Th2 imbalances [27]. Toll-like receptors are the innate immune cell receptors that act as sensors for bacterial flagellae [28]. However, during the neonatal period in mice TLR5 facilitated the counter-selection of flagellated bacterial colonies and this process structured the composition of gut microbiota affecting health and immune homeostasis during adult life [29].

3 Interplay between gut microbiota, immune system, and homeostasis

The intestinal mucosa is the best model for studying the host-microbial interaction interface. The most significant feature of this immune system is its tendency to create an immune tolerance network against changing harmless microbial colonies and preserving the immune reactions in parallel against pathogenic microbial invasion [30]. In a healthy gut environment, the microbiota in the intestines are firmly aligned to the mucosal membrane [31]. The intestinal lumen is separated from underlying tissues by single-layer epithelia. Several mechanisms are involved in microbiota alignment. The intestinal epithelia get separated from the residing gut microbes with the help of the dense mucosal layer [32]. MUC2 (hyperglycosylated mucin) is surrounded by a mucus barrier. MUC2 not only protects the membrane by static shielding but also restricts the immunogenic reactions caused by antigens present in the intestine by targeting enteric DC (dendritic cells) in the antiinflammatory condition [33]. The membrane has tight junctions that restrict trans-epithelial penetration. Signals from microbes such as metabolic indole cause protection of the epithelial barrier by related cytoskeletal proteins and upregulation of tight junctions [34]. Also, the mucosal barrier function is regulated by IgA antibodies' secretion and antimicrobial peptides [35]. Dendritic cells in the intestines play a major role in enteric microbiota alignment to the mucosal surface by a mechanism including gut microbe sampling for antigen demonstration [36].

The innate immune system and gut microbiota share a bidirectional route. Antimicrobial peptides are one of the important components of the innate immune system. The majority of them are produced by small intestinal specialized secretory cells known as Paneth cells [37]. These AMPs display multiple interactions with gut microbes and are found to be important in determining their configuration [38]. In addition to this mechanism, AMPs secreted from the acini of pancreas are reported to be important for maintaining homeostasis of intestines as determine in a mice model featuring lesser secretion of cathelicidin-associated AMPs derived from pancreas because of potassium channel Orai1 deficiency. This deficiency leads to increased microbial translocation and inflammation in systemic circulation causing high mortality [39]. TLRs come under the category of pattern recognition receptors (PRRs); during any infection, they sense signals and elicit immune system protection. Gut microbiota produce ligands that bind TLRs and therefore they are involved in regulating immune reactions and maintaining tissue integrity [40]. TLR expression is determined by diversity in their pattern, i.e., cell-specific, spatial, and temporal in the intestines [41]. TLR5 influences the gut composition [42] that may be critical at the time of birth and neonatal life [29]. The bacterial polysaccharide produced by *B. fragilis* is identified by TLRs in assistance with a C-type lectin PPP, Dectin-160 [43].

Downstream regulation of TLRs and Dectin activates the PI3K (phosphoinositide-3-kinase) pathway that leads to inhibition of GSK3β (glycogen synthase kinase 3β) and finally induces expression of CREB (cAMP response element binding protein)-dependent anti-inflammatory genes [44]. Dectin-1 controls Treg cellular differentiation by modulating microbial configuration and thus regulates the intestinal immune system [45]. In addition, other PRRs, i.e., NOD-like receptors (NLRs) shape the gut microbial composition and nucleotide-binding oligomerization domain-containing protein 1 (NOD1) acts as a sensor for the innate immune system that assist in lymphoid tissue production in response to adaptive response and maintain homeostasis of intestines [46]. The sensor NOD2 from bacteria protects the small intestine from inflammation by inhibiting the growth of the bacteria, *Bacteroides vulgates* [47]. Activation of this NOD2 by gut bacteria stimulates intestinal epithelia stem cell survival and regeneration of epithelia [48]. MyD88 acts on many innate immune cell receptors that sense bacterial signals and its signaling pathways are activated by interleukins (IL-1 and 18) by acting on their relevant receptors [49]. Mice model lacking this MyD99 show alterations in gut microbiota composition [50]. The main function of MyD88 is to control the AMP gene expression in epithelia involving RegIIIγ that restricts the number of Gram-positive bacteria associated with the surface epithelium and limits the stimulation of the adaptive immune system [51]. In addition, MyD88 performs other functions such as promoting microbial homeostasis by the activation of IgA, regulating the differentiation of T cells, and controlling the T17 cell expansion by inhibiting the SFB growth observed in mice models [52]. Inflammasomes are NLRs that after assembly into multiprotein complexes activate the inflammatory cascade and promote IL-1β and IL-18 maturation and pyroptosis (cell lysis) [53]. The (NLRP6) NOD, LRR (leucine-rich repeat), and pyrin domain-containing 6 are inflammasomes present in the intestinal mucosa linked with homeostatic regulation and maintenance of microbial composition [54]. Interestingly, it was observed that NLRP6 has an impact on microbial colonies and is dependent on the vivarium in the microbiota; dysbiosis is seen in mice devoid of NLRP6 and is present only in microbial configurations possessing *Helicobacter* sp., a pathobiont [55]. NLRP3 is an inflammasome, regulation of this signaling is essential in maintaining intestinal homeostasis. During an intestinal injury, certain bacteria of gut microbes such as *Proteus mirabilis* activate monocytes and induce NLRP3-dependent interleukin release, i.e., IL-1β that plays an important role in intestinal inflammation [56]. Absent in melanoma-2 (AIM2) inflammasome regulates the homeostasis of the intestine by the IL-18/22/STAT3 signaling pathway [57]. Another NOD-LRR family protein, IPAF, identifies the flagellin protein and stimulates caspases-1, inflammasomes, and interleukin production (IL-1β) in macrophages infected by *Salmonella* [58]. Other pattern-recognition receptors indicated in maintaining gut microbiome and host body symbiosis are OLRs (OAS-like receptors) [59] and RLRs (RIG-I-like receptors) [60], where further exploration is required in these pathways. Macrophages and monocytes are important innate immune cells

that play a vital role in homeostasis [61]. Bacteria-derived polysaccharides induce antiinflammatory gene expression in murine intestinal macrophages [62]. In addition, butyrate produced by gut microbes drives the differentiation of monocyte to macrophages with the inhibition of HDAC3 (histone deacetylase 3), further amplifying the host defense against microbes [63]. A recent study suggested that trimethylamine N-oxide (TMAO), a soluble metabolite produced by the gut microbiome, can facilitate the polarization of murine macrophages as per an NLRP3-dependent manner [64].

Lymphoid cells of the innate immune system are currently discovered innate immune cells important in the rapid production of chemokines and cytokines to fight against infection and induce repair of mucosal tissues [65]. The host lymphoid cells of innate immune system's functional plasticity and diversity (phenotypic) are aligned by the signals obtained from gut microbes [66].

Recent research uncovered the facts showing association between the adaptive immune system and gut microbiome (Fig. 1). An important example of the adaptive immune system is the beta cell modulators of gut homeostasis that produce a large amount of IgA antibodies in response to gut microbial signals [35]. IgA antibodies are produced by T cell in either a dependent or an independent manner. In the T-cell-dependent manner, IgA performs an important role in shaping the composition of gut microbes [67]. There is a mutual relationship observed between microbiota and IgA antibodies where a specific IgA antibody contributes in the maintenance of balanced and diversified microbiota that drives the extension of Foxp^{3+} regulatory T cells showing IgA-mediated homeostasis in the regulatory pathway [68]. The IgA antibodies secreted from the intestines coat the bacteria, which is colitogenic, and thus prevent the perturbations of inflammation and homeostasis [69]. It was observed that when there is a lack of B cells and IgA antibodies in the intestinal epithelium it causes upregulation of the epithelium-derived immune defense pathway facilitated by an induced interferon response mechanism that is related to successive changes in gut microbial alignment. Simultaneously, Gata4 repression-related metabolic performances in this scenario causes impaired absorption of nutrients through the intestines and metabolic impairment [70]. Researchers have identified new subepithelial cells of the mesenchyma expressing the RANKL cytokine function to serve as M cell activators in the intestines and thus producing IgA antibodies and causing diversification of the gut microbiota [71]. A cross-talk between CD^{4+} regulatory T cells and gut microbiota was investigated in several studies. In GF mice, the CD^{4+} regulatory T cells were absent because of the lack of bacterial colonies that cause production of short-chain fatty acids (SCFAs) by fermenting dietary fibers and undigested carbohydrates [72]. In healthy individuals, intestinal bacteria reactivity seems

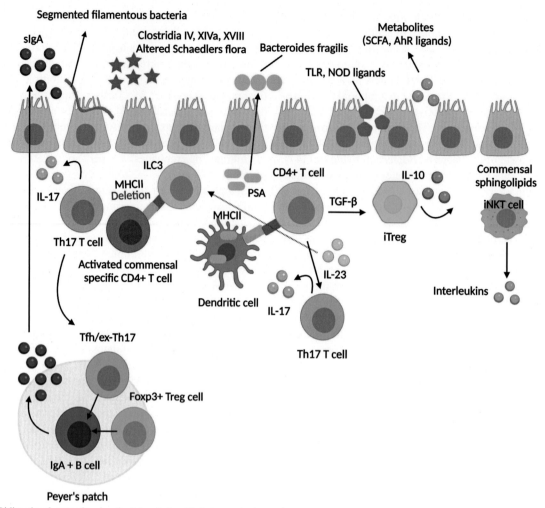

FIG. 1 Bidirectional route showing the interrelationship between the innate immune system and gut microbiota.

to support homeostasis by providing an abundant amount of immune cells that are active against pathogenic infections [73]. Among these immune cells, the Th17 subset is the important one which was intensely investigated by researchers as it shows an ambiguous role in inflammation and host protection [74]. Th17 cells activated by *Citrobacter* are important producers of inflammatory cytokines while Th17 cells induced by SFB function as antiinflammatory mediators [75]. Another important example of gut microbiota regulation by T-cell adaptive response includes cytotoxic CD^{8+} T cells that function in the elimination of cancerous cells and infectious pathogens. Antigen presenting cells (APC) are required for priming of these cells and are CD^{4+} cells amplify these signals [76]. APC-activated CD^{8+} T cells represent no changes in memory cells, observed in the GF mice model, as SCFA produced by gut microbiota are required for promoting their memory potential [77].

4 Interplay between gut microbiota and inflammatory diseases

Gut microbiota and their various metabolites are a important part of the microbial ecological community and help in the regulation of host inflammatory conditions [78,79]. They contain several organisms such as bacteria, fungi, archaea, and protozoa, and can be changed by the host genetics, excess overuse of antibiotics, dietary changes, and habits [80,81]. The human intestine contains many organisms such as *Firmicutes*, *Bacteroidetes*, *Proteobacteria*, and *Actinobacteria* [82]. Some are beneficial for human health and few cause diseases or infection, for example, *Firmicutes* are Gram-positive bacteria, a large class of lactic acid, and *Clostridia*. Lactic acid is one of the marketed probiotic formulations and useful for human health whereas *Bacteroidetes* and *Proteobacteria* are Gram-negative bacteria and trigger the stimulation of macrophages toward the proinflammatory phenotype resulting in inflammation/ infection or many health-related issues [83]. Inflammation is a natural physiological behavior toward unknown invasive microorganisms and plays two contradictory roles in human health [84]. Inflammation is an automatic self-protection response and helps or promotes wound healing conditions whereas in some cases it produces an extreme inflammatory response resulting in immune-mediated inflammatory diseases such as inflammatory bowel diseases, rheumatoid arthritis, cancer, ulcerative colitis (UC), obesity, multiple sclerosis (MS), cardiometabolic disease, asthma and allergic diseases, etc. [85–87]. In case of acute inflammation, only neutrophils are enlisted at the inflamed site and in chronic inflammation conditions macrophages, lymphocytes, and plasma cells accumulate and infiltrate at tissue junctions [88]. Various prevalent chronic inflammation-related conditions are associated with the gut microbiota and contribute to several diseases and their regulatory role in immune system function. Here, in this chapter we have discussed the interaction between gut microbiota in various inflammatory diseases.

4.1 Gut microbiota and inflammatory bowel diseases (IBD)

Inflammatory bowel disease includes both "ulcerative colitis (UC) and Crohn's disease (CD)" and is defined as a chronic, persistent inflammatory disorder of the intestine, and reduction in the microbial diversity or disruption in microbial homeostasis is associated with the pathogenesis of IBD [89]. Under normal conditions, the mucosal immune system protects the intestines from the microorganisms (bacteria) and maintains the immunological environment, and thus benefits the gut microbiota [90]; however, under abnormal conditions, disruption in mucosal immunity contributes to severe intestine inflammation followed by stimulation of an incessant microbial antigenic response [83]. Intestinal inflammation changes the gut microbiota composition and promotes intensifies inflammation [91]. Under IBD condition copious symbiotic bacteria, mainly *Firmicutes* and *Bacteroidetes* and the level of the microbiota metabolites (SCFAs) including butyrate-producing bacteria (*Clostridium* IXa and IV groups), were reduced and limited inflammation of the intestine by regulating colonic T-cell function [92]. Further, a number of facultative anaerobic bacterium such as (family of *Enterobacteriaceae*) were increased in IBD [93]. The first line of defense against foreign pathogens is intestinal macrophages, which is most abundant in the gut immune cells [94]; they do not interact with lipopolysaccharide (LPS) activation due to absence of CD^{14+} cells, which is important for proinflammatory cytokine production (IL-1, IL-6, IL-8, and TNF-α) [94–96]. The advantage of inflammatory macrophages is

they produce an antiinflammatory cytokine, i.e., interleukin (IL-10), and regulate the differentiation of T cells to avert mucosal self-inflammation [97]. Moreover, they execute some necessary functions for maintaining intestinal homeostasis and have strong phagocytic activity [83]. The correlation between IBD and role of several inflammatory mediators' pathways with the gut microbiota are as described in Fig. 2. Therefore, it is clear that intestinal macrophages are well recognized as innate immune system cells and demonstrate bactericidal and phagocytic activity [98].

4.2 Gut microbiota, asthma, and allergic diseases

Asthma is a chronic inflammatory disease characterized by airflow obstruction and airway hyperresponsiveness (AHR). With medical advancement, numerous studies showed a close correlation between the gut microbiome and asthma. According to the "hygiene hypothesis", exposure to microbiota constituents in early life is vital for the development and maturity of immune-related functions and their absence led to increased vulnerability to asthma and allergic diseases [99]. Gut microbiota are different in both healthy as well as in asthmatic individuals and higher microbial community is regarded as favorable, suggested by one study that documented a link between low gut microbial diversity in early life, and a higher chance of asthma in childhood [100]. Further, specific gut bacteria such as *Clostridium* and *Eggerthella lenta* are more prevalent in the gut of asthmatic patients as compared to healthy individuals. Moreover, there is decrease in the concentration of *Bifidobacterium*, *Akkermansia*, and *Faecalibacterium* whereas *Candida* and *Rhodotorula* levels are increased in the gut and there is risk of developing asthma and allergies in a child [101,102]. In some cases, intestinal colonization by *Clostridium difficile* is also associated in the specific age of the child (6–7 years) [103]. Consequently, healthy microbiota community in the gastrointestinal (GI) tract may be useful to the host and reduction in microbial diversity can possibly be a marker for primary underlying pathological conditions. Numerous studies have been demonstrated by researchers to treat or manage the condition of asthma by improving gut microbiota via a significant decrease in the abundances of some bacteria such as *Lachnospira*, *Veillonella*, *Faecalibacterium*, and *Rothia* in the gut of asthmatic infants and inoculations of these microorganisms in immaculate mice mitigate inflammation of airways, thus preventing the development of asthma [104]. Other studies indicated that after oral administration of some bacteria, i.e., *Lactobacillus rhamnosus*, *Lactobacillus casei*, and *Bifidobacterium breve* probably treated allergies in asthmatic patients [105,106]. Further, a randomized, double blind, and placebo controlled trial recruited 160 asthmatic children and

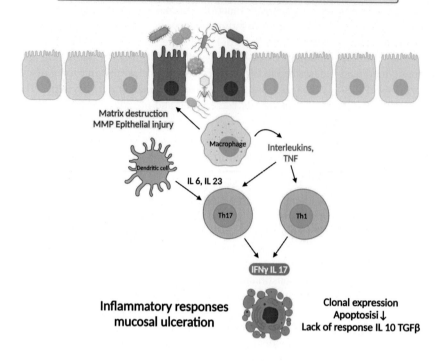

IBD MICROBIOTA
Bacteria diversity ↓, Caudovirales richness ↑

Matrix destruction
MMP Epithelial injury

Macrophage

Interleukins,
TNF

Dendritic cell

IL 6, IL 23

Th17

Th1

IFNy IL 17

Inflammatory responses
mucosal ulceration

Clonal expression
Apoptosisi ↓
Lack of response IL 10 TGFβ

FIG. 2 Correlation between IBD and role of several inflammatory mediator pathways with the gut microbiota.

recommended that *Lactobacillus* was capable of reducing symptoms and severity in asthmatic patients [107].

4.3 Gut microbiota and rheumatoid arthritis (RA)

Rheumatoid arthritis, also known as autoimmune arthritis, is a systemic chronic inflammatory disease described by production of auto-antibodies and primarily affects multiple joints [108]. Several studies in animals demonstrated that gut microbiota are is one of the primary reasons for arthritis symptoms. Previous studies have reported that germ-free mice gut microbiota are responsible for shaping the intestinal immune system [109,110]. It has been reported in earlier studies that intestinal microbiota is altered in recent-onset RA patients, e.g., segmented filamentous bacteria (SFB) stimulate intestine T helper 17 (Th17) cells, thus activating arthritis in mice [109,111]. Further, in few reports it has been noticed that RA patients in Japan reported increased levels of *Prevotellacopri* bacteria within the intestines, which is responsible for inducing Th17 cell-dependent arthritis in animals whereas *P.histicola* inhibit the augmentation of arthritis [112,113]. Therefore, all the above studies supported that species of *Prevotella* were involved in pathogenesis and shown different effects on rheumatoid arthritis [110]. Fig. 3 represents the interrelationship between environmental factors, gut microbiota,

and production of inflammatory mediators in causing rheumatoid arthritis.

4.4 Gut microbiota and multiple sclerosis (MS)

Multiple sclerosis is a degenerative, demyelinating, and chronic inflammatory disease of the central nervous system (CNS) [114]. Numerous studies reported the interaction of gut microbiota in the alteration of the inflammatory activation of the immune system [115]. Kadowaki et al. reported that gut microbiota influence the contact between T-cell C—C chemokine receptor type 9 (CCR9) and its ligand chemokine (CCL25) and plays as a key role in the development of T-cells and immunity of the small intestinal epithelium [116]. They also demonstrated that functionality of type 9 receptor (CCR9) was decreased in relapsing–remitting multiple sclerosis and secondary progressive MS patients. In addition, they also showed involvement of CCR9+ cells in MS, by inducing experimental autoimmune encephalomyelitis (EAE) in wild-type mice along with consequent treatment with antibiotics. They reported that antibiotics treatment increased CCR9+[+] Tm cells and subsequently decreased the severity of EAE. All these data suggested that alteration in the gut-systemic immune axis could be involved in the pathogenesis of MS and thus is considered as a possible diagnostic marker in the management of MS [115,116].

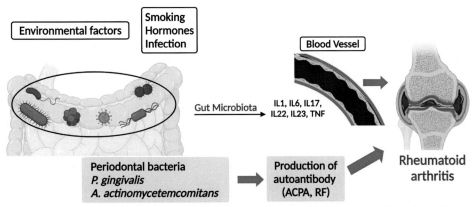

FIG. 3 Interrelationship between environmental factors, gut microbiota, and production of inflammatory mediators in causing rheumatoid arthritis.

Further, a research team compared the microbiota of healthy groups with those of MS patients. They found that MS patients have a impecunious microbiota community comprising *Pedobacteria, Flavobacterium, Pseudomonas, Mycoplana, Acinetobacter, Eggerthella, Dorea, Blautia, Streptococcus,* and *Akkermansia* compared to healthy groups having a higher amount of microbiota populations; and restitution of the microbial community in MS patients lessens inflammatory events, thus, reactivating the immune system [117].

4.5 Gut microbiota and cancer

Cancer is the second leading cause of death and has a multifactorial pathology. Recently, several studies reported the dual nature of the gut microbiota in the host organism leading to cancer development. During gut dysbiosis bacteria can produce several toxins triggers both oncogenesis and inflammation by interfering with host cell growth as described in Fig. 4. In the meantime, many gut resident bacteria able to produce metabolites, by products, called probiotics, and has been recognized as protective against the formation of tumors for e.g., *Lactobacillus rhamnosus* (LGG) [118]. Further, anticancer therapy such as antineoplastic agents (cytotoxic drugs), radiation therapy, and chemotherapeutic agents (topoisomerase I inhibitor or 5-fluorouracil) alters the composition of gut microbiota via a direct or immunological response [119,120]. Additionally, these cancer therapies produce unjustifiable side effects, which directly change the functionality of the intestinal barrier and gut microbial community [121].

4.6 Gut microbiota and diabetes mellitus or obesity

Obesity leads to multifaceted diseases such as type-2 diabetes, cardiometabolic diseases, etc. It has been demonstrated that type-2 diabetes connects with butyrate-producing microbes and higher quantity of

Lactobacillus species in humans [122,123]. Numerous studies have shown that type-2 diabetic patients have fewer *Firmicutes* (*Clostridia*) and abundant *Betaproteobacteria* when compared to control groups. They also observed that Gram-negative *bacterioidetes* and *Proteobacteria* induce type-2 diabetes [124]. Further, a European study recruited obese patients with mild–moderate metabolic syndrome which had overexpressed of *A. muciniphila*. These augments increased microbial diversity as compared to those who were metabolically compromised and type 2 diabetes mellitus may be specific to the population [123].

Recently, there have been only a few reports suggesting connection between type 1 diabetes and the gut microbiota. A study in Finland reported children with type-1 diabetes mellitus have shown minor abundances of *Firmicutes* and higher level of *Bacteroidetes* (Diabetic Prediction and Prevention study) [125]. Further, poor intestinal permeability and impaired gut functionality was reported in the pathogenesis of type-1 diabetes mellitus by Bosi and his research team [126]. Research is currently ongoing and finds the underlying pharmacokinetic and pharmacodynamic alterations in the composition of gut microbiota, which leads to onset of type-1 diabetes mellitus [124].

4.7 Gut microbiota and cardiovascular diseases (CVD)

Cardiovascular disease is the major widespread important cause of mortality in several countries due to significant increase in the common risk factors related to CVD or changes in the lifestyle pattern such as obesity, type 2 diabetes, and others such as metabolic syndrome [127]. Moreover, some of the studies showed gut microbiota have been associated as a contributing factor in the development of several diseases such as atherosclerosis, cardiac failure, hypertension, obesity, type-2 diabetes mellitus, and kidney diseases [128]. A large number of microorganisms such as Chlamydophila pneumoniae, *Porphyromonas gingivalis*, *Helicobacter pylori*, Influenza A virus, Hepatitis C virus,

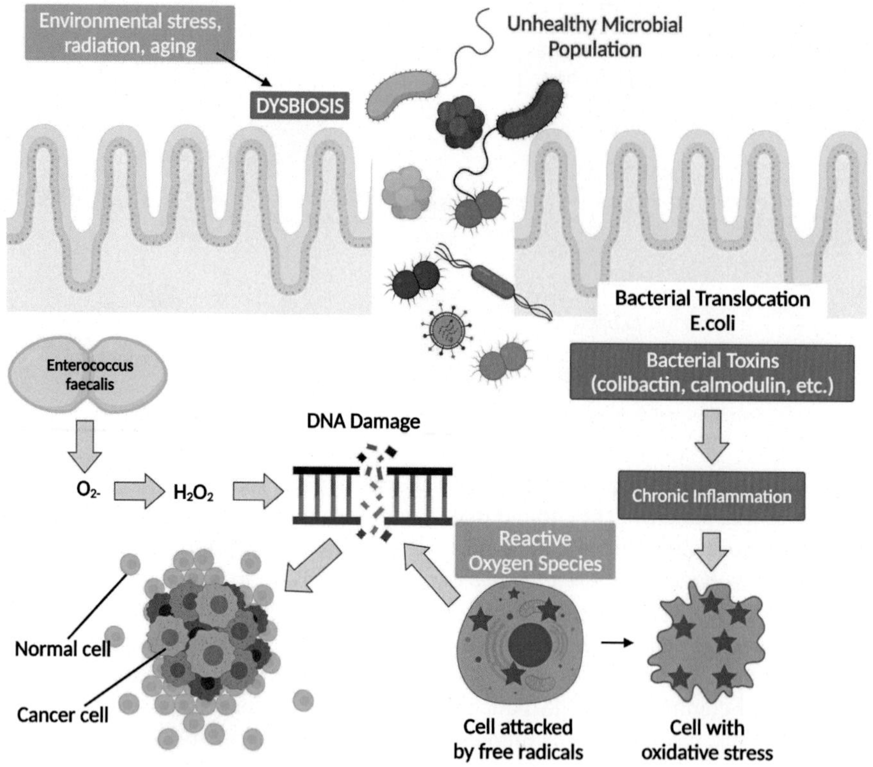

FIG. 4 Gut dysbiosis bacteria can produce several toxins that trigger both oncogenesis and inflammation by interfering with host cell growth.

Cytomegalovirus, and HIV virus were responsible for enhanced risk factors for cardiovascular diseases [129]. All are connected with intestinal inflammation by reducing the integrity of the gut barrier and resulting in the increased level of microbial components and their metabolites such as trimethylamine-N-oxide and short-chain fatty acids, thus aiding in the development of CVD [130]. In previous research studies, many bacteria especially *Firmicutes* belonging to the *Betaproteobacteria* and *Bacteriodales* class were found to be extensively higher in plasma-cholesterol models [131]. Moreover, recent studies showed *Firmicutes* levels are higher in obese patients' gut. Consequently, all these factors contribute to CVD [132].

5 Conclusions

For better immune development, it is important to maintain healthy gut microbiota. Improper microbial signaling and their metabolic products can cause dysregulation of the immune system and result in many chronic inflammatory diseases (autoimmune diseases) such as rheumatoid arthritis, multiple sclerosis, diabetes mellitus, obesity, and cancer. Based on some evidence, it is suggested that any changes in intestinal microbiota may reduce inflammatory diseases. The composition of gut microbiota can be manipulated by use of antibiotics, probiotics, and essential dietary supplements. In this chapter, we have described the role and interaction of gut microbiota with immune homeostasis and various inflammatory diseases. Some microbial organism (bacterial species) in the gut is responsible for the deterrence of diseases and few directly or indirectly contribute to the onset or worsening of the autoimmune disorders. Thus, for that reason healthier intestinal functionality or permeability is necessary to promote intact immune development (host immunity) and reverse gut-microbiota-induced inflammation and associated defects.

References

[1] M.E. Icaza-Chávez, Microbiota intestinal en la salud y la enfermedad, Rev. Gastroenterol. Mex. 78 (2013) 240–248.

[2] S. Hacquard, et al., Microbiota and host nutrition across plant and animalkingdoms, Cell Host Microbe 17 (2015) 603–616.

[3] J.B. Lynch, E.Y. Hsiao, Microbiomes as sources of emergent host phenotypes, Science 365 (2019) 1405–1409.

[4] L. Dethlefsen, M. McFall-Ngai, D.A. Relman, An ecological and evolutionaryperspective on human-microbe mutualism and disease, Nature 449 (2007) 811–818.

[5] A.J. Macpherson, M.B. Geuking, K.D. McCoy, Immune responses that adaptthe intestinal mucosa to commensal intestinal bacteria, Immunology 115 (2005) 153–162.

[6] F. Valitutti, S. Cucchiara, A. Fasano, Celiac disease and the microbiome, Nutrients 11 (2019) 2403.

[7] M. Zhang, et al., Interactions between intestinal microbiota and host immuneresponse in inflammatory bowel disease, Front. Immunol. 8 (2017) 942.

[8] B.S. Main, M.R. Minter, Microbial immuno-communication in neurodegenerative diseases, Front. Neurosci. 11 (2017) 151.

[9] J.E. Belizario, J. Faintuch, M. Garay-Malpartida, Gut microbiome dysbiosis andimmunometabolism: new frontiers for treatment of metabolic diseases, Mediators Inflamm. 2018 (2018) 2037838.

[10] Y. Maeda, K. Takeda, Host-microbiota interactions in rheumatoid arthritis, Exp. Mol. Med. 51 (2019) 150.

[11] V. Gopalakrishnan, B.A. Helmink, C.N. Spencer, A. Reuben, J.A. Wargo, Theinfluence of the gut microbiome on cancer, immunity, and cancer immunotherapy, Cancer Cell 33 (2018) 570–580.

[12] T. Gensollen, S.S. Iyer, D.L. Kasper, R.S. Blumberg, How colonization by microbiota in early life shapes the immune system, Science 352 (2016) 539–544.

[13] F. Backhed, et al., Dynamics and stabilization of the human gut microbiomeduring the first year of life, Cell Host Microbe 17 (2015) 690–703.

[14] S.L. Russell, et al., Early life antibiotic-driven changes in microbiota enhance susceptibility to allergic asthma, EMBO Rep. 13 (2012) 440–447.

[15] X. Zhang, D. Zhivaki, R. Lo-Man, Unique aspects of the perinatal immunesystem, Nat. Rev. Immunol. 17 (2017) 495–507.

[16] J. Neu, W.A. Walker, Necrotizing enterocolitis, N. Engl. J. Med. 364 (2011) 255–264.

[17] M. Gomez de Aguero, et al., The maternal microbiota drives early postnatalinnate immune development, Science 351 (2016) 1296–1302.

[18] M.G. Dominguez-Bello, et al., Delivery mode shapes the acquisition and structure of the initial microbiota across multiple body habitats in newborns, Proc. Natl. Acad. Sci. U. S. A. 107 (2010) 11971–11975.

[19] G. Caballero-Flores, et al., Maternal immunization confers protection to the offspring against an attaching and effacing pathogen through delivery of IgG inbreast milk, Cell Host Microbe 25 (2019) 313–323.

[20] W. Zheng, et al., Microbiota-targeted maternal antibodies protect neonates fromenteric infection, Nature 577 (2020) 543–548.

[21] H. Bauer, R.E. Horowitz, S.M. Levenson, H. Popper, The response of the lymphatic tissue to the microbial flora. Studies on germfree mice, Am. J. Pathol. 42 (1963) 471–483.

[22] Y. Umesaki, H. Setoyama, S. Matsumoto, Y. Okada, Expansion of alpha beta Tcell receptor-bearing intestinal intraepithelial lymphocytes after microbialcolonization in germ-free mice and its independence from thymus, Immunology 79 (1993) 32–37.

[23] S. Hapfelmeier, et al., Reversible microbial colonization of germ-free mice revealsthe dynamics of IgA immune responses, Science 328 (2010) 1705–1709.

[24] T.G. Tan, et al., Identifying species of symbiont bacteria from the human gutthat, alone, can induce intestinal Th17 cells in mice, Proc. Natl. Acad. Sci. U. S. A. 113 (2016) E8141–E8150.

[25] K. Atarashi, et al., Th17 cell induction by adhesion of microbes to intestinal epithelial cells, Cell 163 (2015) 367–380.

[26] S.K. Mazmanian, C.H. Liu, A.O. Tzianabos, D.L. Kasper, An immunomodulatory molecule of symbiotic bacteria directs maturation of the host immunesystem, Cell 122 (2005) 107–118.

[27] D.R. Wesemann, et al., Microbial colonization influences early B-lineage development in the gut lamina propria, Nature 501 (2013) 112–115.

[28] J. Cahenzli, Y. Koller, M. Wyss, M.B. Geuking, K.D. McCoy, Intestinal microbialdiversity during early-life colonization shapes long-term IgE levels, Cell Host Microbe 14 (2013) 559–570.

[29] M. Fulde, et al., Neonatal selection by toll-like receptor 5 influences long-termgut microbiota composition, Nature 560 (2018) 489–493.

[30] A.M. Mowat, To respond or not to respond - a personal perspective of intestinal tolerance, Nat. Rev. Immunol. 18 (2018) 405–415.

[31] A. Konrad, Y. Cong, W. Duck, R. Borlaza, C.O. Elson, Tight mucosal compartmentation of the murine immune response to antigens of the entericmicrobiota, Gastroenterology 130 (2006) 2050–2059.

[32] Y. Belkaid, S. Naik, Compartmentalized and systemic control of tissue immunity by commensals, Nat. Immunol. 14 (2013) 646–653.

[33] M. Shan, et al., Mucus enhances gut homeostasis and oral tolerance by delivering immunoregulatory signals, Science 342 (2013) 447–453.

[34] T. Bansal, R.C. Alaniz, T.K. Wood, A. Jayaraman, The bacterial signal indole increases epithelial-cell tight-junction resistance and attenuates indicators of inflammation, Proc. Natl. Acad. Sci. U. S. A. 107 (2010) 228–233.

[35] D.A. Peterson, N.P. McNulty, J.L. Guruge, J.I. Gordon, IgA response to symbiotic bacteria as a mediator of gut homeostasis, Cell Host Microbe 2 (2007) 328–339.

[36] A.J. Macpherson, T. Uhr, Induction of protective IgA by intestinal dendriticcells carrying commensal bacteria, Science 303 (2004) 1662–1665.

[37] C.L. Bevins, N.H. Salzman, Paneth cells, antimicrobial peptides and maintenance of intestinal homeostasis, Nat. Rev. Microbiol. 9 (2011) 356–368.

[38] D. Ehmann, et al., Paneth cell α-defensins HD-5 and HD-6 display differentialdegradation into active antimicrobial fragments, Proc. Natl. Acad. Sci. U. S. A. 116 (2019) 3746–3751.

[39] M. Ahuja, et al., Orai 1-mediated antimicrobial secretion from pancreatic acini shapes the gut microbiome and regulates gut innate immunity, Cell Metab. 25 (2017) 635–646.

[40] S. Rakoff-Nahoum, J. Paglino, F. Eslami-Varzaneh, S. Edberg, R. Medzhitov, Recognition of commensal microflora by toll-like receptors is required forintestinal homeostasis, Cell 118 (2004) 229–241.

[41] A.E. Price, et al., A map of toll-like receptor expression in the intestinal epithelium reveals distinct spatial, cell type-specific, and temporal patterns, Immunity 49 (2018) 560–575.

[42] F.A. Carvalho, et al., Transient inability to manage proteobacteria promotes chronic gut inflammation in TLR5-deficient mice, Cell Host Microbe 12 (2012) 139–152.

[43] G.D. Brown, Dectin-1: a signalling non-TLR pattern-recognition receptor, Nat. Rev. Immunol. 6 (2006) 33–43.

[44] D. Erturk-Hasdemir, et al., Symbionts exploit complex signaling to educate theimmune system, Proc. Natl. Acad. Sci. U. S. A. (2019), https://doi.org/10.1073/pnas.1915978116.

[45] G.D. Brown, Dectin-1: a signalling non-TLR pattern-recognition receptor, Nat. Rev. Immunol. 6 (2006) 33–43.

[46] C. Tang, et al., Inhibition of Dectin-1 signaling ameliorates colitis by inducing lactobacillus-mediated regulatory T cell expansion in the intestine, Cell Host Microbe 18 (2015) 183–197.

[47] D. Bouskra, et al., Lymphoid tissue genesis induced by commensals through NOD1 regulates intestinal homeostasis, Nature 456 (2008) 507–510.

[48] D. Ramanan, M.S. Tang, R. Bowcutt, P. Loke, K. Cadwell, Bacterial sensor Nod2 prevents inflammation of the small intestine by

restricting the expansion of the commensal Bacteroides vulgatus, Immunity 41 (2014) 311–324.

[49] C.A. Janeway Jr., R. Medzhitov, Innate immune recognition, Annu. Rev. Immunol. 20 (2002) 197–216.

[50] L. Wen, et al., Innate immunity and intestinal microbiota in the development of type 1 diabetes, Nature 455 (2008) 1109–1113.

[51] S. Vaishnava, et al., The antibacterial lectin RegIII gamma promotes the spatial segregation of microbiota and host in the intestine, Science 334 (2011) 255–258.

[52] S. Wang, et al., MyD88 adaptor-dependent microbial sensing by regulatory T cells promotes mucosal tolerance and enforces commensalism, Immunity 43 (2015) 289–303.

[53] P. Broz, V.M. Dixit, Inflammasomes: mechanism of assembly, regulation and signalling, Nat. Rev. Immunol. 16 (2016) 407–420.

[54] M. Levy, et al., Microbiota-modulated metabolites shape the intestinal microenvironment by regulating NLRP6 inflammasome signaling, Cell 163 (2015) 1428–1443.

[55] E.J.C. Gálvez, A. Iljazovic, A. Gronow, R. Flavell, T. Strowig, Shaping of intestinal microbiota in Nlrp6- and Rag2-deficient mice depends on community structure, Cell Rep. 21 (2017) 3914–3926.

[56] S.U. Seo, et al., Distinct commensals induce interleukin-1beta via NLRP3inflammasome in inflammatory monocytes to promote intestinal inflammation in response to injury, Immunity 42 (2015) 744–755.

[57] R.A. Ratsimandresy, M. Indramohan, A. Dorfleutner, C. Stehlik, The AIM2inflammasome is a central regulator of intestinal homeostasis through the IL-18/IL-22/STAT3 pathway, Cell. Mol. Immunol. 14 (2017) 127–142.

[58] L. Franchi, et al., Cytosolic flagellin requires Ipaf for activation of caspase-1 and interleukin 1beta in salmonella-infected macrophages, Nat. Immunol. 7 (2006) 576–582.

[59] V. Hornung, R. Hartmann, A. Ablasser, K.P. Hopfner, OAS proteins and cGAS: unifying concepts in sensing and responding to cytosolic nucleic acids, Nat. Rev. Immunol. 14 (2014) 521–528.

[60] H. Zhu, et al., RNA virus receptor rig-I monitors gut microbiota and inhibitscolitis-associated colorectal cancer, J. Exp. Clin. Cancer Res. 36 (2017) 2.

[61] D.M. Mosser, J.P. Edwards, Exploring the full spectrum of macrophage activation, Nat. Rev. Immunol. 8 (2008) 958–969.

[62] C. Danne, et al., A large polysaccharide produced by helicobacter hepaticus induces an anti-inflammatory gene signature in macrophages, Cell Host Microbe 22 (2017) 733–745.

[63] J. Schulthess, et al., The short chain fatty acid butyrate imprints an antimicrobial program in macrophages, Immunity 50 (2019) 432–445.

[64] K. Wu, et al., Gut microbial metabolite trimethylamine N-oxide aggravates GVHD by inducing M1 macrophage polarization in mice, Blood (2020), https://doi.org/10.1182/blood.2019003990.

[65] M.G. Constantinides, B.D. McDonald, P.A. Verhoef, A. Bendelac, A committed precursor to innate lymphoid cells, Nature 508 (2014) 397–401.

[66] M. Gury-Ben Ari, et al., The spectrum and regulatory landscape of intestinal innate lymphoid cells are shaped by the microbiome, Cell 166 (2016) 1231–1246.

[67] D.B. Sutherland, K. Suzuki, S. Fagarasan, Fostering of advanced mutualismwith gut microbiota by immunoglobulin a, Immunol. Rev. 270 (2016) 20–31.

[68] S. Kawamoto, et al., Foxp3+ T cells regulate immunoglobulin a selection and facilitate diversification of bacterial species responsible for immune homeostasis, Immunity 41 (2014) 152–165.

[69] N.W. Palm, et al., Immunoglobulin a coating identifies colitogenic bacteria in inflammatory bowel disease, Cell 158 (2014) 1000–1010.

[70] N. Shulzhenko, et al., Crosstalk between B lymphocytes, microbiota and the intestinal epithelium governs immunity versus metabolism in the gut, Nat. Med. 17 (2011) 1585–1593.

[71] K. Nagashima, et al., Identification of subepithelial mesenchymal cells that induce IgA and diversify gut microbiota, Nat. Immunol. 18 (2017) 675–682.

[72] N. Arpaia, et al., Metabolites produced by commensal bacteria promote peripheral regulatory T-cell generation, Nature 504 (2013) 451–455.

[73] A.N. Hegazy, et al., Circulating and tissue-resident CD4+ T cells with reactivity tointestinal microbiota are abundant in healthy individuals and function is alteredduring inflammation, Gastroenterology 153 (2017) 1320–1337.

[74] P. Miossec, J.K. Kolls, Targeting IL-17 and Th17 cells in chronic inflammation, Nat. Rev. Drug Discov. 11 (2012) 763–776.

[75] S. Omenetti, et al., The intestine harbors functionally distinct homeostatic tissue resident and inflammatory Th17 cells, Immunity 51 (2019) 77–89.

[76] S. Bedoui, W.R. Heath, S.N. Mueller, CD4(+) T-cell help amplifies innate signals for primary CD8(+) T-cell immunity, Immunol. Rev. 272 (2016) 52–64.

[77] A. Bachem, et al., Microbiota-derived short-chain fatty acids promote the memory potential of antigen-activated CD8(+) T cells, Immunity 51 (2019) 285–297.

[78] H.E. Yang, Y. Li, A. Nishimura, H.F. Jheng, A. Yuliana, R. Kitano-Ohue, et al., Synthesized enone fatty acids resembling metabolites from gut microbiota suppress macrophage-mediated inflammation in adipocytes, Mol. Nutr. Food Res. 61 (2017) 1700064, https://doi.org/10.1002/mnfr.201700064.

[79] Q. Feng, W.D. Chen, Y.D. Wang, Gut microbiota: an integral moderator in health and disease, Front. Microbiol. 9 (2018) 151, https://doi.org/10.3389/fmicb.2018.00151.

[80] Y. Belkaid, T.W. Hand, Role of the microbiota in immunity and inflammation, Cell 157 (2014) 121–141, https://doi.org/10.1016/j.cell.2014.03.011.

[81] J.M. Pickard, M.Y. Zeng, R. Caruso, G. Nunez, Gut microbiota: role in pathogen colonization, immune responses, and inflammatory disease, Immunol. Rev. 279 (2017) 70–89, https://doi.org/10.1111/imr.12567.

[82] J. Tap, S. Mondot, F. Levenez, E. Pelletier, C. Caron, J.P. Furet, et al., Towards the human intestinal microbiota phylogenetic core, Environ. Microbiol. 11 (2009) 2574–2584, https://doi.org/10.1111/j.1462-2920.2009.01982.x.

[83] J. Wang, W.D. Chen, Y.D. Wang, The relationship between gut microbiota and inflammatory diseases: the role of macrophages, Front. Microbiol. 11 (2020) 1065.

[84] W. Xie, M. Li, N. Xu, Q. Lv, N. Huang, J. He, et al., MiR-181a regulates inflammation responses in monocytes and macrophages, PLoS One 8 (2013), e58639, https://doi.org/10.1371/journal.pone.0058639.

[85] M.C. Arrieta, L.T. Stiemsma, P.A. Dimitriu, L. Thorson, S. Russell, S. Yurist-Doutsch, et al., Early infancy microbial and metabolic alterations affect risk of childhood asthma, Sci. Transl. Med. 7 (2015) 307ra152, https://doi.org/10.1126/scitranslmed.aab2271.

[86] M. Knip, H. Siljander, The role of the intestinal microbiota in type 1 diabetes mellitus, Nat. Rev. Endocrinol. 12 (2016) 154–167, https://doi.org/10.1038/nrendo.2015.218.

[87] A.S. Meijnikman, V.E. Gerdes, M. Nieuwdorp, H. Herrema, Evaluating causality of gut microbiota in obesity and diabetes in humans, Endocr. Rev. 39 (2018) 133–153, https://doi.org/10.1210/er.2017-00192.

[88] A. Hakansson, G. Molin, Gut microbiota and inflammation, Nutrients 3 (2011) 637–682, https://doi.org/10.3390/nu3060637.

[89] J. Ni, G.D. Wu, L. Albenberg, V.T. Tomov, Gut microbiota and IBD: causation or correlation? Nat. Rev. Gastroenterol. Hepatol. 14 (2017) 573–584, https://doi.org/10.1038/nrgastro.2017.88.

[90] W.W. Agace, K.D. McCoy, Regionalized development and maintenance of the intestinal adaptive immune landscape, Immunity 46 (2017) 532–548, https://doi.org/10.1016/j.immuni.2017.04.004.

[91] J.M. Pickard, M.Y. Zeng, R. Caruso, G. Nunez, Gut microbiota: role in pathogen colonization, immune responses, and inflammatory disease, Immunol. Rev. 279 (2017) 70–89, https://doi.org/10.1111/imr.12567.

[92] P.M. Smith, M.R. Howitt, N. Panikov, M. Michaud, C.A. Gallini, Y. M. Bohlooly, et al., The microbial metabolites, short-chain fatty acids, regulate colonic Treg cell homeostasis, Science 341 (2013) 569–573, https://doi.org/10.1126/science.1241165.

[93] T. Zuo, S.C. Ng, The gut microbiota in the pathogenesis and therapeutics of inflammatory bowel disease, Front. Microbiol. 9 (2018) 2247, https://doi.org/10.3389/fmicb.2018.02247.

[94] L.E. Smythies, M. Sellers, R.H. Clements, M. Mosteller-Barnum, G. Meng, W.H. Benjamin, et al., Human intestinal macrophages display profound inflammatory anergy despite avid phagocytic and bacteriocidal activity, J. Clin. Invest. 115 (2005) 66–75, https://doi.org/10.1172/jci19229.

[95] R.J. Ulevitch, P.S. Tobias, Receptor-dependent mechanisms of cell stimulation by bacterial endotoxin, Annu. Rev. Immunol. 13 (1995) 437–457, https://doi.org/10.1146/annurev.iy.13.040195.002253.

[96] P.D. Smith, L.E. Smythies, M. Mosteller-Barnum, D.A. Sibley, M. W. Russell, M. Merger, et al., Intestinal macrophages lack CD14 and CD89 and consequently are down-regulated for LPS- and IgA-mediated activities, J. Immunol. 167 (2001) 2651–2656, https://doi.org/10.4049/jimmunol.167.5.2651.

[97] T.L. Denning, Y.C. Wang, S.R. Patel, I.R. Williams, B. Pulendran, Lamina propria macrophages and dendritic cells differentially induce regulatory and interleukin 17-producing T cell responses, Nat. Immunol. 8 (2007) 1086–1094, https://doi.org/10.1038/ni1511.

[98] C.A. Janeway Jr., R. Medzhitov, Innate immune recognition, Annu. Rev. Immunol. 20 (2002) 197–216, https://doi.org/10.1146/annurev.immunol.20.083001.084359.

[99] D. Daley, The evolution of the hygiene hypothesis: the role of early-life exposures to viruses and microbes and their relationship to asthma and allergic diseases, Curr. Opin. Allergy Clin. Immunol. 14 (5) (2014) 390–396.

[100] T.R. Abrahamsson, H.E. Jakobsson, A.F. Andersson, B. Björkstén, L. Engstrand, M.C. Jenmalm, Low gut microbiota diversity in early infancy precedes asthma at school age, Clin. Exp. Allergy 44 (6) (2014) 842–850.

[101] Q. Wang, F. Li, B. Liang, et al., A metagenome-wide association study of gut microbiota in asthma in UK adults, BMC Microbiol. 18 (1) (2018) 114.

[102] K.E. Fujimura, A.R. Sitarik, S. Havstad, et al., Neonatal gut microbiota associates with childhood multisensitized atopy and T cell differentiation, Nat. Med. 22 (10) (2016) 1187–1191.

[103] F.A. van Nimwegen, J. Penders, E.E. Stobberingh, et al., Mode and place of delivery, gastrointestinal microbiota, and their influence on asthma and atopy, J. Allergy Clin. Immunol. 128 (5) (2011) 948–955.e3.

[104] M.C. Arrieta, L.T. Stiemsma, P.A. Dimitriu, L. Thorson, S. Russell, S. Yurist-Doutsch, B. Kuzeljevic, M.J. Gold, H.M. Britton, D.L. Lefebvre, P. Subbarao, Early infancy microbial and metabolic alterations affect risk of childhood asthma, Sci. Transl. Med. 7 (307) (2015) 307ra152.

[105] E.J. Raftis, M.I. Delday, P. Cowie, et al., *Bifidobacterium breve* MRx0004 protects against airway inflammation in a severe asthma model by suppressing both neutrophil and eosinophil lung infiltration, Sci. Rep. 8 (1) (2018) 12024.

[106] L. Chunxi, L. Haiyue, L. Yanxia, P. Jianbing, S. Jin, The gut microbiota and respiratory diseases: new evidence, J. Immunol. Res. 2020 (2020). Article ID: 2340670.

[107] C.-F. Huang, W.-C. Chie, I.-J. Wang, Efficacy of lactobacillus administration in school-age children with asthma: a randomized, placebo-controlled trial, Nutrients 10 (11) (2018) 1678. article e1678.

[108] E.D. Harris Jr., Rheumatoid arthritis. Pathophysiology and implications for therapy, N. Engl. J. Med. 322 (1990) 1277–1289.

[109] H.-J. Wu, I.I. Ivanov, J. Darce, K. Hattori, T. Shima, Y. Umesaki, D. R. Littman, C. Benoist, D. Mathis, Gut-residing segmented filamentous bacteria drive autoimmune arthritis via T helper 17 cells, Immunity 32 (2010) 815–827, https://doi.org/10.1016/j.immuni.2010.06.001.

[110] Y. Maeda, K. Takeda, Role of gut microbiota in rheumatoid arthritis, J. Clin. Med. 6 (6) (2017) 60.

[111] I.I. Ivanov, K. Atarashi, N. Manel, E.L. Brodie, T. Shima, U. Karaoz, D. Wei, K.C. Goldfarb, C.A. Santee, S.V. Lynch, et al., Induction of intestinal Th17 cells by segmented filamentous bacteria, Cell 139 (2009) 485–498, https://doi.org/10.1016/j.cell.2009.09.033.

[112] Y. Maeda, T. Kurakawa, E. Umemoto, D. Motooka, Y. Ito, K. Gotoh, K. Hirota, M. Matsushita, Y. Furuta, M. Narazaki, et al., Dysbiosis contributes to arthritis development via activation of autoreactive T cells in the intestine, Arthritis Rheumatol. 68 (2016) 2646–2661, https://doi.org/10.1002/art.39783.

[113] E.V. Marietta, J.A. Murray, D.H. Luckey, P.R. Jeraldo, A. Lamba, R. Patel, H.S. Luthra, A. Mangalam, V. Taneja, Suppression of inflammatory arthritis by human gut-derived *Prevotella histicola* in humanized mice, Arthritis Rheumatol. 68 (2016) 2878–2888, https://doi.org/10.1002/art.39785.

[114] C.A. Dendrou, L. Fugger, M.A. Friese, Immunopathology of multiple sclerosis, Nat. Rev. Immunol. 15 (9) (2015) 545–558.

[115] S.K. Shahi, S.N. Freedman, A.K. Mangalam, Gut microbiome in multiple sclerosis: the players involved and the roles they play, Gut Microbes 8 (6) (2017) 607–615.

[116] A. Kadowaki, R. Saga, Y. Lin, W. Sato, T. Yamamura, Gut microbiota-dependent CCR9+ CD4+ T cells are altered in secondary progressive multiple sclerosis, Brain 142 (4) (2019) 916–931.

[117] G. Schepici, S. Silvestro, P. Bramanti, E. Mazzon, The gut microbiota in multiple sclerosis: an overview of clinical trials, Cell Transplant. 28 (12) (2019) 1507–1527.

[118] S. Vivarelli, R. Salemi, S. Candido, L. Falzone, M. Santagati, S. Stefani, F. Torino, G.L. Banna, G. Tonini, M. Libra, Gut

microbiota and cancer: from pathogenesis to therapy, Cancers 11 (1) (2019) 38.

[119] Y.D. Nam, H.J. Kim, J.G. Seo, S.W. Kang, J.W. Bae, Impact of pelvic radiotherapy on gut microbiota of gynecological cancer patients revealed by massive pyrosequencing, PLoS One 8 (2013), e82659.

[120] R.R. Jenq, C. Ubeda, Y. Taur, C.C. Menezes, R. Khanin, J.A. Dudakov, C. Liu, M.L. West, N.V. Singer, M.J. Equinda, A. Gobourne, L. Lipuma, L.F. Young, O.M. Smith, A. Ghosh, A. M. Hanash, J.D. Goldberg, K. Aoyama, B.R. Blazar, E.G. Pamer, M.R. van den Brink, Regulation of intestinal inflammation by microbiota following allogeneic bone marrow transplantation, J. Exp. Med. 209 (2012) 903–911.

[121] L. Zitvogel, L. Galluzzi, S. Viaud, M. Vétizou, R. Daillère, M. Merad, G. Kroemer, Cancer and the gut microbiota: an unexpected link, Sci. Transl. Med. 7 (271) (2015) 271ps1.

[122] J. Qin, Y. Li, Z. Cai, et al., A metagenome-wide association study of gut microbiota in type 2 diabetes, Nature 490 (2012) 55–60.

[123] F.H. Karlsson, V. Tremaroli, I. Nookaew, et al., Gut metagenome in European women with normal, impaired and diabetic glucose control, Nature 498 (2013) 99–103.

[124] W. Aw, S. Fukuda, Understanding the role of the gut ecosystem in diabetes mellitus, J. Diabet. Invest. 9 (1) (2018) 5–12.

[125] N. Tai, F.S. Wong, L. Wen, The role of gut microbiota in the development of type 1, type 2 diabetes mellitus and obesity, Rev. Endocr. Metab. Disord. 16 (1) (2015) 55–65.

[126] E. Bosi, L. Molteni, M.G. Radaelli, et al., Increased intestinal permeability precedes clinical onset of type 1 diabetes, Diabetologia 49 (2006) 2824–2827.

[127] GBD 2013 Mortality and Causes of Death Collaborators, Global, regional, and national age-sex specific all-cause and cause-specific mortality for 240 causes of death, 1990–2013: a systematic analysis for the global burden of disease study 2013, Lancet 385 (2015) 117–171.

[128] W.W. Tang, T. Kitai, S.L. Hazen, Gut microbiota in cardiovascular health and disease, Circ. Res. 120 (7) (2017) 1183–1196.

[129] M.E. Rosenfeld, L.A. Campbell, Pathogens and atherosclerosis: update on the potential contribution of multiple infectious organisms to the pathogenesis of atherosclerosis, Thromb. Haemost. 106 (11) (2011) 858–867.

[130] M. Novakovic, A. Rout, T. Kingsley, R. Kirchoff, A. Singh, V. Verma, R. Kant, R. Chaudhary, Role of gut microbiota in cardiovascular diseases, World J. Cardiol. 12 (4) (2020) 110.

[131] T. Le Roy, E. Lécuyer, B. Chassaing, M. Rhimi, M. Lhomme, S. Boudebbouze, F. Ichou, J.H. Barceló, T. Huby, M. Guerin, P. Giral, The intestinal microbiota regulates host cholesterol homeostasis, BMC Biol. 17 (1) (2019) 1–18.

[132] D. Kumar, S.S. Mukherjee, R. Chakraborty, R.R. Roy, A. Pandey, S. Patra, S. Dey, The emerging role of gut microbiota in cardiovascular diseases, Indian Heart J. 73 (3) (2021), https://doi.org/10.1016/j.ihj.2021.04.008.

Chapter 12

Advanced drug delivery system for treating inflammation

Ananya Bishnoi[a], Silpi Chanda[b], Gunjan Vasant Bonde[a], and Raj Kumar Tiwari[a]

[a]School of Health Sciences and Technology, University of Petroleum and Energy Studies, Energy Acres Bidholi, Dehradun, Uttarakhand, India, [b]Amity Institute of Pharmacy, Lucknow, Amity University Uttar Pradesh, Noida, UP, India

1 Introduction

Cancer genesis and progression are known to be characterized by inflammation. Many cancer experts, especially those who specialize in basic science or immunology, believe that cancer-related information mostly refers to the local immune response that occurs at the tumor's site and frequently precedes and contributes to its growth. Cancer-related inflammation is viewed by doctors as a long-term, possibly inappropriate systemic response to cancer that causes fever, sweats, weight loss (the so-called B symptoms), and a variety of other paraneoplastic symptoms. The tumor stage (i.e., early vs metastatic illness) and clinical context influence the perception of cancer-related inflammation (good vs bad prognosis). Inflammation can serve as not only beneficial effects such as T-cell-mediated cytotoxicity leading to tumor inhibition but also as negative systemic effects, such as cachexia. Such reverse impacts of cancer-associated inflammation within the body pose the most difficult obstacles in the cancer treatment [1].

Inflammation has been linked to the development of cancer, according to studies. Cancer is a serious public health issue in the United States, with an estimated 1.6 million new cancer diagnoses and 5.8 million cancer deaths in 2013. Colorectal cancer is the third major cause of cancer-related morbidity and mortality in the United States, after lung cancer and prostate cancer. Recently, cancer chemoprevention has gotten a lot of press, and medicinal plants have been touted as powerful anticancer agents [2–5].

Although chemotherapy and radiotherapy are stronger treatment options for cancers, the involvement of herbal medicines reduces side effects to a great extent. There are several herbal medicines such as root bark of mulberry that possess antiinflammatory and anticancerous activities. On the other hand, Chinese herbal medicines containing some bioactive compounds or a variety of phytochemicals, such as *Coptis chinensis* (Huang lian), *Scutellaria baicalensis* (Huang qin), *Camellia sinensis* (Lu cha), *Wedelia chinensis* (Peng qi ju), and Songyou Yin (a Chinese herbal compound), may reverse EMT and reduce metastasis. As a result, these herbs can be used as complementary and alternative treatments, as well as adjuvant therapy for cytotoxic treatments [6].

The future of medicine is anchored in the past when chemists set out to create synthetic silver bullets for all of life's ills, and before pharmaceutical companies tethered our collective health to a multibillion-dollar wagon. Herbal medicines have been widely utilized all over the world since ancient times, and physicians and patients alike have acknowledged their superior therapeutic value because they have fewer side effects than contemporary pharmaceuticals. Herbal medicine has been practiced since the dawn of time, and throughout the last century, chemical and pharmacological investigations have been conducted on a variety of plant extracts in an attempt to determine their chemical makeup and corroborate traditional medical indications [7]. Historically, practically all medications were derived from plants, with the plant serving as man's sole chemist. Herbs are making a comeback; a herbal 'renaissance' is taking place all over the world, and an increasing number of individuals are turning to herbal therapies to cure a variety of maladies instead of conventional medication. What makes herbal medicine so popular?

- The reliance on medications and surgery, as well as their safety, is causing increasing concern.
- Many of the most prevalent health problems are not properly treated by modern medicine.
- Many natural remedies have been demonstrated to be more effective than medicines or surgery without the negative side effects [8].

Furthermore, there is mounting evidence that current medication therapy only masks symptoms while ignoring the underlying illness processes. On the other hand, many natural products appear to treat the root causes of many ailments and produce better clinical outcomes. Unfortunately,

Recent Developments in Anti-Inflammatory Therapy. https://doi.org/10.1016/B978-0-323-99988-5.00009-7

most doctors and patients are unaware that natural alternatives are available. However, a study in this sector is never-ending.

With novel ways of identifying active molecules and lower drug development costs, Ayurveda has made a significant contribution to the drug discovery process through reverse pharmacology [9]. Another Ayurveda-based technology, this time aimed at increasing drug absorption, has resulted in a paradigm shift in the way medicines are administered. Although phytochemical and phytopharmacological studies have long developed the overall health-promoting abilities of various plant products, there is a growing interest and medical need to strengthen the bioavailability of a huge number of herbal drugs and plant extracts that are poorly lipid-soluble and thus less bioavailable [10]. Despite their amazing potential in vitro, many herbal medications and herbal extracts have low lipid solubility, inappropriate molecular size, or both, leading to poor absorption and bioavailability.

Treatments such as purification and separation might result in a partial loss of specific activity due to the removal of chemically related molecules that contribute to the activity of the major components. The chemical complexity of the extract appears to be quite essential for the bioavailability of the active ingredients in many cases.

Because most plant elements, particularly phenolics, are water-soluble, the inability to pass the lipid membranes of the colon is the primary cause of low bioavailability. Different new delivery systems, such as liposomes, macropinosomes, niosomes, and lipid-based systems, can improve bioavailability by increasing the rate of release and the ability to traverse lipid-rich biomembranes [11].

The way medicine is administered can have a big impact on its effectiveness. Some medications have an optimal concentration range within which they provide the most benefit, whereas quantities outside of this range might be harmful or provide no therapeutic benefit at all. But from the other hand, limited progress within the efficacy of severe illness treatment has revealed an increasing need for a holistic approach to therapeutic delivery to tissue targets. New approaches for managing pharmacokinetics, pharmacodynamics, nonspecific toxicity, immunogenicity, biorecognition, and drug efficacy arose as a result of this. These novel techniques, known as drug delivery systems (DDS), combine polymer science, pharmaceutics, bioconjugate chemistry, and molecular biology in interdisciplinary approaches [12].

The term "novel drug delivery system" refers to a new technique to drug distribution that overcomes the constraints of established drug administration methods. Modern medicine treats a disease by pinpointing the afflicted location inside a patient's body and delivering the medicament directly there. A drug delivery system is a means of administering an optimal amount of a drug to a patient in such a way that it reaches the drug's "site of action" and begins functioning right away. The goal of a novel medication delivery system is to eliminate all of the drawbacks of traditional drug delivery systems. Novel drug delivery can be accomplished through a variety of methods [13].

Therefore, phospholipid-based drug delivery systems have been demonstrated to be effective and efficient in the delivery of herbal drugs. Delivering an effective level of the active component is critical to the success of any herbal product (or pharmaceutical) [14].

2 How is cancer related to inflammation?

There is a substantial link between chronic inflammatory disorders and organ-specific malignancy. Epidemiological data suggest a link between inflammation and cancer susceptibility, i.e., long-term inflammation causes dysplasia. Various variables have been shown to produce persistent inflammatory reactions, which can lead to cancer, for example, infections (e.g., *Helicobacter pylori*, Epstein-Barr virus, human immunodeficiency virus, flukes, schistosomes), chemical irritants (e.g., tumor promoters such as phorbol ester 12-O-tetradecanoyl-13-phorbol acetate, also known as phorbol myristate acetate), and nondigestible particles (e.g., asbestos). Microbial infection is thought to be responsible for roughly 15% of all cancer cases globally, according to epidemiological research [2,3,15].

Inflammation creates reactive oxygen and nitrogen species (ROS and RNS), as per scientific evidence. ROS and RNS, in particular, cause oxidative damage and nitration of DNA bases, which raises the likelihood of DNA mutations and, ultimately, cancer [16]. Chronic inflammatory bowel disease, increased risk of colorectal cancer, chronic gastritis caused by *H. pylori* infection, gastric adenocarcinoma, chronic hepatitis, and liver cancer are the most well-studied instances of inflammation and cancer. Chronic hepatitis B infection increases the risk of liver cancer by roughly 10-fold [17,18].

Inflammation causes leukocytes to flock to the site of tissue damage, secreting a range of proliferative cytokines and angiogenic proteins. These cytokines are recognized to be necessary for wound healing and to drive epithelial cell proliferation, but if they are not regulated, they can cause dysplasias and eventually cancer. Tumor cells also create a variety of cytokines and chemokines that attract leukocytes, which then produce cytokines and chemokines that promote tumor cell growth.

Surprisingly, cytokine shortage (e.g., GM-CSF, IL-2, and IFN) can promote tumor growth. A series of pro- and antiinflammatory signals govern immune homeostasis. Chronic inflammation and proliferative signaling result from the loss of antiinflammatory signals.

Tumor-associated macrophages and leukocytes produce cytokines and chemokines, which induce cancer metastasis and angiogenesis. These cytokines and chemokines stimulate cell motility and tumor-associated vascular expansion. Angiogenesis is also aided by leukocytes, which cause arterial dilatation and tumor cell extravasation. Inflammation also encourages the spread of metastases.

3   Cancer and antiinflammatory herbal treatments

3.1   Breast cancer

IBC (inflammatory breast cancer) is distinguished from other types of primary breast cancer by a distinct phenotype that includes quickly progressing breast inflammation and a high proclivity to spread. Inflammatory breast cancer has a 3-year survival rate of around 40%, compared to 85% in noninflammatory breast cancer. The biological processes that underpin these traits are largely understood, but their discovery might aid diagnosis, patient classification, and medication development [19].

The introduction of new analytical technologies such as DNA microarrays has aided in the identification of genetic signatures for a variety of cancers. DNA microarray-based investigations in noninflammatory breast cancer have identified tumor subclasses with different prognoses [20,21]. In IBC, only a few DNA microarray-based investigations have been conducted [22,23]. One research found a list of 109 genes that distinguished 37 IBCs from 44 non-IBCs based on their expression. Signal transduction, cell motility, invasion, angiogenesis, and local inflammatory processes were all connected with these 109 genes, some of which were NF-B related. A high number of overexpressed NF-B-related genes were discovered in another genome-wide expression profiling research comparing 16 IBCs with 18 nonstage-matched non-IBCs [24]. The same authors recently verified the involvement of several of these NF-B-related genes in IBC using real-time RT-PCR, immunohistochemistry, and NF-B-DNA-binding tests. Researchers found aberrant expression of many NF-B-associated genes in a prior IBC investigation in which they used real-time RT-PCR to assess the expression of 538 cancer genes. As a result, NF-B has been linked to inflammatory breast cancer illness [23,25,26].

Role of curcumin:
Curcumin (diferuloylmethane) is one of the most important components of the famous Indian spice turmeric (Curcuma longa L., a ginger family member). Colon cancer, breast cancer [27], lung metastases, and brain tumors have all been examined for their anticancer properties [28].

Curcumin's anticancer properties are ascribed to its capacity to trigger apoptosis in cancer cells without causing cytotoxicity in healthy cells, which is appealing to cancer researchers. Curcumin inhibits NF-B [16], a protein linked to inflammatory disorders such as cancer. Nuclear transcription factor kappaB activation has now been related to a number of inflammatory illnesses, including cancer. Phytochemicals originating from spices such as turmeric (curcumin), red pepper (capsaicin), cloves (eugenol), and ginger have been found to disrupt the route that activates this transcription factor in recent years (gingerol) [29].

3.2   Cervical cancer

Cervical cancer is the second most prevalent cause of cancer-related death in women globally, with an estimated 450,000 new cases identified each year and a 50% fatality rate. Cervical cancer affects women in most poor nations, accounting for around one-fourth of all female malignancies. As a result, researchers are discovering novel approaches to treat cervical cancer. Because of their low toxicity and considerable chemopreventive efficacies, dietary fruits and vegetables have been extensively studied as possible sources of chemopreventive chemicals. Epidemiological research continues to back up the idea that eating cruciferous vegetables can help lower the incidence of a variety of cancers. Organic isothiocyanates (ITCs) found in a range of edible cruciferous vegetables such as broccoli, watercress, and cabbage may be responsible for their anticarcinogenic activity.

Role of cruciferous vegetables:
One of these veggies' components, phenylethyl isothiocyanate (PEITC), has been shown to help fight a variety of cancers. PEITC's apoptotic effects and molecular mechanism in human cervical cancer cell lines (HEp-2 and KB) were investigated in this work. PEITC inhibited cell growth by inducing apoptosis. PEITC enhanced the expression of death receptors (DR4 and DR5) and cleaved caspase-3 in comparison to the DMSO treatment group, according to the protein chip test. PEITC also caused caspase-8 and truncated BID to be produced. PEITC decreased phosphorylation of extracellular-related kinase (ERK)1/2 but did not affect phosphorylation of c-Jun NH2-terminal kinases (JNK) or phosphorylation of p38 MAPK. MEK inhibitors were used to look into the function of ERK in PEITC-induced apoptosis (PD98059). The expression of DR4 and DR5, as well as activated caspase-3 and cleaved PARP, was enhanced by PD98059. MEK phosphorylation was also reduced by PEITC. As a result, the stimulation of DR4 and DR5 via inactivating ERK and MEK is part of PEITC's apoptotic mechanism in cervical cancer cells. Several ITCs have been discovered to be strong Nrf2 inducers. In cultured murine fibroblasts, the ITCs AITC, 2-phenylethyl isothiocyanate (PEITC), and butyl ITC activated phase II and antioxidant enzymes via Nrf2,

which was accompanied by the activation of the higher MAPK ERK1/2. SFN is the most extensively researched ITC and a well-known plant-derived Nrf2 inducer in vitro and in vivo, with antiinflammatory properties [30].

3.3 Brain cancer

The incidence of primary central nervous system cancers is 27.86 per 100,000 [1]. Glioblastoma (GBM) is the most prevalent malignant primary CNS tumor, with 3.19 per 100,000 yearly incidences. GBM makes for 15.4% of all primary brain tumors and 45.6% of malignant brain tumors [31,32]. Surgical resection followed by the Stupp regimen (adjuvant chemotherapy and radiation) is the current standard of treatment for GBM, and it has been in use for over a decade with no significant improvements.

Because complementary medicine and nutraceuticals are often associated with low toxicity profiles, they have been widely investigated as anticancer treatments. This permits them to be used at large dosages or as an adjuvant treatment to existing chemotherapy regimens.

Role of curcumin:
Curcumin is present in the rhizomes of turmeric (Curcuma longa), a ginger family member [33]. It has long been used in Ayurvedic treatment in India and traditional Chinese medicine to treat infections, liver and skin diseases, wound dressing, burns, and inflammation reduction [34].

Curcumin has been discovered to have remarkable anti-inflammatory properties.

Curcumin's natural antiinflammatory effect is comparable to that of steroidal and nonsteroidal medications such as indomethacin and phenylbutazone, both of which have potentially severe side effects. It appears to have antiinflammatory properties via inhibiting COX-2, LOX, iNOS, and the generation of cytokines like interferon and tumor necrosis factor, as well as activating transcription factors like NF-B and AP-1 [35].

3.4 Lung cancer

Cancer is a diverse collection of illnesses caused by aberrant, uncontrolled cell proliferation and differentiation, which promote tumor development and spread. Lung cancer is the leading cause of cancer-related deaths in both men and women. According to the European Cancer Observatory's (ECO) 2012 estimates, lung cancer was responsible for one-fifth of all cancer-related deaths [36]. Tobacco smoking (direct or indirect, accounting for more than 85% of lung cancer cases), asbestos, ionizing radiation (e.g., radon), and other air pollutants are the leading causes of lung cancer.

Lung cancer is classified into two kinds on a histological level: small-cell lung carcinoma (SCLC) and nonsmall-cell

lung carcinoma (NSCLC). SCLC makes up 12%–15% of all cases, although it is more aggressive and metastatic than NSCLC. NSCLC is less aggressive and spreads more slowly than other types of lung cancer, but it is more prevalent, accounting for 85%–88% of all lung cancer occurrences. Adenocarcinoma (50%), squamous cell carcinoma (30%), and giant cell carcinoma (10%) are the three subtypes of NSCLC. Human cancer-derived cell lines provide a nearly limitless and self-replicating source of tumor cells for study [37–39].

Role of naringenin:
Naringenin-LCNs were tested against human airway epithelium-derived basal cells (BCi-NS1.1) and human lung epithelial carcinoma (A549) cell lines for antiinflammatory and anticancer properties. In lipopolysaccharide-induced BCi-NS1.1 cells, the antiinflammatory activity of Naringenin-LCNs was assessed by qPCR, which indicated a reduction in the levels of IL-6, IL-8, IL-1, and TNF-.

Naringenin was encased in liquid crystalline nanoparticles, resulting in their long-term release. Furthermore, Naringenin-loaded LCNs effectively decreased proinflammatory indicators such as IL-1, IL-6, TNF-, and IL-8. Furthermore, when evaluated in the A549 cell line, the Naringenin-loaded LCNs had significant anticancer action, as evidenced by the suppression of cell proliferation and migration. In A549 cells, they also inhibited colony formation and caused death [40].

3.5 Pancreatic cancer

By 2030, pancreatic cancer (PC) is expected to be the second largest cause of cancer-related fatalities in the United States, after only lung cancer. For individuals with pancreatic ductal adenocarcinoma (PDAC), the most prevalent type of PC, surgery remains the sole possibly curative therapy. Several recent preclinical research have focused on finding effective therapies for PDAC; however, the models used in these studies frequently fail to replicate the tumor's heterogeneity. The clinical use of the data provided by such models is uncertain. In vitro and in vivo human cell line-based models, as well as nonhuman origin models, patient-derived xenograft (PDX) models, have numerous benefits.

Role of triptolide:
Triptolide induces apoptosis in pancreatic cancer cells in vitro and in vivo, and its mode of action is mediated through the inhibition of HSP70. Triptolide is a possible therapeutic drug for the prevention of pancreatic cancer development and metastasis. In both cell lines, triptolide reduced HSP70 mRNA and protein levels and caused apoptosis (as measured by Annexin V, caspase-3, and terminal nucleotidyl transferase-mediated nick end labeling). In vivo administration of triptolide (0.2 mg/kg/d for 60 days)

reduced pancreatic cancer development and dramatically reduced local-regional tumor spread [41].

In another study, scientists looked at the NF-jB inhibitor triptolide as a potential therapeutic target. Triptolide is a diterpenoid triepoxide that inhibits NF-jB and has antiinflammatory properties. Triptolide treatment of BxPc-3, AsPC-1, and MIA-PaCa2 cells for 24 hours significantly reduced hypoxia-induced NF-jB binding activity, as measured by EMSA [42,43].

4 Need for novel drug delivery systems

It is apparent from the literature that herbal medicines have pharmacological activity owing to a single ingredient or a combination of constituents. However, due to ecological variables and the time of plant harvest, the number of components fluctuates from batch to batch. Only when the drug's concentration falls under the therapeutic range can it have a pharmacological impact. Any changes in the therapeutic concentration, whether above or below the therapeutic level, result in harmful consequences or no reaction. As a result, both dosage titration and dose determination are required.

Novel Drug Delivery System (NDDS), which is a unique combination of many areas of research such as polymer technology, pharmaceutics, immunology, molecular biology, and others, plays a significant role in overcoming such instances and improving the efficacy of herbal drugs. Professionals in the field understand the problems associated with the use of herbal products (such as poor stability in the gastric environment, the high extent of first past metabolism, etc.) that create a barrier to their frequent use over synthetic molecules by using nanotechnology, where vesicular systems aid in targeted delivery of the desired constituents.

They have the ability to improve the solubility of the components.

(a) They can reduce the toxicity of the related effects.
(b) Enhancement of pharmacological effects.
(c) The absorption of components by tissue macrophages can be improved due to the lipoidal content [44,45].

The development of new drug delivery methods for herbal medicines has received a lot of interest in recent decades. NDDS is beneficial in delivering the herbal medication at a fixed rate and delivering drugs at the site of action, which reduces the adverse effects by improving bioavailability of the pharmaceuticals. Controlling the distribution of medication is accomplished using the NDDS technology by integrating the drug into altering the structure of the drug at the molecular level. For the delivery of herbal medicines, many new drug delivery systems such as liposomes, niosomes, microspheres, and phytosomes have been described. Liposomes, for example, function as a possible transporter for anticancer drugs, increasing the quantity of drug in the cancer region while decreasing drug accumulation in normal cells/tissues, minimizing tissue damage [7]. Many drug delivery and drug targeting systems are presently being developed in order to decrease drug elimination and loss, prevent undesirable side effects, and improve drug bioavailability and the percentage of the drug accumulated in the target zone [46–48].

Advantages of novel drug delivery system:

(1) A greater level of solubility.
(2) Bioavailability has improved.
(3) Toxic-free protection.
(4) Pharmacological activity has increased.
(5) Stability has improved.
(6) Better dispersion of tissue macrophages.
(7) Consistent delivery.
(8) Resistance to physical and chemical deterioration [49].

5 How are nanotechnology-based drugs most effective as cancer cures?

Cancer is a complicated and developing illness that has been a continual fight across the world, with many advances in treatments and preventative medicines. There is currently no cancer medication that is both specific and decisive. Tumor blood arteries are "leaky" because they include holes ranging from 200 to 2000 nm, allowing nanoparticles to escape into the tumor. Nanoparticles smaller than 500 nm can assist in the delivery of low-solubility medicines and enhance tumor selectivity. In today's cancer treatment, hypothermia is more frequently utilized in conjunction with chemotherapy and radiation therapy than as a stand-alone treatment.

Researchers have been researching novel phytochemicals and their synthetic equivalents to see whether they can fight cancer and mitigate the negative effects of existing chemo and radiation treatments. Nanotechnology has the potential to eradicate cancer tumors while causing little harm to healthy tissue and organs, as well as identify and eliminate cancer cells before they form tumors. Another phytochemical under research for its anticancer properties is paclitaxel, which is similar to curcumin, camptothecin, and paclitaxel. Andrographolide Andrographis paniculata, an Acanthaceae family plant, contains a diterpenoid lactone, which is one of the plant's significant bioactive components. It has been studied for its beneficial properties such as antiinflammatory, analgesics, anti-HIV effects, immune regulation, neuroprotective, choleretic cardiovascular, antihyperglycemic, and antitumor, and is extensively used in clinics for fever, inflammation, and other infectious illnesses treatment. Because of its limited oral bioavailability, which makes it difficult to manufacture, it is critical to create and develop composite derivatives of Andrographolide as first-line anticancer chemotherapeutic medicines [50].

6 Future of nanomedicine in drug delivery

The study of herbal medicines is becoming more popular across the world. This would not only alleviate undesirable side effects such as toxicity and hypersensitivity responses, but it would also improve the patient's internal strength, which is desired. Herbal treatments are also a rich source of useful products that include antioxidants and components that may be used in meals [51]. The notion of herbal nanoparticles for the treatment of essential diseases such as cancer, diabetes mellitus, and anemia medication delivery may attract certain possible study groups in the future, resulting in possibly eye-catching outcomes [52,53].

7 Conclusions

As a result, utilizing "herbal therapy" in the form of nanocarriers will undoubtedly improve its potential for treating a variety of chronic conditions and providing health advantages. This sort of study using traditional "herbal cures" with newer methods to contemporary drug delivery systems, such as "nanotechnology," has the potential to provide pharmaceutical companies with attractive medicines in the near future that will improve people's health. The efficacy and value of natural goods and herbal treatments used in conjunction with the nanocarrier are expected to boost the importance of existing medication delivery methods.

References

[1] C.I. Diakos, K.A. Charles, D.C. McMillan, and S.J. Clarke, "Cancer-related inflammation and treatment effectiveness," Lancet Oncol., vol. 15, no. 11, pp. e493–e503, Oct. 2014, https://doi.org/10.1016/S1470-2045(14)70263-3.

[2] F. Balkwill, A. Mantovani, "Inflammation and cancer: back to Virchow?," Lancet (London, England), vol. 357, no. 9255, pp. 539–545, Feb. 2001, https://doi.org/10.1016/S0140-6736(00)04046-0.

[3] L.M. Coussens and Z. Werb, "Inflammation and cancer," Nature, vol. 420, no. 6917, pp. 860–867, Dec. 2002, https://doi.org/10.1038/NATURE01322.

[4] R. Siegel, D. Naishadham, and A. Jemal, Cancer statistics, 2013, CA, Cancer J. Clin., vol. 63, no. 1, pp. 11–30, Jan. 2013, https://doi.org/10.3322/CAAC.21166.

[5] S. Wang et al., "Fighting fire with fire: poisonous Chinese herbal medicine for cancer therapy," J. Ethnopharmacol., vol. 140, no. 1, pp. 33–45, Mar. 2012, https://doi.org/10.1016/J.JEP.2011.12.041.

[6] J. Zhang et al., "Targeting cancer-related inflammation: chinese herbal medicine inhibits epithelial-to-mesenchymal transition in pancreatic cancer," PLoS One, vol. 8, no. 7, p. e70334, Jul. 2013, https://doi.org/10.1371/JOURNAL.PONE.0070334.

[7] N.S. Acharya, G.V. Parihar, S.R. Acharya, Phytosomes: novel approach for delivering herbal extract with improved bioavailability, 2011. https://www.cabdirect.org/cabdirect/abstract/20113172051. (Accessed 30 August 2021).

[8] P. Goldman, Herbal medicines today and the roots of modern pharmacology, Ann. Intern. Med., vol. 135, no. 8 Pt 1, pp. 594–600, Oct. 2001, https://doi.org/10.7326/0003-4819-135-8_PART_1-200110160-00010.

[9] B. Patwardhan, R.A. Mashelkar, Traditional medicine-inspired approaches to drug discovery: can Ayurveda show the way forward?, Drug Discov. Today, vol. 14, no. 15–16, pp. 804–811, Aug. 2009, https://doi.org/10.1016/J.DRUDIS.2009.05.009.

[10] C. Manach, A. Scalbert, C. Morand, C. Remesy, L. Jimenez, Polyphenols: food sources and bioavailability, Am. J. Clin. Nutr. 79 (5) (2004) 727–747, https://doi.org/10.1093/AJCN/79.5.727.

[11] I.F. Uchegbu, S.P. Vyas, Non-ionic surfactant based vesicles (niosomes) in drug delivery, Int. J. Pharm., vol. 172, no. 1–2, pp. 33–70, Oct. 1998, https://doi.org/10.1016/S0378-5173(98)00169-0.

[12] W.N. Charman, H.-K. Chan, B.C. Finnin, S.A. Charman, Drug delivery: a key factor in realising the full therapeutic potential of drugs, 1999 - Drug Dev. Res. - Wiley Online Library. https://onlinelibrary.wiley.com/doi/abs/10.1002/(SICI)1098-2299(199903/04)46:3/4%3C316::AID-DDR18%3E3.0.CO;2-E (Accessed 30 August 2021).

[13] S. Roy, Why is a Novel Drug Delivery System Important for Herbal or Ayurvedic Medicines?, 2008. http://souravroy.articlealley.com/why-is-a-novel-drug-delivery-system-important-for-herbal-or-ayurvedic-medicines-673669.html. (Accessed 30 August 2021).

[14] N. Moussaoui, M. Cansell, and A. Denizot, "Marinosomes, marine lipid-based liposomes: physical characterization and potential application in cosmetics," Int. J. Pharm., vol. 242, no. 1–2, pp. 361–365, Aug. 2002, https://doi.org/10.1016/S0378-5173(02)00217-X.

[15] H. Kuper, H.O. Adami, D. Trichopoulos, Infections as a major preventable cause of human cancer, J. Intern. Med. 248 (3) (2000) 171–183, https://doi.org/10.1046/J.1365-2796.2000.00742.X.

[16] B.E. Bachmeier et al., Curcumin downregulates the inflammatory cytokines CXCL1 and -2 in breast cancer cells via NFkappaB, Carcinogenesis, vol. 29, no. 4, pp. 779–789, Apr. 2008, https://doi.org/10.1093/CARCIN/BGM248.

[17] K.E. de Visser, A. Eichten, and C.M. Lisa, Paradoxical roles of the immune system during cancer development, Nat. Rev. Cancer, vol. 6, no. 1, pp. 24–37, Jan. 2006, https://doi.org/10.1038/NRC1782.

[18] S.P. Hussain, L.J. Hofseth, C.C. Harris, Radical causes of cancer, Nat. Rev. Cancer 3 (4) (2003) 276–285, https://doi.org/10.1038/NRC1046.

[19] I.A. Jaiyesimi, A.U. Buzdar, G. Hortobagyi, Inflammatory breast cancer: a review, J. Clin. Oncol. 10 (6) (1992) 1014–1024, https://doi.org/10.1200/JCO.1992.10.6.1014.

[20] T. Sørlie et al., "Repeated observation of breast tumor subtypes in independent geneexpression data sets," Proc. Natl. Acad. Sci. U. S. A., vol. 100, no. 14, p. 8418, Jul. 2003, https://doi.org/10.1073/PNAS.0932692100.

[21] C. Sotiriou et al., "Breast cancer classification and prognosis based on gene expression profiles from a population-based study," Proc. Natl. Acad. Sci. U. S. A., vol. 100, no. 18, pp. 10393–10398, Sep. 2003, https://doi.org/10.1073/PNAS.1732912100.

[22] F. Bertucci et al., "Gene expression profiling for molecular characterization of inflammatory breast cancer and prediction of response to chemotherapy," Cancer Res., vol. 64, no. 23, pp. 8558–8565, Dec. 2004, https://doi.org/10.1158/0008-5472.CAN-04-2696.

[23] S.V. Laere et al., "Distinct molecular signature of inflammatory breast cancer by cDNA microarray analysis," Breast Cancer Res. Treat., vol. 93, no. 3, pp. 237–246, Oct. 2005, https://doi.org/10.1007/S10549-005-5157-Z.

[24] D.M. Nguyen et al., "Molecular heterogeneity of inflammatory breast cancer: a hyperproliferative phenotype," Clin. Cancer Res., vol. 12, no. 17, pp. 5047–5054, Sep. 2006, https://doi.org/10.1158/1078-0432.CCR-05-2248.

[25] I. Bieche, F. Lerebours, S. Tozlu, M. Espie, M. Marty, R. Lidereau, Molecular profiling of inflammatory breast cancer: identification of a poor-prognosis gene expression signature, Clin. Cancer Res., vol. 10, no. 20, pp. 6789–6795, Oct. 2004, https://doi.org/10.1158/1078-0432.CCR-04-0306.

[26] S.J. Van Laere et al., Nuclear factor-kappaB signature of inflammatory breast cancer by cDNA microarray validated by quantitative real-time reverse transcription-PCR, immunohistochemistry, and nuclear factor-kappaB DNA-binding, Clin. Cancer Res., vol. 12, no. 11 Pt 1, pp. 3249–3256, Jun. 2006, https://doi.org/10.1158/1078-0432.CCR-05-2800.

[27] B.E. Bachmeier, et al., Reference profile correlation reveals estrogen-like trancriptional activity of Curcumin, Cell. Physiol. Biochem. 26 (3) (2010) 471–482, https://doi.org/10.1159/000320570.

[28] C. Senft, M. Polacin, M. Priester, V. Seifert, D. Kogel, and J. Weissenberger, The nontoxic natural compound Curcumin exerts anti-proliferative, anti-migratory, and anti-invasive properties against malignant gliomas, BMC Cancer, vol. 10, Sep. 2010, https://doi.org/10.1186/1471-2407-10-491.

[29] B.B. Aggarwal, S. Shishodia, Suppression of the nuclear factor-kappaB activation pathway by spice-derived phytochemicals: reasoning for seasoning, Ann. N. Y. Acad. Sci. 1030 (2004) 434–441, https://doi.org/10.1196/ANNALS.1329.054.

[30] C. Sturm, A.E. Wagner, Brassica-derived plant bioactives as modulators of chemopreventive and inflammatory signaling pathways, Int. J. Mol. Sci. 18 (9) (2017) 1890, https://doi.org/10.3390/IJMS18091890.

[31] S.-P. Weathers, M.R. Gilbert, Faculty opinions: advances in treating glioblastoma, 2014. https://facultyopinions.com/prime/reports/m/6/46/. (Accessed 30 August 2021).

[32] Q.T. Ostrom, et al., CBTRUS statistical report: primary brain and central nervous system tumors diagnosed in the United States in 2007–2011, Neuro Oncol. 16 (Suppl. 4) (2014), https://doi.org/10.1093/NEUONC/NOU223. pp. iv1–iv63.

[33] B.B. Aggarwal, Y.-J. Surh, S. Shishodia, 2007. The Molecular Targets and Therapeutic Uses of Curcumin in Health and Disease | SpringerLink, https://link.springer.com/book/10.1007%2F978-0-387-46401-5 (Accessed 01 September 2021).

[34] N.V. Klinger, S. Mittal, Therapeutic potential of curcumin for the treatment of brain tumors, Oxid. Med. Cell. Longev (2016). https://www.hindawi.com/journals/omcl/2016/9324085/. (Accessed 30 August 2021).

[35] V.P. Menon, A.R. Sudheer, Antioxidant and anti-inflammatory properties of curcumin, Adv. Exp. Med. Biol. 595 (2007) 105–125, https://doi.org/10.1007/978-0-387-46401-5_3.

[36] T. Norfleet, 2022. https://www.goodrx.com/blog/surprising-benefits-metformin-diabetes-fertility-cancer/. (Accessed 1 July 2021).

[37] D.J. Giard, et al., In vitro cultivation of human tumors: establishment of cell lines derived from a series of solid tumors, J. Natl. Cancer Inst. 51 (5) (1973) 1417–1423, https://doi.org/10.1093/JNCI/51.5.1417.

[38] W.D. Travis, Update on small cell carcinoma and its differentiation from squamous cell carcinoma and other non-small cell carcinomas, Mod. Pathol. 25 (Suppl. 1) (2012) 18–30, https://doi.org/10.1038/MODPATHOL.2011.150.

[39] L. Korrodi-Gregório, V. Soto-Cerrato, R. Vitorino, M. Fardilha, and R. Pérez-Tomás, "From proteomic analysis to potential therapeutic targets: functional profile of two lung cancer cell lines, A549 and SW900, widely studied in pre-clinical research," PLoS One, vol. 11, no. 11, p. 165973, Nov. 2016, https://doi.org/10.1371/JOURNAL.PONE.0165973.

[40] R. Wadhwa et al., "Anti-inflammatory and anticancer activities of Naringenin-loaded liquid crystalline nanoparticles in vitro," J. Food Biochem., vol. 45, no. 1, Jan. 2021, https://doi.org/10.1111/JFBC.13572.

[41] S. Ziaei and R. Halaby, Immunosuppressive, anti-inflammatory and anti-cancer properties of triptolide: a mini review, Avicenna J. Phytomed., vol. 6, no. 2, p. 149, 2016, Accessed 30 August 2021. [Online]. Available: /pmc/articles/PMC4877967/.

[42] L. Liu, A.V. Salnikov, N. Bauer, et al., Triptolide reverses hypoxia-induced epithelial–mesenchymal transition and stem-like features in pancreatic cancer by NF-κB downregulation, Int. J Cancer 134 (10) (2014) 2489–2503.

[43] P.A. Phillips, et al., "Triptolide induces pancreatic cancer cell death via inhibition of heat shock protein 70," Cancer Res., vol. 67, no. 19, pp. 9407–9416, Oct. 2007, https://doi.org/10.1158/0008-5472.CAN-07-1077.

[44] H. Verma, S.B. Prasad, H. Singh, Herbal drug delivery system: a modern era prospective, Int. J. Curr. Pharm. Res. 4 (3) (2013) 88–101.

[45] E. Terreno, et al., Paramagnetic liposomes as innovative contrast agents for magnetic resonance (MR) molecular imaging applications, Chem. Biodivers. 5 (10) (2008) 1901–1912, https://doi.org/10.1002/CBDV.200890178.

[46] S.S. Biju, S. Talegaonkar, P.R. Mishra, R.K. Khar, Vesicular systems: an overview, 2006. https://www.ijpsonline.com/articles/vesicular-systems-an-overview.html. (Accessed 30 August 2021).

[47] M. Uhumwangho and R. Okor, "Current trends in the production and biomedical applications of liposomes: a review," J. Med. Biomed. Res., vol. 4, no. 1, Mar. 2009, https://doi.org/10.4314/jmbr.v4i1.10663.

[48] N.D. Jasuja, P.R. Sharma, S. Jain, S.C. Joshi, Development of non-invasive transdermal patch of Emblica officinalis for anti atherosclerotic activity, Int. J. Drug Deliv. 5 (4) (2013) 402.

[49] S.G. Bhokare, et al., Herbal novel drug delivery: a review, World J. Pharm. Pharm. Sci. 5 (8) (2016) 593–611.

[50] M. Greenwell and P.K. Rahman, "Medicinal plants: their use in anticancer treatment," Int. J. Pharm. Sci. Res., vol. 6, no. 10, pp. 4103–4112, Oct. 2015, doi:10.13040/IJPSR.0975-8232.6(10).4103-12.

[51] N.K. Sethiya, A. Trivedi, M.B. Patel, and S.H. Mishra, "Comparative pharmacognostical investigation on four ethanobotanicals traditionally used as Shankhpushpi in India," J. Adv. Pharm. Technol. Res., vol. 1, no. 4, pp. 388–395, Oct. 2010, https://doi.org/10.4103/0110-5558.76437.

[52] S.H. Ansari, F. Islam, and M. Sameem, "Influence of nanotechnology on herbal drugs: a review," J. Adv. Pharm. Technol. Res., vol. 3, no. 3, p. 142, Jul. 2012, https://doi.org/10.4103/2231-4040.101006.

[53] V. Baskar, S.I. Meeran, A. Subramani, Shruti, J. Ali, T.K. Shabeer, Historic review on modern herbal nanogel formulation and delivery methods, Int. J. Pharm. Pharm. Sci., vol. 10, no. 10, pp. 1–10, Oct. 2018, doi:10.22159/IJPPS.2018V10I10.23071.

Chapter 13

Advanced nanoparticulate system for the treatment of antiinflammatory diseases

Nitin Verma[a], Neha Kanojia[a], Vivek Puri[a], Ameya Sharma[a], Komal Thapa[a], Lata Rani[a], Mahesh Gupta[b], Dinesh Kumar Chellappan[c], and Kamal Dua[d]

[a]*Chitkara University School of Pharmacy, Chitkara University, Baddi, Solan, Himachal Pradesh, India,* [b]*Department of Biology, University of Saskatchewan, Saskatoon, SK, Canada,* [c]*Department of Life Sciences, School of Pharmacy, International Medical University (IMU), Kuala Lumpur, Malaysia,* [d]*Discipline of Pharmacy, Graduate School of Health, University of Technology Sydney, Sydney, NSW, Australia*

1 Introduction

Inflammation seems to be a defense mechanism that arose in higher species in reaction to harmful shocks like viral invasion, tissue damage, as well as other unpleasant situations. This is a necessary host immunological response which allows for the elimination of unwanted stimuli and the regeneration of tissue [1]. As a result, acute inflammation has been seen as a component of innate immunity, the host's initial line of defense toward external pathogens and dangerous chemicals. Chronic inflammation is thought to occur when the initiating event is not eliminated including a prolonged infection or persistent cellular damage. The greatest harm done to a host in chronic inflammatory disorders is caused first by host's immune response, not from outside attackers like bacteria. It is still a major contributing factor to a wide range of health problems, involving acute and potentially fatal cardiac, respiratory, and cerebral disorders like myocardial injury, severe lung damage, and heart attack. Inflammation medication seems to be a globally significant and complicated target. A plethora of antiinflammatory agents (AIAs) have been discovered, produced, and authorized for therapeutic reasons since the introduction of acetylsalicylic acid. These include all recognized medications like nonsteroidal antiinflammatory drugs (NSAIDs), steroids, and novel molecules like proteins and nucleic acids. Inflamed tissue gets disorganized, resulting in "enhanced permeability and retention effect" (EPR) of an inflammatory barrier, and that is an extra benefit for passive nanoparticulate delivery [2]. Because some cell receptors become mutated in an immune response, these could be utilized during active medication targeting. The acute phase would be the initial nonspecific stage marked by localized vasodilation, enhanced permeability, liquid and protein deposition, neutrophil movement out from the capillary, as well as the release of inflammatory mediators (like histamine, lymphokines, and cytokines) [3]. However, if an underlying cause of the injury is just not addressed, the inflammatory response progresses to chronic inflammation, which is marked by pathological alterations; some of the characteristics are shown in Fig. 1. Chronic inflammation plays an essential part in the development of a variety of illnesses, such heart disease, neurological illnesses, hypertension, malignancy, obesity, allergies, and typical inflammatory maladies [4]. The main therapeutic strategies for inflammatory illnesses have been the inhibition or suppression of inflammatory/proinflammatory facilitators utilizing synthesized antiinflammatory drugs (like nonsteroidal and steroidal). Moreover, the usage of synthetic chemicals has been linked to a few frequent adverse effects such as gastrointestinal irritation, ulcers, clotting, and kidney failure.

However, these innovative therapies could be expensive, unstable, possess poor pharmacokinetic attributes, and need to be delivered to regions inside the tissues that must be targeted. The usage of nanomedicines might aid in overcoming these kinds of obstacles.

2 Inflammation causes

A disease or damage to the body would almost certainly generate a series of physical responses by immune cells, which could finally lead to inflammation. Inflammation at any portion of body does not often indicate a virus contamination [3].

Recent Developments in Anti-Inflammatory Therapy. https://doi.org/10.1016/B978-0-323-99988-5.00020-6

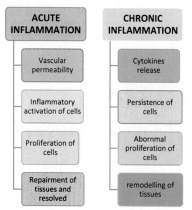

FIG. 1 Acute and chronic inflammation-based characteristics.

The following are the most prevalent causes of infection:

- pathogenic microorganisms such as bacteria, fungus, or virus,
- external wounds or cuts are examples of injuries,
- chemical or radiotherapy that harm the lungs.

Inflammatory diseases or disorders include:

- cystitis: bladder inflammation,
- bronchitis: inflammation of the airways of the lungs,
- otitis media: middle ear inflammation,
- dermatitis: skin inflammation.

3 Inflammation therapies

Inflammatory disorders must be treated using targets found in damaged tissues. To accomplish the desired therapeutic effect on inflammatory cells, substantial medication dosages would be necessary, which might sometimes have negative consequences on normal tissue. Antiinflammatory medicines are classified either as nonsteroidal antiinflammatory drugs (NSAIDS) (naproxen, ibuprofen, and aspirin) or steroidal (dexamethasone prednisone and betamethasone). NSAIDs are available as OTC in modest dosages to treat inflammation-related pain, whereas high dosages of NSAIDs and steroidal medicine are accessible as prescription therapy. Both of these are employed in the treatment of acute and chronic inflammatory disorders. However, long-term usage is connected with a slew of adverse effects. Adrenaline atrophy, water retention, bone loss, that can cause osteoporosis, as well as a higher risk of complications or damage are all side effects of steroidal medicines. Ulcers, allergy, hypertension, and liver and renal disorders can all be caused by NSAIDs. As a result, the research for novel antiinflammatory medicines is becoming increasingly popular, with the goal of achieving higher safety, effectiveness, and a more cost-effective method of treating inflammation. The demand for new treatment for inflammatory, viral, and neurodegenerative system illnesses

has fueled significant growth in nanoscience [5]. Because of the rising group of participants impacted, the intensity of a condition, as well as the economic burden, such illnesses represent a considerable load. As a result, there seems to be an urgent need for the better management and therapy.

4 Nanocarrier-based drug delivery systems

While compared to standard preparations, use of nanocarriers for delivery of drugs provide important benefits, including more effective functioning of hydrophobic drugs at larger doses, medication protection from dangerous conditions (like acidic pH within the digestive system), and sustained delivery for targeted delivery to the tissue within a specified period [5]. There are several kinds of nano-based carriers that are manufactured and selected. Metallic nanoparticles, polymeric nanoparticles, liposomes, solid lipid nanoparticles (SLNs), and dendrimers are examples of nanocarriers as shown in Fig. 2.

4.1 Polymeric nanoparticles

Polymeric nanoparticles are created from organic or inorganic biodegradable and biocompatible polymers; these are an effective drug delivery composition [6]. These act as drug transporters, controlling release of the drug and directing it to areas. In comparison to standard preparations, polymeric nanoparticles may enhance medication solubility, improving absorption and lowering the dose. Polymeric nanoparticles could be created utilizing a variety of

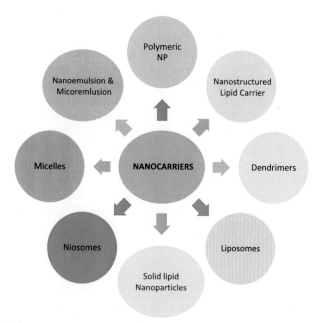

FIG. 2 Different nanocarrier-based drug delivery systems.

synthesis processes, designed for a specific use. These range in diameter between 10 and 1000 nm and are varied in structure and functional arrangement [7]. Polymers which have been widely employed for nanomaterials are poly-lactic-co-glycolic acid (PLGA) and polylactic acid (PLA).

In one study, chitosan/hyaluronic acid nanoparticles were investigated for the chondroprotective effects in a rat-based model. The nanoparticles that efficiently encapsulated DNA plasmid were of suitable size (100–300 nm) but also spherical in form. In a more than a three week of period, the NPs synovial and discharged the DNA appropriately [8]. The researchers identified a nanoparticle-gel combination medication delivery device for locating drugs at the injury site. Polycaprolactone-based nanoparticles were added and entrapped in a fibrin gel. The proposed nanoparticle loaded gel technology produced results that were remarkably like a systemically higher dose of medication [9]. Budesonide-encapsulated PLGA NPs with tailored efficiency were created for therapy of IBD. These averaged in size range 200 ± 05 nm and had a smooth, spherical form. The entrapment efficiency was about $85 \pm 3.5\%$. Drug release from NPs exhibited a biphasic emission characteristic, with an early burst succeeded by continuous release [10]. In this current study, NPs encapsulating TNF-siRNA targeting macrophages were produced for oral treatment preventing administration to prevent hepatic damage in rats. At low dosages, significant TNF reduction was noted, as well as relief of inflammatory symptoms within the liver (clogged central vein, swelling, disorderly hepatocytes, and damaged cytolemma) [11]. Chitosan-loaded poly(glutamic acid) (γ-PGA) nanoparticles as a carrier for diclofenac were developed. The NPs were 315 ± 50 nm in size and had a PDI of 0.36 ± 0.06. The medication was delivered at physiological pH, and then this drug-delivery mechanism was shown to be nontoxic, as well as being promptly absorbed [12].

4.2 Liposomes

Liposomes are round, small-sized particles made up of a natural or manufactured phospholipid bilayer divided via an aqueous phase in its center. Aqueous soluble substances are contained within the liquid segment, whereas lipophilic chemicals are deposited or integrated within the bilayers. A cationic, anionic, or neutral interfacial charge is possible. These are characterized as small, medium, or large, and uni-, or multilamellar, depending on their size [13]. These have assisted in reducing the negative effects of several medications, like antitumor and antimicrobial medications, while also boosting overall efficacy.

An evaluation of liposomes following kidney ischemia damage in rats and their influence on macrophages has been investigated. The build-up of a specific substance in an inflammatory kidney and with increased activation of anti-inflammatory macrophages was also reported [14]. Liposomes encapsulating phosphatidylserine (PS) were designed to serve as a biocompatible transporter for the administration of IL-10 to macrophages. PSL, coupled with IL-10, has a significant affinity for macrophages. The data imply that PSL-IL10 has macrophage-targeting potential as well as improved antiinflammatory benefits due to synergistic antiinflammatory actions [15]. Xu et al. (2019) used a minocycline-encapsulated liposome to modify polyether-etherketone (PEEK) with dexamethasone. In vitro and in vivo tests revealed that the NPs have improved antibacterial, antiinflammatory, and osseointegrative properties, indicating that it has tremendous promise as a restorative dentistry nanostructured material for medical use [16]. Liposomes were produced to improve cerebral injuries by delivering peptides and proteins. In this work, a liposomal preparation at a concentration of 2.5 mg/kg was produced to examine brain injury effects in treatment rats after 90 min continued by 48 h of reperfusion. The findings demonstrate that such a lower dose of medicine in NPs is more efficacious than a higher dosage of medication in its pure form [17].

4.3 Solid lipid nanoparticles

These are colloid-based carrier systems containing highly pure triglycerides, which are mostly made of lipids. Surfactants help to stabilize such nanostructures, which are made of lipids. These incorporate the benefits of various colloid-based systems, like lipid nanoparticles and polymeric nanoparticles, in terms of biocompatibility and biodegradability, with low cytotoxicity. These are mass-produced, have great physicochemical consistency, and provide full protection from drug deterioration. These sizes range between 50 and 1000 nm and could be employed within the healthcare market for medication delivery via various modes of administration including parental and orally administered methods [18].

For the management of RA, a directed solid lipid nanoparticle (SLN) containing prednisolone covered with hyaluronic acid (HA), was created. HA interacts with a CD44 receptor, which is overexpressed upon the external periphery of lymphocytes, fibroblasts, and macrophages. This decreased joint inflammation, bone degradation, and blood levels of inflammatory cytokines. Furthermore, the findings imply that enclosing them may make them safe and useful for the management of inflammatory illnesses [19]. Dexamethasone-loaded cholesteryl butyrate-SLNs have been created. Furthermore, SLN induced a plasma level of $61.7 \pm 3.19\%$, whereas drug-packed SLNs produced a plasma level of $30.8 \pm 8.9\%$ [20].

4.4 Dendrimer

Dendrimers are polymeric materials with continuously branching units ranging in size between 1 and 100 nm, making it among the most intriguing groups of NPs. They are symmetrical compounds with well-defined, homogenous structure composed of tree-like branches. A dendrimer is made up of many elements, including a core structure encircled by repeating units, which begin from inner and grow outward as branches, with many groups [21]. The groups do have greater degree of structural homogeneity and may be tailored in terms of size, valence state, solubility, and biodegradability.

The authors tested the effectiveness of three poly(amidoamine) (PAMAM) dendrimers for transdermal medication administration throughout this investigation. They discovered that neutral and cationic dendrimers improve drug permeability. It was determined that increased indomethacin penetration was attributable to a larger drug payload inside the cationic dendrimer [22,23]. Within this work, enhancement in dithranol absorption is attributable to a greater water solubility as well as an improvement there in diffusion coefficient into skin by a fifth generation dendrimer, which improves drug diffusion throughout the skin [24]. Another method for controlling inflammation is always to eliminate key production of cytokines. This was investigated in an animal model of psoriasis via topical administration of a suppressing RNA against a TNF transcript. This experiment demonstrated an improvement in both the clinical and histological characteristics of the condition, as well as a decrease in the levels of inflammatory interleukin and cytokines [25].

4.5 Nanostructured lipid carriers (NLCs)

NLCs are lipid-based nanoparticles of the second generation. The lipid-based matrix is made up of a combination of lipids with extremely varied structural properties, such as solid lipids containing saturated fatty acids or liquid lipids having a shorter chain of fatty acids. These have several benefits comparable to SLNs, like the utilization of compatible lipids, massive synthesis, and medication deterioration prevention. In contrast to SLNs, which are constituted entirely of solid-based lipids, the entry of liquid-based lipids further into matrices results in a decrease within the sequence of lipids and, as a result, an irregular crystalline structure, which may allow for the incorporation of drug with increased space [26]. It allows for greater encapsulating levels as well as longer term stabilization for NLCs. Surprisingly, the API mometasone furoate, which was encapsulated in SLNs, was also enclosed in NLCs [27]. In comparison, the entrapment percentages are almost the same (56% in SLNs against 60% in NLCs). In comparison to an API commercial cream preparation, skin deposition of

drug is 2.5-fold and is 2.67-fold greater with NLCs and SLNs, respectively. In comparison to the SLN composition, the NLC preparation has also been studied in the in vivo animal model of psoriasis and demonstrated therapeutic potential [27]. Viegas et al. have shown the capability of NLCs for the simultaneous administration of siRNA targeted toward TNF as well as the API tacrolimus. The combination's antipsoriatic efficacy when combined to NLCs is being confirmed in vivo [28].

4.6 Nanoemulsions and microemulsions

Emulsions are heterogeneous-based systems made up of two immiscible fluids, oil and water, one being the dispersed phase (indicated by tiny droplets) and another is the continuous phase. Surfactants, typically in conjunction with cosurfactants, help to stabilize particles. The size of particles can differ based on the characteristics of an emulsion (choice of cosurfactant, oil, and surfactant) as well as the fabrication method, giving lead to various kinds of emulsions: macroemulsions (size scale from 1 to 10 m), nanoemulsions (size below 100 or 200 nm), and multiple emulsions (O/W/O or W/O/W) [29]. Microemulsions and nanoemulsions are macroscopic in nature; however, they are distinct forms of colloid–based dispersions because microemulsions are thermally stable, but nanoemulsions are not [30]. Microemulsions are simple to make since they occur spontaneously, and they are affordable.

A hydrogel-loaded microemulsion was created and tested for antiinflammatory and skin-irritant properties. The proportion of edema suppression decreased there in the order listed: drug-loaded hydrogel ($44.56 \pm 8.08\%$) > NLC-entrapped hydrogel ($35.93 \pm 7.22\%$) > SLN-loaded hydrogel ($25.68 \pm 9.05\%$) [31]. A W/O microemulsion comprising vitamin E and A functions as a nanosystem for acute skin irritation were studied. This demonstrated stability as well as reduced toxicity in a cell line. In comparison to the empty microemulsion-treated group, in vivo interventions providing α-tocopherol decreased cutaneous production of TNF- about 1.3-fold [32]. Authors created a curcumin-nanoemulsion to test for wound healing and antiinflammatory activities. The size was 93.64 ± 6.48 nm, and the PDI is 0.263 ± 0.021. A uniform and circular form of nanoparticles was discovered using microscopic examination. They aided in wound healing and have antiinflammatory properties as a harmless and safe transdermal drug delivery system [33]. The current study aims to build a diclofenac sodium-loaded nanoemulgel for the treatment of chronic pain and inflammation. The size was determined to be 64.07 ± 2.65 nm with PDI of 0.238 ± 0.02 and ZP of (39.0 ± 06 mV). The study's overall results suggest that a new nanoemulgel composition of API might be employed as a possible strategy for inflammation control [34]. The article describes the creation of nanoemulsions for the topical delivery of ibuprofen, an NSAID. For 6 months, it displayed good stability without any separation or deposition. API penetration into human abdominal skin was studied using Franz diffusion cells. The median percentage of absorbed amounts at 24 h did not vary significantly [35]. The current work used etoricoxib to create a nanoemulsion for the administration of COX-2 inhibitors. Following 6 h, the antiinflammatory effects of preparation in rats demonstrated a considerable increase as in % inhibition level (84.61% with nanoemulsion loaded gel and 92.30% with nanoemulsion) in comparison to marketed gel (69.23%) [36].

4.7 Micelles

Micelles are colloidal particles that are in equilibrium with molecules in the solution through which they are generated. They make a slightly soluble material more soluble. In an aqueous phase, a micelle consists of a hydrophobic tail and hydrophilic head, with the head facing the water molecule and thus the tail forms a center. The aggregation numbers, which is the average amount of monomers able to construct a micelle, can vary between 50 and 200.

A micelle-based system for controlled release to inflamed joints was developed, and the strategy was validated in an arthritic rat model. The micelles remained in the bloodstream for even a prolonged period and collected selectively in inflammatory joints. API given through micelles significantly decreased joint edema, bone eroding, and cytokine production for both blood and joint tissue [37]. The purpose of this study is to assess the capacity of FK506 micelles to promote permeability upon an ocular surface. In both ex vivo and in vivo settings, our findings demonstrated that positively charged nanomicelles may dramatically extend FK506 persistence upon the surface of the eye and improve its ocular permeability [38]. Furthermore, in mouse models, poly (ethylene glycol)-poly(caprolactone) micelles coupled with anti-TNFα siRNA were delivered intranasally. When contrasted to a therapy utilizing bare anti-TNFα siRNA, the rats given micelles had lower TNF expression and a marked increase in overall neuropsychological grade [39]. Ibuprofen-loaded, amphiphilic, diblock copolymer micelles were developed. The manufacture and self-association activity of di-block copolymers with aqueous PEG blocks and a water-insoluble drug-containing prodrug blocks were studied. The hydrolysis release characteristics of IBU from micelles were investigated [40]. The characteristics of poly(ethylene oxide)-b-poly(n-butyl acrylate)-b-poly(acrylic acid) polymeric-loaded micelles as transporters for budesonide and prednisolone were investigated in this work. The size distribution of the micelles with a hydrophobic center was less than 40 nm. The size of drug-loaded micelles would not change after 8 h in physiological fluid-like medium, demonstrating remarkable colloidal stability.

This work demonstrated the ability of the terpolymer to act as a transporter of nanosized micelles suited for antiinflammatory medication delivery orally [41]. Micelle-loaded nanocarriers made of chitosan were created to transport ibuprofen to cancer cells. Our findings show that compositions formed into sphere micelles of appropriate sizes (108–252 nm). According to cell uptake experiments, ibuprofen-loaded micelles are easily swallowed by cancer cells and transport their contents throughout the inner membrane, as proven by confocal microscopy [42].

4.8 Niosomes

A niosome is composed of a carrier-generating amphiphilic nature like the Span-60 nonionic surfactant, which is normally maintained by cholesterol addition and a little quantity of anionic surfactant, like dicetyl phosphate, which also aids in vesicle stabilization. The particles can operate as a store to gradually deliver the medicine and provide a targeted release. Because the design of the niosome allows for the incorporation of lipophilic, hydrophilic, and amphiphilic drug components, these may be employed for a wide range of medicines. Because the particle solution is liquid, it provides a therapeutic effect compared to oil-based solutions. They improve the trapped medication's stability. Furthermore, this could improve medication absorption via the skin [43].

Gaafar et al. created ethoniosomes that were also prednisolone-loaded for ocular administration. In rabbits treated to a clove oil-induced acute ocular inflammation, ethoniosomes consisting of cholesterol and Span60 were examined, with ethanol 20% v/v used as a hydrating liquid to a surfactant component. A decrease in the period required for full healing was noticed, as well as a drop in IOP, which the most common adverse effects noticed with standard antiinflammatory therapy. Furthermore, this method displayed great physical durability with at least 2 months at cold temperatures, with acceptable ocular tolerance and low ocular discomfort, indicating a high possibility for use [44]. The extraction of *Zingiber cassumunar* was encapsulated in niosomes and used to create a topical gel. These considerably slowed the thermal-accelerated breakdown of component D throughout the gel (p < 0.05) but had no effect on substance D's activation energy. They accelerated the amount of component D penetration from gel in an in vitro study. Thus, encapsulating material in niosomes improved chemical stabilization and skin permeability while providing topical antiinflammatory benefits equivalent to NSAID and steroids [45]. The goal of this research was to create transdermal delivery of Meloxicam in niosomes. The findings indicated that these had the highest %EE effectiveness (>55%) and size (187.3 nm). The percent inhibition of edema in treated animals with drug-loaded vesicular gel was much higher than in treated animals to free drug gels. The relationship among size of vesicle and cholesterol concentration was inverse. The bilayer strength and penetration improved even as cholesterol molar ratio rose, resulting in effective drug entrapment. The higher skin penetration of drug niosomal gel might account for its inhibitory action [46].

References

[1] Medzhitov, Origin and physiological roles of inflammation, Nature 454 (7203) (2008) 428–435.

[2] Y.H. Bae, Drug targeting and tumor heterogeneity, J. Control. Release 133 (2009) 2–3.

[3] I. Tabas, C.K. Glass, Anti-inflammatory therapy in chronic disease: challenges and opportunities, Science 339 (2013) 166–172, https://doi.org/10.1126/science.1230720.

[4] G.B. Ryan, G. Majno, Acute inflammation: a review, Am. J. Pathol. 86 (1977) 183–276.

[5] T. Sun, Y.S. Zhang, B. Pang, D.C. Hyun, M. Yang, Y. Xia, Engineered nanoparticles for drug delivery in cancer therapy, Angew. Chem. Int. Ed. 53 (2014) 12320–12364, https://doi.org/10.1002/anie.201403036.

[6] I.M. Oliveira, C. Gonçalves, R.L. Reis, J.M. Oliveira, Engineering nanoparticles for targeting rheumatoid arthritis: past, present, and future trends, Nano Res. 11 (9) (2018) 4489–4506.

[7] S.L. Pal, U. Jana, P.K. Manna, G.P. Mohanta, R. Manavalan, Nanoparticle: an overview of preparation and characterization, J. Appl. Pharmaceut. Sci. 1 (6) (2011) 228–234.

[8] P.H. Zhou, B. Qiu, R.H. Deng, H.J. Li, X.F. Xu, X.F. Shang, Chondroprotective effects of hyaluronic acid-chitosan nanoparticles containing plasmid DNA encoding cytokine response modifier A in a rat knee osteoarthritis model, Cell. Physiol. Biochem. 47 (2018) 1207–1216.

[9] Y. Karabey-Akyurek, A.G. Gurcay, O. Gurcan, O.F. Turkoglu, S. - Yabanoglu-Ciftci, H. Eroglu, M.F. Sargon, E. Bilensoy, L. Oner, Localized delivery of methylprednisolone sodium succinate with polymeric nanoparticles in experimental injured spinal cord model, Pharm. Dev. Technol. 22 (2017) 972–981.

[10] H. Ali, B. Weigmann, E.M. Collnot, S.A. Khan, M. Windbergs, C.M. Lehr, Budesonide loaded PLGA nanoparticles for targeting the inflamed intestinal mucosa–pharmaceutical characterization and fluorescence imaging, Pharm. Res. 33 (2016) 1085–1092.

[11] C. He, L. Yin, Y. Song, C. Tang, C. Yin, Optimization of multifunctional chitosansiRNA nanoparticles for oral delivery applications, targeting TNF-alpha silencing in rats, Acta Biomater. 17 (2015) 98–106.

[12] R.M. Goncalves, A.C. Pereira, I.O. Pereira, M.J. Oliveira, M.A. Barbosa, Macrophage response to chitosan/poly-(gamma-glutamic acid) nanoparticles carrying an anti-inflammatory drug, J. Mater. Sci. Mater. Med. 26 (2015) 167.

[13] S. Murthy, E. Papazoglou, N.M.N.S. Kanagarajan, Nanotechnology: towards the detection and treatment of inflammatory diseases, in: C.S. Stevenson, L.A. Marshall, D.W. Morgan (Eds.), Vivo Models of Inflammation. Progress in Inflammation Research, Birkhäuser Basel, Switzerland, 2006.

[14] C.M.A. van Alem, M. Boonstra, J. Prins, T. Bezhaeva, M.F. van Essen, J.M. Ruben, A.L. Vahrmeijer, E.P. van der Veer, J.W. de Fijter, M.E. Reinders, O. Meijer, J.M. Metselaar, C. van Kooten, J.I.

Rotmans, Local delivery of liposomal prednisolone leads to an anti-inflammatory profile in renal ischaemia-reperfusion injury in the rat, Nephrol. Dial. Transplant. 33 (2018) 44–53.

[15] R. Toita, T. Kawano, M. Murata, J.H. Kang, Anti-obesity and anti-inflammatory effects of macrophage-targeted interleukin-10-conjugated liposomes in obese mice, Biomaterials 110 (2016) 81–88.

[16] X. Xu, Y. Li, L. Wang, Y. Li, J. Pan, X. Fu, et al., Triplefunctional polyetheretherketone surface with enhanced bacteriostasis and anti-inflammatory and osseointegrative properties for implant application, Biomaterials 212 (2019) 98–114, https://doi.org/10.1016/j.biomaterials.2019.05.014.

[17] A. Partoazar, S. Nasoohi, S.M. Rezayat, K. Gilani, S.E. Mehr, A. Amani, N. Rahimi, A.R. Dehpour, Nanoliposome containing cyclosporine A reduced neuroinflammation responses and improved neurological activities in cerebral ischemia/reperfusion in rat, Fundam. Clin. Pharmacol. 31 (2017) 185–193.

[18] S. Naahidi, M. Jafari, F. Edalat, K. Raymond, A. Khademhosseini, P. Chen, Biocompatibility of engineered nanoparticles for drug delivery, J. Control. Release 166 (2) (2013) 182–194.

[19] M. Zhou, J. Hou, Z. Zhong, N. Hao, Y. Lin, C. Li, Targeted delivery of hyaluronic acidcoated solid lipid nanoparticles for rheumatoid arthritis therapy, Drug Deliv. 25 (2018) 716–722.

[20] C. Dianzani, F. Foglietta, B. Ferrara, A.C. Rosa, E. Muntoni, P. Gasco, C. Della Pepa, R. Canaparo, L. Serpe, Solid lipid nanoparticles delivering anti-inflammatory drugs to treat inflammatory bowel disease: effects in an in vivo model, World J. Gastroenterol. 23 (23) (2017) 4200–4210.

[21] J.M. Oliveira, N. Kotobuki, A.P. Marques, R.P. Pirraco, J. Benesch, M. Hirose, et al., Surface engineered carboxymethylchitosan/poly (amidoamine) dendrimer nanoparticles for intracellular targeting, Adv. Funct. Mater. 18 (12) (2008) 1840–1853.

[22] V.V.K. Venuganti, O.P. Perumal, Poly(amidoamine) dendrimers as skin penetration enhancers: influence of charge, generation, and concentration, J. Pharm. Sci. 98 (2009) 2345–2356, https://doi.org/10.1002/jps.21603.

[23] A.S. Chauhan, S. Sridevi, K.B. Chalasani, A.K. Jain, S.K. Jain, N.K. Jain, P.V. Diwan, Dendrimer-mediated transdermal delivery: enhanced bioavailability of indomethacin, J. Control. Release 90 (2003) 335–343, https://doi.org/10.1016/S0168-3659(03)00200-1.

[24] U. Agrawal, N.K. Mehra, U. Gupta, N.K. Jain, Hyperbranched dendritic nano-carrier for topical delivery of dithranol, J. Drug Target. 21 (2013) 497–506, https://doi.org/10.3109/1061186X.2013.771778.

[25] P. Pandi, A. Jain, M. Kommineni, M. Ionov, M. Bryszewska, W. Khan, Dendrimer as a new potential carrier for topical delivery of siRNA: a comparative study of dendriplex vs. lipoplex for delivery of TNF-α siRNA, Int. J. Pharm. 550 (2018) 240–250, https://doi.org/10.1016/j.ijpharm.2018.08.024.

[26] Y. Zhai, G. Zhai, Advances in lipid-based colloid systems as drug carrier for topic delivery, J. Control. Release 193 (2014) 90–99, https://doi.org/10.1016/j.jconrel.2014.05.054.

[27] N. Kaur, K. Sharma, N. Bedi, Topical nanostructured lipid carrier based hydrogel of mometasone furoate for the treatment of psoriasis, Pharm. Nanotechnol. 6 (2018) 133–143, https://doi.org/10.2174/2211738506666180523112513.

[28] J.S.R. Viegas, F.G. Praça, A.L. Caron, I. Suzuki, A.V.P. Silvestrini, W.S.G. Medina, J.O. Del Campio, M. Kravicz, M.V.L.B. Bentley, Nanostructured lipid carrier co-delivering tacrolimus and TNF-α siRNA as an innovate approach to psoriasis, Drug Deliv. Transl. Res. 10 (2020) 646–660, https://doi.org/10.1007/s13346-020-00723-6.

[29] G.W. Lu, P. Gao, Emulsions and microemulsions for topical and transdermal drug delivery, in: V.S. Kulkarny (Ed.), Handbook of Non-Invasive Drug Delivery Systems, first ed., Elsevier Inc.; Amsterdam, The Netherland, 2010, pp. 59–94.

[30] D.J. McClements, Nanoemulsions versus microemulsions: terminology, differences, and similarities, Soft Matter 8 (2012) 1719–1729, https://doi.org/10.1039/C2SM06903B.

[31] N.T. Tung, V.D. Vu, P.L. Nguyen, DoE-based development, physicochemical characterization, and pharmacological evaluation of a topical hydrogel containing betamethasone dipropionate microemulsion, Colloids Surf. B Biointerfaces 181 (2019) 480–488,- https://doi.org/10.1016/j.colsurfb.2019.06.002.

[32] F.G. Praça, J.S.R. Viegas, H.Y. Peh, T.N. Garbin, W.S.G. Medina, M.V.L.B. Bentley, Microemulsion co-delivering vitamin A and vitamin E as a new platform for topical treatment of acute skin inflammation, Mater. Sci. Eng. C Mater. Biol. Appl. 110 (2020), 110639, https://doi.org/10.1016/j.msec.2020.110639.

[33] N. Ahmad, R. Ahmad, A. Al-Qudaihi, S. Alaseel, I. Fita, M. Khalid, F. Pottoo, Preparation of a novel curcumin nanoemulsion by ultrasonication and its comparative effects in wound healing and the treatment of inflammation, RSC Adv. 9 (2019) 20192–20206,- https://doi.org/10.1039/C9RA03102B.

[34] Shadab, N.A. Alhakamy, H. Aldawsari, S. Kotta, J. Ahmad, S. Akhter, S. Alam, M. Khan, Z. Awan, P. Sivakumar, Improved analgesic and anti-inflammatory effect of diclofenac sodium by topical nanoemulgel: formulation development—in vitro and in vivo studies, J. Chem. 2020 (2020) 1–10.

[35] N. Salim, M. García-Celma, E. Escribano, J. Nolla, M. Llinàs, M. Basri, C. Solans, J. Esquena, T. Tadros, Formation of nanoemulsion containing ibuprofen by PIC method for topical delivery, Mater. Today: Proc. 5 (2018) S172–S179, https://doi.org/10.1016/j.matpr.2018.08.062.

[36] R.R. Lala, N.G. Awari, Nanoemulsion-based gel formulations of COX-2 inhibitors for enhanced efficacy in inflammatory conditions, Appl. Nanosci. 4 (2014) 143–151, https://doi.org/10.1007/s13204-012-0177-6.

[37] Q. Wang, J. Jiang, W. Chen, H. Jiang, Z. Zhang, X. Sun, Targeted delivery of low-dose dexamethasone using PCL-PEG micelles for effective treatment of rheumatoid arthritis, J. Control. Release 230 (2016) 64–72.

[38] C.G. Sen Lin, D. Wang, Q. Xie, W. Biao, J. Wang, K. Nan, Q. Zheng, W. Chen, Overcoming the anatomical and physiological barriers in topical eye surface medication using a peptide-decorated polymeric micelle, ACS Appl. Mater. Interfaces 11 (2019) 39603–39612.

[39] T. Kanazawa, T. Kurano, H. Ibaraki, Y. Takashima, T. Suzuki, Y. Seta, Therapeutic effects in a transient middle cerebral artery occlusion rat model by nose-to-brain delivery of anti-TNF-alpha siRNA with cell-penetrating peptide-modified polymer micelles, Pharmaceutics 11 (2019) 478.

[40] U. Hasegawa, A.J. van der Vlies, C. Wandrey, J.A. Hubbell, Preparation of well-defined ibuprofen prodrug micelles by RAFT polymerization, Biomacromolecules 14 (9) (2013) 3314–3320, https://doi.org/10.1021/bm4009149.

[41] K. Yoncheva, P. Petrov, I. Pencheva, S. Konstantinov, Triblock polymeric micelles as carriers for anti-inflammatory drug delivery, J. Microencapsul. 32 (3) (2015) 224–230, https://doi.org/10.3109/02652048.2014.995729.

[42] J. Marques, V. Gaspar, E. Costa, C. Paquete, I. Correia, Synthesis and characterization of micelles as carriers of non-steroidal anti-inflammatory drugs (NSAID) for application in breast cancer therapy, Colloids Surf. B Biointerfaces 113C (2013) 375–383, https://doi.org/10.1016/j.colsurfb.2013.09.037.

[43] J.N. Khandare, G. Madhavi, B.M. Tamhankar, Niosomes novel drug delivery system, Eastern Pharm. 37 (1994) 61–64.

[44] P.M. Gaafar, O.Y. Abdallah, R.M. Farid, H. Abdelkader, Preparation, characterization and evaluation of novel elastic nano-sized niosomes (ethoniosomes) for ocular delivery of prednisolone, J. Liposome Res. 24 (2014) 204–215.

[45] A. Priprem, K. Janpim, S. Nualkaew, et al., Topical niosome gel of *Zingiber cassumunar* Roxb. extract for anti-inflammatory activity enhanced skin permeation and stability of compound D, AAPS PharmSciTech 17 (2016) 631–639, https://doi.org/10.1208/s12249-015-0376-z.

[46] S.F. El-Menshawe, A.K. Hussein, Formulation and evaluation of meloxicam niosomes as vesicular carriers for enhanced skin delivery, Pharm. Dev. Technol. 18 (4) (2013) 779–786, https://doi.org/10.3109/10837450.2011.598166.

Chapter 14

Role of theranostics in targeting inflammation in chronic diseases

C. Sarath Chandran[a], Alan Raj[a,b], K. Sourav[a], and K.K. Swathy[a]

[a]Department of Pharmaceutics, College of Pharmaceutical Sciences, Government Medical College Kannur, Pariyaram, Kerala, India, [b]Department of Pharamceutical Biotechnology, Manipal College of Pharmaceutical Sciences, Manipal Academy of Higher Education, Manipal, Karnataka, India

1 Introduction

Inflammation is considered as a part of the defensive mechanism to protect our body from the invasion of viruses/bacteria or any other foreign body [1–3]. Not only external pathogens but also autoimmune disorders may play a crucial role in triggering the inflammations [4]. Based on the time of progression, inflammation is classified into two types: acute and chronic. In acute inflammation, the reaction may vanish within hours [5]. It is associated with conditions such as acute dermatitis, acute meningitis, bronchitis, etc. The inflammatory cells involved in acute inflammations include neutrophil, basophil, eosinophil, monocyte, and macrophages [6]. On the other hand, chronic inflammation may last for months or even for years [7]. The mediators that trigger chronic inflammation are reactive oxygen species, hydrolytic enzymes, cytokines, interferon-γ (INF-γ), and few other growth factors [8,9]. Along with these mediators, pro-inflammatory cytokinin like tumor necrosis factor-alpha (TNF-α) plays a pivotal role in disease progression. It can regulate the genes that are present in the adipose tissues [10]. Moreover, it may induce certain cytokines like interleukin-1β (IL-1β) and IL-8 from the Caco-2 cell lines [11]. IL, nuclear factor kappa (NF-$\kappa\beta$), C-reactive protein (CRP), cyclooxygenases, and lipoxygenases are involved in the progression of chronic inflammations [12,13].

The genesis of chronic inflammation is from acute inflammation, in which it gradually converts into chronic with early-stage symptoms similar to an acute condition. Along with that, vasodilation leads to increased blood flow, high capillary permeability, and possible diapedesis [14]. Admittedly, the change happens in the white blood cells (WBCs) and, the ephemeral neutrophil was replaced with macrophages and lymphocytes [15]. To be specific, the inflammation is characterized by infiltration of macrophages, plasma cells, inflammatory cytokines, growth factors, and specific enzymes, which guides toward the damage of tissues and finally end up with the formation of fibrous tissues [16–19]. To treat these symptoms, the mechanism involved in inflammation should be studied first.

IL-1 and TNF-α are secreted from macrophages and dendritic cells, which further trigger the release of selectins and integrins from the site of endothelial cell injury [20,21]. Moreover, these may potentially stimulate chemotaxis and diapedesis. The leukocyte will migrate to the site along with macrophages and dendritic cells. After the activation of leukocytes, it gradually releases cytokinin and inflammatory mediators [5]. Neutrophils also play a pivotal role in inflammation as it releases reactive oxygen species (ROS), cytokines such as IL-1, IL-6 and TNF-α [22–24]. Similarly, the role of circulating platelets in inflammation was also studied. It induces platelet aggregation, thrombus formation, and finally degranulation by the release of chemokines and inflammatory mediators [25–27]. There are various diseases that are accompanied by inflammation, in that chronic diseases are more affected by inflammation.

The inflammation associated with chronic diseases includes cancer, cardiovascular disease, diabetes, asthma, chronic obstructive pulmonary disease (COPD), and so on (Fig. 1). In cancer, TNF-α is involved not only in carcinogenesis but also in the destruction of cancer cells at an elevated concentration [28]. Similarly IL-1β, a pro-inflammatory cytokinin that comes under the IL-1 family, shows a concentration-dependent activity [29,30]. Due to the immune response, it shows a local inflammatory response at low concentration whereas at elevated concentration, it induces inflammation rather than protection [31].

Atherosclerosis is an inflammatory disease and rheumatoid arthritis patients are more susceptible to this disease than healthy individuals [32]. The elevated levels of IL-6 and C-reactive protein (CRP) are reported in these patients [33]. In diabetic patients, the invasion of macrophages into adipose tissue leads to the release of pro-inflammatory cytokines to reduce insulin sensitivity [34–36]. Moreover, the elevated levels of CRP and inflammatory cytokinin, viz.

Recent Developments in Anti-Inflammatory Therapy. https://doi.org/10.1016/B978-0-323-99988-5.00002-4

FIG. 1 Inflammation associated with chronic diseases.

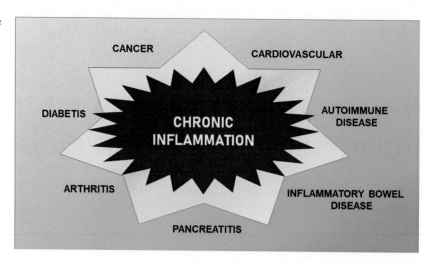

IL-1, IL-6, and TNF-α increase the vascular permeability and attachment of leukocytes in the endothelial tissues. As a result, plasminogen activator inhibitor-1 (PAI-1) is released, to suppress the fibrinolysis and leads to thrombus formation [37–39]. On the other hand, obesity is considered as an integration of various metabolic disorders such as asthma, atherosclerosis, type-2 diabetes mellitus (T2DM), cancer, etc. [40]. The high level of TNF-α in obesity retards the antiinflammatory cytokinin adiponectin and enhances the secretion of pro-inflammatory cytokinin like IL-6, which plays a pivotal role in the pathogenesis of inflammation [41–43]. These cytokinins play a crucial role in triggering inflammation in chronic disease conditions.

Traditionally, the inflammation is treated with antiinflammatory drugs, viz. nonsteroidal antiinflammatory drugs (NSAIDs), corticosteroids, and disease-modifying antirheumatic drugs (DMARDs) [44]. NSAIDs and steroids are commonly used to relieve pain and swelling whereas the tissue damage by inflammation may be avoided by DMARDs, especially when administered in the early stages of the disease. DMARDs are broadly classified into two groups, namely nonbiologic and biologic DMARDs. The nonbiologic DMARDs include low dose methotrexate, thalidomide, etc. [45–47]. Apart from that, the biologic DMARDs were used to block a particular molecule involved in the signaling pathways such as TNF-α and IL-6, which trigger inflammation [45]. Biologic DMARDs are recombinant proteins, which includes rapidly accelerated fibrosarcoma (FAS) protein, IL-6 and IL-1β inhibitors, monoclonal antibodies, etc. [48–50].

But there are few challenges associated with targeting these inflammations because these are triggered by multiple inflammatory mediators and targeting any one of the mediators may not be sufficient to control the inflammation. Targeting any one of the signaling pathways in the inflammation may result in the trigger of another pro-inflammatory cytokinin in other pathways associated with the inflammation, which may finally lead to more complex inflammatory reactions [45,51]. TNF-α has a potential role in triggering inflammation, but on the other hand, patients with anti-TNF-α therapy are at high risk of reoccurrence of tuberculosis (TB) [52]. The above statement was justified by the study conducted among the French patients, in which the patients with anti-TNF-α therapy were found to be more susceptible to TB [53]. Similar results were reported in the case of Hepatitis B infection and demyelinating disorders such as multiple sclerosis, optic neuritis, etc. [54–57]. In contrast, TNF-α plays a pivotal role in cell differentiation, proliferation, and apoptosis, hence the inhibition of TNF may result in hematological problems [58,59]. Anakinra is an IL-1β antagonist used as an antiinflammatory agent, but it impairs the immune system of the body and the patients are at high risk of inflammations such as cellulitis, bursitis, osteomyelitis, etc. [60].

According to World Health Organization (WHO), chronic diseases are a major threat to the global health. The death rate due to chronic inflammatory diseases such as cancer, heart disorders, diabetes, stroke is high. A survey conducted in the United States in 2015 revealed that approximately 125 million people had chronic conditions and 20% of the population had multiple inflammatory diseases [61,62]. These data suggest that the current treatment with biological and nonbiological DMARDs may be ineffective and induce serious problems. Accurately made early diagnosis and treatment can prevent the inflammations associated with chronic diseases. "Theranostics" can play an important role in this condition, and it is a novel treatment strategy recently developed for the effective management of inflammations in chronic disease conditions.

2 Theranostic approach

It is considered as a new treatment strategy to personalize the medication rather than opting for a generalized

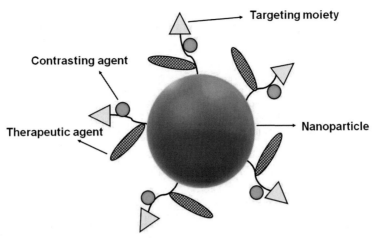

FIG. 2 Theranostic nanoparticle.

approach. It is a type of molecular-based treatment approach for the effective minimization of unwanted systemic side effects due to the intersubject variability [63]. The theranostic approach is a unification of therapy and diagnosis within a single window [64,65]. The introduction of nanotechnology in theranostics, i.e., theranostic nanoparticles (TNPs), has strengthened the outcomes. It offers a wide variety of applications including active and passive targeting, molecular imaging, environmentally sensitive drug release, etc. [66]. A typical TNP contains three elements, namely a targeting moiety, a contrasting agent, and a therapeutic molecule (Fig. 2).

A TNP contains a targeting moiety that binds with the targeting organ and releases the medicament, meanwhile, due to the presence of a contrasting agent, its circulation can be detected [67]. TNPs can be prepared in two ways:

(1) by the incorporation of a contrasting agent into the existing nanoparticles like micelles, polymer-drug conjugate liposomes, etc., and (2) using nanoparticles having intrinsic imaging properties so no need of an external contrasting agent [68]. Nanoparticles used for theranostic purposes include liposomes, dendrimers, drug-polymer conjugate, carbon-based nanoparticles, etc. (Fig. 3) [68,69].

The nanoparticles can be conjugated with drugs as well as imaging agents such as NIR-infrared dyes like IR-783 for optical imaging purposes, ^{19}F compounds for MRI imaging, gold nanoparticles for computed tomography, etc. [70]. Table 1 shows the different imaging methods for the detection of TNPs.

These agents are functionalized nanoparticles in which they have established unique properties. The majority of the TNPs are hydrophobic which limits their use, so surface

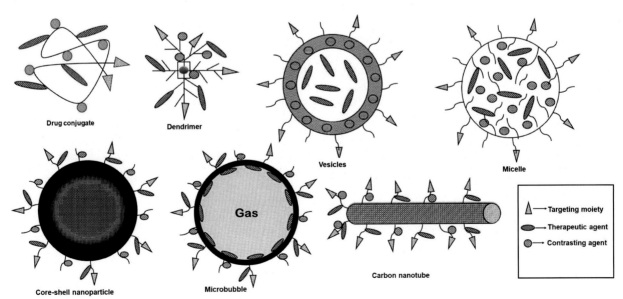

FIG. 3 Functionalized nanoparticles for theranostic approach.

TABLE 1 Examples for contrasting agents and their imaging techniques.

Imaging modality	Contrasting agent
MRI	Gadolinium, iron oxide, magnetic oxide, ^{19}F labeled compounds
PET	^{18}F, ^{64}Cu, ^{11}C, ^{15}O-labeled compounds
SPECT	99mTc, ^{111}In chelates
Optical imaging	Flurochrome, photoproteins
Ultrasound	Nano/microbubbles

modifications with hydrophilic polymers such as polyethylene glycol (PEG) and vitamin E tocopheryl polyethylene glycol succinate (TPGS) are suggested. The chain length of PEG also plays a crucial role in the cellular uptake of TNPs. The shorter PEG chain length are reported with the highest cellular uptake [71,72]. Table 2 summarizes the variety of TNP platforms.

2.1 Liposomes

Liposomes are lipid-based vesicular systems with a hydrophilic core and a hydrophobic outer membrane. Because of its amphiphilic nature, it can accommodate both hydrophilic and hydrophobic active ingredients [78,79]. It generates great interest because of its unique properties such as biocompatibility, biodegradability, low toxicity, and immunogenicity. Liposomes of small molecular size in the range 50–200 nm with neutral/negative charge are selected for theranostic purposes [80,81]. TNPs such as carbon nanotubes, quantum dots, gold nanoparticles and therapeutic agents can be either encapsulated or embedded in the liposomes. Along with these, its targetability can be improved by attaching molecular biomarkers on its surface. The circulation in the blood can be improved by surface modification with PEG. PEGylated liposomes possess better stability and have long $t_{1/2}$ [82,83]. By blocking the inflammatory mediators such as macrophages ILs, and so on the inflammation can be effectively reduced to a great extent.

Glucocorticoids are commonly used as antiinflammatory agents especially in rheumatoid arthritis. But it has serious side effects such as cataracts, bone fracture, osteoporosis, etc. The heterogenous property of the disease retards the effectiveness of a treatment, so a personalized approach may be a more effective approach to treat this disease condition [84]. Multifunctional liposome with glucocorticoid was formulated with an attachment of radiolabeled complex [^{89}Zr] Zr(oxinate)$_4$ in the liposomal core (^{89}Zr-NSSL-MPS). Its biodistribution was detected by positron emission tomography (PET) and its efficacy was tested in the K/B$_x$N serum transfer arthritis model. The PET image revealed that it accumulates in the inflamed joints rather than in normal joint cells. PET imaging helps to distinguish the inflamed and noninflamed joints [85]. Inorganic–organic hybrid nanoparticles of [ZrO]$^{2+}$ [(BMP)$_{0.9}$ (FMN)$_{0.1}$]$^{2-}$ was formulated for the treatment of inflammatory diseases. Glucocorticoid was taken as the active ingredient and its biodistribution was detected by fluorescence-activated cell sorting (flow cytometry). It blocks the inflammatory mediators such as macrophages, which were further confirmed in monocytes isolated from humans [86].

Long circulating PEG liposomes of glucocorticoid show a marked reduction in the inflammation in joints after IV administration. Liposomes were labeled with ^{111}In-oxine to determine its biodistribution, and it was found that it accumulated only in the inflamed joints, so systemic toxicity was reduced to a greater extent. It was reported to produce better accumulation in the joints, with a stronger therapeutic effect [87]. Atherosclerosis is an inflammatory disorder in which the pro-inflammatory cytokinin upregulates the intracellular adhesion molecule-1 (ICAM-1) present in the blood vessels [88]. Paramagnetic liposomes linked with contrasting agent gadolinium and anti-ICAM-1 antibody were able to downregulate these inflammatory mediators. MRI imaging gives an idea about the normal

TABLE 2 Applications of theranostics.

Nanocarriers	Therapeutic agent	Contrasting agent	Targeting approach	Reference
Dendrimer	5-Fluorouracil	5-Fluorouracil	Active	[73]
Lipid vesicle	Docetaxel	Tc 99-m	Passive	[74]
Micelle	Doxorubicin	SPIO	Active	[75]
Microbubble	Doxorubicin	PFP	Passive	[76]
Carbon nanotube	Cisplatin	QD	Active	[77]

and upregulated ICAM-1 expression in the blood vessels [89]. Similar work was done in immunoliposomes to target the atherosclerosis plaque. Iohexol was selected as the contrasting agent. Anti-ICAM-1 was specifically bound with the ICAM-1 receptor present on the surface of the blood vessel [90].

2.2 Dendrimers

Dendrimers are hyperbranched macromolecules that contain symmetrical branching around a central core. The end groups of dendrimers can be functionalized to modify their physicochemical and biological properties [91,92]. The terminal group can be modified with therapeutic agents, fluorochromes, nucleic acids, etc. [93]. Polyionic dendrimers have unique properties because of their size and shape and they are highly flexible [94]. Dendrimer consists of three parts: the central core, from which the branches arise; the intermediate zone, which gives an idea about the generation; and the terminal part, where the functional groups are located [95]. It can be synthesized by either divergent method or convergent method. In the divergent approach, the dendrimer is synthesized from its core, whereas in the convergent approach, the synthesis starts from the surface to the core [96–98]. One of the interesting facts is that dendrimer itself has an intrinsic antiinflammatory activity. The most common dendrimers are poly(amidoamine) PAMAM, poly(propylene imine) PPI, and poly(lysine) [99].

Osteoarthritis (OA) is a chronic inflammatory disease characterized by the destruction of cartilage, which leads to serious pain and inflammation in joints [100]. Insulin-like growth factor 1 (I GF-1) is an anabolic growth factor that helps in the regeneration of cartilages. PAMAM dendrimer with different concentrations of PEG was conjugated with I GF-1 as a therapeutic moiety and fluorophore as a contrasting agent. The formulation was injected intraarticularly in the rat synovial fluid. Dendrimer with generation-6, 4% PEG shows higher $t_{1/2}$ than others [101]. Carbosilane dendrimer of the third generation conjugated with infliximab and contrasting agent fluorescein isocyanate (FITC) was formulated for the treatment of rheumatoid arthritis. The dendrimer is reported to improve the biological half-life of DMARDs in the bloodstream. These dendrimer conjugates show high antiinflammatory activity and their biodistribution was detected by the Kaiser test spectroscopy [102]. Beta folate receptors were highly overexpressed in the inflamed cells and methotrexate (MTX) can effectively bind with these folate receptors which helps in reducing the inflammation [103,104]. Generation-5 PAMAM dendrimer-loaded MTX is conjugated with FITC to determine biodistribution and binding efficacy of MTX. The confocal laser scanning microscopical image gives a clear idea about the binding of these

complexes with KB and RAW 264.7 cell lines. It shows a dose-dependent antiinflammatory activity [105]. The studies revealed that gold (Au) nanoparticles have unique properties such as the photothermal effect, which is extended to antiinflammatory therapy. Au nanoparticles were attached to dendrimer (DEN) and IR780, a near-infrared region (NIR) bioactive agent for photothermal therapy. The Au-DEN-MTX shows a photothermal effect, and it generated reactive oxygen species (ROS) which gives a synergistic antiinflammatory response. The cellular uptake of the agent was confirmed by confocal laser microscopy [106].

2.3 Polymer-drug conjugates

The nucleic acids and proteins were previously explored for the delivery of therapeutic as well as an imaging agents to the specific cells. But the poor biodistribution, nonspecific binding, and short half-life limited their use [107]. Later after several modifications, the polymeric drug conjugates with a size in the range of 1–10 nm could bypass the renal and hepatic clearance to provide enhanced biodistribution. High molecular weight conjugates show better biodistribution and half-life [108,109]. It has mainly three components: polymer component, therapeutic moiety, and imaging/contrasting agent, sometimes the therapeutic agent itself can act as a contrasting agent. Therapeutic agents such as doxorubicin, ellipticine, paclitaxel, and bleomycin possess fluorescence properties [110–112]. The preparation of polymeric drug conjugates is illustrated in Fig. 4. Polymers used include poly(lactide-co-glycolide) (PLGA), polylactide (PLA), polyglycolide, polycaprolactone (PCL) and poly (D,L-lactide), and poly N-(2-hydroxypropyl)-methacrylamide-(poly-HPMA) [113].

The inflamed synovial joints are overexpressed with secreted protein acidic and rich in cysteine (SPARC). Human serum albumin (HSA)-conjugated SPARC loaded with methotrexate (MTX) was formulated. Chlorin e6, a naturally occurring photosensitizer, was conjugated to detect the biodistribution. Upon intravenous injection, the HSA-SPARC-MTX complex showed higher accumulation and retention in the inflamed joints with a better antiinflammatory response. It was confirmed by fluorescence/magnetic resonance dual model imaging [114]. NIR-II photoacoustic molecular imaging (PMI) is a new technique developed for the detection and treatment of rheumatoid arthritis (RA). Tocilizumab (TCZ) comes under biological DMARDs, which can effectively block IL-6 inflammatory cells. TCZ was conjugated with indocyanine (ICG) contrasting agent and nanoparticle for theranostic purposes. The PMI imaging revealed the efficient suppression of the inflammation with a better therapeutic half-life [115]. Stealth polymer nanoconjugates can efficiently deliver both drug and contrasting agents in a single platform. The unique

FIG. 4 Preparation of polymeric-drug conjugate theranostics.

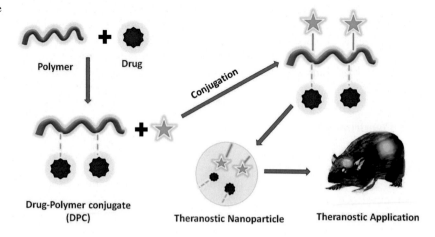

properties of Au were previously discussed. A stimuli-responsive polymeric nanoparticle can effectively release the therapeutic agent upon internal/external stimuli [116]. The MTX-loaded PEG-PLGA nanoparticles suppress IL-1β and IL-6 inflammatory cells. For further confirmation, it was conjugated with FITC, and the confocal fluorescence microscopy revealed that it was successfully taken up by the inflammatory cells [117]. Similarly, MTX was loaded in PEG-hyperbranched semiconducting polymer (HSP)-based nanoparticles along with a 99mTc radioisotope (99mTc-HSP-PEG). The CT image revealed that nanoparticles were highly accumulated in the inflamed joints [118]. MTX and dexamethasone-loaded chitosan polymeric nanoparticle (CHNP) show a high antiarthritic effect. The biodistribution of CHNP-^{99}Tc was determined and a higher level of nanoparticles was found in the inflamed site after IV injection [119].

2.4 Carbon-based theranostic nanoparticles

Carbon-based nanoparticles is a big family comprising carbon nanotubes (CNTs), graphene oxide (GO), graphene quantum dots (GQDs), and fullerene [120]. Each nanoparticle has its unique properties in terms of targeting ability, biosensing, imaging, diagnosis, and so on [121,122]. Physical properties of carbon nanoparticles can be altered by surface modification with hydroxyl, epoxy, and carboxylic acid groups on their surface. Due to their unique size and larger surface area, they can be easily functionalized with contrasting agents, targeting moiety, and therapeutic agents. The potential use of carbon nanoparticles in antiinflammatory therapy was previously studied. They act by generating reactive oxygen species (ROS) which damages the inflamed cells. Due to their intrinsic optical imaging properties, they are extensively used for theranostic purposes [123].

2.4.1 Carbon nanotubes (CNTs)

Carbon nanotubes are cylindrical form of graphene nanomaterials having intrinsic unique properties. Based on the number of layers of graphene sheets CNTs are subdivided into two types: single-walled carbon nanotubes (SWCNTs) and multiwalled carbon nanotubes (MWCNTs) [124]. CNTs possess photothermal, photothermoacoustic, and photoacoustic effects, in which they can absorb NIR radiation and convert it into heat energy, which leads to the destruction of inflammatory mediators. CNTs can be functionalized with gadolinium (Gd), an MRI contrasting agent, for theranostic purpose [125–127]. The drug can be conjugated to CNTs either by a passive approach or by covalent conjugation [128].

As we know that chronic inflammation leads to DNA damage which further induces cancer. SWCNTs are considered an excellent candidate to treat cancer, but the hydrophobic nature limited their use. Hence surface modification with hydrophilic polymers helps in the internalization of nanoparticles into cells and provide a prolonged half-life. SWCNTs were functionalized with asparagine-glycine-arginine (NGR) and tamoxifen (TAM) was prepared for cancer therapy. NGR-SWCNT-TAM complex has synergistic antitumor efficiency with hyperemia effect. The higher intracellular uptake was proved by fluorescence microscopy in the presence of an FITC contrasting agent [129]. In another study, SWCNTs were conjugated with Gd, doxorubicin (DOX), and hyaluronic acid (HA) for cancer targeting (Gd/SWCNTs-HA-DOX). It shows a time-dependent release of DOX in the blood compared with free DOX. The fluorescence microscopy imaging proved that high internalization of nanoconjugate than the free drug. Also, the MRI image gives the exact idea about the biodistribution of the complex. High fluorescent intensity was detected in the tumor sites with a prolonged half-life. Multiple contrasting agents and imaging techniques were used. FITC was detected by fluorescence imaging and confocal laser scanning microscopy to study the redox-sensitive release of DOX. Similarly, IR-783, a near-infrared region (NIR) dye, helps to detect the biodistribution of nanoconjugate by NIR optical imaging technique [130].

The photothermal effect of SWCNTs was explored for the treatment of atherosclerosis. Scavenging the macrophages is one of the effective treatment strategies for atherosclerosis. SWCNTs were conjugated with phenoxylated dextran to improve targetability and aqueous solubility. In this, the SWCNT itself acts as a therapeutic agent. The fluorescence image revealed that it was selectively taken up by the macrophages. Upon laser irradiation, within 700–1100 nm it shows photothermal ablation effect toward macrophages [131]. Conjugation of Cy5.5 fluorescent dye in SWCNTs helps in the treatment of atherosclerosis by photothermal ablation on 808 nm laser irradiation. The uptake of the complex by macrophages was proved by a confocal microscopic image [132].

2.4.2 Quantum dots (QDs)

QDs are luminescent semiconductor nanocrystals having intrinsic fluorescence property which is related to size, functional groups, crystalline nature, etc. The fluorescence property can be enhanced by chemical modification on the surface of QDs with organic functional groups [133]. Hydrophilic carbon QDs are widely used for theranostic purposes rather than hydrophobic QDs [134]. QDs are an excellent vehicle for imaging and diagnosis due to their properties, viz. biocompatibility, low toxicity, plasma clearance, and low immunogenicity. Their surface contains carboxylic acid and alcoholic groups which can easily be modified with contrasting agents [135].

The antiinflammatory action of *Allium sativum*. L (garlic) was previously reported. Luminescent garlic QDs was prepared for macrophage neutralization. The data shows that it selectively binds with macrophages and exhibits antiinflammatory properties. Fluorescence microscopic images showed the presence of QDs in the cytoplasm of cells [136]. QD-aptamer (A10 RNA) complex was conjugated with doxorubicin (DOX) for prostate cancer therapy, QD-Apt (DOX). Aptamer A10 can bind with prostate tumor cells and release DOX. A time-dependent release was obtained, which was confirmed by the difference in fluorescence intensity, i.e., as the time increases the intensity of fluorescence increases, which is directly proportional to DOX release [137]. Methotrexate (MTX) is a well-known anticancer drug, but the upregulated efflux transport system act as a barrier resulting in lower accumulation of the drug in tissues. The multifunctional properties of QDs have been explored for anticancer drug delivery along with imaging [138]. The MTX-QD conjugate was effectively accumulated in tumor cells via receptor-mediated endocytosis, as revealed by fluorescence image [139].

3 Conclusions

The theranostic approach toward inflammation management helps in personalized medication rather than the traditional approach. One of the major problems associated with chronic disease is its heterogenicity and the application of theranostic nanoparticles can effectively overcome this problem. The scale-up of the theranostic nanoparticles may be a challenging task, but the latest advanced methodologies could overcome this challenge in scale-up to enable its application in wider mode. The future for theranostic nanoparticles is great, which can be extended from the successful management of inflammatory diseases to much-complicated disease conditions.

References

[1] J. Fritsch, M.T. Abreu, The microbiota and the immune response: what is the chicken and what is the egg? Gastrointest. Endosc. Clin. N. Am. 29 (3) (2019) 381–393, https://doi.org/10.1016/j.giec.2019.02.005.

[2] D. Michels da Silva, H. Langer, T. Graf, Inflammatory and molecular pathways in heart failure-ischemia, HFpEF and transthyretin cardiac amyloidosis, Int. J. Mol. Sci. 20 (9) (2019), https://doi.org/10.3390/ijms20092322.

[3] X. Zhang, X. Wu, Q. Hu, J. Wu, G. Wang, Z. Hong, J. Ren, Lab for Trauma and Surgical Infections, Mitochondrial DNA in liver inflammation and oxidative stress, Life Sci. 236 (November) (2019), 116464, https://doi.org/10.1016/j.lfs.2019.05.020.

[4] I.B. McInnes, G. Schett, The pathogenesis of rheumatoid arthritis, N. Engl. J. Med. 365 (23) (2011) 2205–2219, https://doi.org/10.1056/NEJMra1004965.

[5] C.-O. Sahlmann, P. Ströbel, Pathophysiology of inflammation, Nuklearmedizin. Nuclear Medicine 55 (1) (2016) 1–6.

[6] D. Laveti, M. Kumar, R. Hemalatha, R. Sistla, V. Naidu, V. Talla, V. Verma, N. Kaur, R. Nagpal, Anti-inflammatory treatments for chronic diseases: a review, Inflamm. Allergy Drug Targets 12 (5) (2013) 349–361, https://doi.org/10.2174/18715281113129990053.

[7] D. Placha, J. Jampilek, Chronic inflammatory diseases, anti-inflammatory agents and their delivery Nanosystems, Pharmaceutics 13 (1) (2021) 64, https://doi.org/10.3390/pharmaceutics13010064.

[8] L.A. Abdulkhaleq, M.A. Assi, R. Abdullah, M. Zamri-Saad, Y.H. Taufiq-Yap, M.N.M. Hezmee, The crucial roles of inflammatory mediators in inflammation: a review, Veterinary World 11 (5) (2018) 627–635, https://doi.org/10.14202/vetworld.2018.627-635.

[9] S. Anwikar, M. Bhitre, Study of the synergistic anti-inflammatory activity of solanum Xanthocarpum Schrad and Wendl and *Cassia fistula* Linn, Int. J. Ayurveda Res. 1 (3) (2010) 167–171, https://doi.org/10.4103/0974-7788.72489.

[10] H. Ruan, P.D.G. Miles, C.M. Ladd, K. Ross, T.R. Golub, J.M. Olefsky, H.F. Lodish, Profiling gene transcription in vivo reveals adipose tissue as an immediate target of tumor necrosis factor-alpha: implications for insulin resistance, Diabetes 51 (11) (2002) 3176–3188, https://doi.org/10.2337/diabetes.51.11.3176.

[11] A. Lang, M. Lahav, E. Sakhnini, I. Barshack, H.H. Fidder, B. Avidan, E. Bardan, R. Hershkoviz, S. Bar-Meir, Y. Chowers, Allicin inhibits spontaneous and TNF-alpha induced secretion of proinflammatory cytokines and chemokines from intestinal epithelial cells, Clin. Nutr. (Edinburgh, Scotland) 23 (5) (2004) 1199–1208, https://doi.org/10.1016/j.clnu.2004.03.011.

[12] G.R. Souza, T.M. Cunha, R.L. Silva, C.M. Lotufo, W.A. Verri, M.I. Funez, C.F. Villarreal, et al., Involvement of nuclear factor kappa B in the maintenance of persistent inflammatory hypernociception, Pharmacol. Biochem. Behav. 134 (July) (2015) 49–56, https://doi.org/10.1016/j.pbb.2015.04.005.

[13] J.R. Thiele, J. Zeller, H. Bannasch, G.B. Stark, K. Peter, S.U. Eisenhardt, Targeting C-reactive protein in inflammatory disease by preventing conformational changes, Mediat. Inflamm. 2015 (2015) 1–9, https://doi.org/10.1155/2015/372432.

[14] J.S. Pober, W.C. Sessa, Inflammation and the blood microvascular system, Cold Spring Harb. Perspect. Biol. 7 (1) (2015), https://doi.org/10.1101/cshperspect.a016345.

[15] P. Libby, Inflammatory mechanisms: the molecular basis of inflammation and disease, Nutr. Rev. 65 (1) (2008) 140–146, https://doi.org/10.1111/j.1753-4887.2007.tb00352.x.

[16] M. Cutolo, S. Soldano, V. Smith, Pathophysiology of systemic sclerosis: current understanding and new insights, Expert. Rev. Clin. Immunol. 15 (7) (2019) 753–764, https://doi.org/10.1080/1744666X.2019.1614915.

[17] V.M. Milenkovic, E.H. Stanton, C. Nothdurfter, R. Rupprecht, C.H. Wetzel, The role of chemokines in the pathophysiology of major depressive disorder, Int. J. Mol. Sci. 20 (9) (2019) 2283, https://doi.org/10.3390/ijms20092283.

[18] E.J. Needham, A. Helmy, E.R. Zanier, J.L. Jones, A.J. Coles, D.K. Menon, The immunological response to traumatic brain injury, J. Neuroimmunol. 332 (July) (2019) 112–125, https://doi.org/10.1016/j.jneuroim.2019.04.005.

[19] A. Yousuf, W. Ibrahim, N.J. Greening, C.E. Brightling, T2 biologics for chronic obstructive pulmonary disease, J Allergy Clin Immunol Pract 7 (5) (2019) 1405–1416, https://doi.org/10.1016/j.jaip.2019.01.036.

[20] W.A. Muller, Getting leukocytes to the site of inflammation, Vet. Pathol. 50 (1) (2013) 7–22, https://doi.org/10.1177/0300985812469883.

[21] W.A. Muller, Leukocyte-endothelial cell interactions in the inflammatory response, Lab. Investig. 82 (5) (2002) 521–534, https://doi.org/10.1038/labinvest.3780446.

[22] E. Mortaz, S.D. Alipoor, I.M. Adcock, S. Mumby, L. Koenderman, Update on neutrophil function in severe inflammation, Front. Immunol. 9 (2) (2018) 2171, https://doi.org/10.3389/fimmu.2018.02171.

[23] C. Rosales, Neutrophil: a cell with many roles in inflammation or several cell types? Front. Physiol. 9 (1) (2018) 113, https://doi.org/10.3389/fphys.2018.00113.

[24] C. Rosales, C.A. Lowell, M. Schnoor, E. Uribe-Querol, Neutrophils: their role in innate and adaptive immunity 2017, J Immunol Res 2017 (November) (2017), e9748345, https://doi.org/10.1155/2017/9748345.

[25] A. Margraf, A. Zarbock, Platelets in inflammation and resolution, J. Immunol. 203 (9) (2019) 2357–2367, https://doi.org/10.4049/jimmunol.1900899.

[26] O. Sonmez, M. Sonmez, Role of platelets in immune system and inflammation, Porto Biomed. J. 2 (6) (2017) 311–314, https://doi.org/10.1016/j.pbj.2017.05.005.

[27] M.R. Thomas, R.F. Storey, The role of platelets in inflammation, Thromb. Haemost. 114 (3) (2015) 449–458, https://doi.org/10.1160/TH14-12-1067.

[28] A. Mantovani, P. Allavena, A. Sica, F. Balkwill, Cancer-related inflammation, Nature 454 (7203) (2008) 436–444, https://doi.org/10.1038/nature07205.

[29] K.J. Baker, A. Houston, E. Brint, IL-1 family members in cancer; two sides to every story, Front. Immunol. 10 (June) (2019), https://doi.org/10.3389/fimmu.2019.01197.

[30] S. Tu, G. Bhagat, G. Cui, S. Takaishi, E.A. Kurt-Jones, B. Rickman, K.S. Betz, et al., Overexpression of interleukin-1β induces gastric inflammation and cancer and mobilizes myeloid-derived suppressor cells in mice, Cancer Cell 14 (5) (2008) 408–419, https://doi.org/10.1016/j.ccr.2008.10.011.

[31] R.N. Apte, E. Voronov, Interleukin-1—a major pleiotropic cytokine in tumor-host interactions, Semin. Cancer Biol. 12 (4) (2002) 277–290, https://doi.org/10.1016/s1044-579x(02)00014-7.

[32] I.C. van Eijk, M.J.L. Peters, E.H. Serné, I.E. van der Horst-Bruinsma, B.A.C. Dijkmans, Y.M. Smulders, M.T. Nurmohamed, Microvascular function is impaired in ankylosing spondylitis and improves after tumour necrosis factor alpha blockade, Ann. Rheum. Dis. 68 (3) (2009) 362–366, https://doi.org/10.1136/ard.2007.086777.

[33] I. Ford, G.J. Blauw, M.B. Murphy, J. Shepherd, S.M. Cobbe, E.L.E. M. Bollen, B.M. Buckley, et al., A prospective study of pravastatin in the elderly at risk (PROSPER): screening experience and baseline characteristics, Curr. Controll. Trials Cardiovasc. Med. 3 (1) (2002) 8, https://doi.org/10.1186/1468-6708-3-8.

[34] J.-P. Bastard, M. Maachi, C. Lagathu, M.J. Kim, M. Caron, H. Vidal, J. Capeau, B. Feve, Recent advances in the relationship between obesity, inflammation, and insulin resistance, Eur. Cytokine Netw. 17 (1) (2006) 4–12.

[35] E.E. Kershaw, J.S. Flier, Adipose tissue as an endocrine organ, J. Clin. Endocrinol. Metab. 89 (6) (2004) 2548–2556, https://doi.org/10.1210/jc.2004-0395.

[36] J.C. Pickup, G.D. Chusney, S.M. Thomas, D. Burt, Plasma Interleukin-6, tumour necrosis factor alpha and blood cytokine production in type 2 diabetes, Life Sci. 67 (3) (2000) 291–300, https://doi.org/10.1016/s0024-3205(00)00622-6.

[37] A.R. Folsom, W.D. Rosamond, E. Shahar, L.S. Cooper, N. Aleksic, F.J. Nieto, M.L. Rasmussen, K.K. Wu, Prospective study of markers of hemostatic function with risk of ischemic stroke. The atherosclerosis risk in communities (ARIC) study investigators, Circulation 100 (7) (1999) 736–742, https://doi.org/10.1161/01.cir.100.7.736.

[38] A.J. Grau, F. Buggle, H. Becher, E. Werle, W. Hacke, The Association of Leukocyte Count, fibrinogen and C-reactive protein with vascular risk factors and ischemic vascular diseases, Thromb. Res. 82 (3) (1996) 245–255, https://doi.org/10.1016/0049-3848(96)00071-0.

[39] R. Shurtz-Swirski, S. Sela, A.T. Herskovits, S.M. Shasha, G. Shapiro, L. Nasser, B. Kristal, Involvement of peripheral polymorphonuclear leukocytes in oxidative stress and inflammation in type 2 diabetic patients, Diabetes Care 24 (1) (2001) 104–110, https://doi.org/10.2337/diacare.24.1.104.

[40] G.S. Hotamisligil, Inflammation and metabolic disorders, Nature 444 (7121) (2006) 860–867, https://doi.org/10.1038/nature05485.

[41] G.S. Hotamisligil, P. Peraldi, A. Budavari, R. Ellis, M.F. White, B. M. Spiegelman, IRS-1-mediated inhibition of insulin receptor tyrosine kinase activity in TNF-alpha- and obesity-induced insulin

resistance, Science (New York, N.Y.) 271 (5249) (1996) 665–668, https://doi.org/10.1126/science.271.5249.665.

[42] A.D. Pradhan, J.E. Manson, N. Rifai, J.E. Buring, P.M. Ridker, C-reactive protein, interleukin 6, and risk of developing type 2 diabetes mellitus, JAMA 286 (3) (2001) 327–334, https://doi.org/10.1001/jama.286.3.327.

[43] K. Stenlöf, I. Wernstedt, T. Fjällman, V. Wallenius, K. Wallenius, J.-O. Jansson, Interleukin-6 levels in the central nervous system are negatively correlated with fat mass in overweight/obese subjects, J. Clin. Endocrinol. Metab. 88 (9) (2003) 4379–4383, https://doi.org/10.1210/jc.2002-021733.

[44] J.A. Singh, D.E. Furst, A. Bharat, J.R. Curtis, A.F. Kavanaugh, J.M. Kremer, L.W. Moreland, et al., 2012 update of the 2008 American College of Rheumatology Recommendations for the use of disease-modifying antirheumatic drugs and biologic agents in the treatment of rheumatoid arthritis, Arthritis Care Res. 64 (5) (2012) 625–639, https://doi.org/10.1002/acr.21641.

[45] I. Tabas, C.K. Glass, Anti-inflammatory therapy in chronic disease: challenges and opportunities, Science (New York, N.Y.) 339 (6116) (2013) 166–172, https://doi.org/10.1126/science.1230720.

[46] T. Liu, F. Guo, X. Zhu, X. He, L. Xie, Thalidomide and its analogues: a review of the potential for immunomodulation of fibrosis diseases and Opthalmopathy (review), Exp. Therapeut. Med. 14 (1) (2017), https://doi.org/10.3892/etm.2017.5209.

[47] D. Millrine, T. Kishimoto, A brighter side to thalidomide: its potential use in immunological disorders, Trends Mol. Med. 23 (4) (2017) 348–361, https://doi.org/10.1016/j.molmed.2017.02.006.

[48] A.B. Beshir, G. Ren, A.N. Magpusao, L.M. Barone, K.C. Yeung, G. Fenteany, Raf kinase inhibitor protein suppresses nuclear factor-KB-dependent cancer cell invasion through negative regulation of matrix metalloproteinase expression, Cancer Lett. 299 (2) (2010) 137–149, https://doi.org/10.1016/j.canlet.2010.08.012.

[49] B. Ferger, A. Leng, A. Mura, B. Hengerer, J. Feldon, Genetic ablation of tumor necrosis factor-alpha (TNF-alpha) and pharmacological inhibition of TNF-synthesis attenuates MPTP toxicity in mouse striatum, J. Neurochem. 89 (4) (2004) 822–833, https://doi.org/10.1111/j.1471-4159.2004.02399.x.

[50] Q. Wang, X.-r. Zuo, Y.-y. Wang, W.-p. Xie, H. Wang, M. Zhang, Monocrotaline-induced pulmonary arterial hypertension is attenuated by TNF-α antagonists via the suppression of TNF-α expression and NF-KB pathway in rats, Vasc. Pharmacol. 58 (1–2) (2013) 71–77, https://doi.org/10.1016/j.vph.2012.07.006.

[51] L. Chen, H. Deng, H. Cui, J. Fang, Z. Zuo, J. Deng, Y. Li, X. Wang, L. Zhao, Inflammatory responses and inflammation-associated diseases in organs, Oncotarget 9 (6) (2017) 7204–7218, https://doi.org/10.18632/oncotarget.23208.

[52] P.L. Lin, H.L. Plessner, N.N. Voitenok, J.A.L. Flynn, Tumor necrosis factor and tuberculosis, J. Investig. Dermatol. Symp. Proc. 12 (1) (2007) 22–25, https://doi.org/10.1038/sj.jidsymp.5650027.

[53] F. Tubach, D. Salmon, P. Ravaud, Y. Allanore, P. Goupille, M. Bréban, B. Pallot-Prades, et al., Risk of tuberculosis is higher with anti-tumor necrosis factor monoclonal antibody therapy than with soluble tumor necrosis factor receptor therapy: the three-year prospective French research axed on tolerance of biotherapies registry, Arthritis Rheum. 60 (7) (2009) 1884–1894, https://doi.org/10.1002/art.24632.

[54] S. Bernatsky, C. Renoux, S. Suissa, Demyelinating events in rheumatoid arthritis after drug exposures, Ann. Rheum. Dis. 69 (9) (2010) 1691–1693, https://doi.org/10.1136/ard.2009.111500.

[55] E. Kaltsonoudis, P.V. Voulgari, S. Konitsiotis, A.A. Drosos, Demyelination and other neurological adverse events after anti-TNF therapy, Autoimmun. Rev. 13 (1) (2014) 54–58, https://doi.org/10.1016/j.autrev.2013.09.002.

[56] D. Pugliese, L. Guidi, P.M. Ferraro, M. Marzo, C. Felice, L. Celleno, R. Landi, et al., Paradoxical psoriasis in a large cohort of patients with inflammatory bowel disease receiving treatment with anti-TNF alpha: 5-year follow-up study, Aliment. Pharmacol. Ther. 42 (7) (2015) 880–888, https://doi.org/10.1111/apt.13352.

[57] D. Vassilopoulos, L.H. Calabrese, Management of rheumatic disease with comorbid HBV or HCV infection, Nat. Rev. Rheumatol. 8 (6) (2012) 348–357, https://doi.org/10.1038/nrrheum.2012.63.

[58] V. Baud, M. Karin, Signal transduction by tumor necrosis factor and its relatives, Trends Cell Biol. 11 (9) (2001) 372–377, https://doi.org/10.1016/s0962-8924(01)02064-5.

[59] A.C. Mackey, L. Green, C. Leptak, M. Avigan, Hepatosplenic T cell lymphoma associated with infliximab use in young patients treated for inflammatory bowel disease: update, J. Pediatr. Gastroenterol. Nutr. 48 (3) (2009) 386–388, https://doi.org/10.1097/mpg.0b013e3181957a11.

[60] L.D. Settas, G. Tsimirikas, G. Vosvotekas, E. Triantafyllidou, P. Nicolaides, Reactivation of pulmonary tuberculosis in a patient with rheumatoid arthritis during treatment with IL-1 receptor antagonists (anakinra), J. Clin. Rheumatol.: Pract. Rep. Rheum. Muscoloskel. Dis. 13 (4) (2007) 219–220, https://doi.org/10.1097/RHU.0b013e31812e00a1.

[61] I.P. de Barcelos, R.M. Troxell, J.S. Graves, Mitochondrial dysfunction and multiple sclerosis, Biology 8 (2) (2019), https://doi.org/10.3390/biology8020037.

[62] D.-H. Tsai, M. Riediker, A. Berchet, F. Paccaud, G. Waeber, P. Vollenweider, M. Bochud, Effects of short- and long-term exposures to particulate matter on inflammatory marker levels in the general population, Environ. Sci. Pollut. Res. Int. 26 (19) (2019) 19697–19704, https://doi.org/10.1007/s11356-019-05194-y.

[63] F. Pene, E. Courtine, A. Cariou, J.-P. Mira, Toward theragnostics, Crit. Care Med. 37 (1 Suppl) (2009) S50–S58, https://doi.org/10.1097/CCM.0b013e3181921349.

[64] S. Mura, P. Couvreur, Nanotheranostics for personalized medicine, Adv. Drug Deliv. Rev. 64 (13) (2012) 1394–1416, https://doi.org/10.1016/j.addr.2012.06.006.

[65] P. Rai, S. Mallidi, X. Zheng, R. Rahmanzadeh, Y. Mir, S. Elrington, A. Khurshid, T. Hasan, Development and applications of photo-triggered theranostic agents, Adv. Drug Deliv. Rev. 62 (11) (2010) 1094–1124, https://doi.org/10.1016/j.addr.2010.09.002.

[66] S.M. Janib, Imaging and drug delivery using theranostic nanoparticles, Adv. Drug Deliv. Rev. 62 (11) (2010) 1052–1053, https://doi.org/10.1016/j.addr.2010.08.004.

[67] E. Haglund, M.-M. Seale-Goldsmith, J.F. Leary, Design of multifunctional nanomedical systems, Ann. Biomed. Eng. 37 (10) (2009) 2048–2063, https://doi.org/10.1007/s10439-009-9640-2.

[68] F. Chen, E.B. Ehlerding, W. Cai, Theranostic nanoparticles, J. Nucl. Med.: Off. Publ. Soc. Nucl. Med. 55 (12) (2014) 1919–1922, https://doi.org/10.2967/jnumed.114.146019.

[69] M. Gorabi, N.K. Armita, Ž. Reiner, F. Carbone, F. Montecucco, A. Sahebkar, The therapeutic potential of nanoparticles to reduce inflammation in atherosclerosis, Biomol. Ther. 9 (9) (2019), https://doi.org/10.3390/biom9090416.

[70] D.N. Heo, K.H. Min, G.H. Choi, I.K. Kwon, K. Park, S.C. Lee, Chapter 24—Scale-up production of theranostic nanoparticles, in:

X. Chen, S. Wong (Eds.), Cancer Theranostics, Academic Press, Oxford, 2014, pp. 457–470, https://doi.org/10.1016/B978-0-12-407722-5.00024-4.

[71] K.Y. Win, S.-S. Feng, Effects of particle size and surface coating on cellular uptake of polymeric nanoparticles for Oral delivery of anticancer drugs, Biomaterials 26 (15) (2005) 2713–2722, https://doi.org/10.1016/j.biomaterials.2004.07.050.

[72] L. Zhao, S.-S. Feng, Enhanced oral bioavailability of paclitaxel formulated in vitamin E-TPGS emulsified nanoparticles of biodegradable polymers: in vitro and in vivo studies, J. Pharm. Sci. 99 (8) (2010) 3552–3560, https://doi.org/10.1002/jps.22113.

[73] S.D. Konda, M. Aref, S. Wang, M. Brechbiel, E.C. Wiener, Specific targeting of folate-dendrimer MRI contrast agents to the high affinity folate receptor expressed in ovarian tumor xenografts, Magma (New York, N.Y.) 12 (2–3) (2001) 104–113, https://doi.org/10.1007/BF02668091.

[74] D.A. Christian, S. Cai, D.M. Bowen, Y. Kim, J.D. Pajerowski, D.E. Discher, Polymersome carriers: from self-assembly to siRNA and protein therapeutics, Eur. J. Pharmaceut. Biopharmaceut.: Off. J. Arbeitsgemeinschaft Fur Pharmazeutische Verfahrenstechnik e. V. 71 (3) (2009) 463–474, https://doi.org/10.1016/j.ejpb.2008.09.025.

[75] M. Talelli, C.J.F. Rijcken, C.F. van Nostrum, G. Storm, W.E. Hennink, Micelles based on HPMA copolymers, Adv. Drug Deliv. Rev. 62 (2) (2010) 231–239, https://doi.org/10.1016/j.addr.2009.11.029.

[76] Z. Gao, A.M. Kennedy, D.A. Christensen, N.Y. Rapoport, Drug-loaded nano/microbubbles for combining ultrasonography and targeted chemotherapy, Ultrasonics 48 (4) (2008) 260–270, https://doi.org/10.1016/j.ultras.2007.11.002.

[77] S. Dhar, Z. Liu, J. Thomale, H. Dai, S.J. Lippard, Targeted single-wall carbon nanotube-mediated Pt(IV) prodrug delivery using folate as a homing device, J. Am. Chem. Soc. 130 (34) (2008) 11467–11476, https://doi.org/10.1021/ja803036e.

[78] J.T. Cole, N.B. Holland, Multifunctional nanoparticles for use in theranostic applications, Drug Delivery Transl. Res. 5 (3) (2015) 295–309, https://doi.org/10.1007/s13346-015-0218-2.

[79] Y. Malam, M. Loizidou, A.M. Seifalian, Liposomes and nanoparticles: nanosized vehicles for drug delivery in cancer, Trends Pharmacol. Sci. 30 (11) (2009) 592–599, https://doi.org/10.1016/j.tips.2009.08.004.

[80] C. Grange, S. Geninatti-Crich, G. Esposito, D. Alberti, L. Tei, B. Bussolati, S. Aime, G. Camussi, Combined delivery and magnetic resonance imaging of neural cell adhesion molecule-targeted doxorubicin-containing liposomes in experimentally induced Kaposi's sarcoma, Cancer Res. 70 (6) (2010) 2180–2190, https://doi.org/10.1158/0008-5472.CAN-09-2821.

[81] V.P. Torchilin, Recent advances with liposomes as pharmaceutical carriers, Nat. Rev. Drug Discov. 4 (2) (2005) 145–160, https://doi.org/10.1038/nrd1632.

[82] W.T. Al-Jamal, K. Kostarelos, Liposomes: from a clinically established drug delivery system to a nanoparticle platform for theranostic nanomedicine, Acc. Chem. Res. 44 (10) (2011) 1094–1104, https://doi.org/10.1021/ar200105p.

[83] M.S. Muthu, S.A. Kulkarni, J. Xiong, S.-S. Feng, Vitamin E TPGS coated liposomes enhanced cellular uptake and cytotoxity of docetaxel in brain cancer cells, Int. J. Pharm. 421 (2) (2011) 332–340, https://doi.org/10.1016/j.ijpharm.2011.09.045.

[84] T. Lammers, L.Y. Rizzo, G. Storm, F. Kiessling, Personalized nanomedicine, Clin. Cancer Res.: Off. J. Am. Assoc. Cancer Res. 18 (18) (2012) 4889–4894, https://doi.org/10.1158/1078-0432.CCR-12-1414.

[85] P.J. Gawne, F. Clarke, K. Turjeman, A.P. Cope, N.J. Long, Y. Barenholz, S.Y.A. Terry, R.T.M. de Rosales, PET imaging of liposomal glucocorticoids using 89Zr-Oxine: theranostic applications in inflammatory arthritis, Theranostics 10 (9) (2020) 3867–3879, https://doi.org/10.7150/thno.40403.

[86] E. Montes-Cobos, S. Ring, H.J. Fischer, J. Heck, J. Strauß, M. Schwaninger, S.D. Reichardt, C. Feldmann, F. Lühder, H.M. Reichardt, Targeted delivery of glucocorticoids to macrophages in a mouse model of multiple sclerosis using inorganic-organic hybrid nanoparticles, J. Controll. Release: Off. J. Controll. Release Soc. 245 (January) (2017) 157–169, https://doi.org/10.1016/j.jconrel.2016.12.003.

[87] J.M. Metselaar, M.H.M. Wauben, J.P.A. Wagenaar-Hilbers, O.C. Boerman, G. Storm, Complete remission of experimental arthritis by joint targeting of glucocorticoids with long-circulating liposomes, Arthritis Rheum. 48 (7) (2003) 2059–2066, https://doi.org/10.1002/art.11140.

[88] B. Rossi, S. Angiari, E. Zenaro, S.L. Budui, G. Constantin, Vascular inflammation in central nervous system diseases: adhesion receptors controlling leukocyte-endothelial interactions, J. Leukoc. Biol. 89 (4) (2011) 539–556, https://doi.org/10.1189/jlb.0710432.

[89] L.E.M. Paulis, I. Jacobs, N.M. van den Akker, T. Geelen, D.G. Molin, L.W.E. Starmans, K. Nicolay, G.J. Strijkers, Targeting of ICAM-1 on vascular endothelium under static and shear stress conditions using a liposomal Gd-based MRI contrast agent, J. Nanobiotechnol. 10 (June) (2012) 25, https://doi.org/10.1186/1477-3155-10-25.

[90] D. Danila, R. Partha, D.B. Elrod, S. Melinda Lackey, W. Casscells, J.L. Conyers, Antibody-labeled liposomes for CT imaging of atherosclerotic plaques, Tex. Heart Inst. J. 36 (5) (2009) 393–403.

[91] E. Abbasi, S. Aval, A. Akbarzadeh, M. Milani, H. Nasrabadi, S. Joo, Y. Hanifehpour, K. Nejati-Koshki, R. Pashaei-Asl, Dendrimers: synthesis, applications, and properties, Nanoscale Res. Lett. 9 (1) (2014) 247, https://doi.org/10.1186/1556-276X-9-247.

[92] S.-E. Stiriba, H. Frey, R. Haag, Dendritic polymers in biomedical applications: from potential to clinical use in diagnostics and therapy, Angew. Chem. (Int. Ed. Engl.) 41 (8) (2002) 1329–1334, https://doi.org/10.1002/1521-3773(20020415)41:8<1329::aid-anie1329>3.0.co;2-p.

[93] A.-M. Caminade, J.-P. Majoral, Which dendrimer to attain the desired properties? Focus on phosphorhydrazone dendrimers, Molecules (Basel, Switzerland) 23 (3) (2018) E622, https://doi.org/10.3390/molecules23030622.

[94] M.K. Bhalgat, J.C. Roberts, Molecular modeling of polyamidoamine (PAMAM) starburst™ dendrimers, Eur. Polym. J. 36 (3) (2000) 647–651, https://doi.org/10.1016/S0014-3057(99)00088-9.

[95] N. Martinho, H. Florindo, L. Silva, S. Brocchini, M. Zloh, T. Barata, Molecular modeling to study dendrimers for Biomedical applications, Molecules (Basel, Switzerland) 19 (12) (2014) 20424–20467, https://doi.org/10.3390/molecules191220424.

[96] S.M. Grayson, J.M. Fréchet, Convergent dendrons and dendrimers: from synthesis to applications, Chem. Rev. 101 (12) (2001) 3819–3868, https://doi.org/10.1021/cr990116h.

[97] L. Palmerston Mendes, J. Pan, V.P. Torchilin, Dendrimers as nanocarriers for nucleic acid and drug delivery in cancer therapy,

Molecules: J. Synth. Chem. Nat. Prod. Chem. 22 (9) (2017) 1401, https://doi.org/10.3390/molecules22091401.

[98] D.A. Tomalia, Birth of a new macromolecular architecture: dendrimers as quantized building blocks for nanoscale synthetic polymer chemistry, Prog. Polym. Sci. 30 (3–4) (2005) 294–324, https://doi.org/10.1016/j.progpolymsci.2005.01.007.

[99] Leiro, V., P. Garcia, H. Tomas, and A.P. Peg. n.d. "The present and the future of degradable dendrimers and derivatives in theranostics." Bioconjug. Chem., 16.

[100] J.A. Buckwalter, C. Saltzman, T. Brown, The impact of osteoarthritis: implications for research, Clin. Orthop. Relat. Res. 427 (Suppl (October)) (2004) S6–S15, https://doi.org/10.1097/01. blo.0000143938.30681.9d.

[101] B.C. Geiger, S. Wang, R.F. Padera, A.J. Grodzinsky, P.T. Hammond, Cartilage penetrating nanocarriers improve delivery and efficacy of growth factor treatment of osteoarthritis, Sci. Transl. Med. 10 (469) (2018) eaat8800, https://doi.org/10.1126/scitranslmed.aat8800.

[102] T. Rodríguez-Prieto, B. Hernández-Breijo, M.A. Ortega, R. Gómez, J. Sánchez-Nieves, L.G. Guijarro, Dendritic nanotheranostic for the delivery of infliximab: a potential carrier in rheumatoid arthritis therapy, Int. J. Mol. Sci. 21 (23) (2020) 9101, https://doi.org/10.3390/ijms21239101.

[103] E.S.L. Chan, B.N. Cronstein, Mechanisms of action of methotrexate, Bull. Hosp. Joint Disease 71 (Suppl. 1) (2013) S5–S8.

[104] B. Jekic, N. Maksimovic, T. Damnjanovic, Methotrexate pharmacogenetics in the treatment of rheumatoid arthritis, Pharmacogenomics 20 (17) (2019) 1235–1245, https://doi.org/10.2217/pgs-2019-0121.

[105] R. Qi, I. Majoros, A. Misra, A. Koch, P. Campbell, H. Marotte, I. Bergin, et al., Folate receptor-targeted dendrimer-methotrexate conjugate for inflammatory arthritis, J. Biomed. Nanotechnol. 11 (8) (2015) 1431–1441, https://doi.org/10.1166/jbn.2015.2077.

[106] P.K. Pandey, R. Maheshwari, N. Raval, P. Gondaliya, K. Kalia, R.K. Tekade, Nanogold-core multifunctional dendrimer for pulsatile chemo-, photothermal- and photodynamic- therapy of rheumatoid arthritis, J. Colloid Interface Sci. 544 (May) (2019) 61–77, https://doi.org/10.1016/j.jcis.2019.02.073.

[107] N. Ahmed, H. Fessi, A. Elaissari, Theranostic applications of nanoparticles in cancer, Drug Discov. Today 17 (17–18) (2012) 928–934, https://doi.org/10.1016/j.drudis.2012.03.010.

[108] S. Sadekar, A. Ray, M. Janàt-Amsbury, C.M. Peterson, H. Ghandehari, Comparative biodistribution of PAMAM dendrimers and HPMA copolymers in ovarian-tumor-bearing mice, Biomacromolecules 12 (1) (2011) 88–96, https://doi.org/10.1021/bm101046d.

[109] L.W. Seymour, D.R. Ferry, D.J. Kerr, D. Rea, M. Whitlock, R. Poyner, C. Boivin, et al., Phase II studies of polymer-doxorubicin (PK1, FCE28068) in the treatment of breast, lung and colorectal cancer, Int. J. Oncol. 34 (6) (2009) 1629–1636, https://doi.org/10.3892/ijo_00000293.

[110] A.-K. Heinrich, H. Lucas, L. Schindler, P. Chytil, T. Etrych, K. Mäder, T. Mueller, Improved tumor-specific drug accumulation by polymer therapeutics with PH-sensitive drug release overcomes chemotherapy resistance, Mol. Cancer Ther. 15 (5) (2016) 998–1007, https://doi.org/10.1158/1535-7163.MCT-15-0824.

[111] P. Mohan, N. Rapoport, Doxorubicin as a molecular nanotheranostic agent: effect of doxorubicin encapsulation in micelles or nanoemulsions on the ultrasound-mediated intracellular delivery and nuclear trafficking, Mol. Pharm. 7 (6) (2010) 1959–1973, https://doi.org/10.1021/mp100269f.

[112] N.S. Motlagh, P.P. Hosseini, F. Ghasemi, F. Atyabi, Fluorescence properties of several chemotherapy drugs: doxorubicin, paclitaxel and bleomycin, Biomed. Opt. Express 7 (6) (2016) 2400–2406, https://doi.org/10.1364/BOE.7.002400.

[113] C.-M.J. Hu, R.H. Fang, B.T. Luk, L. Zhang, Polymeric nanotherapeutics: clinical development and advances in stealth functionalization strategies, Nanoscale 6 (1) (2014) 65–75, https://doi.org/10.1039/c3nr05444f.

[114] L. Liu, H. Fanlei, H. Wang, W. Xiaoli, A.S. Eltahan, S. Stanford, N. Bottini, et al., Secreted protein acidic and rich in cysteine mediated biomimetic delivery of methotrexate by albumin-based nanomedicines for rheumatoid arthritis therapy, ACS Nano 13 (5) (2019) 5036–5048, https://doi.org/10.1021/acsnano.9b01710.

[115] J. Chen, J. Qi, C. Chen, J. Chen, L. Liu, R. Gao, T. Zhang, et al., Tocilizumab–conjugated polymer nanoparticles for NIR-II photoacoustic-imaging-guided therapy of rheumatoid arthritis, Adv. Mater. 32 (37) (2020) 2003399, https://doi.org/10.1002/adma.202003399.

[116] H. Park, J. Yang, J. Seo, K. Kim, J. Suh, D. Kim, S. Haam, K.-H. Yoo, Multifunctional nanoparticles for photothermally controlled drug delivery and magnetic resonance imaging enhancement, Small (Weinheim an Der Bergstrasse, Germany) 4 (2) (2008) 192–196, https://doi.org/10.1002/smll.200700807.

[117] S.A. Costa Lima, S. Reis, Temperature-responsive polymeric nanospheres containing methotrexate and gold nanoparticles: a multidrug system for theranostic in rheumatoid arthritis, Colloids Surf. B: Biointerfaces 133 (September) (2015) 378–387, https://doi.org/10.1016/j.colsurfb.2015.04.048.

[118] Q. Zhang, D. Li, J. Zhong, W. Yanglin, Y. Shi, H. Yang, L. Zhao, K. Yang, J. Lin, SPECT imaging and highly efficient therapy of rheumatoid arthritis based on hyperbranched semiconducting polymer nanoparticles, Biomater. Sci. 9 (5) (2021) 1845–1854, https://doi.org/10.1039/d0bm02037k.

[119] V. Kumar, A. Leekha, A. Tyagi, A. Kaul, A.K. Mishra, A.K. Verma, Preparation and evaluation of biopolymeric nanoparticles as drug delivery system in effective treatment of rheumatoid arthritis, Pharm. Res. 34 (3) (2017) 654–667, https://doi.org/10.1007/s11095-016-2094-y.

[120] A. Mostofizadeh, Y. Li, B. Song, Y. Huang, Synthesis, properties, and applications of low-dimensional carbon-related nanomaterials, J. Nanomater. 2011 (December) (2010) e685081, https://doi.org/10.1155/2011/685081.

[121] K. Bhattacharya, S.P. Mukherjee, A. Gallud, S.C. Burkert, S. Bistarelli, S. Bellucci, M. Bottini, A. Star, B. Fadeel, Biological interactions of carbon-based nanomaterials: from coronation to degradation, Nanomedicine 12 (2) (2016) 333–351, https://doi.org/10.1016/j.nano.2015.11.011.

[122] G. Hong, S. Diao, A.L. Antaris, H. Dai, Carbon nanomaterials for biological imaging and nanomedicinal therapy, Chem. Rev. 115 (19) (2015) 10816–10906, https://doi.org/10.1021/acs.chemrev.5b00008.

[123] A.M. Pinto, I.C. Gonçalves, F.D. Magalhães, Graphene-based materials biocompatibility: a review, Colloids Surf. B: Biointerfaces 111 (November) (2013) 188–202, https://doi.org/10.1016/j.colsurfb.2013.05.022.

[124] A. Eatemadi, H. Daraee, H. Karimkhanloo, M. Kouhi, N. Zarghami, A. Akbarzadeh, M. Abasi, Y. Hanifehpour, S.W. Joo, Carbon nanotubes: properties, synthesis, purification, and medical applications,

Nanoscale Res. Lett. 9 (1) (2014) 393, https://doi.org/10.1186/1556-276X-9-393.

[125] L. Golubewa, I. Timoshchenko, O. Romanov, R. Karpicz, T. Kulahava, D. Rutkauskas, M. Shuba, A. Dementjev, Y. Svirko, P. Kuzhir, Single-walled carbon nanotubes as a photo-thermo-acoustic cancer theranostic agent: theory and proof of the concept experiment, Sci. Rep. 10 (1) (2020) 22174, https://doi.org/10.1038/s41598-020-79238-6.

[126] N. Kuźnik, M.M. Tomczyk, Multiwalled carbon nanotube hybrids as MRI contrast agents, Beilstein J. Nanotechnol. 7 (July) (2016) 1086–1103, https://doi.org/10.3762/bjnano.7.102.

[127] A. Servant, I. Jacobs, C. Bussy, C. Fabbro, T. da Ros, E. Pach, B. Ballesteros, M. Prato, K. Nicolay, K. Kostarelos, Gadolinium-functionalised multi-walled carbon nanotubes as a T1 contrast agent for MRI cell labelling and tracking, Carbon Biomed. Appl. Carbon Nanomater. 97 (February) (2016) 126–133, https://doi.org/10.1016/j.carbon.2015.08.051.

[128] L.M. Kaminskas, B.D. Kelly, V.M. McLeod, G. Sberna, D.J. Owen, B.J. Boyd, C.J.H. Porter, Characterisation and tumour targeting of PEGylated polylysine dendrimers bearing doxorubicin via a PH labile linker, J. Controll. Release: Off. J. Controll. Release Soc. 152 (2) (2011) 241–248, https://doi.org/10.1016/j.jconrel.2011.02.005.

[129] C. Chen, L. Hou, H. Zhang, L. Zhu, H. Zhang, C. Zhang, J. Shi, L. Wang, X. Jia, Z. Zhang, Single-walled carbon nanotubes mediated targeted tamoxifen delivery system using Aspargine-glycine-arginine peptide, J. Drug Target. 21 (9) (2013) 809–821, https://doi.org/10.3109/1061186X.2013.829071.

[130] L. Hou, X. Yang, J. Ren, Y. Wang, H. Zhang, Q. Feng, Y. Shi, X. Shan, Y. Yuan, Z. Zhang, A novel redox-sensitive system based on single-walled carbon nanotubes for chemo-photothermal therapy and magnetic resonance imaging, Int. J. Nanomedicine 11 (1) (2016) 607–624, https://doi.org/10.2147/IJN.S98476.

[131] S. Han, T. Kwon, J.-E. Um, S. Haam, W.-J. Kim, Highly selective photothermal therapy by a phenoxylated-dextran-functionalized smart carbon nanotube platform, Adv. Healthc.

Mater. 5 (10) (2016) 1147–1156, https://doi.org/10.1002/adhm.201600015.

[132] H. Kosuge, S.P. Sherlock, T. Kitagawa, R. Dash, J.T. Robinson, H. Dai, M.V. McConnell, Near infrared imaging and photothermal ablation of vascular inflammation using single-walled carbon nanotubes, J. Am. Heart Assoc.: Cardiovasc. Cerebrovasc. Disease 1 (6) (2012), e002568, https://doi.org/10.1161/JAHA.112.002568.

[133] H. Lin, J. Huang, L. Ding, Preparation of carbon dots with high-fluorescence quantum yield and their application in dopamine fluorescence probe and cellular imaging, J. Nanomater. 2019 (1) (2019) 1–9, https://doi.org/10.1155/2019/5037243.

[134] J.C.G. Esteves da Silva, H.M.R. Gonçalves, Analytical and bioanalytical applications of carbon dots, TrAC Trends Anal. Chem. Clim. Change Impacts Water Chem. 30 (8) (2011) 1327–1336, https://doi.org/10.1016/j.trac.2011.04.009.

[135] K.O. Boakye-Yiadom, S. Kesse, Y. Opoku-Damoah, M.S. Filli, M. Aquib, M.M.B. Joelle, M.A. Farooq, et al., Carbon dots: applications in bioimaging and theranostics, Int. J. Pharm. 564 (June) (2019) 308–317, https://doi.org/10.1016/j.ijpharm.2019.04.055.

[136] C. Yang, R. Ogaki, L. Hansen, J. Kjems, B. Teo, Theranostic carbon dots derived from garlic with efficient anti-oxidative effect towards macrophages, RSC Adv. 5 (November) (2015), https://doi.org/10.1039/C5RA16874K.

[137] V. Bagalkot, L. Zhang, E. Levy-Nissenbaum, S. Jon, P.W. Kantoff, R. Langer, O.C. Farokhzad, Quantum dot-aptamer conjugates for synchronous cancer imaging, therapy, and sensing of drug delivery based on bi-fluorescence resonance energy transfer, Nano Lett. 7 (10) (2007) 3065–3070, https://doi.org/10.1021/nl071546n.

[138] B. Seruga, A. Ocana, I.F. Tannock, Drug resistance in metastatic castration-resistant prostate cancer, Nat. Rev. Clin. Oncol. 8 (1) (2011) 12–23, https://doi.org/10.1038/nrclinonc.2010.136.

[139] M. Johari-Ahar, J. Barar, A.M. Alizadeh, S. Davaran, Y. Omidi, M.-R. Rashidi, Methotrexate-conjugated quantum dots: synthesis, characterisation and cytotoxicity in drug resistant cancer cells, J. Drug Target. 24 (2) (2016) 120–133, https://doi.org/10.3109/1061186X.2015.1058801.

Chapter 15

Natural product-based antiinflammatory agents

Vimal Arora[a], Lata Rani[b], Ajmer Singh Grewal[c], and Harish Dureja[d]

[a]*University Institute of Pharma Sciences, Chandigarh University, Gharuan, India,* [b]*Chitkara University School of Pharmacy, Chitkara University, Baddi, Solan, Himachal Pradesh, India,* [c]*Guru Gobind Singh College of Pharmacy, Yamunanagar, Haryana, India,* [d]*Faculty of Pharmaceutical Sciences, Maharshi Dayanand University, Rohtak, Haryana, India*

1 Introduction

Inflammation is treated as one of the very important physiological phenomenon representing the series of events taking place during interaction of foreign matters, environment and/or any stimulus with body's defense mechanism. It can also be treated as the first signal initiation on the site of infection, representing the activation of response toward any invading foreign substance or a stimulus like itching, etc., as illustrated in Fig. 1. It is a natural immune response of the body against any injury, toxins, and pathogens. It can also be treated as the first step in the process of homeostasis (a body is returned to its original state) where antibodies and other fighter proteins (immunogens) inhabit to fight infectious diseases, stimulus/injury, and invade foreign substances [1]. Inflammation most of the time is associated with redness, swelling, warmth, and pain, which can range from mild to moderate levels [2]. On the other hand, if this state of inflammation is persistent, not treated in time (in a chronic state), or it starts affecting the infection site or host tissue, then it may lead to some other severe disorders called inflammatory disease like rheumatoid arthritis or even tissue damage. Generally, the inflammation is categorized as acute, subacute, and chronic with varying time of an inflammatory episode and the severity of the associated events like pain, swelling, and tissue damage, etc. [3], as illustrated in Fig. 2.

2 Etiology and pathophysiology of inflammation

Inflammation is generally observed in various pathological conditions such as mild infections, arthritis, cancer, autoimmune diseases, and organ transplant rejections. The inflammatory response is also accompanied with a variety of vascular events at the inflammation site, such as vasodilation and augmented vascular permeability [4]. The second important feature of inflammatory response is the porous endothelial barrier, i.e., at inflammation sites, proteins, tissue/intercellular fluid, and cells (leukocytes) diffuse out of the vasculature and accumulate in the interstitial space [5]. Moreover, during inflammation, specialized cells like mast cells, macrophages, mediators as well as plasma proteins accrue and play a very vital role in the process of tissue repair and regeneration; more specifically, the phagocytic action of macrophages is dominant, especially in the areas of wounds, infection, and injury [6,7]. The mechanism of inflammation and the series of events are shown in Fig. 3.

3 Treatment and its limitations

The two predominantly used treatments available for the management of inflammatory diseases are the drugs belonging to the class of corticosteroids and the Nonsteroidal antiinflammatory drugs (NSAIDs). The NSAIDS are further classified into various groups based on their chemical structure [8], as shown in Fig. 4. NSAIDs show antiinflammatory action by inhibiting enzymes, namely cyclooxygenase (COX) and lipoxygenase (LOX), which aids in the conversion of arachidonic acid to prostaglandins as illustrated in Fig. 5. Recently, it has been reported in one of the studies that the high concentrations of some of the conventional NSAIDs like diclofenac and indomethacin can induce apoptosis, especially in the synovial fibroblasts in the case of rheumatoid arthritis [9]. Different classes of NSAIDs have certain limitations or adverse effects, which restricts their frequent and prolonged use; some of them are discussed in the next section.

There are many adverse effects and/or complications associated with the long-term administration of NSAIDs such as gastrointestinal complications, renal impairment, and myocardial infarction, as described below.

Recent Developments in Anti-Inflammatory Therapy. https://doi.org/10.1016/B978-0-323-99988-5.00011-5

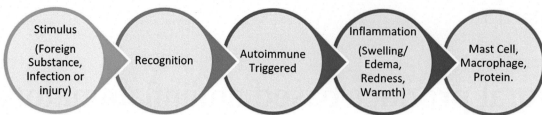

FIG. 1 Events in the process of inflammation.

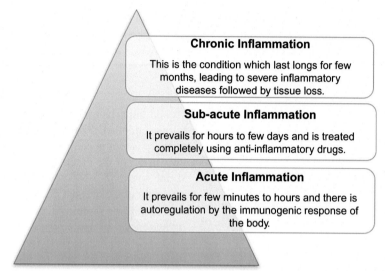

FIG. 2 Types of inflammation.

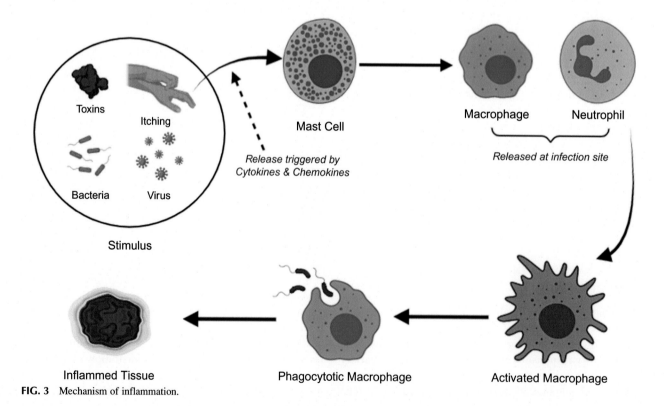

FIG. 3 Mechanism of inflammation.

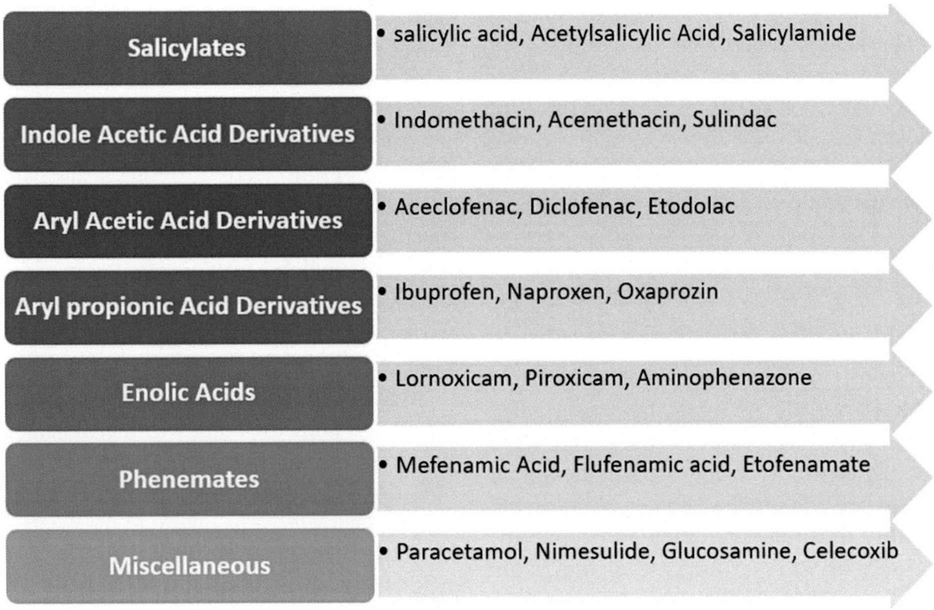

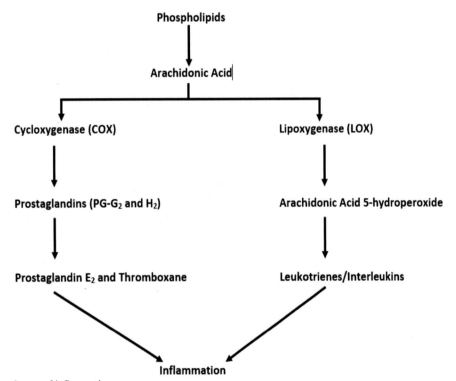

FIG. 4 Types of nonsteroidal antiinflammatory drugs (NSAIDs).

FIG. 5 Enzymatic pathways of inflammation.

3.1 Gastrointestinal complications

In various preclinical and clinical studies, it has been reported that the incidences of mild-to-severe gastrointestinal complications are normally observed in almost all the classes of NSAIDs [10]. The GIT complications are also reported to be associated with gastroduodenal ulcers, after a moderate time duration. Among these two different COX pathways, COX-2 has been reported to be present in the tissue comprising gastric ulcer in some experimental studies conducted in rats. As COX-2 is reported to be participating in the healing of ulcers, certain COX-2 inhibitors are administered for the treatment of ulcer and they in turn cause prolonged ulcer healing. It has also been suggested by some researchers that selective COX-2 inhibitors never lead to a significant reduction in the gastric complications as compared to other drugs used conventionally. On the other hand, in many of the research studies, it has also been reported that selective cyclooxygenase-2 inhibitors result in lowering the rate of gastric complications in comparison to NSAIDs [11,12].

3.2 Myocardial infarction and other thrombotic diseases

Research studies have revealed that the incidences of ischemic heart disease were elevated in the cases when COX-2 antiinflammatory drugs like celecoxib were used [13]. However, the incidence of thrombosis after treatment with such drugs have been reported a number of times and there is the possibility of thrombus formation or amplification of clotting may be there in the case of utilization of these drugs, as compared to the other conventional NSAIDs. In one of the studies, Whelton et al. reported that there is increase in blood pressure (systolic) in the case of aged patients especially suffering from osteoarthritis; and it is more commonly seen in patients treated with rofecoxib than those treated with celecoxib [14]. In 2004, Merck announced the withdrawal of rofecoxib because of increased incidences of myocardial infarction in a long-term clinical investigation, which was designed to investigate polyps' prevention. Therefore, the safety of selective COX-2 inhibitors, especially celecoxib along with some other commonly used NSAIDs, is debatable [8].

3.3 Renal impairment

In various clinical studies, it has been reported that the selective COX-2 inhibitor may cause impaired renal blood flow and accumulation of sodium. It has also been stated that the COX-2 enzyme is specifically expressed by certain renal cells and, therefore, it could be considered as a major factor leading to the state of renal impairment [15].

4 Natural products as antiinflammatory agents

There are a variety of drugs available to treat the state of inflammation or to provide a sort of symptomatic treatment, which commonly belongs to the class of either opioids or NSAIDs. Even though these two classes of drugs are being used from the past many decades around the globe, their use is restricted due to their associated side effects, and this led to a continuous approach to either discover new drug molecules or to explore various natural resources, especially plants, based up on the facts available in the traditional literature. The phytoconstituents are reported to be very

helpful in lowering the inflammation without any significant side effects [16,17].

According to the Indian traditional system of medicine, i.e., "Ayurveda," all the three doshas are involved in the process of development of inflammation; "Kapha" causes swelling, "Pitta" leads to redness and warmth (increased temperature at the site of infection/injury), whereas "Vata" lead to the initiation of pain on the site of inflammation. This system of medicine proposes its treatment via balanced diet (deprived of allergens) and natural medicines, majorly comprising of plants and minerals, based on the source of initiation of inflammation and associated symptoms [18].

Medicinal plants are the most frequently and abundantly explored natural resources in the management of various health conditions since ancient times. Another reason for exploring the plants is the diversity of plant types with varying characteristics owing to their varied chemical constituents, climatic conditions, etc. Furthermore, it is estimated that more than 1,50,000 species of plants have been explored till date; that resulted in the discovery of a good number of chemical constituents having remarkable therapeutic value. The field of plant sciences, in conjunction with various other novel technologies, has been in demand since the past few years; and there is a manifold increase in the number of scientists and researchers working in this field of drug discovery [19,20]. As per the traditional literature, the plants have an adaptation for tackling pathogens and environmental stress, due to which they either produce or release various biologically active chemicals, commonly belonging to the class of secondary metabolites [17,21].

Another name in the list of natural resources is marine resources. These are treated as a bio-diversified group of living organisms comprising of fish, crabs, coral reefs, and microorganisms found in big water bodies like seas and oceans. These resources are explored for their medicinal uses from time to time and it has been reported that many of the taxonomic groups like Arthropoda, Mollusca, Cnidaria, Porifera, Echinodermata, and various others are used in treatment of different ailments such as inflammation, cancer, microbial infections, hypertension, coagulation, etc. [3,22]. These marine resources are rich in biologically active natural products predominantly metabolites from the class of isoprenoid derivatives, especially sesterterpenes; a few examples from the group of sponges having analgesic and antiinflammatory potential [23] are given in Table 1.

Another active source of providing bioactive compounds is animal-based food that can offer a wide variety of micronutrients that are otherwise not provided adequately by the plant source foods alone. Animal-based materials and their metabolites have been explored extensively for their medicinal potential and even few are used traditionally for the treatment number of ailments in various parts of the globe. One of the biggest evidence of such utilizations is "zootherapy" which is being practiced exhaustively in

TABLE 1 Sponges with antiinflammatory activity.

S. no.	Source	Chemical compound	Activity	Reference
	Luffariella variabilis	Monalide and variabilins	Inhibition of phospholipase A_2	[24]
	Ircinia campana	Terpenoids	Inhibition of phospholipase A_2	[25]
	Callyspongia siphonella	Callysterol	Inhibits of release of superoxide anion and thromboxane B2	[26]
	Theonella swinhoei	Solomonsterol-A	Reduces the expression of IL-17, TNFα, IFNγ, and MIP1α (chemokine)	[27]
	Spongia officinalis	Spongidines A–D	Inhibition of phospholipase A_2	[3]
	Axinella Sps	Cycloamphilectene-2	Inhibits the NFκB pathway	[3]

almost all parts of the world [24]. In Chhattisgarh, India, more than 500 species of spiders, insects, and mites are reported to be utilized for the management of number of common and complicated ailments. In one of the studies, it has been reported that melittin (tetrameric polypeptide), one of the major constituents of bee venom, has shown antiinflammatory and antiarthritic potential [28]. From ancient times, leeches are being used in the treatment of conditions like inflammatory abscess, skin diseases, blood infections, rheumatoid arthritis, and poisonous bites [3].

It is a well-known fact that inflammation is considered a very useful process of immunogenic response of the body for its protection and survival against the pathogens or other invading foreign substances. It is defined as the complex sequence of changes or biological responses taking place in any tissue to eradicate the cause of infection at the site of injury; occurring due to either infectious agents or their metabolites, i.e., either the microorganisms or their toxins, and other physical, chemical, or biological agents such as radiation, trauma, and burn. Inflammation is a process of complex biological response leading to tissue repair and regeneration or is simply called homeostasis. The process of inflammation is induced and propagated through inflammatory mediators namely cytokines and chemokines. However, the continuous release of these inflammatory mediators along with the activation of pathways of signal transduction in turn leads to different levels of inflammation (mild to chronic) [29].

The capability of plants to produce secondary metabolites with clinically proven therapeutic effects makes them the most reliable resource for exploring new opportunities in combating and successful treatment of the inflammatory disorders [30,31]. Another advantage of using plant-derived drugs is their capability to interact with the microbiome of the gut. Certain bacteria present in the GIT cause intensive metabolism of the drug molecules and convert them a to

low-molecular-mass metabolites, which are highly bioavailable, and significantly bioactive, and thus can be used successfully in the treatment various metabolic disorders [32]. Some of the widely explored plants for their antiinflammatory potential are cited in Table 2.

4.1 Plant extracts

In the investigation of the biological potential of any plant part, the extraction is the first key step, presenting numerous advantages in comparison to the isolation of an active compound [33]. The use of the extracted fraction has an advantage that it may exhibit synergism between two or more active components, which might get lost during the process of their isolation. On the other hand, the availability or the mixing of various active components together may exhibit an inhibitory effect; for instance, one component or constituent may lower or antagonize the biological potential of another. Some studies revealed that the antiinflammatory potential of some isolated constituents like pseudohypericin, amentoflavone, and hyperforin has shown better results as compared to the extracts of the plants containing these active constituents [33–35].

4.2 Phytoconstituents as antiinflammatory agents

A diverse variety of secondary metabolites is also present in plants; most of them do not seem to contribute directly for plant growth and development. Phytoconstituents are active secondary metabolites, which occur naturally in the plants; but, they do not have essential nutrient value. They are accountable for the defensive mechanism of plants in contrast to infections, invasions, or predation by microorganisms, insects, germs, or predators [36,37]. Many of

TABLE 2 Plants explored for their antiinflammatory activity.

S. no.	Botanical name	Family	Common name (Hindi)	Plant part(s) used	Chemical constituents
01	*Acacia catechu*	Mimosaceae	Khair	Bark, wood, flowering tops, gum	Catechuic acid, gum, tannin
02	*Azadirachta indica*	Meliaceae	Neem	Leaf, root, oil, seed, gum, fruit, flower	Azadirachtin, margosine, bitter oil
03	*Caesalpinia crista*	Caesalpiniaceae	Kantkarej	Seeds, root, leaf, root bark	Oleic acid, linoleic acid, palmitic acid, stearic acid, phytosterols
04	*Cassia angustifolia*	Caeasalpinaceae	Sanaya	Pods, dried leaves	Emodin, eatharitin, senna-picrin, mucilage, opleanic acid
05	*Coriandrum sativum*	Umbelliferaeapiaceae	Dhaniya	Leaf, bark, flower	Cathartin, malic acid, albuminoids, Tannin
06	*Curcuma longa*	Zingiberaceae	Haldi	Rhizome	Curcumin
07	*Cuscuta reflexa*	Convolvulaceae	Amar Bel	Plant, seed, fruit, stem	Cuscutine, bergenin, coumarin, glucoside, flavonoids
08	*Enicostema littorale*	Gentianaceae	Chhota Chirayat	Whole plant	Alkaloids, gentiocrucine
09	*Euphorbia tirucalli*	Euphorbiaceae	Charmkasha	Root, plant (milk, juice)	β-Sitosterol, malic acid, ellagic acid, citric acid, eupholglucose
10	*Fagonia cretica*	Zygophyllaceae	Dhamasa	Leaves, twigs, bark	Betulin
11	*Ficus carica*	Moraceae	Anjeer	Fruit, root	β-Carotene, lutein, Alkaloids, caffeic acid, linoleic acid, pantothenic acid, β-amyrin
12	*Ficus religiosa*	Moraceae	Peepal	Bark, leaves, fruits, tender shoots, seeds	Tannins, rubber, wax
13	*Foeniculum vulgare*	Apiaceae	Saunf	Fruit, root, seeds, leaves	Estragole, coumaric acid, caffeic acid, α-terpinene, scoparone, scopoletin, cynarin, D-limonene, α-phellandrene
14	*Gaultheria fragrantissima*	Ericaceae	Gandhpura	Leaves and fruits	Ursolic acid, methyl salicylate, β-sitosterol
15	*Gentiana kuroo*	Gentianaceae	Chireta	Rhizomes (roots)	Gentiopicrine, gentianic acid
16	*Gloriosa superba*	Liliaceae	Bachnag	Rhizome, tuber, leaves, flower	Choline, colchicine, stigmasterol, salicylic acid, 2-methylcolchicine
17	*Glycyrrhiza glabra*	Papilionaceae	Mulethi	Roots, leaves	Genistein, eugenol, bergapten, glycyrrhizin, acetophenone, estragole, apigenin, anethole
18	*Gmelina arborea*	Verbenaceae	Gamhar	Whole plant	Betulin

TABLE 2 Plants explored for their antiinflammatory activity—cont'd

S. no.	Botanical name	Family	Common name (Hindi)	Plant part(s) used	Chemical constituents
19	*Grewia asiatica*	Tiliaceae	Phalsa	Leaves, roots, fruits, bark	Betulin
20	*Hibiscus rosa-Sinensis*	Malvaceae	Gurhal	Buds, roots, leaves, flower	Quercetin
21	*Martynia annua*	Pedaliaceae	Ulat Kanta	Fruits, leaves	Pelargonidin-3,5-diglucoside, cyanidin-3-galactosidel
22	*Momordica charantia*	Cucurbitaceae	Karela	Whole plant	5-Hydroxytryptamine, ascorbic acid, β-carotene, cholesterol, lutein, diosgenin, lanosterol, lycopene, momordicin, charantin, momordicoside, and alkaloids
23	*Moringa oleifera*	Moringaceae	Senjana	Roots, bark, leaves, seeds	Choline, moringinine, myristic, ascorbic acid, β-carotene, niacin, oleic acid, spirochin, stearic acid, tocopherol, vanillin
24	*Nelumbo nucifera*	Nymphaeaceae	Kamal	Whole plant	Anonaine, ascorbic acid, β-carotene, copper, erucic acid, glutathione, hyperoside, myristic acid, nuciferine, oxoushinsunine, rutin, stearic acid, trigonelline, kaempferol, D-catechin
25	*Nicotiana tobacum*	Solanaceae	Tambaku	Leaves	1,8-Cineole, 4-vinylguaiacol, acetaldehyde, acetophenone, alkaloids, anabasine, nicotinic acid, nicotine, scopoletin, quercitrin, sorbitol, tocopherol stigmasterol, trigonelline
26	*Nigella sativa*	Ranunculaceae	Kalonji	Seeds	α-Spinasterol, ascorbic acid, β-sitosterol, carvone, D-limonene, linoleic acid, myristic acid, methionine, nigellone, stearic acid, stigmasterol, tannin, thymoquinone, hederagenin
27	*Ocimum basilicum*	Laminaceae	Tulsi	Whole plant	Acetic acid, aspartic acid, apigenin, arginine
28	*Plumbago zeylanica*	Plumbaginaceae	Chitrak	Root, leaves, root, bark	Plumbagin, droserone, 3-chloroplumbagin, chitranone, zeylinone, elliptione, isozeylinone
29	*Portulaca oleraceae*	Portulaceae	Nonia	Stem, leaves, seeds	Oleracins I and II, acylated betacyanins, carbohydrate, galacturonic acid, mucilage
30	*Pterocarpus marsupium*	Fabaceae	Vijayasar	leaves, flower, gum Heartwood	Alkaloids, gum, essential oil, semi-drying fixed oil
31	*Solanum melongena*	Solanaceae	Baingan	Roots, leaves, tender fruits	Ascorbic acid, alanine, arginine, caffeic acid
32	*Solanum nigrum*	Solanaceae	Makoi	Whole plant	Solenin, solasodine
33	*Stereopermum suaveolens*	Bignoniaceae	Patala	Roots, flower	Lapachol, dehydrotectol, β-sitosterol, n-triacontanol

Continued

TABLE 2 Plants explored for their antiinflammatory activity—cont'd

S. no.	Botanical name	Family	Common name (Hindi)	Plant part(s) used	Chemical constituents
34	*Tephrosia purpurea*	Fabaceae	Sarpanka	Whole plant	Tephrosin, betulinic acid, lupeol, rutin
35	*Terminalia chebula*	Combretaceae	Harad	Mature, immature fruits	Gallic acid, ellagic acid, chebulic acid
36	*Thespesia populneoides*	Malvaceae	Paras-pipal	Whole plant	Populneol, gossypol, kaempferol, quercetin-5-glucoside, calycopterin, kaempferol-5-glucoside, kaempferol-3-gluoside
37	*Vernonia cinerea*	Asteraceae	Sahadevi	Whole plant	Linoleic acid, lupeol, vernolic acid

them are accountable for the shade, odor, and additional organoleptic characteristics. It has been documented that since prehistoric era, the herbs, herbal medicinal products or simply phytotherapeutic agents, are being used successfully because of their minimum or insignificant side effects [38–40]. Phytoconstituents reported with potential antiinflammatory activity can be classified as alkaloids, phenolic compounds, terpenoids, steroids, polysaccharides, peptides, lectins, fatty acids, and miscellaneous compounds, illustrated in Fig. 6.

4.2.1 Alkaloids

Alkaloids are the basic nitrogen-containing compounds and epitomize the major solitary class of secondary metabolites. They generally possess an outstanding variety of pharmacotherapeutic effects and are frequently poisonous to humans too [41]. A broad variety of pharmacological actions were documented for alkaloids, comprising vomitive, anticancer, parasympatholytic, diuretic, cholinomimetic, antiviral, hypotensive, pain relieving, antidepressant, muscle-tranquilizing, antitussive, antibacterial, and antiinflammatory action [42]. Plants from the *Berberis* genus are employed as conventional therapy for the treatment of numerous inflammation-related ailments [43]. The most significant families of plants possessing alkaloids accountable for inflammation reducing properties consist of *Liliaceae, Lamiaceae, Lauraceae, Aristolochiaceae, Apocynaceae, Ranunculaceae, Malvaceae, Monimiaceae, Rutaceae, Solanaceae, Leguminosae, Menispermaceae, Piperaceae, Berberidaccae, Loganiaceae, Simaroubaceae, Ephedraceae, Annonaceae, Papaveraceae,* and Brassicaceae [44]. Quinoline, isoquinoline, and indole derivatives were the utmost investigated alkaloids for inflammation-reducing effects [39]. Some of the most

important alkaloids reported with potential antiinflammatory activity are presented in Table 3.

4.2.2 Flavonoids and other phenolic compounds

Phenolic compounds are a heterogeneous cluster of phytoconstituents comprising aromatic rings having at least one hydroxyl functional group and are universally found in most plant tissues, like vegetables, fruits, cereals, roots, and leaves [90]. These are a diversified group of secondary metabolites, synthesized by the shikimic acid and phenylpropanoid pathways. These compounds are usually associated with defense responses in plants [91]. However, phenolic compounds show a significant role in more operations, such as integrating striking compounds to quicken cross-pollination, shading for disguise and protection from herbivore animals, in addition to bactericidal and fungicidal effects [92]. Phenolic compounds comprise flavonoids (including flavanols, flavonols, flavones, flavanones, isoflavones, and anthocyanidins), phenolic acids, tannins, anthocyanins, stilbenes, xanthines, lignans, and coumarins [93]. Phenolic compounds were of growing curiosity to scientists and food chemists owing to their advantageous effects on human health in the past decade. Epidemiology studies had correlated excessive consumption of phenolic compound-rich diet with decline in the proportion of long-lasting ailments including cardiovascular disorders, neuromuscular disorders (Alzheimer's and Parkinson's disease), metabolic syndrome, and inflammatory diseases [93,94]. Phenolic derivatives are the most popular in regular human diets among the dietary antioxidants. Some of them have exhibited antiinflammatory properties [95]. Some of the important phenolic compounds reported with potential antiinflammatory activity in vivo and/or in vitro are listed in Table 4.

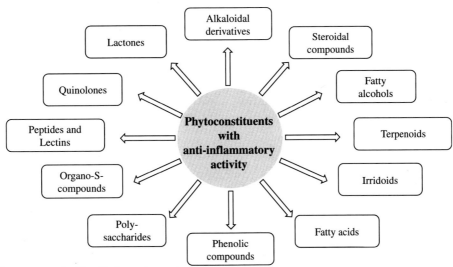

FIG. 6 Phytoconstituents reported with antiinflammatory potential.

TABLE 3 Alkaloids with antiinflammatory potential.

Compound	Chemical structure	Source	Reference
Ailanthamide		*Zanthoxylum ailanthoides* (Rutaceae)	[45]
Akuammigine (pseudo)		*Picralima nitida* (Apocynaceae)	[46]
Aristolochic acid		*Aristolochia kaempferi* (Aristolochiaceae)	[47]
Berbamine		*Berberis crataegina* (Berberidaceae)	[48]

Continued

TABLE 3 Alkaloids with antiinflammatory potential—cont'd

Compound	Chemical structure	Source	Reference
Berberine		*Berberis crataegina* (Berberidaceae), *Rhizoma coptidis* (Ranunculaceae)	[49]
Boldine		*Peumus boldus* (Monimiaceae)	[50]
Brucine		*Strychnos nux-vomica* (Loganiaceae)	[51]
Brucine-*N*-oxide		*Caulerpa racemosa* (Caulerpaceae)	[51]
β-Carboline		*Picrasma quassioides* (Simaroubaceae)	[52]
Caulerpin		*Caulerpa racemosa* (Caulerpaceae)	[53]

TABLE 3 Alkaloids with antiinflammatory potential—cont'd

Compound	Chemical structure	Source	Reference
Colchicine		*Colchcum autumnale* (Colchicaceae)	[54]
Columbamine		*Berberis crataegina* (Berberidaceae)	[48]
Decarine		*Chrysophyllum albidum* (Sapotaceae)	[45]
Dehydroevodiamine		*Evodia fructus* (Rutaceae)	[55]
7'-(3',4'-Dihydroxy-phenyl)-N-[(4-methoxyphenyl) ethyl] propenamide		*Fissistigma oldhamii* (Annonaceae)	[56]
Eleagnine		*Chrysophyllum albidum* (Sapotaceae)	[57]
Ephedrine		*Ephedra sinica* (Ephedraceae)	[58]

Continued

TABLE 3 Alkaloids with antiinflammatory potential—cont'd

Compound	Chemical structure	Source	Reference
13-Ethylberberine		*Berberis vulgaris* (Berberidaccae)	[59]
Evodiamine		*Evodia rutaecarpa* (Rutaceae)	[60]
Evolitrine		*Euodia lunuankenda* (Rutaceae)	[61]
Fangochinoline		*Stephania tetrandrae* (Menispermaceae)	[62]
Guanidine diisopentenyl		*Alchornea cordifolia* (Euphorbiaceae)	[63]
Guanidine triisopentenyl		*Alchornea cordifolia* (Euphorbiaceae)	[63]
Hederacine A		*Glechoma hederaceae* (Lamiaceae)	[64]

TABLE 3 Alkaloids with antiinflammatory potential—cont'd

Compound	Chemical structure	Source	Reference
Hederacine B		*Glechoma hederaceae* (Lamiaceae)	[64]
Indigo		*Indigofera tinctoria* (Fabaceae)	[65]
Indirubin		*Indigofera tinctoria* (Fabaceae)	[65]
Indole-3-carbinol		*Brassica oleracea* (Brassicaceae)	[66]
N-Isobutyl-6-oxohepta-2,4-dienamide		*Zanthoxylum ailanthoides* (Rutaceae)	[45]
Laurotetanine		*Litsea cubeba* (Lauraceae)	[67]
Ligustrazine		*Ligusticum chuanxiong* (Apiaceae)	[68]
Magnoflorine		*Berberis crataegina* (Berberidaccae)	[48]

Continued

TABLE 3 Alkaloids with antiinflammatory potential—cont'd

Compound	Chemical structure	Source	Reference
Matrine		*Sophora subprostrata* (Fabaceae)	[69]
11-Methoxy henningsamine		*Strychnos cathayensis* (Loganiaceae)	[70]
13-Methylberberine		*Berberis vulgaris* (Berberidaccae)	[71]
Norisoboldine		*Radix linderae* (Lauraceae)	[72]
Oxyacanthine		*Berberis crataegina* (Berberidaceae)	[48]
Palmatine		*Berberis crataegina* (Berberidaccae)	[48]

TABLE 3 Alkaloids with antiinflammatory potential—cont'd

Compound	Chemical structure	Source	Reference
Persicaside		*Prunus persica* (Rosaceae)	[73]
Picrinine		*Alstonia scholaris* (Apocynaceae)	[74]
Piperine		*Piper* spp. (Piperaceae)	[75]
Piperlactam S		*Piper betle* (Piperaceae)	[76]
Quinine		*Cinchona* spp. (Rubiaceae)	[77]
Riparin I		*Aniba riparia* (Lauraceae)	[78]
Riparin II		*Aniba riparia* (Lauraceae)	[79]
Rutaecarpine		*Evodia rutaecarpa* (Rutaceae)	[60]

Continued

TABLE 3 Alkaloids with antiinflammatory potential—cont'd

Compound	Chemical structure	Source	Reference
Scholaricine		*Alstonia scholaris* (Apocynaceae)	[72]
Sinomenine		*Sinomenium acutum* (Menispermaceae)	[80]
Skimmianine		*Decatropis bicolor* (Rutaceae)	[81]
Strychnine		*Strychnus nux-vomica* (Loganiaceae)	[82]
Swatinine		*Aconitum leave* (Ranunculaceae)	[82]
Terandrine		*Stephania tetrandra* (Menispermaceae)	[83]
Theacrine		*Camellia sinensis* (Theaceae)	[84]

TABLE 3 Alkaloids with antiinflammatory potential—cont'd

Compound	Chemical structure	Source	Reference
Toddaliopsin A		*Toddaliopsis bremekampii* (Rutaceae)	[85]
Toddaliopsin B		*Toddaliopsis bremekampii* (Rutaceae)	[85]
Toddaliopsin C		*Toddaliopsis bremekampii* (Rutaceae)	[85]
Toddaliopsin D		*Toddaliopsis bremekampii* (Rutaceae)	[85]
Tryptanthrin		*Isatis tinctoria* (Brassicaceae)	[86]
Tylophorine		*Tylophora asthamatica* (Apocynaceae)	[87]
Vallesamine		*Alstonia scholaris* (Apocynaceae)	[74]

Continued

TABLE 3 Alkaloids with antiinflammatory potential—cont'd

Compound	Chemical structure	Source	Reference
Vasicine		*Sida cordifolia* (Malvaceae)	[88]
Warifteine		*Cissampelos sympodialis* (Menispermaceae)	[89]

TABLE 4 Flavonoids and other phenolic compounds with antiinflammatory activity.

Compound	Chemical structure	Source	Reference
(−)-Bornyl caffeate		*Verbenisa turbacensis* (Verbenaceae)	[96]
3-Hydroxy-anthranilic acid		*Hibiscus tilliaceus* (Malvaceae)	[97]
3-Methyl kaempferol		*Zingiber zerumbet* (Zingiberaceae)	[98]
5-Demethyl-nobiletin		*Sideretis tragoriganum* (Lamiaceae)	[99]
Aciculatin		*Chrysopogon aciculatis* (Poaceae)	[100]
Aiphanol		*Aiphanes aculeata* (Arecaceae)	[101]

TABLE 4 Flavonoids and other phenolic compounds with antiinflammatory activity—cont'd

Compound	Chemical structure	Source	Reference
Anthocyanin		*Colocasia esculenta* (Araceae)	[102]
Apigenin		*Justicia gendarussa* (Acanthaceae)	[103]
Arctigenin		*Trachelospermum jasminoides* (Apocynaceae)	[104]
Artocarpesin		*Artocarpus heterophyllus* (Moraceae)	[105]
Atroviridine		*Garcinia atroviridis* (Clusiaceae)	[106]
Axillarin		*Artemisia copa* (Asteraceae)	[107]
Caffeic acid		*Sambucus ebulus* (Caprifoliaceae)	[108]
Calanolide		*Calophyllum teysmanii* (Calophyllaceae)	[109]
Canniprene		*Cannabis sativa* (Cannabinaceae)	[110]
Capillarisin		*Artemisia capillaris* (Asteraceae)	[111]

Continued

TABLE 4 Flavonoids and other phenolic compounds with antiinflammatory activity—cont'd

Compound	Chemical structure	Source	Reference
Capsaicin		*Capsicum annuum* (Solanaceae)	[112]
Catechin		*Camellia sinensis* (Theaceae)	[113]
Chrysoeriol		*Artemisia copa* (Asteraceae)	[107]
Coumaric acid		*Cynodon dactylon* (Poaceae)	[36]
Curcumin		*Curcuma longa* (Zingiberaceae)	[87]
Cyanidin		*Robus plicatus* (Rosaceae)	[114]
Daidzein		*Glycine max* (Fabaceae)	[115]
Delphinidin		*Vitis labrusca* (Vitaceae)	[116]
Desoxy-rhapontigenin		*Rheum undulatum* (Polygonaceae)	[117]
Ent-Gallocatechin 4'-methyl ether		*Atuna racemose* (Chrysobalanaceae)	[118]

TABLE 4 Flavonoids and other phenolic compounds with antiinflammatory activity—cont'd

Compound	Chemical structure	Source	Reference
Epigallocatechin-3-gallate		*Camellia sinensis* (Theaceae)	[119]
Eupalitin-3-glucoside		*Tephrosia spinosa* (Leguminosae)	[120]
Ferulic acid		*Lolium multiflorum* (Poaceae)	[121]
Flavone velutin		*Euterpe oleracea* Mart (Arecaceae)	[122]
Forsythoside A		*Fructus forsythia* (Oleaceae)	[123]
Gallic acid		*Terminalia chebula* (Combretaceae)	[124]
Gallocatechin		*Eugenia brasiliensis* (Myrtaceae)	[125]

Continued

TABLE 4 Flavonoids and other phenolic compounds with antiinflammatory activity—cont'd

Compound	Chemical structure	Source	Reference
Genistein		*Glycine max* (Fabaceae)	[115]
Gigantol		*Cymbidium goeringii* (Orchidaceae)	[126]
Hesperetin		*Cordia sebestena* (Boraginaceae)	[127]
Hypericin		*Hypericum perforatum* (Hypericaceae)	[128]
Isorhapontigenin		*Aiphanes aculeata* (Arecaceae)	[101]
Jaceosidin		*Artemisia copa* (Asteraceae)	[107]
Kaempferol		*Andrographis paniculata* (Acanthaceae)	[115]
Kuwanon C		*Morus alba* (Moraceae)	[129]

TABLE 4 Flavonoids and other phenolic compounds with antiinflammatory activity—cont'd

Compound	Chemical structure	Source	Reference
Lapachol		*Handroanthus impetiginosus* (Bignoniaceae)	[130]
Luteolin		*Apium graveolens* (Apiaceae)	[131]
Malvidin		*Vaccinium ashei* (Ericaceae)	[132]
Monodesmoside		*Kalopanax pictus* (Araliaceae)	[133]
Morin		*Maclura pomifera* (Moraceae)	[44]
Morusin		*Morus alba* (Moraceae)	[129]
Myricetin		*Myrica rubra* (Myricaceae)	[134]
Myricetin glucuronide		*Epilobium angustifolium* (Onagraceae)	[135]

Continued

TABLE 4 Flavonoids and other phenolic compounds with antiinflammatory activity—cont'd

Compound	Chemical structure	Source	Reference
Naringenin		*Citrus maxima* (Rutaceae)	[115]
Narirutin		*Citrus unshiu* (Rutaceae)	[136]
Niranthin		*Phyllanthus amarus* (Euphorbiaceae)	[137]
Nirtetralin		*Phyllanthus amarus* (Euphorbiaceae)	[137]
Ochnaflavone		*Lonicera japonica* (Caprifoliaceae)	[138]
Olivetol		*Cannabis sativa* (Cannabinaceae)	[139]
Olivetolic acid		*Cannabis sativa* (Cannabinaceae)	[110]

TABLE 4 Flavonoids and other phenolic compounds with antiinflammatory activity—cont'd

Compound	Chemical structure	Source	Reference
Oroxylin A		*Scutellaria baicalensis* (Lamiaceae)	[140]
Ouratea-catechin		*Vantanea peruviana* (Humiriaceae)	[118]
Oxy-resveratrol		*Artocarpus heterophyllus* (Moraceae)	[105]
Pelargonidin		*Ficus benghalensis* (Moraceae)	[115]
Penduletin		*Artemisia copa* (Asteraceae)	[107]
Phyllanthin		*Phyllanthus amarus* (Euphorbiaceae)	[137]
Phyltetralin		*Phyllanthus amarus* (Euphorbiaceae)	[137]
Pinosylvin		*Hovenia dulcis* (Rhamnaceae)	[141]

Continued

TABLE 4 Flavonoids and other phenolic compounds with antiinflammatory activity—cont'd

Compound	Chemical structure	Source	Reference
Polyzellin		*Polyozellus multiplex* (Thelephoraceae)	[142]
Proanthocynidin A		*Vantanea peruviana* (Humiriaceae)	[118]
Protocatechuic acid		*Hibiscus sabdariffa* (Malvaceae)	[143]
Quercetin		*Drosera madagascariensis* (Droseraceae)	[144]
Resveratrol		*Polygonum cuspidatum* (Polygonaceae)	[145]
Robustaflavone		*Selaginella tamariscina* (Selaginellaceae)	[146]
Rosmarinic acid		*Rosmarinus officinalis* (Lamiaceae)	[147]

TABLE 4 Flavonoids and other phenolic compounds with antiinflammatory activity—cont'd

Compound	Chemical structure	Source	Reference
Salicin		*Salix alba* (Salicaceae)	[148]
Scopoletin		*Artemisia feddei* (Asteraceae)	[149]
Secoisolariciresinol		*Linum usitatissimum* (Linaceae)	[150]
Spinacetin		*Artemisia copa* (Asteraceae)	[115]
Sumantoflavone		*Selaginella tamariscina* (Selaginellaceae)	[146]
Taxifolin		*Larix gmelinii* (Pinaceae)	[151]
Tectoridin		*Belamcanda chinensis* (Iridaceae)	[152]
Tectorigenin		*Belamcanda chinensis* (Iridaceae)	[152]
Tricin		*Artemisia copa* (Asteraceae)	[107]

Continued

TABLE 4 Flavonoids and other phenolic compounds with antiinflammatory activity—cont'd

Compound	Chemical structure	Source	Reference
Wogonin		*Scutellaria baicalensis* (Lamiaceae)	[132]
Yakuchinone A		*Zingiber officinale* (Zingiberaceae)	[153]

4.2.3 Terpenoids

Terpenoids (or isoprenoids) are a huge and assorted group of naturally distributed organic compounds derived from isoprene (a 5-C moiety), and the polymers of isoprene are known as terpenes. Even though occasionally used conversely with "terpenes," "terpenoids" consist of added functional moieties, generally containing oxygen. Terpenoids can be categorized into hemiterpenes, monoterpenes, sesqui-terpenes, diterpenes, sesterpenes, tri-terpenes, and tetra-terpenoids (or carotenoids) containing one, two, three, four, five, six, and eight C-5 isoprenoid units, correspondingly [154]. Terpenoids obtained from plants are employed owing to their fragrant abilities and portray a significant part in conventional plant-based therapy. Many terpenoids possess considerable pharmacotherapeutic activity and have attracted much attention of the scientific community [92,155,156]. Terpenoids' significant therapeutic effects include antibacterial, anticancer, antimalarial, and inflammation-suppressing actions in severe and long-lasting inflammatory ailments such as "chronic obstructive pulmonary disease" and "osteo-arthritis." [157,158]. Mono-terpenoids and sesquiterpenoids are frequently distributed in the essential oils of remedial herbs; and higher molecular weight terpenoids with higher molecular mass are mostly distributed in balsam and the resin part of herbs [157,159]. Plant families rich in terpenoids include Acanthaceae, Anacardiaceae, Apocynaceae, Araliaceae, Aristolochiaceae, Asteraceae, Betulaceae, Cannabaceae, Celastraceae, Compositae, Cucurbitaceae, Cupressaceae, Cyperaceae, Dilleniaceae, Hypericaceae, Labiatae, Lamiaceae, Lauraceae, Magnoliaceae, Meliaceae, Oleaceae, Pinaceae, Pteridaceae, Rutaceae, Salicaceae, Taxaceae, and Zingiberaceae. Terpenoids reported with antiinflammatory activity are presented in Table 5.

TABLE 5 Terpenoids having potential antiinflammatory activity.

Compound	Chemical structure	Source	Reference
Acanthoic acid		*Acanthopanax kiusianus* (Araliaceae)	[160]
1-O-Acetyl britannilactone		*Inula britannica* (Asteraceae)	[161]
β-Acoradiene		*Casearia sylvestris* (Salicaceae)	[162]

TABLE 5 Terpenoids having potential antiinflammatory activity—cont'd

Compound	Chemical structure	Source	Reference
Agnuside		*Vitex peduncularis* (Lamiaceae)	[163]
α-Amyrin acetate		*Alstonia boonei* (Apocynaceae)	[164]
β-Amyrin acetate		*Alstonia boonei* (Apocynaceae)	[164]
Andrographolide		*Andrographis paniculate* (Acanthaceae)	[165]
Artemisinin		*Artemisia sinica* (Asteraceae)	[166]
Azadiradione		*Azadirachta indica* (Meliaceae)	[167]
Betulinic acid		*Betula pubescens* (Betulaceae)	[168]

Continued

TABLE 5 Terpenoids having potential antiinflammatory activity—cont'd

Compound	Chemical structure	Source	Reference
Bicyclo-germacrene		*Casearia sylvestris* (Salicaceae)	[162]
Boswellic acid		*Boswellia serrata* (Burseraceae)	[169]
Cacalol		*Psacalium decompositum* (Asteraceae)	[170]
Cacalone		*Psacalium decompositum* (Asteraceae)	[170]
Calamenene		*Casearia sylvestris* (Salicaceae)	[162]
Carnosic acid		*Rosmarinus officinalis* (Lamiaceae)	[171]
Carnosol		*Rosmarinus officinalis* (Lamiaceae)	[171]
Caryophyllene		*Casearia sylvestris* (Salicaceae)	[162]
Celastrol		*Tripterygium wilfordii* (Celastraceae)	[172]

TABLE 5 Terpenoids having potential antiinflammatory activity—cont'd

Compound	Chemical structure	Source	Reference
Costunolide		*Laurus nobilis* (Lauraceae)	[173]
Costunolide		*Magnolia grandiflora* (Magnoliaceae)	[174]
Cucurbitacin B		*Cucumis callosus* (Cucurbitaceae)	[175]
Cumanin		*Ambrosia psilostachya* (Asteraceae)	[176]
Curdione		*Curcuma zedoaria* (Zingiberaceae)	[177]
α-Cyperone		*Cyperus rotundus* (Cyperaceae)	[178]
Dehydrocostus lactone		*Saussurea lappa* (Asteraceae)	[179]
Deoxymikanolide		*Mikania cordata* (Asteraceae)	[180]
Eupatolide		*Inula britannica* (Asteraceae)	[181]

Continued

TABLE 5 Terpenoids having potential antiinflammatory activity—cont'd

Compound	Chemical structure	Source	Reference
Filicene		*Adiantum cuneatum* (Pteridaceae)	[182]
Ganoderal A		*Ganoderma lucidum* (Ganodermataceae)	[183]
Ganoderal B		*Ganoderma lucidum* (Ganodermataceae)	[183]
Germacrene-B		*Casearia sylvestris* (Salicaceae)	[162]
Germacrene-D		*Casearia sylvestris* (Salicaceae)	[162]
Gingkolide A		*Ginkgo biloba* (Ginkgoaceae)	[184]
Gingkolide B		*Ginkgo biloba* (Ginkgoaceae)	[184]
Globulol		*Casearia sylvestris* (Salicaceae)	[162]
Glycyrrhizin		*Glycyrrhiza glabra* (Papilionaceae)	[185]

TABLE 5 Terpenoids having potential antiinflammatory activity—cont'd

Compound	Chemical structure	Source	Reference
Helenalin		*Arnicae flos* (Asteraceae)	[186]
Hinkitiol		*Thuja plicata* (Cupressaceae)	[187]
α-Humulene		*Casearia sylvestris* (Salicaceae)	[162]
7-Hydroxy-costunolide		*Podachaenium eminens* (Asteraceae)	[188]
Hyperforin		*Hypericum perforatum* (Hypericaceae)	[128]
Inuviscolide		*Inula viscosa* (Asteraceae)	[189]
Koetjapic acid		*Dillenia serrata* (Dilleniaceae)	[190]
Labdane F2		*Sideritis javalambrensis* (Labiateae)	[191]
Linderalactone		*Neolitsea parvigemma* (Lauraceae)	[192]

Continued

TABLE 5 Terpenoids having potential antiinflammatory activity—cont'd

Compound	Chemical structure	Source	Reference
Mikanolide		*Mikania cordata* (Asteraceae)	[180]
Molephantin		*Elephantopus mollis* (Asteraceae)	[193]
(−)-Myrtenol		*Rhodiola rosea* (Crassulaceae)	[194]
Nimbin		*Azadirachta indica* (Meliaceae)	[195]
Cis-α-Ocimene		*Litsea cubeba* (Lauraceae)	[196]
Oleanolic acid		*Rosmarinus officinalis* (Lamiaceae)	[197]
Oleanonic acid		*Pistacia terebinthus* (Anacardiaceae)	[198]
3-Oxoolean-12-en-30-oic		*Dillenia serrata* (Dilleniaceae)	[190]

TABLE 5 Terpenoids having potential antiinflammatory activity—cont'd

Compound	Chemical structure	Source	Reference
Parthenolide		*Magnolia grandiflora* (Magnoliaceae)	[174]
(+)-α-Pinene		*Pinus longaeva* (Pinaceae)	[199]
Pseudo-neolinderane		*Neolitsea parvigemma* (Lauraceae)	[192]
Spathulenol		*Casearia sylvestris* (Salicaceae)	[162]
Styraxoside A		*Styrax japonica* (Asteraceae)	[200]
Sugiol		Calocedrus formosana (Cupressaceae)	[201]
Taraxasteryl acetate		*Pluchea sagittalis* (Compositeae)	[202]
Δ-Tetrahydro cannabinol		*Cannabis sativa* (Cannabaceae)	[139]
Thujopsene		*Casearia sylvestris* (Salicaceae)	[162]

Continued

TABLE 5 Terpenoids having potential antiinflammatory activity—cont'd

Compound	Chemical structure	Source	Reference
Tripdiolide		*Tripterygium wilfordii* (Celastraceae)	[203]
Triptolide		*Tripterygium wilfordii* (Celastraceae)	[203]
Tsugaric acid A		*Ganoderma lucidum* (Ganodermataceae)	[183]
Ursolic acid		*Plantago major* (Plantaginaceae)	[204]
Zedoarondiol		*Curcuma heyneana* (Zingiberaceae)	[177]
Zerumbone		*Zingiber zerumbet* (Zingiberaceae)	[98]

4.2.4 Phytosterols

Phytosterols or phytosteroids (also denoted as "plant sterols" and "stanol esters") are a cluster of phytochemicals present in the cell membranes of plants. They are important structural components that stabilize the biological membranes of plants [205]. There is growing logical indicator endorsing the idea that phytosterols and their analogs possess numerous therapeutic effects, such as human well-being indorsing capacities. These well-being effects consist of the capability to decrease "total" and "low-density lipoprotein cholesterol" concentrations, so diminishing the danger of various ailments [206]. Additionally, phytosteroids regulate inflammatory processes; possess antioxidant, antiulcer, immune-modulatory, antimicrobial, and fungicidal properties; and intercede in the promotion of wound healing and inhibition of platelet aggregation as well [207]. Phytosterols reported with antiinflammatory effects belong to plant families such as Apocynaceae, Asparagaceae, Burseraceae, Fabaceae, Fomitopsidaceae, Meripilaceae, Oleaceae, Onagraceae, and Solanaceae. Steroidal derivatives obtained from plants possessing antiinflammatory activity are listed in Table 6.

TABLE 6 Phytosterols/phytosteroids with antiinflammatory activity.

Compound	Chemical structure	Source	Reference
Antcin M		*Antrodia salmonea* (Fomitopsidaceae)	[208]
Campesterol		*Lopezia racemosa* (Onagraceae)	[209]
Diosgenin		*Trigonella foenum graecum* (Fabaceae)	[210]
Ergosterol		*Grifola frondosa* (Meripilaceae)	[211]
Ergostra-4,6,8(14),22-tetraen-3-one		*Grifola frondosa* (Meripilaceae)	[211]
Guggulsterol		*Commiphora mukul* (Burseraceae)	[212]
Guggulsterone		*Commiphora mukul* (Burseraceae)	[213,214]
Methyl antcinate K		*Antrodia salmonea* (Fomitopsidaceae)	[208]

Continued

TABLE 6 Phytosterols/phytosteroids with antiinflammatory activity—cont'd

Compound	Chemical structure	Source	Reference
Methyl antcinate L		*Antrodia salmonea* (Fomitopsidaceae)	[208]
Neridienone A		*Nerium oleander* (Apocynaceae)	[215]
Physalin F		*Physalis alkekengi* (Solanaceae)	[216]
Sarsasapogenin		*Rhizoma anemarrhenae* (Asparagaceae)	[91]
β-Sitosterol		*Olea europaea* (Oleaceae)	[217]
Solasodine		*Solanum xanthocarpum* (Solanaceae)	[218]
Velutinol A		*Mandevilla velutina* (Apocynaceae)	[219]
Withaferin A		*Withania sominifera* (Solanaceae)	[220]

4.2.5 Polysaccharides

In recent years, polysaccharides having antiinflammatory potential, obtained majorly from natural resources have gathered extensive attention owing to their safety and accessibility [221]. Polysaccharides obtained from *Bletilla striata* promoted platelet aggregation with an antiinflammatory effect in a gingivitis rat model [222]. *Asarum* polysaccharide isolated from *Asarum heterotropoides* showed a significant antitussive effect in a guinea pig model of cigarette smoke-induced chronic cough hypersensitivity [223]. The polysaccharide fraction (F1) of *Curcuma longa* extract (NR-INF-02) significantly inhibited carrageenan-induced paw edema in rats and xylene-induced ear edema in mice [224]. The polysaccharide fraction isolated from *Sargentodoxa cuneata* demonstrated antiinflammatory activities in vitro (suppressed nitric oxide release in LPS-induced RAW264.7 cells by downregulating the inducible nitric oxide synthase (iNOS) level) and in vivo (inhibited carrageenan-induced rat hind paw edema, decreased in the hind paw, serum and liver malondialdehyde levels and prostaglandin E2 levels) [225]. Polysaccharides isolated from *Dendrobium officinale* leaves remarkably repressed "toll-like receptor-4," "myeloid differentiation factor," and "tumor necrosis factor" receptor-associated factor-6 mRNA and protein expression in LPS-stimulated THP-1 cells [226]. A water-soluble polysaccharide isolated from purple sweet potato roots showed an antiinflammatory effect in vitro (lipopolysaccharide-induced inflammatory RAW264.7 macrophages) as well as in vivo (mice model) [227]. Polysaccharides from *Zizyphus jujube cv. Muzao* showed significant in vitro antioxidant and antiinflammatory effects in lipopolysaccharide-treated RAW264.7 cells [228]. Water-soluble polysaccharides isolated from

Tripterygium wilfordii showed an antiinflammatory effect in lipopolysaccharide-treated RAW264.7 cells with an IC_{50} value of 32.1 µg/mL [229]. Comaruman, a pectin isolated from *Comarum palustre* showed preventive effect in acetic acid-induced colitis in a mice model [230].

4.2.6 Miscellaneous compounds

Some other types of phytoconstituents including fatty acids, fatty alcohols, lectins, peptides, irridoids, quinolones, lactones, and organo-sulfur compounds showed antiinflammatory activity (Table 6). *Daucus carota* is the utmost extensively used herb globally. In some areas of the Earth, this herb is used as ornate therapy for the treatment of gastrointestinal ailments, cardiovascular conditions, convulsions, and fertility issues [231]. Galactolipids are a type of phytoconstituents broadly distributed in the flora, including eatable herbs, and are significant constituents of their cell membranes. Numerous galactolipids had demonstrated significant antiinflammatory properties in vitro and in animal models [232]. In an investigation, "monogalactosyldiacylglycerol," which is a principal lipid of the cell membrane of seed plants and the utmost distributed polar lipid, displayed a powerful antiinflammatory effect in "12-*O*-tetradecanoylphorbol-13-acetate" induced edema development on mice ears [233]. Furthermore, phenethyl isothiocyanate distributed in herbs of the Crucifereae family demonstrated an encouraging effect on enduring inflammatory ailments, which are arbitrated via inflection of a Toll/IL-1 receptor domain containing "adapter-inducing interferon-β-dependent" signaling pathway of Toll-like receptors [234]. A few miscellaneous phytoconstituents with antiinflammatory potential are discussed in the Table 7.

TABLE 7 Miscellaneous phytoconstituents reported with antiinflammatory activity.

Compound	Chemical structure	Source	Reference
Fatty acids			
γ-Linolenic acid		*Ocimum sanctum* (Lamiaceae)	[235]
α-Linolenic acid		*Ocimum sanctum* (Lamiaceae)	[236]
Docosahexaenoic acid		*Plantago major* (Plantaginaceae)	[237]

Continued

TABLE 7 Miscellaneous phytoconstituents reported with antiinflammatory activity—cont'd

Compound	Chemical structure	Source	Reference
Eicosapentaenoic acid		*Plantago major* (Plantaginaceae)	[237]
5-Thia-8,11,14,17-eicosatetraenoic acid		*Plantago major* (Plantaginaceae)	[237]
(*S*)-Coriolic acid		*Hernandia ovigera* (Hernandiaceae)	[238]
9-Oxo-octadecadienoic acid		*Solanum lycopersicum* (Solanaceae)	[239]
Oleic acid		*Daucus carota* (Apiaceae)	[231]
Palmitic acid		*Hernandia ovigera* (Hernandiaceae)	[240]
Linoleic acid		*Hernandia ovigera* (Hernandiaceae)	[240]
Fatty alcohols			
Tetracosanol		*Clematis brevicaudata* (Ranunculaceae)	[241]
Iridoids			
Verminoside		*Kigelia africana* (Bignoniaceae)	[242]
Harpagoside		Harpagophytum procumbens (Pedaliaceae)	[243]

TABLE 7 Miscellaneous phytoconstituents reported with antiinflammatory activity—cont'd

Compound	Chemical structure	Source	Reference
Quinolones			
Ardisiaquinone G		*Ardisia teysmanniana* (Myrsinaceae)	[244]
Lactones			
Z-Ligustilide		Angelica sinensis (Apiaceae)	[245]
Organo-sulfur compounds			
Allicin		*Allium sativum* (Amaryllidaceae)	[246]

5 Commercial value of natural resources as antiinflammatory agents

Extensive diverse herbal medications are commercially available all over the world. Owing to increasing consumption of plant-based formulations, safety and efficiency of herbal products have become a community well-being worry [247]. Traditional medical practitioners believe that the phytochemicals present in plant-based products have better compatibility with the human system [248]. Numerous kinds of formulations are available commercially based on herbal products or containing phytoconstituents claiming antiinflammatory effects. Some of the commercially available herbal/plant product-based formulations with antiinflammatory effects in humans are listed in Table 8.

6 Conclusions and future prospects

The plant-based antiinflammatory drugs/moieties have a long way to go and this field of research can have some promising outcomes in the times to come if a multidirectional approach is followed to explore this arena effectively. The widely distributed plant wealth with exhaustive

TABLE 8 Commercially available herbal products with antiinflammatory effect.

S. no.	Brand name	Herbal product	Company	Application
1	OraMagic Rx	*Aloe vera*	MPM Medical Inc., USA	Treatment of eczema and angular cheilitis
2	Bioderma Cicabio Arnica+	*Arnica chamissonis*	Naos Skin Care India Pvt. Ltd., India	Treatment for acne, boils, bruises, rashes, sprains, pains and wounds
3	Curcuma plus	*Curcuma longa* and *Piper longum*	Nisarga Herbs, India	Antioxidant and antiinflammatory

Continued

TABLE 8 Commercially available herbal products with antiinflammatory effect—cont'd

S. no.	Brand name	Herbal product	Company	Application
4	Aloweda Turmeric Curcumin	Turmeric root and curcumin	Madhur Pharma & Research Laboratories (P) Ltd., India	Antiinflammatory supplement
5	Dezcumin	Curcumin and piperine	Desons Therapeutics Pvt. Ltd., India	Antiinflammatory supplement
6	Turmeric, Inflammation Response	Turmeric, carrot, ginger and pepper	MegaFood, USA	Antiinflammatory supplement
7	Antiinflammatory	Green tea, ginger, sage leaf, turmeric, cinnamon, black pepper, and cayenne pepper	Khroma Herbal Products, USA	Antiinflammatory supplement
8	Inflame-X	Willow bark, turmeric, bromelain, yucca, and ginger	Zahlers, USA	Inflammation reducer
9	Ultra-Pure Sea Buckthron	Sea Buckthron	Saisir Global Technologies Pvt. Ltd., India	Antiinflammatory supplement
10	D-Flame	Basil, ursolic acid, turmeric, ginger, green tea, boswelin, bromelain, resveratrol and berberine	NOW, USA	Treatment of minor aches and pains due to overexertion

research studies on more than 150,000 species for their utilization in the management of number of ailments clearly reflects the potential of drugs from the plant origin for their utilization in various therapies. The two different categories of drug products, which are widely used in the management of inflammation and pain, are orally administered products (tablets, capsules, etc.) and the locally applied pain-killer products (sprays, ointment, and gel). Interestingly, both these categories cover a good number of plant-based drugs. Now with the increasing use of novel and sophisticated technologies, it is easier to isolate one specific bioactive compound and formulate newer products comprising of one or more such moieties. Furthermore, the use of nanotechnology can further help in making such formulation more effective and efficient; in this direction, a very exhaustive work is already in progress in the domain of liposomal drug delivery of natural antiinflammatory drugs. Another approach that may be utilized or explored is the synthesis of analogs and their derivatization.

References

[1] C.M.A. Van Alem, J.M. Metselaar, C. van Kooten, J.I. Rotmans, Recent advances in liposomal-based anti-inflammatory therapy, Pharmaceutics 13 (2021) 1004.

[2] J.C. Maroon, J.W. Bost, A. Maroon, Natural anti-inflammatory agents for pain relief, Surg. Neurol. Int. 1 (2010) 80.

[3] P. Jain, R. Pandey, S.S. Shukla, Inflammation: Natural Resources and Its Applications, vol. 6, Springer, 2015, p. 14.

[4] D.L. Wilhelm, Mechanisms responsible for increased vascular permeability in acute inflammation, Agents Actions 3 (1973) 297–306.

[5] J.S. Pober, W.C. Sessa, Inflammation and the blood microvascular system, Cold Spring Harb. Perspect. Biol. (2015) 7.

[6] Y. Oishi, I. Manabe, Macrophages in inflammation, repair and regeneration, Int. Immunol. 30 (2018) 511–528.

[7] C.M.A. Van Alem, M. Boonstra, J. Prins, T. Bezhaeva, M.E. van Essen, J.M. Ruben, A.L. Vahrmeijer, E.P. van der Veer, J.W. deFijter, M.E. Reinders, et al., Local delivery of liposomal prednisolone leads to an anti-inflammatory profile in renal ischaemia-reperfusion injury in the rat, Nephrol. Dial. Transplant. 33 (2018) 44–53.

[8] S. Kawai, F. Kojima, N. Kusunoki, Recent advances in nonsteroidal anti-inflammatory drugs, Allergol. Int. 54 (2005) 209–215.

[9] R. Yamazaki, N. Kusunoki, T. Matsuzaki, S. Hashimoto, S. Kawai, Nonsteroidal anti-inflammatory drugs induce apoptosis in association with activation of peroxisome proliferator-activated receptor γ in rheumatoid synovial cells, J. Pharmacol. Exp. Ther. 302 (2002) 18–25.

[10] S. Kawai, Cyclooxygenase selectivity and the risk of gastrointestinal complications of various nonsteroidal anti-inflammatory drugs: a clinical consideration, Inflamm. Res. 47 (Suppl. 2) (1998) S102–S106.

[11] J. Shigeta, S. Takahashi, S. Okabe, Role of cyclooxygenase-2 in the healing of gastric ulcers in rats, J. Pharmacol. Exp. Ther. 286 (1998) 1383–1390.

[12] P. Juni, A.W. Rutjes, P.A. Dieppe, Are selective COX 2 inhibitors superior to traditional non steroidal anti-inflammatory drugs, BMJ 324 (2002) 1287–1288.

[13] D. Mukherjee, S.E. Nissen, E.J. Topol, Risk of cardiovascular events associated with selective COX-2 inhibitors, JAMA 286 (2001) 954–959.

[14] A. Whelton, W.B. White, A.E. Bello, J.A. Puma, J.G. Fort, SUCCESS-VII Investigators, Effects of celecoxib and rofecoxib on blood pressure and edema in patients > or = 65 years of age with systemic hypertension and osteoarthritis, Am. J. Cardiol. 90 (2002) 959–963.

[15] R.C. Harris, J.A. Mckanna, Y. Akai, H.R. Jacobson, R.N. Dubois, M.D. Breyer, Cyclooxygenage-2 is associated with the macula densa of rat kidney and increases with salt restriction, J. Clin. Invest. 94 (1994) 2504–2510.

[16] C. dos Reis Nunes, et al., Plants as sources of anti-inflammatory agents, Molecules 25 (2020) 3726.

[17] S.J. Virshette, M.K. Patil, A.P. Somkuwar, A review on medicinal plants used as anti-inflammatory agents, J. Pharmacogn. Phytochem. 8 (2019) 1641–1646.

[18] P.N. Vinaya, Inflammation in ayurveda and modern medicine, Int. Ayurv. Med. J. (2013) 2–4.

[19] J.A. Shazhni, A. Renu, P. Vijayaraghavan, Insights of antidiabetic, anti-inflammatory and hepatoprotective properties of antimicrobial secondary metabolites of corm extract from Caladium x hortulanum, Saudi J. Boil. Sci. 25 (2018) 1755–1761.

[20] Z. Cao, Z. Deng, De novo assembly, annotation, and characterization of root transcriptomes of three caladium cultivars with a focus on necrotrophic pathogen resistance/defense-related genes, Int. J. Mol. Sci. 18 (2017) 712.

[21] C. Locatelli, G.M. Nardi, A.d.F. Anuario, C.G. Freire, F. Megiolaro, K. Schneider, M.R.A. Perazzoli, S.R.D. Nascimento, A.C. Gon, L.N.B. Mariano, et al., Anti-inflammatory activity of berry fruits in mice model of inflammation is based on oxidative stress modulation, Pharmacog. Res. 8 (2016) S42–S49.

[22] M. De Zoysa, Medicinal benefits of marine invertebrates: sources for discovering natural drug candidates, Adv. Food Nutr. Res. 65 (2012) 153–169.

[23] G. Yuan, M.L. Wahlqvist, G. He, M. Yang, D. Li, Natural products and anti-inflammatory activity, Asia Pac. J. Clin. Nutr. 15 (2) (2006) 143–152.

[24] E.M. Costa-Neto, Animal-based medicines: biological prospection and the sustainable use of zootherapeutic resources, Acad. Bras. Cienc. 77 (1) (2005) 33–43.

[25] S. Jirge Supriya, Y.S. Chaudhari, Marine: the ultimate source of bioactives and drug metabolites, IJRAP 1 (1) (2010) 55–62.

[26] D.T.A. Youssefa, A.K. Ibrahim, S.I. Khalifa, M.K. Mesbah, A.M.S. Mayer, R.W.M. van Soest, New anti-inflammatory sterols from the Red sea sponges Scalarispongia aqabaensis and Callyspongia siphonella, Nat. Prod. Commun. 5 (1) (2010) 27–31.

[27] A. Mencarelli, C. D'Amore, B. Renga, S. Cipriani, A. Carino, V. Sepe, E. Perissutti, M.V. D'Auria, A. Zampella, E. Distrutti, S. Fiorucci, Solomonsterol A, a marine Pregnane-X-receptor agonist, attenuates inflammation and immune dysfunction in a mouse model of arthritis, Mar. Drugs 12 (2014) 36–53.

[28] P. Oudhia, Traditional knowledge about medicinal insects, mites and spiders in Chhattisgarh, India, Insect Environ. 4 (1995) 57–58.

[29] C.H. Liu, N. Abrams, D.M. Carrick, P. Chander, J. Dwyer, M.R.J. Hamlet, F. Macchiarini, M. Prabhudas, G.L. Shen, P. Tandon, et al., Biomarkers of chronic inflammation in disease development and prevention: challenges and opportunities, Nat. Immunol. 18 (2017) 1175–1180.

[30] Y. Li, D. Kong, Y. Fu, M.R. Sussman, H. Wu, The effect of developmental and environmental factors on secondary metabolites in medicinal plants, Plant Physiol. Biochem. 148 (2020) 80–89.

[31] M. Zaynab, M. Fatima, S. Abbas, Y. Sharif, M. Umair, M.H. Zafar, K. Bahadar, Role of secondary metabolites in plant defense against pathogens, Microb. Pathog. 124 (2018) 198–202.

[32] T.A. Thumann, E.-M. Pferschy-Wenzig, C. Moissl-Eichinger, R. Bauer, The role of gut microbiota for the activity of medicinal plants traditionally used in the European Union for gastrointestinal disorders, J. Ethnopharmacol. 245 (2019) 112–153.

[33] A.N. Azab, A. Nassar, A.N. Azab, Anti-inflammatory activity of natural products, Molecules 21 (2016) 13–21.

[34] F. Maione, R. Russo, H. Khan, N. Mascolo, Medicinal plants with anti-inflammatory activities, Nat. Prod. Res. 30 (2015) 1343–1352.

[35] K. Rtibi, S. Selmi, M.-A. Jabri, G. Mamadou, N. Limas-Nzouzi, H. Sebai, J. El-Benna, L. Marzouki, B. Eto, M. Amri, Effects of aqueous extracts from Ceratonia siliqua L. pods on small intestinal motility in rats and jejunal permeability in mice, RSC Adv. 6 (2016) 44345–44353.

[36] F. Zhu, B. Du, B. Xu, Anti-inflammatory effects of phytochemicals from fruits, vegetables, and food legumes: a review, Crit. Rev. Food Sci. Nutr. 58 (8) (2018) 1260–1270.

[37] R. Direito, J. Rocha, B. Sepodes, M. Eduardo-Figueira, Phenolic compounds impact on rheumatoid arthritis, inflammatory bowel disease and microbiota modulation, Pharmaceutics 13 (2) (2021) 145.

[38] Y. Bellik, L. Boukraâ, H.A. Alzahrani, B.A. Bakhotmah, F. Abdellah, S.M. Hammoudi, M. Iguer-Ouada, Molecular mechanism underlying anti-inflammatory and anti-allergic activities of phytochemicals: an update, Molecules 18 (1) (2012) 322–353.

[39] M. Ghasemian, S. Owlia, M.B. Owlia, Review of anti-inflammatory herbal medicines, Adv. Pharmacol. Sci. 2016 (2016) 913–979.

[40] F. Shahidi, J. Yeo, Bioactivities of phenolics by focusing on suppression of chronic diseases: a review, Int. J. Mol. Sci. 19 (6) (2018) 1573.

[41] W.H. Talib, A.M. Mahasneh, Antimicrobial, cytotoxicity and phytochemical screening of Jordanian plants used in traditional medicine, Molecules 15 (2010) 1811–1824.

[42] A.L. Souto, J.F. Tavares, M.S. da Silva, F. Diniz Mde, P.F. de Athayde-Filho, J.M. Barbosa Filho, Anti-inflammatory activity of alkaloids: an update from 2000 to 2010, Molecules 16 (10) (2011) 8515–8534.

[43] E. Yesilada, E. Küpeli, Berberis crataegina DC. root exhibits potent anti-inflammatory, analgesic and febrifuge effects in mice and rats, J. Ethnopharmacol. 79 (2002) 237–248.

[44] S. Beg, S. Swain, H. Hasan, M.A. Barkat, M.S. Hussain, Systematic review of herbals as potential anti-inflammatory agents: recent advances, current clinical status and future perspectives, Pharmacogn. Rev. 5 (10) (2011) 120–137.

[45] J.J. Chen, C.Y. Chung, T.L. Hwang, J.F. Chen, Amides and benzenoids from Zanthoxylum ailanthoides with inhibitory activity on superoxide generation and elastase release by neutrophils, J. Nat. Prod. 72 (2009) 107–111.

[46] M. Duwiejua, E. Woode, D.D. Obiri, Pseudo-akuammigine, an alkaloid from Picralima nitida seeds, has anti-inflammatory and analgesic actions in rats, J. Ethnopharmacol. 81 (2002) 73–79, https://doi.org/10.1016/S0378-8741(02)00058-2.

[47] T.S. Wu, Y.L. Leu, Y.Y. Chan, Aristofolin-A, a denitro-aristolochic acid glycoside and other constituents from Aristolochia kaempferi, Phytochemistry 49 (1998) 2509–2510.

[48] E. Kupeli, M. Kosar, E. Yesilada, K.H.C. Baser, C. Baser, A comparative study on the anti-inflammatory, antinociceptive and antipyretic effects of isoquinoline alkaloids from the roots of turkish berberis species, Life Sci. 72 (2002) 645–657.

[49] I. Orhan, E. Kupeli, B. Sener, E. Yesilada, Appraisal of anti-inflammatory potential of the clubmoss, Lycopodium clavatum L, J. Ethnopharmacol. 109 (2007) 146–150.

[50] M.C. Lanhers, J. Fleurentin, F. Mortier, A. Vinche, C. Younos, Anti-inflammatory and analgesic effects of an aqueous extract of Harpagophytum procumbens, Planta Med. 58 (1992) 117–123.

[51] W. Yin, T.S. Wang, F.Z. Yin, B.C. Cai, Analgesic and anti-inflammatory properties of brucine and brucine N-oxide extracted from seeds of Strychnos nux-vomica, J. Ethnopharmacol. 88 (2–3) (2003) 205–214.

[52] F. Zhao, Z. Gao, W. Jiao, L. Chen, L. Chen, X. Yao, In vitro anti-inflammatory effects of beta-carboline alkaloids, isolated from Picrasma quassioides, through inhibition of the iNOS pathway, Planta Med. 78 (18) (2012) 1906–1911.

[53] E.T. Souza, D.P. de Lira, A.C. de Queiroz, D.J. da Silva, A.B. de Aquino, E.A. Mella, V.P. Lorenzo, G.E. de Miranda, J.X. de Araújo-Júnior, M.C. Chaves, J.M. Barbosa-Filho, P.F. de Athayde-Filho, B.V. Santos, M.S. Alexandre-Moreira, The antinociceptive and anti-inflammatory activities of caulerpin, a bisindole alkaloid isolated from seaweed of the genus Caulerpa, Mar. Drugs 7 (2009) 689–704.

[54] S.K. Das, S. Ramakrishnan, K. Mishra, R. Srivastava, G.G. Agarwal, R. Singh, A.R. Sircar, A randomized controlled trial to evaluate the slow acting symptom-modifying effects of colchicine in osteoarthritis of the knee: a preliminary report, Arthritis Care Res. 47 (2002) 280–284.

[55] E.J. Noh, K.S. Ahn, E.M. Shin, S.H. Jung, Y.S. Kim, Inhibition of lipopolysaccharide-induced iNOS and COX-2 expression by dehydroevodiamine through suppression of NF-kappaB activation in RAW 264.7 macrophages, Life Sci. 79 (2006) 695–701.

[56] Z. Yang, W. Lu, X. Ma, D. Song, Bioassay-guided isolation of an alkaloid with antiangiogenic and antitumor activities from the extract of Fissistigma cavaleriei root, Phytomedicine 19 (2012) 301–305.

[57] T.O. Idowu, E.O. Iwalewa, M.A. Aderogba, B.A. Akinpelu, A.O. Ogundaini, Antinociceptive, anti-inflammatory and antioxidant activities of eleagnine: an alkaloid isolated from Chrysophyllum albidum seed cotyledons, J. Biol. Sci. 6 (2006) 1029–1034.

[58] C.D.R. Nunes, M. Barreto Arantes, M. de Faria, S. Pereira, L. Leandro da Cruz, P.M. de Souza, L. Pereira de Moraes, I.J.C. Vieira, D. Barros de Oliveira, Plants as sources of anti-inflammatory agents, Molecules 25(16):3726 (2020).

[59] H. Jin, Y.S. Ko, S.W. Park, K.C. Chang, H.J. Kim, 13-Ethylberberine induces apoptosis through the mitochondria-related apoptotic pathway in radiotherapy-resistant breast cancer cells, Molecules 24 (13) (2019) 2448.

[60] Y.H. Choi, E.M. Shin, Y.S. Kim, X.F. Cai, J.J. Lee, H.P. Kim, Anti-inflammatory principles from the fruits of Evodia rutaecarpa and their cellular action mechanisms, Arch. Pharm. Res. 29 (2006) 293–297.

[61] B. Lal, N.B. Bhise, R.M. Gidwani, A.D. Lakdawala, J. Kalpana, S. Patvardhan, Isolation, synthesis and biological activity of evolitrine and analogs, ARKIVOC 11 (2005) 77–97.

[62] H.S. Choi, H.S. Kim, K.R. Min, Y. Kim, H.K. Lim, Y.K. Chang, M. W. Chung, Anti-inflammatory effects of fangchinoline and tetrandrine, J. Ethnopharmacol. 69 (2) (2000) 173–179.

[63] H.M. Manga, M. Haddad, L. Pieters, C. Baccelli, A. Penge, J.Q. Leclercq, Anti-inflammatory compounds from leaves and root bark of Alchornea cordifolia (Schumach. & Thonn.) Müll. Arg, J. Ethnopharmacol. 115 (2008) 25–29.

[64] K. Yashodharan, P.J. Cox, M. Jaspars, N. Lutfun, D.S. Satyajit, Isolation, structure elucidation and biological activity of hederacine A and B, two unique alkaloids from Glechoma hederaceae, Tetrahedron 59 (2003) 6403–6407.

[65] Y.L. Ho, H.Y. Tsai, Y.S. Chang, Studies on the antinociceptive and anti-inflammatory effects of indigo and indirubin in mice, J. Chin. Med. Sci. 2 (2001) 263–271.

[66] J. Jiang, T.B. Kang, D.W. Shim, N.H. Oh, T.J. Kim, K.H. Lee, Indole-3-carbinol inhibits LPS-induced inflammatory response by blocking TRIF-dependent signaling pathway in macrophages, Food Chem. Toxicol. 57 (2013) 256–261.

[67] W.Y. Chen, F.N. Ko, Y.C. Wu, S.T. Lu, C.M. Teng, Vasorelaxing effect in rat thoracic aorta caused by laurotetanine isolated from Litsea cubeba Persoon, J. Pharm. Pharmacol. 46 (1994) 380–382.

[68] Z. Peng, Z.X. Zhang, Y.J. Xu, Effect of ligustrazine on CD11c and CD14 content on alveolar macrophages from patients with chronic bronchitis, Zhongguo Yaolixue Yu Dulixue Zazhi 14 (2000) 157–160.

[69] C.W. Ao, N. Araki, S. Tawata, Cyclooxygenase inhibitory compounds with antioxidant activities from Sophora subprostrata, Asian J. Chem. 21 (2009) 745–754.

[70] J.J. Chen, Y.T. Luo, T.L. Hwang, P.J. Sung, T.C. Wang, I.S. Chen, A new indole alkaloid and anti-inflammatory constituents from Strychnos cathayensis, Chem. Biodivers. 5 (2008) 1345–1352.

[71] Z. Peng, H. Zhan, Y. Shao, Y. Xiong, L. Zeng, C. Zhang, Z. Liu, Z. Huang, H. Su, Z. Yang, 13-Methylberberine improves endothelial dysfunction by inhibiting NLRP3 inflammasome activation via autophagy induction in human umbilical vein endothelial cells, Chin. Med. 15 (2020) 8.

[72] Y. Luo, M. Liu, Y. Xia, Y. Dai, G. Chou, Z. Wang, Therapeutic effect of norisoboldine, an alkaloid isolated from Radix Linderae, on collagen-induced arthritis in mice, Phytomedicine 17 (2010) 726–731.

[73] J.R. Rho, C.S. Jun, Y.A. Ha, M.J. Yoo, M.X. Cui, H.S. Baek, J.A. Lim, Y.H. Lee, K.Y. Chai, Isolation and characterization of a new alkaloid from seed of Prunus persica L. and its anti-inflammatory activity, Bull. Korean Chem. Soc. 28 (2007) 1289–1293.

[74] J.H. Shang, X.H. Cai, T. Feng, Y.L. Zhao, J.K. Wang, L.Y. Zhang, M. Yan, X.D. Luo, Pharmacological evaluation of Alstonia scholaris: anti-inflammatory and analgesic effects, J. Ethnopharmacol. 129 (2010) 174–181.

[75] M.B. Daware, A.M. Mujumdar, S. Ghaskabdi, Reproductive toxicity of piperine in swiss albino mice, Planta Med. 66 (2000) 231–236,- https://doi.org/10.1055/s-2000-8560.

[76] S.A. Amin, P. Bhattacharya, S. Basak, S. Gayen, A. Nandy, A. Saha, Pharmacoinformatics study of Piperolactam A from Piper betle root as new lead for non steroidal anti fertility drug development, Comput. Biol. Chem. 67 (2017) 213–224.

[77] L. Williamson, H. Illingworth, D. Smith, A. Mowat, Oral quinine in ankylosing spondylitis: a randomized placebo controlled double blind crossover trial, J. Rheumatol. 27 (2000) 2054–2055.

[78] F.L. Araújo, C.T. Melo, N.F. Rocha, B.A. Moura, C.P. Leite, J.F. Amaral, J.M. Barbosa-Filho, S.J. Gutierrez, S.M. Vasconcelos, G. S. Viana, F.C. de Sousa, Antinociceptive effects of (O-methyl)-N-benzoyl tyramine (riparin I) from Aniba riparia (Nees) Mez

(Lauraceae) in mice, Naunyn Schmiedeberg's Arch. Pharmacol. 380 (2009) 337–344.

[79] F.C.F. Sousa, A.M.R. Carvalho, C.P. Leite, N.F.M. Rocha, E.R.V. Rios, L.F. Vasconcelos, C.T.V. Melo, S.T. Lima, J.M. Barbosa-Filho, S.M.M. Vasconcelos, Anti-inflammatory activity of riparin II (N-2-hydroxybenzoyl tyramine) in rats, Inflamm. Res. 60 (2011) 206.

[80] Z. Zhao, J. Xiao, J. Wang, W. Dong, Z. Peng, D. An, Anti-inflammatory effects of novel sinomenine derivatives, Int. Immuno-pharmacol. 29 (2) (2015) 354–360.

[81] A. García-Argáez, M. Apan, H. Parra-Delgado, G. Velázquez, M. -Martinez-Vazquez, Anti-inflammatory activity of coumarins from *Decatropis bicolor* on TPA ear mice model, Planta Med. 66 (2009) 279–281.

[82] F. Shaheen, M. Ahmad, T.H. Khan, S. Jalil, A. Ejaz, M.N. Sultankhodjaev, M. Arfan, M.I. Choudhary, A.U. Rahman, Alkaloids of *Aconitum laeve* and their anti-inflammatory, antioxidant and tyrosinase inhibition activities, Phytochemistry 66 (2005) 935–940.

[83] T. Liu, X. Liu, W. Li, Tetrandrine, a Chinese plant-derived alkaloid, is a potential candidate for cancer chemotherapy, Oncotarget 7 (26) (2016) 40800–40815.

[84] Y. Wang, X. Yang, X. Zheng, J. Li, C. Ye, X. Song, Theacrine, a purine alkaloid with anti-inflammatory and analgesic activities, Fitoterapia 81 (2010) 627–631.

[85] D. Naidoo, P.H. Coombes, D.A. Mulholland, N.R. Crouch, A.J.J. van Den Bergh, N-substituted acridone alkaloids from *Toddaliopsis bremekampii* (Rutaceae: Toddialoideae) of South-Central Africa, Phytochemistry 66 (2005) 1724–1728.

[86] H. Danz, S. Stoyanova, P. Wippich, A. Brattström, M. Hamburger, Identification and isolation of the cyclooxygenase-2 inhibitory principle in *Isatis tinctoria*, Planta Med. 67 (2001) 411–416.

[87] A.P. Singh, Promising phytochemicals from Indian medicinal plants, Ethnobot. Leafl. 9 (2005) 15–23.

[88] R.K. Sutradhar, A.M. Rahman, M. Ahmad, S.C. Bachar, A. Saha, T. G. Roy, Antiinfl ammatory and analgesic alkaloid from *Sidacordifolia* Linn, Pak. J. Pharm. Sci. 20 (2007) 185–188.

[89] H.F. Costa, C.R. Bezerra-Santos, J.M. Barbosa Filho, M.A. Martins, M.R. Piuvezam, Warifteine, a bisbenzylisoquinoline alkaloid, decreases immediate allergic and thermal hyperalgesic reactions in sensitized animals, Int. Immunopharmacol. 8 (2008) 519–525.

[90] D. Tungmunnithum, A. Thongboonyou, A. Pholboon, A. Yangsabai, Flavonoids and other phenolic compounds from medicinal plants for pharmaceutical and medical aspects: an overview, Medicines (Basel) 5 (3) (2018) 93.

[91] S.M. Lim, J.J. Jeong, G.D. Kang, K.A. Kim, H.S. Choi, D.H. Kim, Timosaponin AIII and its metabolite sarsasapogenin ameliorate colitis in mice by inhibiting NF-κB and MAPK activation and restoring Th17/Treg cell balance, Int. Immunopharmacol. 25 (2) (2015) 493–503.

[92] T. Acamovic, J.D. Brooker, Biochemistry of plant secondary metabolites and their effects in animals, Proc. Nutr. Soc. 64 (3) (2005) 403–412.

[93] L. Bravo, Polyphenols: chemistry, dietary sources, metabolism, and nutritional significance, Nutr. Rev. 56 (1988) 317–333.

[94] S. Mohamed, Functional foods against metabolic syndrome (obesity, diabetes, hypertension and dyslipidemia) and cardiovascular disease, Trends Food Sci. Technol. 35 (2014) 114–128.

[95] C. Alarcón de la Lastra, I. Villegas, Resveratrol as an anti-inflammatory and anti-aging agent: mechanisms and clinical implications, Mol. Nutr. Food Res. 49 (2005) 405–430.

[96] C.B. Yang, W.J. Pei, J. Zhao, Y.Y. Cheng, X.H. Zheng, J.H. Rong, Bornyl caffeate induces apoptosis in human breast cancer MCF-7 cells via the ROS- and JNK-mediated pathways, Acta Pharmacol. Sin. 35 (1) (2014) 113–123.

[97] K. Lee, J.H. Kwak, S. Pyo, Inhibition of LPS-induced inflammatory mediators by 3-hydroxyanthranilic acid in macrophages through suppression of PI3K/NF-κβ signaling pathways, Food Funct. 7 (2016) 3073–3082.

[98] T.Y. Chien, L.G. Chen, C.J. Lee, F.Y. Lee, C.C. Wang, Anti-inflammatory constituents of *Zingiber zerumbet*, Food Chem. 110 (2008) 584–589.

[99] E. Bas, M.C. Recio, R.M. Giner, S. Manez, M.C. Nicholas, J.L. Rios, Anti-inflammatory activity of 5-O-demethylnobiletin, a poly-methoxyflavone isolated from *Sideretis tragoriganum*, Planta Med. 72 (2006) 136–142 (PubMed, Google Scholar).

[100] I.N. Hsieh, A.S. Chang, C.M. Teng, C.C. Chen, C.R. Yang, Aciculatin inhibits lipopolysaccharide-mediated inducible nitric oxide synthase and cyclooxygenase-2 expression via suppressing NF-kappaB and JNK/p38 MAPK activation pathways, J. Biomed. Sci. 18 (2011) 28.

[101] D. Lee, M. Cuendet, J.S. Vigo, J.G. Graham, F. Cabieses, H.H. Fong, J.M. Pezzuto, A.D. Kinghorn, A novel cyclooxygenase-inhibitory stilbenolignan from the seeds of *Aiphanes aculeata*, Org. Lett. 3 (2001) 2169–2171.

[102] L.S. Wang, G.D. Stoner, Anthocyanins and their role in cancer prevention, Cancer Lett. 269 (2) (2008) 281–290.

[103] K.S. Kumar, V. Sabu, G. Sindhu, A.A. Rauf, A. Helen, Isolation, identification and characterization of apigenin from *Justicia gendarussa* and its anti-inflammatory activity, Int. Immunopharmacol. 59 (2018) 157–167.

[104] I. Inagaki, A. Sakushima, N. Sueo, H. Sansei, Flavones and flavone glucosides from the leaves of *Trachelospermum asiaticum*, Phytochemistry 12 (1973) 1498.

[105] S.C. Fang, C.L. Hsu, G.C. Yen, Anti-inflammatory effects of phenolic compounds isolated from the fruits of *Artocarpus heterophyllus*, J. Agric. Food Chem. 56 (2008) 4463–4468.

[106] I. Nursakinah, H.A. Zulkhairi, M. Norhafizah, B. Hasnah, M.S. Zamree, S.I. Farrah, D. Razif, F.H. Hamzah, Nutritional content and in vitro antioxidant potential of *Garcinia atroviridis* (*Asam gelugor*) leaves and fruits, Malays. J. Nutr. 18 (3) (2012) 363–371.

[107] V. Moscatelli, O. Hnatyszyn, C. Acevedo, M. Javier, M.J. Alcaraz, G. Ferraro, Flavonoids from Artemesia copa with anti-inflammatory activity, Planta Med. 72 (2006) 72–74.

[108] E. Sezik, M. Tabata, E. Yeşilada, G. Honda, K. Goto, Y. Ikeshiro, Traditional medicine in Turkey: I, Folk medicine in northeast Anatolia, J. Ethnopharmacol. 35 (1991) 191–196.

[109] K. Nakatani, N. Norimichi, A. Tsutomu, Y. Hideyuki, O. Yasushi, Inhibition of cyclooxygenase and prostaglandin E2 synthesis by γ-mangostin, a xanthone derivative in mangosteen, in C6 rat glioma cells, Biochem. Pharmacol. 63 (2002) 73–79.

[110] R.B. Zurier, Prospects for cannabinoids as anti-inflammatory agents, J. Cell Biochem. (2003) 20.

[111] S. Khan, R.J. Choi, O. Shehzad, H.P. Kim, M.N. Islam, J.S. Choi, Y. S. Kim, Molecular mechanism of capillarisin-mediated inhibition of MyD88/TIRAP inflammatory signaling in in vitro and in vivo experimental models, J. Ethnopharmacol. 145 (2) (2013) 626–637.

[112] C.S. Kim, T. Kawada, B.S. Kim, I.S. Han, S.Y. Choe, T. Kurata, R. Yu, Capsaicin exhibits anti-inflammatory property by inhibiting IkB-a degradation in LPS-stimulated peritoneal macrophages, Cell. Signal. 15 (3) (2003) 299–306.

[113] F.Y. Fan, L.X. Sang, M. Jiang, Catechins and their therapeutic benefits to inflammatory bowel disease, Molecules 22 (3) (2017) 484.

[114] Y.H. He, C. Xiao, Y.S. Wang, L.H. Zhao, H.Y. Zhao, Y. Tong, J. Zhou, H.W. Jia, C. Lu, X.M. Li, A.P. Lu, Antioxidant and anti-inflammatory effects of cyanidin from cherries on rat adjuvant-induced arthritis, Zhongguo Zhong Yao Za Zhi 30 (20) (2005) 1602–1605.

[115] M. Hamalainen, R. Nieminen, P. Vuorela, M. Heinonen, E. Moilanen, Anti-inflammatory effects of flavonoids: genistein, kaempferol, quercetin, and daidzein inhibit STAT-1 and NF-kappaBactivations, whereas flavone, isorhamnetin, naringenin, and pelargonidin inhibit only NF-kappaB activation along with theirinhibitory effect on iNOS expression and NO production in activated macrophages, Mediat. Inflamm. 2007 (2007) 45673.

[116] C.H. Wang, L.L. Zhu, K.F. Ju, J.L. Liu, K.P. Li, Anti-inflammatory effect of delphinidin on intramedullary spinal pressure in a spinal cord injury rat model, Exp. Ther. Med. 14 (6) (2017) 5583–5588.

[117] R. Joo Choi, M.S. Cheng, K.Y. Shik, Desoxyrhapontigenin up-regulates Nrf2-mediated heme oxygenase-1 expression in macrophages and inflammatory lung injury, Redox Biol. 2 (2014) 504–512.

[118] Y. Noreen, G. Serrano, P. Perera, L. Bohlin, Flavan-3-ols isolated from some medicinal plants inhibiting COX-1 and COX-2 catalysed prostaglandin biosynthesis, Planta Med. 64 (6) (1998) 520–524.

[119] P.C. Chen, D.S. Wheeler, V. Malhotra, K. Odoms, A.G. Denenberg, H.R. Wong, A green tea-derived polyphenol, epigallocatechin-3-gallate, inhibits IκB kinase activation and IL-8 gene expression in respiratory epithelium, Inflammation 26 (5) (2002) 233–241.

[120] V. Chakradhar, Y.H. Babu, S. Ganapaty, Y.R. Prasad, N.K. Rao, Anti-inflammatory activity of a flavonol glycoside from *Tephrosia spinosa*, Nat. Prod. Sci. 11 (2005) 63–66.

[121] K.C. Choi, Y.O. Son, J.M. Hwang, B.T. Kim, M. Chae, J.C. Lee, Antioxidant, anti-inflammatory and anti-septic potential of phenolic acids and flavonoid fractions isolated from *Lolium multiflorum*, Pharm. Biol. 55 (1) (2017) 611–619.

[122] J. Kang, C. Xie, Z. Li, S. Nagarajan, A.G. Schauss, T. Wu, X.L. Wu, Flavonoids from acai (*Euterpe oleracea* Mart.) pulp and their antioxidant and anti-inflammatory activities, Food Chem. 128 (2011) 152–157.

[123] J. Han, Y. Zhang, C. Pan, Z. Xian, C. Pan, Y. Zhao, C. Li, Y. Yi, L. Wang, J. Tian, S. Liu, D. Wang, J. Meng, A. Liang, Forsythoside A and Forsythoside B contribute to shuanghuanglian injection-induced pseudoallergic reactions through the RhoA/ROCK signaling pathway, Int. J. Mol. Sci. 20 (24) (2019) 6266.

[124] B.H. Kroes, A.J. van den Berg, H.C. Quarles van Ufford, H. van Dijk, R.P. Labadie, Anti-inflammatory activity of gallic acid, Planta Med. 58 (6) (1992) 499–504.

[125] D. Siebert, C. Paganelli, G. Queiroz, M. Alberton, Anti-inflammatory activity of the epicuticular wax and its isolated compounds catechin and gallocatechin from *Eugenia brasiliensis* Lam. (Myrtaceae) leaves, Nat. Prod. Res. (2020) 1–4, https://doi.org/10.1080/14786419.2019.1710707.

[126] J.H. Won, J.Y. Kim, K.J. Yun, J.H. Lee, N.I. Back, H.G. Chung, S.A. Chung, T.S. Jeong, M.S. Choi, K.T. Lee, Gigantol isolated from the whole plants of *Cymbidium goeringii* inhibits the LPS-induced INOS and COX-2 expression via NF-kB inactivation in RAW 264.7 macrophages cells, Planta Med. 72 (2006) 1181–1187.

[127] H. Parhiz, A. Roohbakhsh, F. Soltani, R. Rezaee, M. Iranshahi, Antioxidant and anti-inflammatory properties of the citrus flavonoids hesperidin and hesperetin: an updated review of their molecular mechanisms and experimental models, Phytother. Res. 29 (3) (2015) 323–331.

[128] S. Gadzovska, S. Maury, S. Ounnar, M. Righezza, S. Kascakova, M. Refregiers, M. Spasenoski, C. Joseph, D. Hagège, Identification and quantification of hypericin and pseudohypericin in different *Hypericum perforatum* L. in vitro cultures, Plant Physiol. Biochem. 43 (6) (2005) 591–601.

[129] Y.S. Chi, H.G. Jong, K.H. Son, H.W. Chang, S.S. Kang, H.P. Kim, Effects of naturally occurring prenylated flavonoids on enzymes metabolizing arachidonic acid: cyclooxygenases and lipoxygenases, Biochem. Pharmacol. 62 (2001) 1185–1191.

[130] E.R. De Almeida, A.A. da Silva Filho, E.R. dos Santos, C.A. Lopes, Anti-inflammatory action of lapachol, J. Ethnopharmacol. 29 (1990) 239–241.

[131] G. Seelinger, I. Merfort, C.M. Schempp, Antioxidant, anti-inflammatory and antiallergic activities of luteolin, Planta Med. 74 (2008) 1667.

[132] W.-Y. Huang, X.-N. Wang, J. Wang, Z.-Q. Sui, Malvidin and its glycosides from vaccinium ashei improve endothelial function by anti-inflammatory and angiotensin I-converting enzyme inhibitory effects, Nat. Prod. Commun. 13 (1) (2018) 49–52.

[133] Y.K. Kim, R.G. Kim, S.J. Park, J.H. Ha, J.W. Choi, H.J. Park, K.T. Lee, In vitro anti-inflammatory activity of kalopanaxsaponin A isolated from Kalopanax pictus in murine macrophage RAW 264.7 cells, Biol. Pharm. Bull. 25 (4) (2002) 472–476.

[134] S.J. Wang, Y. Tong, S. Lu, R. Yang, X. Liao, Y.F. Xu, X. Li, Anti-inflammatory activity of myricetin isolated from *Myrica rubra* Sieb. et Zucc. leaves, Planta Med. 76 (14) (2010) 1492–1496.

[135] A. Hiermann, H. Schramm, S. Laufer, Anti-inflammatory activity of myricetin-3-O-ß-D-glucuronide and related compounds, Inflamm. Res. 47 (1998) 421–427.

[136] S.K. Ha, H.Y. Park, H. Eom, Y. Kim, I. Choi, Narirutin fraction from citrus peels attenuates LPS-stimulated inflammatory response through inhibition of NF-k;B and MAPKs activation, Food Chem. Toxicol. 50 (2012) 3498–3504.

[137] C.A. Kassuya, D.F. Leite, L.V. de Melo, V.L. Rohder, J.B. Calixto, Anti-inflammatory properties of extracts, fractions and lignans isolated from *Phyllanthus amarus*, Planta Med. 71 (2005) 721–726.

[138] H.W. Chang, S.H. Baek, K.W. Chung, K.H. Son, H.P. Kim, S.S. Kang, Inactivation of phospholipase A2 by naturally occurring biflavonoid, ochnaflavone, Biochem. Biophys. Res. Commun. 205 (1994) 843–849.

[139] E.A. Formukong, A.T. Evans, F.J. Evans, Analgesic and anti-inflammatory activity of constituents of *Cannabis sativa* L, Inflammation 12 (1988) 361–371.

[140] L. Huang, H. Fuchino, N. Kawahara, Y. Narukawa, N. Hada, F. Kiuchi, Application of a new method, orthogonal projection to latent structure (OPLS) combined with principal component analysis (PCA), to screening of prostaglandin E2 production inhibitory flavonoids in Scutellaria Root, J. Nat. Med. 70 (2016) 731–739.

[141] S.J. Lim, M. Kim, A. Randy, C.W. Nho, Inhibitory effect of the branches of *Hovenia dulcis* Thunb. and its constituent pinosylvin on the activities of IgE-mediated mast cells and passive cutaneous anaphylaxis in mice, Food Funct. 6 (2015) 1361–1370.

[142] X.Y. Jin, S.H. Lee, J.Y. Kim, Y.Z. Zhao, E.J. Park, B.S. Lee, J.X. Nan, K.S. Song, G. Ko, D.H. Sohn, Polyozellin inhibits nitric oxide production by down-regulating LPS-induced activity of NF-kB and SAPK/JNK in RAW 264.7 cells, Planta Med. 72 (2006) 857–859.

[143] C. Kaewmool, P. Kongtawelert, T. Phitak, P. Pothacharoen, S. Udomruk, Protocatechuic acid inhibits inflammatory responses in LPS-activated BV2 microglia via regulating SIRT1/NF-κB pathway contributed to the suppression of microglial activation-induced PC12 cell apoptosis, J. Neuroimmunol. 341 (2020), 577164.

[144] M.F. Melzig, H.H. Pertz, L. Krenn, Anti-inflammatory and spasmolytic activity of extracts from *Droserae herba*, Phytomedicine 8 (2001) 225–229.

[145] N. Elmali, O. Baysal, A. Harma, I. Esenkaya, B. Mizrak, Effects of resveratrol in inflammatory arthritis, Inflammation 30 (2007) 1–6.

[146] J.W. Yang, Y.R. Pokharel, M.R. Kim, E.R. Woo, H.K. Choi, K.W. Kang, Inhibition of inducible nitric oxide synthase by sumaflavone isolated from *Selaginella tamariscina*, J. Ethnopharmacol. 105 (2006) 107–113.

[147] G.P. Amaral, N.R. de Carvalho, R.P. Barcelos, F. Dobrachinski, L. Portella Rde, M.H. da Silva, T.H. Lugokenski, G.R. Dias, S.C. da Luz, A.A. Boligon, M.L. Athayde, M.A. Villetti, F.A. Antunes Soares, R. Fachinetto, Protective action of ethanolic extract of *Rosmarinus officinalis* L. in gastric ulcer prevention induced by ethanol in rats, Food Chem. Toxicol. 55 (2013) 48–55.

[148] E.L. Maistro, P.M. Terrazzas, F.F. Perazzo, I.O.M. Gaivão, A.C.H.F. Sawaya, P.C.P. Rosa, Salix alba (white willow) medicinal plant presents genotoxic effects in human cultured leukocytes, J. Toxicol. Environ. Health A 82 (23-24) (2019) 1223–1234.

[149] H.J. Kim, S.I. Jang, Y.J. Kim, H.T. Chung, Y.G. Yun, T.H. Kang, O. S. Jeong, Y.C. Kim, Scopoletin suppresses pro-inflammatory cytokines and PGE2 from LPS-stimulated cell line, RAW 264.7 cells, Fitoterapia 75 (3–4) (2004) 261–266. 03;88:462–466.

[150] S. Zhang, M. Cheng, Z. Wang, Y. Liu, Y. Ren, S. Rong, X. Wang, Secoisolariciresinol diglucoside exerts anti-inflammatory and antiapoptotic effects through inhibiting the Akt/IκB/NF-κB pathway on human umbilical vein endothelial cells, Mediat. Inflamm. 2020 (2020) 3621261.

[151] M.B. Gupta, T.N. Bhalla, G.P. Gupta, C.R. Mitra, K.P. Bhargava, Anti-inflammatory activity of taxifolin, Jpn. J. Pharmacol. 21 (3) (1971) 377–382.

[152] K.S. Ahn, E.J. Noh, K.-H. Cha, Y.S. Kim, S.S. Lim, K.H. Shin, S.H. Jung, Inhibitory effects of Irigenin from the rhizomes of *Belamcanda chinensis* on nitric oxide and prostaglandin E2 production in murine macrophage RAW 264.7 cells, Life Sci. 78 (20) (2006) 2336–2342.

[153] Y.A. Han, C.W. Song, W.S. Koh, G.H. Yon, Y.S. Kim, S.Y. Ryu, H. J. Kwon, K.H. Lee, Anti-inflammatory effects of the *Zingiber officinale* roscoe constituent 12-dehydrogingerdione in lipopolysaccharide-stimulated Raw 264.7 cells, Phytother. Res. 27 (8) (2013) 1200–1205.

[154] B. De las Heras, B. Rodriguez, L. Bosca, A.M. Villar, Terpenoids: sources, structure elucidation and therapeutic potential in inflammation, Curr. Top. Med. Chem. 3 (2003) 171–185.

[155] P.M. Dewick, Medicinal Natural Products: A Biosynthetic Approach, John Wiley & Sons, 2002, pp. 170–250.

[156] J.W. Rowe, Natural Products of Woody Plants, Springer Science & Business Media, 2012, pp. 691–735.

[157] A. Rufino, M. Ribeiro, F. Judas, L. Salgueiro, M. Lopes, C. Cavaleiro, A. Mendes, Anti-inflammatory and chondroprotective activity of (+)-α-pinene: structural and enantiomeric selectivity, J. Nat. Prod. 77 (2) (2014) 264–269.

[158] J. Ma, H. Xu, J. Wu, C. Qu, F. Sun, S. Xu, Linalool inhibits cigarette smoke-induced lung inflammation by inhibiting NF-κB activation, Int. Immunopharmacol. 29 (2) (2015) 708–713.

[159] W. Yang, X. Chen, Y. Li, S. Guo, Z. Wang, X. Yu, Advances in pharmacological activities of terpenoids, Nat. Prod. Commun. 15 (3) (2020) 1–13.

[160] Y.G. Suh, Y.H. Kim, M.H. Park, Y.H. Choi, H.K. Lee, J.Y. Moon, K. H. Min, D.Y. Shin, J.K. Jung, O.H. Park, R.O. Jeon, H.S. Park, S.A. Kang, Pimarane cyclooxygenase 2 (COX-2) inhibitor and its structure-activity relationship, Bioorg. Med. Chem. Lett. 11 (4) (2001) 559–562.

[161] M. Han, J.K. Wen, J. Zheng, D.Q. Zhang, Acetylbritannilatone suppresses NO and PGE2 synthesis in RAW 264.7 macrophages through the inhibition of iNOS and COX-2 gene expression, Life Sci. 75 (2004) 675–684.

[162] I. Esteves, I.R. Souza, M. Rodrigues, L.G. Cardoso, L.S. Santos, J.A. Sertie, F.F. Perazzo, L.M. Lima, J.M. Schneedorf, J.K. Bastos, J.C. Carvalho, Gastric antiulcer and anti-inflammatory activities of the essential oil from *Casearia sylvestris* Sw, J. Ethnopharmacol. 101 (2005) 191–196.

[163] A. Suksamrarn, S. Kumpun, K. Kirtikara, S.S. Yingyongnarongkul, Iridoids with anti-inflammatory activity from Vitex peduncularis, Planta Med. 68 (2002) 72–73.

[164] N.N. Okoye, D.L. Ajaghaku, H.N. Okeke, E.E. Ilodigwe, C.S. Nworu, F.B. Okoye, beta-Amyrin and alpha-amyrin acetate isolated from the stem bark of *Alstonia boonei* display profound anti-inflammatory activity, Pharm. Biol. 52 (11) (2014) 1478–1486.

[165] S.S. Madav, K. Tadan, J. Lal, H.C. Tripathi, Anti-inflammatory activity of andrographolide, Fitoterapia 67 (1996) 452–458.

[166] K. Kohli, J. Ali, Curcumin: a natural anti-inflammatory agent, Indian J. Pharm. 37 (2005) 141–147.

[167] K. Ilango, G. Maharajan, S. Narasimhan, Anti-nociceptive and anti-inflammatory activities of *Azadirachta indica* fruit skin extract and its isolated constituent azadiradione, Nat. Prod. Res. 27 (2013) 1463–1467.

[168] P. Yogeeswari, D. Sriram, Betulinic acid and its derivatives: a review on their biological properties, Curr. Med. Chem. 12 (6) (2005) 657–666.

[169] U. Dahmen, Y.L. Gu, O. Dirsch, L.M. Fan, J. Li, K. Shen, C.E. Broelsch, Boswellic acid, a potent anti-inflammatory drug, inhibits rejection to the same extent as high dose steroids, Transplant. Proc. 33 (2001) 539–541.

[170] M. Jimenez-Estrada, R.R. Chilpa, T.R. Apan, F. Lledias, W. Hansberg, D. Arrieta, F.J. Aguilar, Anti-inflammatory activity of cacalol and cacalone sesquiterpenes isolated from *Psacalium decompositum*, J. Ethnopharmacol. 105 (2006) 34–38.

[171] C.F. Kuo, J.D. Su, C.H. Chiu, C.C. Peng, C.H. Chang, T.Y. Sung, S. H. Huang, W.C. Lee, C.C. Chyau, Anti-inflammatory effects of supercritical carbon dioxide extract and its isolated carnosic acid from *Rosmarinus officinalis* leaves, J. Agric. Food Chem. 59 (8) (2011) 3674–3685.

[172] G. Sethi, K.S. Ahn, M.K. Pandey, B.B. Aggarwal, Celastrol, a novel triterpene, potentiates TNF-induced apoptosis and suppresses invasion of tumor cells by inhibiting NF-kB-regulated gene products and TAK1-mediated NF-kB activation, Blood 109 (2007) 2727–2735.

[173] H. Matsuda, K. Tadashi, T. Iwao, U. Hiroki, M. Toshio, Y. Masayuki, Inhibitory effects of sesquiterpenes from bay leaf on nitric oxide production in lipopolysaccharide-activated macrophages: structure requirement and role of heat shock protein induction, Life Sci. 66 (2000) 2151–2157.

[174] T.H. Koo, J.-H. Lee, Y.J. Park, Y.-S. Hong, H.S. Kim, K.-W. Kim, J.J. Lee, A sesquiterpene lactone, costunolide, from *Magnolia grandiflora* inhibits NF-kB by targeting IkB phosphorylation, Planta Med. 67 (2001) 103–107.

[175] U. Kaushik, V. Aeri, S.R. Mir, Cucurbitacins—an insight into medicinal leads from nature, Pharmacogn. Rev. 9 (17) (2015) 12–18, https://doi.org/10.4103/0973-7847.156314.

[176] A.L. Lastra, T.O. Ramírez, L. Salazar, M. Martínez, J. Trujillo-Ferrara, The ambrosanolide cumanin inhibits macrophage nitric oxide synthesis: some structural considerations, J. Ethnopharmacol. 95 (2004) 221–227.

[177] W. Cho, J.W. Nam, H.J. Kang, T. Windono, E.K. Seo, K.T. Lee, Zedoarondiol isolated from the rhizoma of *Curcuma heyneana* is involved in the inhibition of iNOS, COX-2 and pro-inflammatory cytokines via the downregulation of NF-kappaB pathway in LPS-stimulated murine macrophages, Int. Immunopharmacol. 9 (9) (2009) 1049–1057.

[178] S.H. Jung, S.J. Kim, B.G. Jun, K.T. Lee, S.P. Hong, M.S. Oh, D.S. Jang, J.H. Choi, α-Cyperone, isolated from the rhizomes of *Cyperus rotundus*, inhibits LPS-induced COX-2 expression and PGE2 production through the negative regulation of NFκB signalling in RAW 264.7 cells, J. Ethnopharmacol. 147 (1) (2013) 208–214.

[179] P.R. Rao Vadaparthi, K. Kumar, V.U. Sarma, Q.A. Hussain, K.S. Babu, Estimation of costunolide and dehydrocostus lactone in *Saussurea lappa* and its polyherbal formulations followed by their stability studies using HPLC-DAD, Pharmacogn. Mag. 11 (41) (2015) 180–190.

[180] M. Ahmed, M.T. Rahman, M. Alimuzzaman, J.A. Shilpi, Analgesic sesquiterpene dilactone from *Mikania cordata*, Fitoterapia 72 (2001) 919–921.

[181] J. Lee, N. Tae, J.J. Lee, T. Kim, J.H. Lee, Eupatolide inhibits lipopolysaccharide-induced COX-2 and iNOS expression in RAW264.7 cells by inducing proteasomal degradation of TRAF6, Eur. J. Pharmacol. 636 (2010) 173–180.

[182] M.M. De Souza, M.A. Pereira, J.V. Ardenghi, T.C. Mora, L.F. Bresciani, R.A. Yunes, F. Delle Monache, V. Cechinel-Filho, Filicene obtained from Adiantum cuneatum interacts with the cholinergic, dopaminergic, glutamatergic, GABAergic, and tachykinergic systems to exert antinociceptive effect in mice, Pharmacol. Biochem. Behav. 93 (2009) 40–46.

[183] H.H. Ko, C.F. Hung, J.P. Wang, C.N. Lin, Anti-inflammatory triterpenoids and steroids from *Ganoderma lucidum* and *G. tsugae*, Phytochemistry 69 (2008) 234–239.

[184] H. Lim, K.H. Son, H.W. Chang, S.S. Sang, H.P. Kim, Effects of anti-inflammatory biflavonoid, ginkgetin on chronic skin inflammation, Biol. Pharm. Bull. 29 (2006) 1046–1049.

[185] E.D. Jesch, T.P. Carr, Food ingredients that inhibit cholesterol absorption, Prev. Nutr. Food Sci. 22 (2017) 67–80.

[186] G. Lyss, T.J. Schmidt, I. Merfort, H.L. Pahl, Helenalin, an anti-inflammatory sesquiterpene lactone from Arnica, selectively inhibits transcription factor NF-kappaB, Biol. Chem. 378 (9) (1997) 951–961.

[187] S.E. Byeon, Y.G. Lee, J.C. Kim, J.G. Han, H.Y. Lee, J.Y. Cho, Hinokitiol: a natural tropolone derivative, inhibits TNF-alpha production

in LPS-activated macrophages via suppression of NF-KB, Planta Med. 74 (2008) 828–833.

[188] V. Castro, R. Murillo, C.A. Klaas, C. Meunier, G. Mora, H.L. Pahl, I. Merfort, Inhibition of the transcription factor NF-kB by sesquiterpene lactones from *Podachaenium eminens*, Planta Med. 66 (2000) 591–595.

[189] S. Manez, V. Hernandez, R.M. Giner, J.L. Rios, R.M. del Carmen, Inhibition of pro-inflammatory enzymes by inuviscolide: a sesquiterpene lactone from Inula viscosa, Fitoterapia 78 (2007) 329–331.

[190] J. Jalil, C.W. Sabandar, N. Ahmat, J.A. Jamal, I. Jantan, N.A. Aladdin, K. Muhammad, F. Buang, H.F. Mohamad, I. Sahidin, Inhibitory effect of triterpenoids from *Dillenia serrata* (Dilleniaceae) on prostaglandin E2 production and quantitative HPLC analysis of its koetjapic acid and betulinic acid contents, Molecules 20 (2) (2015) 3206–3220.

[191] L. Pang, de las Heras B, Hoult JR., A novel diterpenoid labdane from *Sideritis javalambrensis* inhibits eicosanoid generation from stimulated macrophages but enhances arachidonate release, Biochem. Pharmacol. 51 (1996) 863–868.

[192] K.S. Chen, P.W. Hsieh, T.L. Hwang, F.R. Chang, Y.C. Wu, Anti-inflammatory furanogermacrane sesquiterpenes from *Neolitsea parvigemma*, Nat. Prod. Res. 19 (2005) 283–286.

[193] B. Siedle, L. Gustavsson, S. Johansson, R. Murillo, V. Castro, L. Bohlin, I. Merfort, The effect of sesquiterpene lactones on the human neutrophil elastase, Biochem. Pharmacol. 65 (2003) 897–903.

[194] B.S. Gomes, B.P.S. Neto, E.M. Lopes, F.V.M. Cunha, A.R. Araújo, C.W.S. Wanderley, D.V.T. Wong, R.C.P.L. Júnior, R.A. Ribeiro, D.P. Sousa, V.R. Medeiros, J, Oliveira RCM, Oliveira FA., Anti-inflammatory effect of the monoterpene myrtenol is dependent on the direct modulation of neutrophil migration and oxidative stress, Chem. Biol. Interact. 273 (2017) 73–81.

[195] M.A. Alzohairy, Therapeutics role of *Azadirachta indica* (Neem) and their active constituents in diseases prevention and treatment, Evid. Based Complement. Alternat. Med. 2016 (2016) 7382506.

[196] E.M. Choi, J.K. Hwang, Effects of methanolic extract and fractions from Litsea cubeba bark on the production of inflammatory mediators in RAW264.7 cells, Fitoterapia 75 (2004) 141–148.

[197] G. Altinier, S. Sosa, R.P. Aquino, T. Mencherini, R.D. Loggia, A. Tubaro, Characterization of topical anti-inflammatory compounds in *Rosmarinus officinalis* L, J. Agric. Food Chem. 55 (2007) 1718–1723.

[198] E.M. Giner-Larza, S. Manez, M.C. Recio, R.M. Giner, J.M. Prieto, M. Cerda-Nicolas, J.L. Rios, Oleanonic acid, a 3-oxotriterpene from *Pistacia*, inhibits leukotriene synthesis and has anti-inflammatory activity, Eur. J. Pharmacol. 428 (2001) 137–143.

[199] B. Salehi, S. Upadhyay, I. Erdogan Orhan, A. Kumar Jugran, S.L.D. Jayaweera, D.A. Dias, F. Sharopov, Y. Taheri, N. Martins, N. Baghalpour, W.C. Cho, J. Sharifi-Rad, Therapeutic potential of α- and β-pinene: a miracle gift of nature, Biomol. Ther. 9 (11) (2019) 738.

[200] K.J. Yun, B.S. Min, J.Y. Kim, K.T. Lee, Styraxoside A isolated from the stem bark of *Styrax japonica* inhibits lipopolysaccharide-induced expression of inducible nitric oxide synthase and cyclooxygenase-2 in RAW 264.7 cells by suppressing nuclear factor-kappa B activation, Biol. Pharm. Bull. 30 (2007) 139–144.

[201] K.-P. Chao, K.-F. Hua, H.-Y. Hsu, Y.-C. Su, S.-T. Chang, Anti-inflammatory activity of Sugiol, a diterpene isolated from *Calocedrus formosana* bark, Planta Med. 71 (2005) 300–305.

[202] F. Perez-Garcia, E. Martin, T. Parella, T. Adzet, S. Canigueral, Activity of taraxasteryl acetate on inflammation and heat shock protein synthesis, Phytomedicine 12 (2005) 278–284.

[203] J. Ma, M. Dey, H. Yang, A. Poulev, R. Pouleva, R. Dorn, P.E. Lipsky, E.J. Kennelly, I. Raskin, Anti-inflammatory and immunosuppressive compounds from *Tripterygium wilfordii*, Phytochemistry 68 (2007) 1172–1178.

[204] S.M. Jachak, Cyclooxygenase inhibitory natural products: current status, Curr. Med. Chem. 13 (2006) 659–678.

[205] R.A. Moreau, L. Nyström, B.D. Whitaker, J.K. Winkler-Moser, D.J. Baer, S.K. Gebauer, K.B. Hicks, Phytosterols and their derivatives: structural diversity, distribution, metabolism, analysis, and health-promoting uses, Prog. Lipid Res. 70 (2018) 35–61.

[206] J. Plat, S. Baumgartner, T. Vanmierlo, D. Lütjohann, K.L. Calkins, D.G. Burrin, et al., Plant-based sterols and stanols in health and disease: "Consequences of human development in a plant-based environment?", Prog. Lipid Res. 74 (2019) 87–102.

[207] R.J. Ogbe, D.O. Ochalefu, S.G. Mafulul, O.B. Olaniru, A review on dietary phytosterols: their occurrence, metabolism and health benefits, Asian J. Plant Sci. Res. 5 (2015) 10–21.

[208] C.C. Shen, Y.-H. Wang, T.-T. Chang, L.-C. Lin, M.-J. Don, Y.-C. Hou, K.-T. Lio, S. Chang, W.-Y. Wang, H.-C. Ko, Y.-C. Shen, Anti-inflammatory ergostanes from the basidiomata of *Antrodia salmonea*, Planta Med. 73 (2007) 1208–1213.

[209] N.E. Moreno-Anzúrez, S. Marquina, L. Alvarez, A. Zamilpa, P. -Castillo-España, I. Perea-Arango, P.N. Torres, M. Herrera-Ruiz, E.R. Díaz García, J.T. García, J. Arellano-García, A cytotoxic and anti-inflammatory campesterol derivative from genetically transformed hairy roots of *Lopezia racemosa* cav. (Onagraceae), Molecules 22(1):118 (2017).

[210] S. Shishodia, B.B. Aggarwal, Diosgenin inhibits osteoclastogenesis, invasion, and proliferation through the downregulation of Akt, I kappa B kinase activation and NF-kappa B-regulated gene expression, Oncogene 25 (2006) 1463–1473.

[211] Y. Zhang, G.L. Mills, M.G. Nair, Cyclooxygenase inhibitory and antioxidant compounds from the mycelia of the edible mushroom *Grifola frondosa*, J. Agric. Food Chem. 50 (2002) 7581–7585.

[212] N. Manjula, B. Gayathri, K.S. Vinaykumar, N.P. Shankernarayanan, R.A. Vishwakarma, A. Balakrishnan, Inhibition of MAP kinases by crude extract and pure compound isolated from *Commiphora mukul* leads to down regulation of TNF-a, IL-1b and IL-2, Int. Immunopharmacol. 6 (2006) 122–132.

[213] D. Khanna, G. Sethi, K.S. Ahn, M.K. Pandey, A.B. Kunnumakara, B. Sung, A. Aggarwal, B.B. Aggarwal, Natural products as a gold mine for arthritis treatment, Curr. Opin. Pharmacol. 7 (2007) 344–351.

[214] C. Gebhard, S.F. Stampfli, C.E. Gebhard, A. Akhmedov, A. Breitenstein, G.G. Camici, E.W. Holy, T.F. Luscher, F.C. Tanner, Guggulsterone, an anti-inflammatory phytosterol, inhibits tissue factor and arterial thrombosis, Basic Res. Cardiol. 104 (2009) 285–294.

[215] L. Bai, L. Wang, M. Zhao, A. Toki, T. Hasegawa, H. Ogura, T. Kataoka, K. Hiroe, J. Sakai, J. Bai, M. Ando, Bioactive pregnanes from *Nerium oleander*, J. Nat. Prod. 70 (2007) 14–18.

[216] Y.K. Yang, S.D. Xie, W.X. Xu, Y. Nian, X.L. Liu, X.R. Peng, Z.T. Ding, M.H. Qiu, Six new physalins from *Physalis alkekengi* var. *franchetii* and their cytotoxicity and antibacterial activity, Fitoterapia 112 (2016) 144–152.

[217] F. Gelmini, M. Ruscica, C. Macchi, V. Bianchi, R. Maffei Facino, G. Beretta, P. Magni, Unsaponifiable fraction of unripe fruits of *Olea europaea*: an interesting source of anti-inflammatory constituents, Planta Med. 82 (3) (2016) 273–278.

[218] S. Govindana, S.B. Viswanathan, V.B. Vijayasekaran, A.R. Alagappan, Further studies on the clinical efficacy of *Solanum xanthocarpum* and *Solanum trilobatum* in bronchial asthma, Phytother. Res. 18 (2004) 805–809.

[219] R.A. Yunes, M.G. Pizzolatti, A.E.G. Sant'Ana, G.E. Hawkes, J.B. Calixto, The structure of velutinol A, an anti-inflammatory compound with a novel pregnane skeleton, Phytochem. Anal. 4 (2) (1993) 76–81.

[220] E.P. Sabina, S. Chandal, M.K. Rasool, Inhibition of monosodium urate crystal-induced inflammation by withaferin A, J. Pharm. Pharm. Sci. 11 (2008) 46–55.

[221] C. Hou, L. Chen, L. Yang, X. Ji, An insight into anti-inflammatory effects of natural polysaccharides, Int. J. Biol. Macromol. 153 (2020) 248–255.

[222] Q. Guo, B. Li, C. Bao, Y. Li, Y. Cao, C. Wang, W. Wu, *Bletilla striata* polysaccharides improve hemostatic, anti-inflammatory efficacy, and platelet aggregation in gingivitis rat model, Starch 73 (2021) 2000185.

[223] X. Liu, K. Lai, Antitussive, anti-inflammatory and antioxidant activity of polysaccharides from *Asarum heterotropoides* in a guinea pig model for chronic cough induced by cigarette smoke exposure, Chest 149 (4, Supplement) (2016) A537.

[224] R. Illuri, B. Bethapudi, S. Anandakumar, S. Murugan, J.A. Joseph, D. Mundkinajeddu, A. Agarwal, C.V. Chandrasekaran, Anti-inflammatory activity of polysaccharide fraction of *Curcuma longa* extract (NR-INF-02), Antiinflamm. Antiallergy Agents Med. Chem. 14 (1) (2015) 53–62.

[225] L. Guo, R. Ma, H. Sun, A. Raza, J. Tang, Z. Li, Anti-inflammatory activities and related mechanism of polysaccharides isolated from *Sargentodoxa cuneata*, Chem. Biodivers. 15 (11) (2018), e1800343.

[226] M. Zhang, J. Wu, J. Han, H. Shu, K. Liu, Isolation of polysaccharides from *Dendrobium officinale* leaves and anti-inflammatory activity in LPS-stimulated THP-1 cells, Chem. Cent. J. 12 (1) (2018) 109.

[227] J. Sun, Y. Gou, J. Liu, H. Chen, J. Kan, C. Qian, N. Zhang, F. Niu, C. Jin, Anti-inflammatory activity of a water-soluble polysaccharide from the roots of purple sweet potato, RSC Adv. 10 (2020) 39673–39686.

[228] X. Ji, Q. Peng, H. Li, F. Liu, M. Wang, Chemical characterization and anti-inflammatory activity of polysaccharides from *Zizyphus jujube* cv. Muzao, Int. J. Food Eng. 13 (7) (2017) 20160382.

[229] D. Di Shao, W.D. Dunlop, E.M.K. Lui, M.A. Bernards, Immunostimulatory and anti-inflammatory polysaccharides from *Tripterygium wilfordii*: comparison with organic extracts, Pharm. Biol. 46 (1–2) (2008) 8–15.

[230] S.V. Popov, R.G. Ovodova, P.A. Markov, I.R. Nikitina, Y.S. Ovodov, Protective effect of comaruman, a pectin of cinquefoil *Comarum palustre* L., on acetic acid-induced colitis in mice, Dig. Dis. Sci. 51 (9) (2006) 1532–1537.

[231] R.A. Momin, D.L. De Witt, M.G. Nair, Inhibition of cyclooxygenase (COX) enzymes by compounds from *Daucus carota* L. seeds, Phytother. Res. 17 (2003) 976–979.

[232] L.P. Christensen, Galactolipids as potential health promoting compounds in vegetable foods, Recent Pat. Food Nutr. Agric. 1 (2009) 50–58.

[233] A. Murakami, Y. Nakamura, K. Koshimizu, H. Ohigashi, Glyceroglycolipids from *Citrus hystrix*, a traditional herb in Thailand, potently inhibit the tumor-promoting activity of 12-O-tetradecanoylphorbol 13-acetate in mouse skin, J. Agric. Food Chem. 43 (1995) 2779–2783.

[234] H.J. Park, S.J. Kim, S.J. Park, S.H. Eom, G.J. Gu, S.H. Kim, H.S. Youn, Phenethyl isothiocyanate regulates inflammation through suppression of the TRIF-dependent signaling pathway of Toll-like receptors, Life Sci. 92 (2013) 793–798.

[235] A. Kumar, A. Rahal, S. Chakraborty, R. Tiwari, S.K. Latheef, K. Dhama, *Ocimum sanctum* (Tulsi): a miracle herb and boon to medical science—a review, Int. J. Agron. Plant Prod. 4 (7) (2013) 1580–1589.

[236] S. Singh, V. Nair, S. Jain, Y.K. Gupta, Evaluation of anti-inflammatory activity of plant lipids containing alpha-linolenic acid, Indian J. Exp. Biol. 46 (2008) 453–456.

[237] T. Ringbom, U. Huss, A. Stenholm, S. Flock, L. Skattebol, P. Perera, L. Bohlin, COX-2 inhibitory effects of naturally occurring and modified fatty acids, J. Nat. Prod. 64 (2001) 745–749.

[238] D.S. Jang, M. Cuendet, B.-N. Su, S. Totura, S. Riswan, H.H.S. Fong, J.M. Pezzuto, A.D. Kinghorn, Constituents of the seeds of *Hernandia ovigera* with inhibitory activity against cyclooxygenase-2, Planta Med. 70 (2004) 893–896.

[239] S. Mohri, H. Takahashi, M. Sakai, S. Takahashi, N. Waki, K. Aizawa, H. Suganuma, T. Ara, Y. Matsumura, D. Shibata, T. Goto, T. Kawada, Wide-range screening of anti-inflammatory compounds in tomato using LC-MS and elucidating the mechanism of their functions, PLoS ONE 13 (1) (2018), e0191203.

[240] R. Bauer, A. Pröbstle, H. Lotter, W. Wagner-Redecker, U. Matthiesen, Cyclooxygenase inhibitory constituents from *Houttuynia cordata*, Phytomedicine 2 (1996) 305–308.

[241] M. Vergara, A. Olivares, C. Altamirano, Antiproliferative evaluation of tall-oil docosanol and tetracosanol over CHO-K1 and human melanoma cells, Electron. J. Biotechnol. 18 (4) (2015) 291–294.

[242] P. Picerno, G. Autore, S. Marzocco, M. Meloni, R. Sanogo, R.P. Aquino, Anti-inflammatory activity of verminoside from *Kigelia africana* and evaluation of cutaneous irritation in cell cultures and reconstituted human epidermis, J. Nat. Prod. 68 (2005) 1610–1614.

[243] T.H. Huang, V.H. Tran, R.K. Duke, S. Tan, S. Chrubasik, B.D. Roufogalis, C.C. Duke, Harpagoside suppresses lipopolysaccharide-induced iNOS and COX-2 expression through inhibition of NF-kappa B activation, J. Ethnopharmacol. 104 (1-2) (2006) 149–155.

[244] L.K. Yang, C. Khoo-Beattie, K.L. Goh, B.L. Chng, K. Yoganathan, Y.H. Lai, M.S. Butler, Ardisiaquinones from *Ardisia teysmanniana*, Phytochemistry 58 (8) (2001) 1235–1238.

[245] T.T. Dong, K.J. Zhao, Q.T. Gao, Z.N. Ji, T.T. Zhu, J. Li, R. Duan, A. W. Cheung, K.W. Tsim, Chemical and biological assessment of a chinese herbal decoction containing Radix Astragali and Radix Angelicae Sinensis: determination of drug ratio in having optimized properties, J. Agric. Food Chem. 54 (7) (2006) 2767–2774.

[246] S. Bose, B. Laha, S. Banerjee, Anti-inflammatory activity of isolated allicin from garlic with post-acoustic waves and microwave radiation, J. Adv. Pharm. Edu. Res. 3 (2013) 512–515.

[247] C.S.J. Woo, J. See, H. Lau, H. El-Nezami, Herbal medicine: toxicity and recent trends in assessing their potential toxic effects, in: L.F. Shyur, L. ASY (Eds.), Recent Trends in Medicinal Plants Research, vol. 62, 2012, pp. 365–384.

[248] N. Chattopadhyay, R. Maurya, Herbal Medicine. Reference Module in Biomedical Sciences, Elsevier Reference Collection, 2015.

Chapter 16

Mechanisms of antiinflammatory effects of naturally derived secondary metabolites

Ramakrishna Thilagar Uma Maheswari[a], Pradeep Kumar[b], and Mariappan Rajan[a]

[a]Department of Natural Products Chemistry, School of Chemistry, Madurai Kamaraj University, Madurai, Tamil Nadu, India, [b]Wits Advanced Drug Delivery Platform Research Unit, Department of Pharmacy and Pharmacology, School of Therapeutic Sciences, Faculty of Health Sciences, University of the Witwatersrand, Johannesburg, South Africa

1 Introduction

Inflammation is a biological response of the immune system that can be triggered by many factors, like microbes, infections, and damaged cells. Inflammation comes from the Latin word *inflammare*, which means "to set on fire." Inflammation is a response of a tissue to some injury that includes recruiting blood components, such as plasma proteins and leukocytes, to the injured tissue. It brings factors that cause inflammation aggravation, which including hormones, and most significant nutritional factors. The course of inflammation is controlled by immunological, physiological, and behavioral measures induced by intercellular signaling proteins called cytokines. Inflammation can be caused by some infections. While inflammation is needed for healing after injury, understanding the significant job and phases of irritation during the time spent mending is central to keep constant and weakening sicknesses from happening. Because of the circumstance and obsessive provisions, there are two significant types of inflammation: acute and chronic [1].

A physical issue or sickness can include intense, acute irritation that happens quickly upon injury and may remain for a couple of days. Microorganisms, allergens, toxins, burns, and frostbite are some of the causes of acute inflammation. During intense irritation, intrinsic invulnerable cells structure the primary line of safe safeguard and direct actuation of versatile, safe response [2]. On the other hand, chronic inflammation can go on for quite a long time. Inflammation was previously found in 5th century when Hippocrates perceived it as an early reaction to healing after injury and presented terms like edema and sepsis, which are still being used today [3].

Antiinflammatory activity of a bioactive compound essentially decreases the inflammatory responses. These drugs, called antiinflammatories, make up a part of all the "painkiller" drugs, helping relieve pain by lessening inflammation rather than by narcotic effects, which influence the focal apprehension to block pain signals to the brain. These medications are comprehensively grouped into two classifications: steroidal and nonsteroidal antiinflammatory drugs (NSAIDs). Some of them are at this point not utilized any longer due to their serious side effects. Some common examples of NSAIDs are aspirin, ibuprofen, and naproxen. Traditionally, people have been using powerful antiinflammatory medicines from plant sources for many years as a part of their herbal remedies and pharmaceutical arsenal. Additionally, secondary compounds derived from these plants may offer critical sources of antiinflammatory drugs [4]. Natural products are a major source for the discovery of new and potential therapeutic antiinflammatory drugs. A huge number of plant, microbial, and marine sources have been investigated for the purpose of producing bioactive compounds. Currently, the search for novel secondary metabolites is centered around microorganisms isolated from various sources; numerous bioactive metabolites, alluded to simply as novel substances, exhibit a wide variety of natural properties, such as antiinfective, antitumor, antiinflammatory, and antioxidant [2].

1.1 Secondary metabolites

Secondary metabolites are extensively described as organic compounds, synthesized by an organism, that are not critical to supporting that organism's growth and life. These compounds are produced by the organism and they confer some advantage, but are not needed for their primary metabolic action. The expression "secondary" presented by Albrecht Kossel in 1891 implies that, while essential metabolites are available in each living cell fit for cell division, the secondary metabolites are available unexpectedly and are not of vital importance to the lifeform's survival. Secondary metabolites are considered to be the finished results of

Recent Developments in Anti-Inflammatory Therapy. https://doi.org/10.1016/B978-0-323-99988-5.00013-9

essential metabolites, since they are implied by the pathways in which the essential metabolites are included. Secondary metabolites are thus considered the main metabolites' end products, because they are derived from the pathways in which the primary metabolites are involved. They are involved in ecological interaction, but are not required for the organism's survival [5] (Table 1).

Secondary metabolites regularly play a vital role in defense, such as defense against herbivory by plants, and other interspecies defenses. Humans use secondary metabolites as medicines, flavorings, pigments, and recreational drugs. More than 2,140,000 secondary metabolites are known and are normally grouped by their immense variety of design, capacity, and biosynthesis. There are five principal classes of secondary metabolites: terpenoids and steroids; fatty-acid derived substances and polyketides; alkaloids; nonribosomal polypeptides; and enzyme cofactors. This chapter focuses on phenolics, alkaloids, saponins, terpenes, and carbohydrates [5] (Fig. 1).

2 Secondary metabolites and their antiinflammatory activity

Metabolism can be described as the generally large number of biochemical reactions carried out by a living organism to maintain life [5]. Secondary metabolites, also known as toxins, secondary products, or bioactive compounds, are natural compounds produced by bacteria, fungi, plants, and others. Different phytochemical studies have determined that the presence of secondary metabolites, for example, anthraquinones, terpenoids, saponins, phenolic acids, and tannins, is of huge pharmacological value, with some having healing and therapeutic properties. The action of antiinflammatory and pain-relieving products, for example, antiinflammatory medicines such as indomethacin, was not discovered until the mid-1960s. This all changed in the 1970s, when John Vane found the system of activity of antiinflammatory medicines and other nonsteroidal antiinflammatory drugs (NSAIDs), expanding our capacity to develop novel therapeutic treatments [6]. The

achievements of NSAIDs in treating different inflammatory conditions such as rheumatoid joint pain (RA) and osteoarthritis (OA) proved the inhibition of the enzyme prostaglandin H synthase (PGHS) or cyclooxygenase (COX) as an appropriate objective in antianxiety treatments [7]. However, the gastrointestinal (GI) irritation levels related to continuous NSAID use ended up being an important drawback during long-term treatment [8].

All antiinflammatory drugs exert their impacts by reducing prostaglandin (PG) synthesis. PG synthesis is inhibited by impeding the catalyst cyclooxygenase, a chemical in the arachidonic acid (AA) pathway for the synthesis of prostanoids. The AA pathway is a fundamental part of the inflammatory response, because it rapidly causes damaged cell films by the activity of protein phospholipase A2 (PLA2). This film-based arachidonic acid catalyzed by cyclooxygenases (two isoforms: COX-1 and COX-2) brings about the development of prostaglandin G2 (PGG2); in a resulting peroxidase response PGG2 goes through a two-electron decrease to PGH2. PGH2 may then be followed up on by different chemicals to yield prostaglandins (PGD2, PGE2, PGF2), prostacyclin (PGI2), and thromboxane (THA2). Prostaglandins play a key role in the generation of the inflammatory response. The antiinflammatory effects of NSAIDs are carried out through COX-2 inhibitors (Fig. 2) [4].

Nuclear factor-kappa B protein (NF-κB) plays a significant role in bowel irritation, and expression and activation of NF-κB is displayed in human IBD. The expression of NF-κB isn't causative for IBD; however, it appears to assume a significant role in these conditions, so the inhibitors of NF-κB or IKK can be utilized as a treatment strategy for IBD [9]. The NF-κB proteins are confined in the cytoplasm of the cell and are related to a group of inhibitory proteins known as IκB. The IκB proteins are normally bound to NF-κB and block their nuclear localization signal. This load of provocative cytokines assumes a basic role in controlling the majority of inflammatory cycles, with the result that NF-κB acts as a switch for inflammation. Aspirin and different NSAIDs repress the action of the catalyst cyclooxygenase, which prompts the development of prostaglandins (PGs) that cause the irritation, swelling, pain, and fever that represent the inflammatory response.

3 Sources of secondary metabolites

Novel bioactive peptides from plants, animals, marine sponges, bacteria, and microalgae are additionally reported for their pharmacological effects in connection with inflammation. We present here a nondefinitive yet important list of the most important plant sources, depicting their circulation, plant parts utilized, known compound constituents, and pharmacological activity.

TABLE 1 Types of metabolites.

Primary metabolites	Secondary metabolites
Important for the growth and maintenance of cellular function.	Involved in ecological functions.
E.g., Amino acids, Vitamins, Organic acids, Lactic acids, Alcohol.	E.g., Phenolics, Alkaloids, Saponins, Terpenes, Lipids, Steroids, Antibiotics, Pigments.

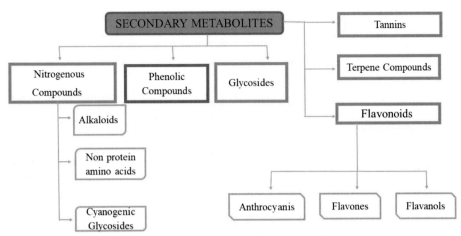

FIG. 1 Classification of secondary metabolites.

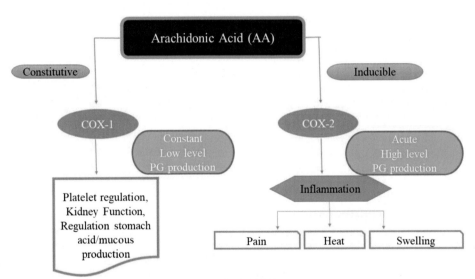

FIG. 2 Antiinflammatory effects of NSAIDs are mediated through COX-2 inhibition.

3.1 Plant sources

The number of plants used traditionally for treating inflammation is quite large, and the antiinflammatory activity of a number of these plants has been well reported [1]. Presently, despite the fact that drug discovery uses modern and innovative technology such as atomic displaying, combinatorial science, and other engineered scientific techniques, natural products are still of great interest as significant sources of drugs for human well-being. Large numbers of the normal compounds isolated from plants have shown powerful antiinflammatory activity in in-vitro and in-vivo animal models. They work by inhibiting the inflammation pathways along the lines of NSAIDs. Examples of major plant sources include *Curcuma longa*, *Camellia sinensis*, *Boswellia serrata*, andrographolide, magnolia species, raspberries, *Helichrysum italicum*, *Centella asiatica*, *Reynoutria*

japonica, *Rosa laevigata*, *Aloe vera*, *Ribes nigrum* L., *Zygophyllum simplex* L., *Gastrodia elata* root, *Fuligo septica*, *Adhatoda vasica*, among many others.

3.2 Marine sources

The marine environment represents one of the richest sources of antiinflammatory compounds; many biological entities living in seas and oceans are very useful to humans. Marine environments contain huge biodiversity, including species of fish, coral reefs, crabs, microorganisms, and parasites, having major therapeutic significance. Sources of potential therapeutic compounds, such as sesquiterpenoids, diterpenes, steroids, polysaccharides, alkaloids, fatty acids, protein, and other chemical compounds found in marine creatures, have shown antiinflammatory properties:

examples include *Enteromorpha prolifera*, *Fucoxanthin*, *Sarcophyton subviride*, *Streptomyces* sp., *Pseudopterogorgia elisabethae*, *Gorgonian Muricella* spp., algae, fungi, sponges, *Cyanobacteria*, *Stypopodium flabelliforme*, diterpenoids, *Psammocinia* spp., Zealand marine sponge, and *Dysidea avara*.

3.3 Microorganism sources

Microorganisms like parasites and microscopic organisms colonize the intercellular spaces of plant tissues. Unicellular creatures like microbes and yeasts incorporate probiotics from the gastrointestinal tract (GIT) that could be valuable for treatment of inflammation and infectious diarrhea. Common commensal microbes include *Bifidobacteria*, *Bacteroides fragilis*, *Escherichia coli*, *Bacillus* sp., *Psychroflexus torquis*, *Psychroflexus pacifica*, *Krokinobacter eikastus*, and *Krokinobacter diaphorus*, *Aureispira marina*, *Enterococcus faecium*, and *Streptomyces* sp.

3.4 Animal sources

The utilization of products from animal species in clinical practice is a long-time practice. The antiquity and persistence in the usage of restorative products from animals is a declaration of the significance of these remedial assets to humans: examples include honeybees, *Balaenoptera acutorostrata*, *Python reticulatus*, and *Sparus aurata* [1].

4 Isolation of secondary metabolites from plants and microorganisms

4.1 Isolation of secondary metabolites from plants

4.1.1 Conventional

The secondary metabolite from plant by various phytochemical strategies together with organic solvents, steam, and supercritical extraction was followed in the conventional methods. The advances in biotechnological strategies like plant tissue culture, enzyme, and fermentation technology have contributed to in-vitro synthesis and the production of plant secondary metabolites. The main processes used are discussed in the following paragraphs.

4.1.2 Immobilization

Generally cells or biocatalysts are held within a matrix by entanglement, adsorption, or covalent linkage. When a suitable substrate is added and optimum active compounds are provided, synthesis of the desired secondary metabolites takes place. Immobilization using a suitable bioreactor system has its benefits, like continuous process operation;

however, for the development of an immobilized plant cell culture process, natural or artificially induced secretion of the product into the encompassing medium is needed.

4.1.3 In-vitro tissue, organ, and cell culture

Under sterile condition plant cell, tissue cultures, and the extraction of secondary metabolites from various parts of the plants (plant leaves, stems, roots) are extracted. Secondary metabolites which are specified located in various tissues can be separated through suspension cultures [10].

4.2 Separation of secondary metabolites from microorganisms

4.2.1 Liquid fermentation

Secondary metabolites from microorganisms are useful products that are normally produced by liquid culture but can be produced by solid-state fermentation (SSF). Generally, fed-batch fermentation is useful for high yields as well as microbial growth so, it will help to production of secondary metabolites. Inoculum is developed after careful strain improvement of producing organism. Shake flask culture has been used for quite a long time to develop microscopic organisms. First, the cultures which are in active growth phase are shifted into a small fermenter and later into a main production medium. Several parameters are controlled the system like medium composition, pH, temperature, and agitation and aeration rate. For example, an inducer like methionine is used in cephalosporin fermentations, phosphate is restricted in chlortetracycline fermentations, and glucose is avoided in penicillin or erythromycin fermentations.

4.2.2 Solid-state fermentation (SSF)

Solid-state fermentation is defined as the fermentation process happens on in the absence of free water, with sufficient moisture to support microbial growth and metabolism, an important potential for the production of secondary metabolites. Mostly used in the food, pharmaceutical, cosmetic, fuel, textile industries. Depending on the nature of solid phase used it is separated into two types of SSF. (a) Solid culture of one support-substrate phase solid phase and (b) solid culture of two substrate-support phase solid phase. The advantages of SSF in connection with submerged fermentation include the fact that the energy requirement is generally low, since oxygen is moved directly to the microorganism. Also, secondary metabolites are normally created in high yields, frequently in a short time, and sterile conditions are frequently not required [10].

5 Mechanisms of secondary metabolite action and their value

5.1 Plant sources

- *B. serrata*: The plant *B. serrata* has been utilized for the treatment of inflammatory conditions for some time. Boswellic acid is isolated from the gum sap of this plant, and it viably inhibits leukotriene synthesis by means of 5-LOX. *Boswellia* helps to inhibit the indications of ongoing inflammatory conditions [11] (Fig. 3A).

- Strawberries, raspberries: A normally occurring phenolic acid (ellagic acid) is a bioactive compound lessening intense lung injury-related inflammation by diminishing COX-2 induced inflammation [10].

- Turmeric: *C. longa* contains polysaccharides and has been investigated in many major and ongoing inflammatory models. Curcumin has the ability to inhibit COX-2, LOX, and iNOS. Improper upregulation of COX-2 or possibly iNOS has been connected to the pathophysiology of explicit types of human cancer as well as inflammatory disorders [10,12].

- *Andrographis paniculata*: Andrographolide is a significant dynamic compound isolated from this plant (14-deoxy-11,12-didehydroandrographolide, neondrographolide). It shows a decrease in the production of proinflammatory arbiters, for example, COX-2, iNOS, and cytokines such as IL-1β, IL-6, and IL-10, and decreases the actuation of record factors such as NF-κB, AP-1, STAT3, and NFAT and inhibits intracellular signaling pathways [11,13].

- *A. vera*: The anthraquinones, including aloe-emodin and chrysophanol, tricyclic sweet-smelling quinones containing salicylic acid, saponins, beta-carotene, nutrient B12, folic acid, and choline, help the skin to heal rapidly [13–15] (Fig. 3B).

- *H. italicum:* New acetophenone subsidiary of 12-acetoxytremetone (4-hydroxy-3-(3-methyl-2-butenyl) acetophenone) is another double inhibitor of arachidonate digestion, and it is utilized in antiinflammatory

and pain-relieving drugs. The acylphloroglucinol arzanol has recently been proposed as a pharmalogically active solution for inhibiting the activation of inflammatory transcription factor NF-κB, HIV replication in T cells, and release of IL-1β, IL-6, IL-8, and TNF-α [11,16].

- *R. japonica:* Another dynamic compound, emodin-6-*O*-β-ᴅ-glucoside, has been shown to provide strong antiinflammatory and barrier protective effects in HUVE cells and also in animal models [17].

- *C. asiatica:* Asiaticoside has been used for some time as a memory enhancer drug in India. Since triterpenoid and flavonoids have antiinflammatory activity, dextropropoxyphene and indomethacin are significant for pain-relieving and antiinflammatory activities. These impacts could be associated with the inhibition of proinflammatory arbiters, including TNF-α and IL-6 levels, COX-2 expression, and PGE2 production, as with MPO action [11,18].

- *R. laevigata*: Bioassay-guided fractionation afforded two new 19-oxo-18,9-seco-ursane-type triterpenes, ursane-type triterpene lactone saponine, and oleanane-type triterpenoids. Isolation of three new kinds of triterpenoids inhibited the LPS-induced NF-κBT transcriptional activity [11,19,20].

- Blackcurrant (*R. nigrum* L.): Contains proanthocyanidins (PACs), the main mechanism of which mostly lies in interference with migration of leukocytes and inhibition of in-vivo nitric oxide [21].

- *Z. simplex* L.: Five significant phenolic compounds were extracted (myricitrin, luteolin, isorhamnetin, and others) from this plant as antiinflammatories [22].

- *G. elata* root (Orchidaceae) showed antiinflammatory properties as well as inhibition of the activity of COX-1, II; results showed that phenolic compounds of GE are antiinflammatory [23].

- *F. septica*: Phenanthroindolizidine alkaloids (tylophorinedehydrotylophorine, ficuseptine-A) were extracted from the leaves of *F. septica*; their calming effects are

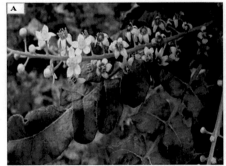
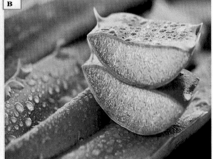

FIG. 3   Image of (A) *Boswellia serrata* and (B) *Aloe barbadensis* Miller.

applied by inhibiting expression of the proinflammatory factors and related signaling pathways [24].

- *A. vasica*: Contains the quinazoline alkaloids vasicine, 7-hydroxyvasicine, vasicinolone, 3-deoxyvasicine, vasicol, vasicoline, vasicolinone, adhatodine, and anisotine as main compounds exhibiting antiinflammatory effects [25].

- Turkish berberis: Roots and bark have isoquinoline alkaloids, to be specific, berberine, berbamine, palmatine, oxyacanthine, magnoflorine, and columbamine, which exhibit antiinflammatory actions [26].

- *Dysoxylum gotadhora*: New terpenoids, cyclolanostane triterpenoids and isopimarane diterpenoids, displayed important inhibition of nitric oxide production incited by lipopolysaccharide [27].

- *Bupleurum rotundifolium* L. (Apiaceae): Saponins isolated from this species were found to have antiinflammatory activity against both 12-O-tetradecanoylphorbol-13-acetic acid derivation (TPA)-induced ear edema and persistent skin inflammation [28].

- *Garcinia cambogia*: Extracts diminished MPO activity, COX-2, and iNOS expression. Moreover, this treatment was able to reduce PGE2 and IL-1β colonic levels. It did not display any mortality or toxicity signals after being given orally [29,30].

- *Inonotus obliquus* (mushroom): Six principal constituents were isolated: lanosterol, 3-hydroxy-8, 24-diene-21-al, ergosterol, inotodiol, ergosterol peroxide, and trametenolic acid, which showed antiinflammatory activity. *Coriolus versicolor* and *Prunus mume* extracts have also been found to have anti-IBD effects, which likely occurred due to the attenuating proinflammatory gene expression, especially that of TNF-α, IL-4, and IL-1ß [29,31] (Table 2).

5.2 Marine sources

- Stypopodium: *Stypopodium zonale* had three antiinflammatory diterpenes extracted, and stypoquinonic acid, taondiol, and atomaric acid were additionally isolated, exhibiting potent effective antiinflammatory action identified with the inhibition of leukocyte amassing [35].

- *P. elisabethae*: This organism contains diterpene pentose glycosides, and seco-pseudopterosins; diterpene glycosides are antiinflammatory, inhibiting PGE2 and LTC4 production in zymosan-invigorated murine peritoneal macrophages. This information suggests that the pseudopterosins may intervene in their

TABLE 2 Plant sources of secondary metabolites.

S. No.	Source	Part	Activity	Reference
1.	*Boswellia serrata*	Gum resin	Antiarthritic, Antiinflammatory	[11,32]
2.	Turmeric	Full part	Antiinflammatory, Anticancer, Antimicrobial, Neuroprotective	[10,12]
3.	*Andrographis paniculata*	Aerial part, root	Antiinflammatory, Diabetes, High blood pressure, Ulcer, Hansen's disease	[10–14,33,34]
4.	*Helichrysum italicum*	Root	Antiinflammatory, Allergies, Wound healing, Muscle and joint inflammation	[11,16]
5.	*Reynoutria japonica*	Full part	Antiinflammatory, Skin disorder, Lung diseases	[17]
6.	*Centella asiatica*	Full part	Antiinflammatory, Skin diseases, Antioxidant, Antimicrobial activity	[11,18]
7.	*Rosa laevigata*	Full part	Antiinflammatory, Antioxidant, Antiproliferative, Antinociceptive, Antimicrobial	[11,19,20]
8.	*Zygophyllum simplex* L.	Leaves, Fruits, Stems	Antiinflammatory, Local anesthetic, Antihistamine, Antidiabetic agent	[22]
9.	*Gastrodia elata*	Root, Tuber	Antiinflammatory, Antiangiogenic, Vertigo, Stroke	[23]
10.	Turkish berberis	Root, Bark	Antiinflammatory, Antinociceptive, Antipyretic, Anticancer, Liver disease, Hyperglycemia	[26]
11.	*Bupleurum rotundifolium* L.	Root	Antiinflammatory, Fever, Malaria, Chronic liver diseases	[28]

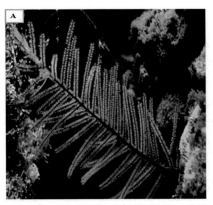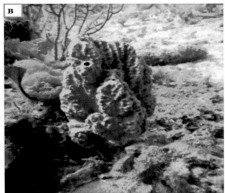

FIG. 4 Image of (A) *Pseudopterogorgia kallos* and (B) *Stylissa caribica.*

antiinflammatory impacts by inhibiting eicosanoid discharge from inflamed cells [35,36] (Fig. 4A).

- *D. avara* marine sponges: Isolation of 4-methyl aminoavaronr regular substance with a sesquiterpenoid subbed quinone exhibited antiinflammatory activity, possibly resulting from the inhibition of eicosanoid delivery and discouragement of superoxide age in leukocytes [37].

- *Stylissa* species: Separation of two new bisimidazopyrano-imidazole bromopyrrole ether alkaloids, stylissadines A and B, for their particular bioactive antiinflammatory action [38].

- *Stylissa* aff. *carteri*: Three new dimeric pyrrole-2-aminoimidazole alkaloids, futunamine, pyrrolo1, 2-imidazole center, have been isolated and have shown antiinflammatory activity [39] (Fig. 4B).

- *E. prolifera*: Pheophytin has been isolated and shown to inhibit 12-*O*-tetradecanoylphorbol-13-acetic acid derivation (TPA)-actuated superoxide extremist ($O_2^{\bullet}$) and inflammatory reactions in mouse macrophages [40].

- Secondary metabolites obtained from marine green growth known to have promising antiinflammatory activity are new cyclic heptapeptides, cyclomarins, which have been isolated from a marine bacterium [40].

- Pheophytin in green alga *E. prolifera* has shown to be an intense suppressive substance against superoxide anion and TPA-induced inflammatory response [41].

- Red-green algae of the class Gracilaria have been shown to be a significant source of antiinflammatory compounds and alkaloids with explained organic activity [38] (Table 3).

5.3 Microorganism sources

P. torquis, P. pacifica, K. eikastus, and *K. diaphorus, A. marina* (a gliding bacterium) produce the main compounds of arachidonic acid (about 40%) that show antiinflammatory activities.

TABLE 3 Marine sources of secondary metabolites.

S. No.	Source	Activity	Reference
1.	*Stypopodium*	Pythiaceous fungi and the human fungal pathogen *Cryptococcus neoformans*	[35]
2.	*Pseudopterogorgia elisabethae*	Antiinflammatory, Antianalgesic	[35,36]
3.	*Dysidea avara* marine sponges	Antiinflammatory, Antimicrobial activity	[37]
4.	*Stylissa* aff. *carteri*	Antiinflammatory, Anticancer	[39]
5.	Marine bacterium	Antiinflammatory, Antifungal, Antidiabetic	[40]

- *Streptomyces* sp.: Isolated from *Ficus benjamina*: 5,7-dimethoxy-4-pmethoxyphenyl coumarin and 5,7-dimethoxy-4-phenyl coumarin were extracted from *Streptomyces aureofaciens* CMUAc130, and had antiinflammatory activities [42].

- *Bacillus subtilis*: Flavonoids can diminish inflammatory reactions by adjusting the NF-κB signaling pathway, just as further developing intestinal boundary integrity, *B. subtilis*-fermented beans are good natural sources for antioxidant and antiinflammatory source [43,44].

- *E. faecium*: *E. faecium, Lactobacillus rhamnosus* GG MTCC 1408, and LCS show an antiinflammatory impact by inhibiting TNF-α production and upregulating IL-10 levels in LPS-induced macrophage cell lines [45].

- *Aspergillus terreus*: An uncommon austinoid, 1,2-dehydro-terredehydroaustin with known meroterpenoids, has been isolated from the fungus, having the capacity to genuinely impact immunocompromised patients who need explicitly resistant cells. Specifically, the patient has prolonged neutropenia and the animal has fungal infectious [46,47].

- *Agaricus bisporus*: An isolated polysaccharide (fucogalactan) showed inhibition of neurogenic and inflammatory phases, antinociceptive effects, and antiinflammatory activity [48].
- *Caripia montagnei*: Glucans from this mushroom diminished inflammatory infiltrate produced by thioglycolate-actuated peritonitis by 75.5%; in addition, NO level, IL-1ra, IL-10, and IFN-γ decreased, showing antiinflammatory actions [49].
- *Agaricus blazei*: This mushroom has polysaccharides that inhibited β-hexosaminidase degranulation and prostaglandin D and leukotriene C production, showing antiinflammatory actions [50,51] (Table 4).

5.4 Animal sources

- *P. reticulatus*: Python snake bile has bile acids, bile salts, proteins, glutathione, nutrient E, and melatonin, which have shown antiinflammatory actions [52] (Fig. 5A).
- *S. aurata*: Inflammatory reaction in gilthead sea bream revealed a sublethal mixture of carbamazepine, cadmium chloride, and polybrominated diphenyl ether [53].

TABLE 4 Microorganism sources of secondary metabolites.

S. No.	Source	Activity	Reference
1.	*Streptomyces* sp.	Pythiaceous fungi and the human fungal pathogen *Cryptococcus neoformans*	[42]
2.	*Bacillus subtilis*	Antiinflammatory, Antioxidant	[43,44]
3.	*Enterococcus faecium*	Antiinflammatory, Antioxidant, Antihypertensive	[45]
4.	*Aspergillus terreus*	Antiinflammatory, Anticancer, Antimicrobial, Antifilarial	[46,47]
5.	*A. bisporus*	Antiinflammatory, Antioxidant, Antinociceptive	[48]

- Honey: Honey has flavonoids (flavanonols, flavonols, flavones, isoflavones, anthocyanins, and anthocyanidins) and phenolic compounds that promoted wound healing, helped the patients to recover from discomfort zone and diminished inflammation response. Hydrogen peroxide is responsible for the antiinflammatory behavior [54,55] (Fig. 5B).
- Fish oil, rich in omega-3 polyunsaturated fats, reduces arachidonic acid content in invulnerable and endothelial cells, prompting lower inflammatory activity [1]. The animal sources of secondary metabolites are presented in Table 5.

6 Current antiinflammatory therapy based on secondary metabolites

Nonsteroidal antiinflammatory drugs in Parkinson's disease (PD) address a remedial methodology opportunity for this neurological issue. In fact, it has been shown that cyclooxygenase type 2 (COX-2) is upregulated in SNc dopaminergic neurons in both PD patients and animal models of PD and, in addition, nonsteroidal antiinflammatory drugs (NSAIDs) pretreatment secures against 1-methyl-4-phenyl-1,2,3,6-tetrahydropyridine (MPTP) or 6-hydroxydopamine (6-OHDA)-actuated nigrostriatal dopamine degeneration. NSAIDs may apply their neuroprotective activities inhibiting COX compounds as well as by following up on NF-κB, iNOS, PPARγ, inhibiting the development of DA quinones, searching ROS, and RNS activity likely by other unknown systems. It has recently been suggested that antiinflammatory compounds may inhibit microglial multiplication, affecting the cell cycle activity and apoptosis; epidemiological information investigating the viability of NSAIDs in anticipation of PD and their conceivable use as adjuvants in the treatment of this neurodegenerative condition will likewise be analyzed.

6.1 Antiinflammatory therapies for atherosclerosis

The utilization of antiinflammatory treatments for atherosclerosis is fundamentally founded on either observational or some interventional studies that assess proxy markers of inflammation action. All things considered, this information is critical to comprehend the role of inflammation in atherosclerosis and to configure randomized controlled studies to assess the impact of explicit antiinflammatory procedures on cardiovascular outcomes. Randomized controlled trials (RCTs) to examine antiinflammatory drugs for the treatment of atherosclerosis are fundamental before the value of such treatment as a feature of secondary cardiovascular counteraction can be anticipated. A few stages are needed for the effective improvement of antiinflammatory

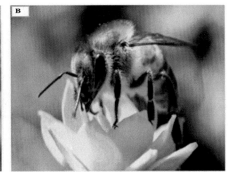

FIG. 5 Image of (A) *Python reticulatus* and (B) *Apidae corbiculate.*

TABLE 5 Animal sources of secondary metabolites.

S. No.	Source	Part	Activity	Reference
1.	*Python reticulatus*	Bodies, Blood	Antiinflammatory, Rheumatism, Broken bones	[52]
2.	*Sparus aurata*	Skin	Antiinflammatory, Antioxidant	[53]
3.	Honeybee	Honey	Antiinflammatory, Antioxidant, Antibacterial, Antiviral	[54,55]

treatments for atherosclerosis tests, to contemplate giving the reasoning and confirmation of ideas regarding expected targets; observational and biomarker concentrates with regard to human disease; and major RCTs to characterize the suitable target population, treatment periods, results, and expectation of potential adverse effects [55].

6.2 Antiinflammatory therapy with canakinumab for atherosclerotic disease

Clinical information suggests that lessening inflammation without influencing lipid levels might reduce the danger of cardiovascular illness. Canakinumab, a restorative monoclonal immunizer focused on interleukin-1β, underwent a randomized trial including 10,061 patients with past myocardial localized necrosis and a high-affectability C-responsive protein level of 2 mg. Antiinflammatory treatment, focused on the interleukin-1β inhibitor with canakinumab at a dosage of 150 mg at regular intervals, prompted a fundamentally lower rate of repeated cardiovascular events than placebo, with no effect on lipid concentrations [56].

- In September 2016, the FDA approved the expanded use of canakinumab for three additional uncommon autoinflammatory diseases, including Tumor Necrosis Factor Receptor-Associated Periodic Syndrome (TRAPS) [57].
- In June 2020, canakinumab was approved in the UK to treat active Still's disease, including Adult-Onset Still's Disease (AOSD).

6.3 Activities of *Malaxis muscifera*

These plants showed promising antiinflammatory maturing action in in-vitro derived plantlets, in which were uncovered numerous bioactive metabolites, such as dietary unsaturated fats, phenolic acids, sterols, and amino acids, which explains the use of this plant as antiaging ingredients in numerous ayurvedic formulations.

6.4 Secondary metabolite profiling, antiinflammatory potential [58]

Nardostachys jatamansi is an esteemed, fragrant spice utilized in Ayurvedic and Unani medicinal practices. Antiinflammatory and antityrosinase (5-lipoxygenase and hyaluronidase) properties of various plant parts used as delivering system for delivering bioactive compounds [59].

6.5 *Garcinia indica* as antiinflammatory

A benzophenone from the natural product has an antiinflammatory impact by means of regulating arachidonic acid metabolism; it serves to inhibit iNOS expression, NF-B action, and COX-2 expression; it has likewise been studied for cell antioxidant and anticancer activity. It also has antiobesity and hepatoprotective effects, and can possibly be utilized in renal disease, endometriosis, and heart failure [60].

6.6 Marine alkaloids with antiinflammatory activity

Compounds can be found in sponges, microorganisms, ascidians, and cnidarians. Very few investigations have distinguished and described them. Specifically, studies on kelp alkaloids should be renewed to clarify the full scope of the natural activities of these compounds, particularly their antiinflammatory potential [61].

6.7 Large-scale bioprospecting of cyanobacteria and micro-/macroalgae from the Aegean Sea

The capacity of cyanobacteria and micro-/macroalgae as sources of antimicrobial, antitumor, and antiinflammatory compounds has been accounted for widely. A concentrate from the earthy colored algae *Dilophus fasciola* showed the most noteworthy antiinflammatory activity as estimated in essential microglial and astrocyte cell cultures and by the decrease of proinflammatory cytokines [62,63].

6.8 Zinc: An antioxidant and antiinflammatory agent

Zinc in humans assumes a significant role in cell-mediated immune functions and is likewise a cancer prevention agent and antiinflammatory. Zinc is used to several signaling roles for immune system and numerous record factors engaged with the quality expression of inflammatory cytokines and adhesion particles are directed by zinc. Zinc concentrate supplementation in older people have shown a diminished frequency of infections, diminished oxidative stress, and diminished generation of inflammatory cytokines [64].

6.9 Onion as antiinflammatory agent

Onions contain strong cancer prevention agents that intensify the inflammatory battle against numerous diseases. The highest content of sodium, zinc, and calcium have been found in red onions. The compounds furfuraldehyde, 2-methyl-2-pentenal, and 1-propanethiol are helping to decrease inflammation and oxidative stresses. Water tests of *Allium cepa* L. show an antiinflammatory reaction in the lipoxygenase inhibitor [65,66].

6.10 Tomatoes as antiinflammatory agent

Tomatoes are a source of abundant lycopene, which provides strong cell protection against inflammation. It decreases the danger of provoking inflammation, so lycopene serves as an antiinflammatory agent, preventing inflammatory cytokine production [67].

7 Conclusion

This chapter examines the significance of secondary metabolic processes from different origins such as plants and microorganisms, including microbes, fungi, and marine organisms, and their antiinflammatory actions, normal synthesis, and segregation guidelines and strategies for different sources. Mechanisms of secondary metabolite activity and current antiinflammatory treatments are examined. The marine environments are rich sources of compounds with currently exhibited antimicrobial, antitumor, anticoagulant, and antiinflammatory activities. Many individuals today are interested in treating inflammation by numerous natural remedies available on the market from natural producers, drugstores, and grocery stores, and self-medicating with these substances is commonplace. The need is great for new sources of bioactive secondary metabolites with novel activity. Specialized metabolites are one of the fundamental sources of such discovery and development, and these metabolites are easily accessible for study. Secondary metabolites with significant organic activity are thus considered an important option for obtaining a major portion of engineered drugs and other economically important compounds. Nowadays, we know that diet and lifestyle changes can assist with forestalling constant inflammation. Eating more natural products from food sources that have omega-3-unsaturated fats, such as salmon, fish, pecans, flax seeds, and soybeans, grapes, celery, blueberries, garlic, olive oil, ginger, rosemary, and turmeric, can help to prevent acute and chronic inflammation.

Acknowledgment

M. Rajan appreciates the financial support under the plan of the Rashtriya Uchchatar Shiksha Abhiyan (Ref. 007-R2/RUSA/MKU/2020-21).

References

[1] J. Parag, P. Ravindra, S. Shivshankar, Inflammation. Natural Resources and Its Applications, Springer, New Delhi, Heidelberg, New York, Dordrecht, London, 2015, pp. 25–102.

[2] D.R. Germolec, K.A. Shipkowski, R.P. Frawley, E. Evans, Markers of inflammation, in: Methods Molecular Biology, vol. 1803, Immunotoxicity Testing, 2018, pp. 57–79.

[3] R. Medzhitov, Origin and physiological roles of inflammation, Nature 454 (7203) (2008) 428–435.

[4] P. Rao, E.E. Knaus, Evolution of nonsteroidal anti-inflammatory drugs (NSAIDs): cyclooxygenase (COX) inhibition and beyond, J. Pharm. Pharm. Sci. 11 (2) (2008) 81–110.

[5] D. Thirumurugan, A. Cholarajan, S.S. Raja, R. Vijayakumar, An introductory chapter: secondary metabolites, in: Second Metabolites—Sources and Application, IntechOpen, 2018, pp. 1–21.

[6] J.R. Vane, Inhibition of prostaglandin synthesis as a mechanism of action for aspirin-like drugs, Nat. New Biol. 43 (1971) 232–235.

[7] J.R. Vane, The mode of action of aspirin and similar compounds, J. Allergy Clin. Immunol. 58 (6) (1976) 691–712.

[8] S. Moncada, S.H. Ferreira, J.R. Vane, Prostaglandins, aspirin-like drugs and the oedema of inflammation, Nature 246 (1973) 217–219.

[9] D. Trishna, D.H. Kim, O.L. Beong, Natural products as a source of anti-inflammatory agents associated with inflammatory bowel disease, Molecules 18 (2013) 7253–7270.

[10] A.L. Demain, Pharmaceutically active secondary metabolites of microorganisms, Appl. Microbiol. Biotechnol. 52 (4) (1999) 455–463.

[11] P. Pushpangadan, T.P. Ijinu, V. George, Plant based anti-inflammatory secondary metabolites, Ann. Phytomed. 4 (1) (2015) 17–36.

[12] N. Chainani-Wu, Safety and anti-inflammatory activity of curcumin: a component of Tumeric (*Curcuma longa*), J. Altern. Complement. Med. 9 (1) (2003) 161–168.

[13] M.D. Boudreau, F.A. Beland, An evaluation of the biological and toxicological properties of *Aloe barbadensis* (Miller), *Aloe vera*, J. Environ. Sci. Health C Environ. Carcinog. Ecotoxicol. Rev. 24 (2006) 103–154.

[14] E. Ernst, Adverse effects of herbal drugs in dermatology, Br. J. Dermatol. 143 (5) (2000) 923–929.

[15] B.K. Vogler, E. Ernst, *Aloe vera*: a systematic review of its clinical effectiveness, Br. J. Gen. Pract. 49 (447) (1999) 823–828.

[16] S. Araceli, R.M. Carmen, R.S. Gillermo, M. Salvador, M.G. Rosa, et al., A new dual inhibitor of arachidonate metabolism isolated from *Helichrysum italicum*, Eur. J. Pharmacol. 460 (2–3) (2003) 219–226.

[17] L. Wonhwa, K. Sae- Kwang, J.-S. Bae, Emodin-6-O-β-D-glucoside down-regulates endothelial protein C receptor shedding, Arch. Pharm. Res. 36 (9) (2013) 1160–1165.

[18] S. Saha, T. Guria, T. Singha, T. Maity, Evaluation of analgesic and anti-inflammatory activity of chloroform and methanol extracts of *Centella asiatica* Linn, ISRN Pharmacol. 2013 (2013) 1–6. Article ID: 789613.

[19] Z. Na, S. Yang, L.-Z. Li, W.-H. Jiao, P.-Y. Gao, S.-J. Song, W.-S. Chen, H.-W. Lin, Anti-inflammatory triterpenes from the leaves of *Rosa laevigata*, J. Nat. Prod. 74 (4) (2011) 732–738.

[20] M. Yan, Y. Zhu, H.-J. Zhang, W.-H. Jiao, B.-N. Han, Z.-X. Liu, Q. Feng, W.-S. Chen, H.-W. Lin, Anti-inflammatory secondary metabolites from the leaves of *Rosa laevigata*, Bioorg. Med. Chem. 21 (11) (2013) 3290–3297.

[21] V. Michael, C. Sean, S. Derek, S.C. Andersson, S. Verrall, E. Johansson, K. Rumpunen, Phenolic compounds in blackcurrant (*Ribes nigrum L.*) leaves relative to leaf position and harvest date. *Journal of*, Food Chem. 172 (2015) 135–142.

[22] M.S. Mohammed, W.J. Osman, E.A. Garelnabi, Z. Osman, B. Osman, H.S. Khalid, M.A. Mohamed, Secondary metabolites as anti-inflammatory agents, J. Phytopharmacol. 3 (4) (2014) 275–285.

[23] R. Al-Halabi, M. Bou Chedid, R. Abou Merhi, H. El-Hajj, H. Zahr, R. Schneider-Stock, A. Bazarbachi, H. Gali-Muhtasib, Gallotannin inhibits NFκB Signaling and growth of human colon cancer xenografts, Cancer Biol. Ther. 12 (1) (2011) 59–68.

[24] C.-W. Yang, W.-L. Chen, P.-L. Wu, H.-Y. Tseng, S.-J. Lee, Anti-inflammatory mechanisms of phenanthroindolizidine alkaloids, Mol. Pharmacol. 69 (2006) 749–758.

[25] A. Chakraborty, A.H. Brantner, Study of alkaloids from *Adhatoda vasica* Nees on their anti-inflammatory activity, Phytother. Res. 15 (2001) 532–534.

[26] J.M. Barbosa-Filho, M.R. Piuvezam, M.D. Moura, M.S. Silva, K.V.B. Lima, E.V.L. da-Cunha, I.M. Fechine, O.S. Takemura, Anti-inflammatory activity of alkaloids: a twenty-century review, Braz. J. Pharmacogn. 16 (1) (2006) 109–139.

[27] J. Kan, L.-L. Chen, F.W. Shu, W. Yi, T. Li, K. Gao, Anti-inflammatory terpenoids from the leaves and twigs of *Dysoxylum gotadhora*, J. Nat. Prod. 78 (5) (2015) 1037–1044.

[28] D.N. Quang, T. Hashimoto, Y. Arakawa, et al., Grifolin derivatives from *Albatrellus caeruleoporus*, new inhibitors of nitric oxide production in RAW264.7 cells, Bioorg. Med. Chem. 14 (1) (2006) 164–168.

[29] S.Y. Choi, S.J. Hur, C.S. An, Y.H. Jeon, Y.J. Jeoung, J.P. Bak, B.O. Lim, Anti-inflammatory effects of *Inonotus obliquus* in colitis induced by dextran sodium sulfate, Biomed. Res. Int. (2010).

[30] S.B. Dos Reis, C.C. de Oliveira, S.C. Acedo, D.D. Miranda, M.L. Ribeiro, J. Pedrazzoli Jr., A. Gambero, Attenuation of colitis injury in rats using *Garcinia cambogia* extract, Phytother. Res. 23 (2009) 324–329.

[31] B.O. Lim, *Coriolus versicolor* suppresses inflammatory bowel disease by inhibiting the expression of STAT1 and STAT6 associated with IFN-γ and IL-4 expression, Phytother. Res. 25 (8) (2011) 1257–1261.

[32] B. Nirit, A. Muhammad, D. Muhammad, K. Hinanit, F. Marcelo, G. Jonathan, Anti-inflammatory potential of medicinal plants: a source for therapeutic secondary metabolites, Adv. Agron. 150 (2018) 131–183.

[33] V.P. Menon, R.S. Adluri, Antioxidant and anti-inflammatory properties of curcumin. The molecular target and therapeutic uses of curcumin in health and disease, Adv. Exp. Med. Biol. (2007) 105–125.

[34] Y.S. Lee, H.K. Ju, Y.J. Kim, T.G. Lim, M.R. Uddin, Y.B. Kim, J.H. Baek, S.W. Kwon, K.W. Lee, H.S. Seo, S.U. Park, Enhancement of anti-inflammatory activity of *Aloe vera* adventitious root extracts through the alteration of primary and secondary metabolites via salicylic acid elicitation, PLoS One 8 (12) (2013) 1–13.

[35] J.A. Maria, M.B. Luis, B. Paulina, Bioactive secondary metabolites from octocoral-associated microbes-new chances for blue growth, Mar. Drugs 16 (2018) 485.

[36] A.L. Saally, F. William, S.J. Robert, C. Jon, The pseudopterosins: anti-inflammatory and analgestic natural products from sea whip *Pseudopterogorgia elisabethae*, Proc. Natl. Acad. Sci. U. S. A. 83 (17) (1986) 6238–6240.

[37] R. Puliti, S. De Rosa, A.M. Carlo, 4-Methylaminoavarone from *Dysidea avara*, Acta Crystallogr. Sect. C Cryst. Struct. Commun. 54 (12) (1998) 1954–1957.

[38] M.K. Renner, Y.C. Shen, X.-C. Cheng, P.R. Jensen, W. Frankmoelle, C.A. Kauffman, et al., Cyclomarins A-C, new anti-inflammatory cyclic peptides produced by a marine bacterium (*Streptomyces* sp.), J. Am. Chem. Soc. 121 (49) (1999) 11273–11276.

[39] M.G. Maria, G. Sandra, K.J. Laurence, G.J. Gregory, C. Kevin, A. Amparo, M.B. Luis, P.T. Oluvier, Futunamine a pyrrole-imidazole alkaloid from sponge *Stylissa* aff. *carteri* collected off the Futuna Islands, J. Nat. Prod. 83 (7) (2020) 2299–2304.

[40] P. Ratih, S.-K. Kim, Biological activities and health benefit effects of natural pigments derived from marine algae, J. Funct. Foods (2011) 255–266.

[41] O. Yasuji, H.O. Kiyoka, Potent anti-inflammatory activity of pheophytin a derived from edible green alga, *Enteromorpha prolifera* (Sujiao-nori), Int. J. Immunopharmacol. 19 (1997) 355–358.

[42] C.L.F. Almeida, H.d.S. Falcao, G.R.d.M. Lima, C.d.A. Montenegro, N.S. Lira, P.F. de Athayde-Filho, et al., Bioactivities from marine algae of the genus *Gracilaria*, Int. J. Mol. Sci. 12 (2011) 4550–4573.

[43] V.L. Hong-Ting, L. Wen-Jung, T. Guo-Jane, H. Pai-An, Enhanced anti-inflammatory activity of brown seaweed *Laminaria japonica* by fermentation using *Bacillus subtilis*, Process Biochem. 51 (12) (2016) 1945–1953.

[44] S.S. Han, et al., A comparison of antioxidative and anti-inflammatory activities of sword beans and soybeans fermented with *Bacillus subtilis*, Food Funct. 6 (8) (2015) 2736–2748.

[45] O. Yasuji, H.-O. Kiyoka, Potent anti-inflammatory activity of pheophytin a derived from edible green alga, *Enteromorpha prolifera*, Int. J. Immunopharmacol. 19 (6) (1997) 355–358.

[46] L. Zhaoming, L. Hongju, C. Yaan, S. Zhigang, A new anti-inflammatory meroterpenoid from the fungus *Aspergillus terreus* H010, Nat. Prod. Res. 32 (22) (2018) 2652–2656.

[47] G. Szakacs, G. Morovjan, R. Tengerdy, Production of lovastatin by a wild strain of *Aspergillus terreus*, Biotechnol. Lett. 20 (4) (1998) 411–415.

[48] A.C. Ruthes, Y.D. Rattmann, S.M. Malquevicz-Paiva, et al., *Agaricus bisporus* fucogalactan structural characterization and pharmacological approaches, Carbohydr. Polym. 92 (1) (2013) 184–191.

[49] L.S. Queiroz, M.S. Nascimento, A.K.M. Cruz, Glucans from the *Caripia montagnei* mushroom present anti-inflammatory activity, Int. Immunopharmacol. 10 (1) (2010) 34–42.

[50] H.-H. Song, H.-S. Chae, S.-R. Oh, H.-K. Lee, Y.-W. Chin, Anti-inflammatory and anti-allergic effect of *Agaricus blazei* extract in bone marrow-derived mast cells, Am. J. Chin. Med. 40 (5) (2012) 1073–1084.

[51] M.P. Marina, A.L. Ana, J.C. Pergentino, G.V. Luis, F. Fabio, Anti-inflammatory activity of aqueous and alkaline extracts from mushrooms (*Agaricus blazei* Murill), J. Med. Food 12 (2) (2009) 359–364.

[52] M.M. Thwin, P. Gopalakrishnakone, R. Manjunathakini, A. Armugam, K. Jeyaseelan, Recombinant antitoxic and anti-inflammatory factor from the nonvenomous snake *Python reticulatus*: phospholipase A2 inhibition and venom neutralizing potential, Biochemistry 39 (31) (2000) 9604–9611.

[53] A. Cuesta, M.A. Esteban, J. Meseguer, Natural cytotoxic activity in seabream (*Sparus aurata* L.) and its modulation by vitamin C, Fish Shellfish Immunol. 13 (2) (2002) 97–109.

[54] C. Sonne, R. Dietz, J.S. Hans, Impairment of cellular immunity in west Greenland sledge dogs (*Canis familiaris*) dietary exposed to polluted minke whale (*Balaenoptera acutorostrata*) blubber, Environ. Sci. Technol. 40 (2006) 2056–2062.

[55] D. Cianciosi, T.Y. Forbes-Hernández, S. Afrin, M. Gasparrini, P. -Reboredo-Rodriguez, P.P. Manna, J. Zhang, L. Bravo Lamas, S. Martínez Flórez, P. Agudo Toyos, J.L. Quiles, Phenolic compounds in honey and their associated health benefits, Molecules 23 (9) (2018) 2322.

[56] B. Magnus, H. Goran, Anti-inflammatory therapies for atherosclerosis, Nat. Rev. Cardiol. 12 (4) (2015) 199–211.

[57] P.M. Ridker, B.M. Everett, T. Thuren, J.G. MacFadyen, W.H. Chang, C. Ballantyne, F. Fonseca, et al., Anti-inflammatory therapy with canakinumab for atherosclerotic disease, N. Engl. J. Med. 377 (2017) 1119–1131.

[58] B. Biswajit, C. Hiranjit, T. Pramod, K. Suman, Studies on secondary metabolite profiling, anti-inflammatory potential, in vitro photo protective and skin-aging related enzyme inhibitory a threatened orchid of nutraceutical importance, J. Photochem. Photobiol. B Biol. 173 (2017) 686–695.

[59] B. Bose, D. Tripathy, A. Chatterjee, P. Tandon, S. Kumaria, Secondary metabolite profiling, cytotoxicity, anti-inflammatory potential and in vitro inhibitory activities of *Nardostachys jatamansi* on key enzymes linked to hyperglycemia, hypertension and cognitive disorders, J. Phytomed. 1 (55) (2019) 58–69.

[60] W. Purnima, B. Kalyani, P. Bala, Anti-arthritic effect of garcinol enriched fraction against adjuvant induced arthritis, Recent Patents Inflamm. Allergy Drug Discov. 13 (1) (2019) 49–58.

[61] C.R.M. Souza, W.P. Bezerra, J.T. Souto, Marine alkaloids with anti-inflammatory activity: current knowledge and future perspectives, Mar. Drugs 18 (2020) 147.

[62] S. Montalvao, Z. Demirel, P. Devi, V. Lombardi, V. Hongisto, M. Perala, J. Hattara, E. Imamogl, S.S. Tilvi, G. Turan, et al., Large-scale bioprospecting of cyanobacteria, micro- and macroalgae from the Aegean Sea, New Biotechnol. 33 (2016) 399–406.

[63] X. Liu, S. Wang, S. Cao, X. He, L. Qin, M. He, Y. Yang, J. Hao, W. Mao, Structural characteristics and anticoagulant property in vitro and in vivo of a seaweed sulfated rhamnan, Mar. Drugs 16 (2018) 243.

[64] S.P. Ananda, Zinc: an antioxidant and anti-inflammatory agent: role of zinc in degenerative disorders of aging, J. Trace Elem. Med. Biol. 28 (4) (2014) 364–371.

[65] S. Rokayya, E. Abeer, A. Mona, A. Manal, B. Nada, et al., In-vitro evaluation of the antioxidant and anti-inflammatory activity of volatile compounds and minerals in five different onion varieties, Separations 8 (5) (2021) 57.

[66] T. Mizuho, S. Takayuki, Chemical compositions and antioxidant and anti-inflammatory activity of stream distillate from freeze-dried onion (*Allium cepa* L.) sprout, J. Agric. Food Chem. 56 (22) (2008) 10462–10467.

[67] G. Mahsa, S. Ahmad, D. Maahmoud, S. Giti, R.E. Mohammad, M. Alimalekshahi, et al., Tomato juice consumption reduces systemic inflammation in overweight and obese females, Br. J. Nutr. 109 (11) (2013) 2031–2035.

Chapter 17

Antiinflammatory activity of herbal bioactive-based formulations for topical administration

Madhu Sharma[a], Ritu Rathi[b], Sukhanpreet Kaur[b], Inderbir Singh[b], Erazuliana Abd Kadir[c], Amir-Modarresi Chahardehi[c], and Vuanghao Lim[c]

[a]Amravati Enclave, Panchkula, Haryana, India, [b]Chitkara College of Pharmacy, Chitkara University, Punjab, India, [c]Advanced Medical and Dental Institute, Universiti Sains Malaysia, Penang, Malaysia

1 Introduction

Pain can be defined as an emotional event that may involve damage to the tissues and various sensory organs. In response to any injury (physical, chemical, or microbial), the tissues provide some immunological response, which is referred to as "inflammation." Mobility of the leukocytes, swelling at the injury site, accumulation of the fluid are some of the characteristic features of inflammation. Interleukins (IL-1, IL-6, IL-8, and IL-10), tumor necrosis factor (TNF-α), reactive oxygen species (ROS), and nitric oxide are some of the mediators that are released during inflammation. The major mediator involved in inflammation is prostaglandin E2 (PGE$_2$) also referred as "pain enhancing mediator." PGE$_2$ is induced by cycloxygenase-2 (COX-2) during inflammation.

Types of inflammation

Inflammation can be classified into two types:

1. Acute inflammation
2. Chronic inflammation

1.1 Acute inflammation

The response of the body toward stimuli that could harm the body is referred to as acute inflammation. It happens immediately after injury and lasts for a few days. It is characterized by increase in the movement of plasma and leukocytes, especially granulocytes, from blood to the injured site. Cytokines and chemokines help in promoting the shift of neutrophils and macrophages to the inflammation site [1]. Toll-like receptors (TLRs) help in the recognition of pathogens. After that, certain biochemical events take place and they help to mature the inflammatory response including the vascular and immune systems. Pathogens, toxins, and burns are some of the causative agents of acute inflammation. Acute inflammation can be a way by which tissues can be protected from injury.

1.2 Chronic inflammation

It is also referred to as prolonged inflammation and involves shifting of the type of cells present at the site where the inflammation took place. It involves the mononuclear cells (monocytes, macrophages, lymphocytes, etc.). The various diseases mediated by chronic inflammation are diabetes, chronic obstructive pulmonary disorder (COPD), etc. [2]. Chronic inflammation is promoted by stress, obesity, and poor diet. The destruction and repair of the tissues take place simultaneously and it is the characteristic feature of chronic inflammation. Various signs of inflammation are redness, swelling, heat, pain, and loss of function.

1.2.1 Inflammation pathway

Prostaglandins are defined as the localized hormones that are released by the cells at the time of any injury (chemical or traumatic). These are generally shortlived. They are responsible for initiating pain and inflammation. Thromboxanes are the activators of hormones and are responsible for regulating the tone of blood vessels, platelet aggregation, etc. An inflammation pathway, if once stimulated by injury, may produce these hormonal activators, pain and destruction of tissues as their initial effect. This is followed by healing of tissues. Arachidonic acid is the main component of the arachidonic acid pathway as shown in Fig. 1. The tissue is traumatized, followed by the release of arachidonic acid. The transformation of arachidonic acid occurs into prostaglandins and thromboxanes. This step is mediated by the action of enzyme cyclooxygenase [3,4].

Recent Developments in Anti-Inflammatory Therapy. https://doi.org/10.1016/B978-0-323-99988-5.00015-2

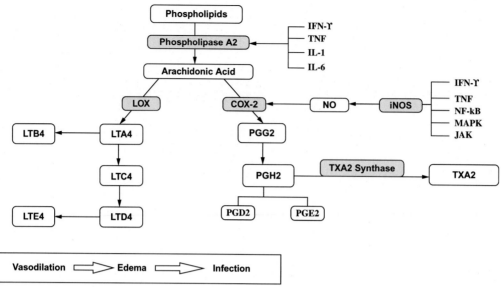

FIG. 1 Diagram illustrating the arachidonic acid inflammation pathway (where *iNOS*, inducible NO synthase; *NF-kB*, nuclear factor; *MAPK*, mitogen activated protein kinase; *JAK*, janus kinase).

Cycloxygenase (COX) enzymes are of two types: COX-1 and COX-2. Nonsteroidal antiinflammatory drugs (NSAIDs) can range from complete blockage of COX-1 and COX-2 to selective inhibition of COX-2 in order to inhibit the inflammation response and decrease the production of prostaglandins and thromboxanes.

The most common drugs used to prevent inflammation are nonsteroidal antiinflammatory drugs (NSAIDs). But, there are various side effects that are associated with these drugs, the most common of which is the formation of gastric ulcers. Under the condition of oxidative stress, reactive oxygen species (ROS) are formed that play a crucial role in certain diseases like aging, Alzheimer's disease, and carcinomas. So, antioxidants are most widely used category of drugs that can be used to scavenge the ROS and hence can be used to treat the inflammation.

Other choices of drugs are immunosuppressants, various biological drugs, and glucocorticoids. Despite the many choices of drugs, therapy is often hampered. The reason is the intolerable side effects of these drugs. So, there is a huge demand for new, antiinflammatory agents in the academia and industry as well. The natural products have played and will continue to play a major role in achieving the milestone of drug discovery and drug development. Plants bear a tendency to synthesize chemical compounds that play a crucial role in defending us from predators like insects and other microbes. For instance, *Emblica officinalis* is a strong antioxidant due to the presence of active constituents like flavonoids (rutin and quercetin) and polyphenols (gallic acid and ellagic acid).

Approximately 80% of the world's total population use either herbal medicine alone or in combination with allopathic medicines for their health issues [5].

2 Anatomy and physiology of skin

Multiple layers of cells and tissues that are linked together with the help of connective tissues constitute the skin. The skin is considered to be the largest organ of the body that comprises about 15% of the total body weight and a surface area of about 20 ft^2. The skin acts as a primary protective organ that acts as a soft cover for the entire external surface. It provides the first-line protection against environmental conditions too. It helps in maintaining vital functions such as regulation of body temperature, protection against disease causing microbes (pathogens), ultraviolet radiations, trauma, toxins, and certain microbes. It provides protection against various physical, chemical, and biological assailants and also prevents the excessive loss of water from the skin [6,7].

The skin may not be considered as a typical organ. It is basically a group of tissues that work unitedly to perform some critical functions, for instance, prevention of excessive loss of water from the skin and to maintain the body temperature. The skin and its accessory structures constitute the integumentary system that helps to maintain healthy structure and to carry out proper functioning of the skin. So to maintain that, it is the first and foremost requirement to understand the basic anatomy and composition of the skin.

The skin is composed of several layers—epidermis, dermis, and subcutaneous tissue, as shown in Fig. 2. The epidermis that constitutes the outermost layer of skin consists of group of cells known as keratinocytes. These cells help to synthesize keratin, which is a long, thread-like protein. The dermis consists of a structural protein referred to as collagen. Below the dermis, a layer of subcutaneous

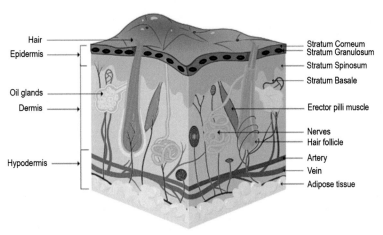

FIG. 2 Structure of the skin.

tissue is present that contains tiny fatty lobes referred as lipocytes. The thickness of all these layers depends on the anatomical location. For instance, the eyelid possesses the thinnest layer of epidermis (0.1 mm), while the palms of hand possess very thick layer of epidermis (1.5 mm). The dermis is around 30–40 times thick at the back as compared to epidermis.

2.1 Epidermis

It is the outermost layer of the skin. It is further differentiated into five types. It may be as thin as 50 cell layers and as thick as having 100 layers of cells. On an average, the thickness of epidermis is around 0.1 mm. The epidermal layer being the outermost layer acts a protective shield for the skin and it has the tendency to regenerate itself after an interval of 28 days.

(i) *Stratum basale*: It is the very first layer of epidermis. This layer possesses cube-shaped cells and it lies directly on the dermal layer. The formation of keratinocytes (i.e., the new epidermal cells) takes place here through cell division and also, these newly formed cells replace the old, worn-out cells. This process of regeneration is referred to as skin cell renewal. As the process of aging goes on, the process of cell renewal also slows down. The production of melanin through melanin-producing cells (melanocytes) also takes place here and once melanin is formed, it is transferred to keratinocytes and then it eventually migrates to the skin surface. Melanin helps in protecting the skin from ultraviolet radiations.

(ii) *Stratum spinosum*: It is the second epidermal layer and comprises of 8–10 layers of polygonal keratinocytes. These keratinocytes then begin to flatten.

(iii) *Stratum granulosum*: It is the third layer of epidermis, which is granular in texture. It possesses 3–5 flattened keratinized layers. The cells being far away from the dermal layer could not receive sufficient nutrition through diffusion; so, they begin to die.

(iv) *Stratum lucidium*: It is also referred to as a clear layer and it contains 3–5 layers that possess only flattened cells and is present in specific areas like finger tips, soles of feet, and palms only.

(v) *Stratum corneum*: It is the fifth epidermal layer which is also referred as horny layer. This outermost epidermal layer consists of 25–30 layers of flattened and dead keratinocytes. This layer is actually responsible for the protective nature of the skin. Keratinocytes present in this layer are continuously shed by friction and the worn-out cells are immediately replaced by the cells present in the deep sections of the skin. Keratinocytes are composed of fatty acids, ceramide, and lipids and act as a cement for the various skin cells. Keratinocytes, when combined with epidermal lipids, form a barrier of moisture which is waterproof in nature. This barrier decreases the transepidermal water loss (TEWL) so as to maintain moisture in the skin. The moisture barrier provides protection against microbes, allergens, and chemical irritants. In case sufficient moisture is not maintained in this moisture barrier, the skin will become more prone to dryness, itching, and other skin issues.

The outer layer of moisture barrier, owing to the presence of various sweat and sebaceous glands, has a pH of 4.5–6.5 that is slightly acidic in nature. These acidic layers of the moisture barrier are referred to as the acid mantle. The major advantage of acidic pH is that it is helpful in maintaining the hardness of keratin protein that further helps in binding them tightly. Also, it inhibits the growth of harmful bacteria and fungi. In the case the pH of acid mantle shifts toward alkalinity, the skin becomes more prone to dehydration, roughness, and flaking. Both the dermal and epidermal layers contain hair, pores, sweat, and sebaceous glands.

If the epidermal layer is folded into the dermal layer, it results in the formation of pores. The cells surrounding the pore continuously shed like the epidermis. But sometimes, during the shedding, the cells mix with the sebum, the result of which is the clogging of pores, which can initiate acne. Hair develops out of the pores and is full of proteins. A bulb-like follicle at the base of every hair gets divided to form new cells. Tiny blood vessels provide nourishment to the follicles. The presence of hair prevents heat loss and provides protection to the epidermis against harmful radiations of the sun and minor abrasions.

Sebaceous glands are responsible for secreting sebum and are attached to the hair follicles. This helps in providing lubrication to the hair follicles. The production of oil within the sebaceous glands is in direct control of androgens, e.g., testosterone. Sweat glands are long, coiled, and hollow tubes of cells. The sweat will be produced in the coiled section. These glands contain a duct that helps in connecting glands to the pores on the skin surface. The perspiration produced by the sweat glands helps to cool down the body, eliminate toxins (e.g., salt), and to hydrate the skin.

2.2 Dermis

It is located in between the epidermal and hypodermal layer. This layer provides structure to the skin owing to the presence of a fibrous network of tissues. The thickness of this layer is about 2 mm and is much thicker than the epidermis. The major role of dermis is that it cushions the deeper structures from any sort of mechanical injury. It helps in fulfillment of the nutritional requirements of the epidermis. It has an important role to play in wound healing. The mesh-like network of fibrous tissues comprises of structural proteins like collagen and elastin. Various specialized cells (for instance, mast cells and fibroblasts) and epidermal appendages are scattered within the dermal layer.

The dermis consists of two different types of layers:

(i) *Superficial papillary dermis*: It is a thin layer that consists of connective tissue having capillaries, some amount of collagen and elastic fibers. While reticular dermis contains a thick layer of comparatively dense connective tissue having large blood vessels, elastic fibers, and thick layers of collagen. Along with that it also contains mast cells, fibroblasts, and some appendages on the epidermis. The structures are surrounded by a viscous gel that helps various hormones, nutrients, and the waste products to pass through the dermal layer. Moreover, it lubricates collagen and elastic fibers. It makes the dermis act as a shock absorber.

(ii) *Specialized dermal cells*: The main types of cells present in dermis are fibroblasts and its main role is to synthesize elastin and collagen within the dermis.

Collagen constitutes the major part of dermis, i.e., approximately 70% of dermis. But, it is broken down in continuation and is replaced. Elastin provides elasticity to the skin.

Both the elastin and collagen are affected by age and exposure toward UV rays. This leads to sagging of the skin as the person ages over if a person is exposed to large amounts of UV radiation. Mast cells help to release histamine, which is involved in moderation of inflammatory response in the skin. Blood vessels in the dermal layer form a complex network and can be divided into two types:

(a) *Superficial plexus*: This consists of interconnecting arterioles and venules that lie close to the border of epidermis and it wraps around the dermis. The function of the superficial plexus is to provide oxygen and other essential nutrients to the cells.

(b) *Deep plexus*: It is found deep inside the border with the subcutaneous layer. Its vessels connect to the superficial plexus vertically. The drainage of skin through lymphatic system is important, the main function of which is to conserve plasma proteins and to scavenge foreign particulates and other antigens.

2.3 Hypodermis

It is a subcutaneous layer that lies below the dermal layer. It contains mainly fat. The main function of the hypodermis is to provide structural support to the skin. Another important function is that it insulates the body from cold and helps in the absorption of shock. It contains various nerves and blood vessels.

2.3.1 Routes of drug transportation
Cell membrane

For a drug to be absorbed in the body, its distribution into various tissues or organs and for its excretion too, it has to pass through various biological membranes. The movement of drug across these biological membranes present in various locations is termed as drug transport. The tissues possess space between the cells. It is through this space that the drug molecules can pass freely. The lining of blood capillaries is an example. For the hydrophilic molecules and ions it is very difficult to pass through the lipophilic region. They need to pass through either by active transportation or by intercellular pores. This is the reason the drug molecules are designed in such a way so as to render them lipophilic. There are six different transport systems by which drugs can be transported in the body as follows:

(1) Passive transcellular transport
(2) Passive paracellular transport
(3) Carrier-mediated transport

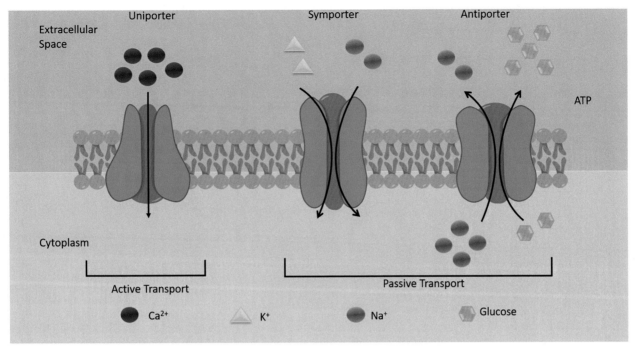

FIG. 3 Diagrammatic representation of carrier-mediated uniporter, symporter, and antiporter systems.

(4) Active transport

(5) Receptor-mediated transcytosis

(6) Absorption-mediated transcytosis

1. Passive transcellular transport

This pathway is followed by lipophilic drugs. Lipid molecules with molecular weight less than 400–500 Da are able to enter the brain with the help of free diffusion, which is mediated by the lipids [8,9]. Abusive drugs for instance, alcohol, caffeine, heroin, etc., are transported by this mechanism. But, the uptake of some drugs transported by this method is increased by peripheral tissues and some of them are sequestered in the brain. This leads to decrease in drug delivery toward the brain.

2. Passive paracellular transport

This transport system is followed by hydrophilic molecules. The tight interendothelial junction microvessels present in the CNS do not let the hydrophilic molecules to enter the CNS freely. Because of this reason, peptides, polysaccharides, and proteins cross the BBB to a very poor extent [8].

3. Carrier-mediated transportation

The mechanism of this transport system is that the drug molecule will bind itself with a transporter protein and will alter its shape. Once the shape is altered, the addition of any other substance, e.g., ATP, will in turn alter the shape of transporter proteins and the drug molecule will be released on the other side of the cellular membrane [10]. The essential nutrients, ions, can be transported using this system depending on the requirement of cells. There are three types of mediated transporters, as shown in Fig. 3.

Uniporter: It is responsible for transportation of a single solute at a time, e.g., GLUT-1. It transports glucose in a single direction of concentration gradient.

Symporter: In this type of system, transportation and counter transportation of the solute takes place at the same time even in the same direction, e.g., SGLT-1. It is a sodium glucose transport protein found in the intestines.

Antiporter: It helps in the transportation of solute in a single direction whereas counter transportation of solute takes place in the opposite direction, for example, sodium calcium antiport system. It transports three Na^+ ions by exchanging single Ca^{2+} molecule. This exchange occurs in the opposite direction and may either take place inside or outside the cell.

4. Primary active transport system

The primary active transport system helps in the active transportation of Na^+ and K^+ ions as well. But, it also allows the secondary transportation to occur. Unlike primary transportation, the secondary transport mechanism is also active, i.e., it also requires energy as done by the primary transport system. A very important example of pumps in animal cells is the Na^+-K^+ ATPase pump (Fig. 4). This pump helps in maintaining the concentration gradient of Na^+ and K^+ ions. This pump helps in moving two K^+ ions inside cells, whereas it allows the movement of three Na^+ ions out of the cells. The existence of Na^+-K^+ ATPase is in

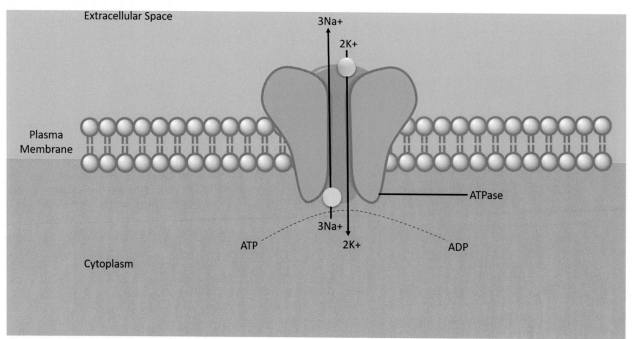

FIG. 4 Diagram explaining the Na⁺ K⁺ ATPase pump.

two forms and is dependent on the orientation toward the interior/exterior of the cells and whether it has affinity for sodium or potassium ions. The process involves the following steps:

(1) If the enzyme is oriented toward the interior side of the cell, the carrier would have more affinity for Na⁺ ions. Three Na⁺ ions would bind to a protein.

(2) The carrier (protein) would hydrolyze ATP and a phosphate group would attach to it. Because of this, the carrier would change its shape and its reorientation would occur. Because of this reorientation, the protein would lose its affinity for Na⁺ ions and three Na⁺ ions would leave the carrier.

(3) Because of alteration in the shape of carriers, their affinity for K⁺ ions would increase and two K⁺ ions would bind themselves to the protein. So, a low energy phosphate group would be detached from the carrier.

(4) Because of the release of the phosphate ions and the attachment of phosphate ions, the repositioning of carrier will take place toward the internal side of the cell.

(5) Now that the carrier has repositioned itself, it would lose its affinity toward potassium ions too. Now, a situation would arise having high amounts of Na⁺ ions outside the cells and more number of K⁺ ions inside the cell. For three ions of Na⁺, two ions of potassium would move inside. As a result of this, more negative ions would be present inside rather

than outside. This difference in the charges creates necessary conditions for the secondary process. Thus, the Na⁺ K⁺ ATPase pump creates a charge imbalance on the membrane.

5. Receptor-mediated transcytosis

This transport mainly occurs for the penetration as well as clearance of proteins and peptides in the brain [8,11]. It deals with the transport of low-density lipoproteins, insulin, transferrin, melanotransferrin, etc. [12]. This transport system can proceed in both the directions, i.e., from the brain to blood and from blood toward the brain. This bidirectional transport mainly occurs in the case of transferrin (Fig. 5). An example of unidirectional transport is the F_c receptor that helps to transport IgG from the brain toward blood [8]. This process can be explained in the following three steps.

(i) Endocytosis that takes place at the lumen of brain endothelial cells.

(ii) Transcytosis that occurs in vesicles through the narrow cytoplasm of cells.

(iii) Exocytosis that occurs in the abluminal site of endothelium [8].

Plasmalemmal vesicles, caveolae control the permeability transcellularly by the regulation of signals in lipid-based microdomains, transcytosis, and endocytosis [12]. The caveolar membrane possesses receptors of insulin, transferrin, etc. [13]. This pathway is useful for the targeting of the larger molecules, for instance, the targeting of nanoparticles to the brain [14].

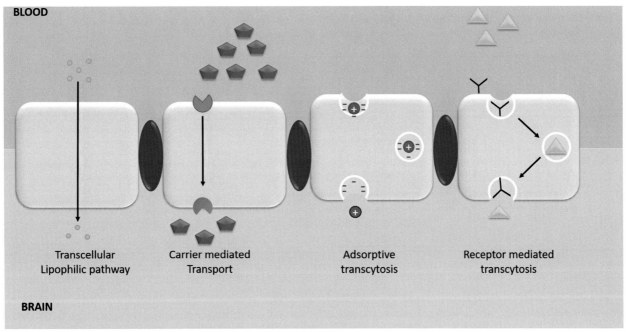

FIG. 5 Various transportation pathways used in blood brain barrier (BBB) transport.

6. Adsorptive-mediated transcytosis

Restriction in the paracellular pathway along with reduction in pinocytosis and lack of endothelial fenestrations results in the leakage of plasma proteins which is not being regulated properly [9]. Adsorptive-mediated transcytosis helps in the transfer of albumin and is present in endothelial cells. It is downregulated at the BBB but it gets reactivated in the case of brain edema, seizures, and medications like histamine [15].

2.3.2 Mechanism of inflammation

It can be explained using two components—vascular and cellular component. The vascular phase happens initially, which is followed by the cellular phase which involves the immune cells.

1. Vascular components

The vascular components include the movement of plasma carrying some important proteins. For example, antibodies and fibrin moving toward inflamed tissue.

(i) *Vasodilation and rise in permeability*

When the macrophages and mast cells come in contact with PAMPs, the release of certain vasoactive amines (e.g., histamine and serotonin) and eicosanoids (e.g., PGE_2 and LTB_4) takes place, so that the remodeling of the local vascular system is done. The release of nitric oxide by the macrophages causes the vasodilation of these mediators. Hence, it makes the blood vessels more permeable. Plasma is distributed from the blood vessels into the tissue space. Because of excessive collection of fluid in the tissues, swelling (edema) takes place. The exudated fluid contains different types of antimicrobial plasma mediators (complement, various antibodies, and lysozyme). These mediators deal with the damage to the microbes and carry out the opsonization of the microbe, so as to prepare them for the cellular phase (Table 1). If the stimulus is a lacerated wound, the platelets, kinin and coagulants that have been exudated can help in the clotting of the wound. These clotting factors help in making the structural framework too at the inflammation site with the help of fibrin for the process of phagocytosis and wound repairing in the later stages. The lymphatic system also flushes out the exudated tissue fluid containing bacteria to the lymph nodes so that the immune system begins the recognization and attacks those bacteria.

Many vascular changes take place during acute inflammation. These include vasodilation, increase in permeability, and increase in blood flow as well. These changes are induced by various inflammatory mediators. Initially, vasodilation takes place at the arterioles, and then slowly progresses to the capillary level. This will increase the net amount of blood and causes the redness of skin and inflammation.

TABLE 1 Various plasma derived mediators involved in vascular phase.

S. no	Mediators	Origin	Function
1	Bradykinin	Kinin system	Helps in induction of vasodilation, pain and contraction of smooth muscles
2	C_3	Complement system	C_3 cleaves itself into C_{3a} and C_{3b}. C_{3a} helps in the release of histamine from mast cells. Hence, results in vasodilation. C_{3b} binds itself to the cell wall of bacterias and opsonise them, so that they are easily marked as foreign bodies and they are targeted by phagocytes for the process of phagocytosis
3	C_5	Complement system	Helps in the release of histamine from the mast cells. Hence it produces vasodilatory effect. It promotes the chemotaxis by directing the cells towards inflammation site
4	Factor XII (Hageman factor)	Liver	This protein is initially inactive, then gets converted to activated form by platelets and collagen etc. When it gets activated, it further activates three plasma systems-kinin system, fibrinolysis system, coagulation system. All these systems are involved in inflammation
5	Membrane attack complex	Complement system	It is a complex formed by C_{5b}, C_6, C_7, C_8, and various units of C_9. This complex has the ability to insert into cell walls of bacteria and undergo cell lysis so as to ensure the death of bacteria
6	Plasmin	Fibrinolysis system	It has the ability to break the clots of fibrin. It can lead to cleavage of complement protein C_3 and helps in activation of factor XII
7	Thrombin	Coagulation system	It helps in cleavage of fibrinogen (soluble) to fibrin (insoluble), the aggregation of which can form blood clot. Thrombin binds to cells through PAR_1 receptors to initiate other inflammatory responses like production of chemokines and nitric oxide as well

The increase in the permeability of vessels causes the plasma to move into tissues. Then, a condition called stasis will occur. This is because the concentration of cells in the blood will increase. Stasis is a condition in which vessels are enlarged and packed with cells. It is because of stasis that the leukocytes move along the endothelium. There are four various plasma systems that are involved in the vascular phase—complement system, kinin system, coagulation system, and fibrinolysis system.

2. Cellular component

Leukocytes are involved as the cellular component as they move toward the inflamed tissue. Some of them start acting as phagocytes and ingest bacteria, viruses, and other cellular debris, while others release the granules that destroy the pathogens. Some inflammatory mediators are also released by leukocytes that help to maintain the inflammatory response. Basically, acute inflammation is controlled by granulocytes. Monocytes and lymphocytes are responsible for mediating the chronic inflammation.

(1) Migration of leukocytes (extravasation)

Leukocytes (neutrophils), in particular, are involved in initiating and maintaining inflammation. These cells migrate from their location toward the site of injury. The process by which leukocytes move from the blood toward tissues through the blood vessels is termed as extravasation.

A number of steps are involved in this process, which are enlisted below:

(i) *Margination of leukocytes and adherence with endothelium*

The centrally located white blood cells move toward the periphery of the walls of blood vessels. The macrophages that are activated release cytokines (IL-1 and TNF-α). This in turn produces chemokines that bind themselves to the proteoglycans. A gradient will be formed between the inflamed tissue and endothelium. Cytokines induce the expression of P-selectin on endothelium and P-selectin makes a slight weak bond with carbohydrates present on the surface of leukocytes. This causes the rolling of leukocytes and the formed bonds will be broken. On the other hand, the injured cells release E-selectin on endothelium. The function of E-selectin is similar to that of P-selectin.

Cytokines also induce the expression of ligands (ICAM-1 and VCAM-1) on the endothelium and mediate the adhesion. The leukocytes would slow down. The weakly bound leukocytes are free to detach themselves, if they are not activated by chemokines after the transduction of signals through G-protein-coupled receptors.

(ii) *Diapedesis*

The difference of the concentration of chemokines leads to the stimulation of leukocytes to move between the endothelial cells that lie adjacent to each other. The retraction of endothelial cells helps the leukocyte to pass into surrounding tissues via the basement membrane. The adhesion molecules (ICAM-1) also helps the leukocytes in their passage to surrounding tissues.

(iii) *Leukocyte movement in the tissue through chemotaxis*

Leukocytes that reach the interstitium of tissues bind themselves with extracellular matrix proteins through integrins so that they can be prevented from leaving the site. In contrast, various chemoattractants (C_{3a} or C_5) are also produced and will make sure that the leukocytes migrate toward the inflammatory source in the direction of a chemotactic gradient (Fig. 6).

(2) Phagocytosis

Neutrophils, after extravasation, usually come in contact with microbes at the inflammation site. Phagocytes lead to the expression of pattern recognition receptors (PRR). These receptors have an affinity for microbe associated molecular patterns (PAMP). PAMPs are nonspecific in nature; peptidoglycan, β-glycans, and mannans are responsible for initiating phagocytosis when the PAMPs bind with the PRRs.

Neutrophils, macrophages, and eosinophils are some of the examples of phagocytes [16]. The function of neutrophils is to patrol the bloodstream. Its rapid movement toward tissues takes place only in the case of certain infections [17]. After ingesting them, neutrophils can efficiently kill the pathogens. Neutrophils aid in phagocytosis with the help of $F_{C\gamma}$ receptors and through complement receptors 1 and 3. The microbicidal ability of neutrophils is because of the presence of granules that contain certain proteases (collagenase, gelatinase, etc.).

Macrophages help in initiating phagocytosis with the help of scavenger receptors, $F_{C\gamma}$ receptors, and complement receptors (1, 3, and 4). Macrophages are capable of phagocytosis with the help of the formation of new lysosomes [17,18]. Dendritic cells also play an important role in phagocytosis. They do not kill the microbes. In fact, they break them and present them as antigens toward the cells of the adaptive immune system [17].

(i) *Initiating receptors*

These are of two types—The first ones are the opsonic receptors which entirely depend on opsonins [19]. These receptors help in the recognition of the F_c segment of the IgG antibody, and deposit complement that helps in the recognition of other opsonins. The second type is of nonopsonic receptors. The examples of nonopsonic receptors are

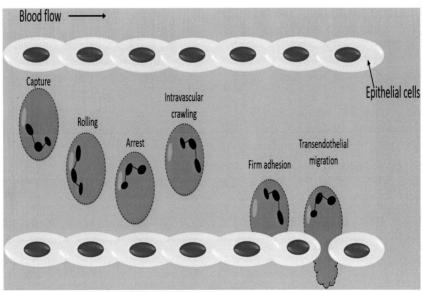

FIG. 6 Diagrammatic representation of various steps of migration of leukocytes.

dectin-type- and lectin-type receptors. But, in some cases, a second signal is required from pattern recognition receptors (PRRs). They get activated on attachment with pathogen-associated molecular patterns (PAMPs), thereby leading to the activation of NF-kB [16].

(ii) *$F_{c\gamma}$ receptors*

$F_{c\gamma}$ receptors are useful in the recognition of targets that are coated with IgG. $F_{c\gamma}$ receptors mediate phagocytosis by the formation of the protrusion of cells (phagocytic cup) and leads to the activation of oxidative bursts in neutrophils.

(iii) *Complement receptors*

The receptors are capable of recognizing C_{3b}-, C_{4b}-, and C_{3bi}-coated targets. A lectin-like complement binding domain is present extracellularly on the domains. Sometimes, recognition by complement receptors is not sufficient. Some additional signals are also needed. For example, macrophages possess CR_1, CR_3, and CR_4 for recognizing the targets. The targets coated with complement sink internally into the phagocytic membrane without protrusion [18].

(iv) *Mannose receptors*

The recognition of mannose and other sugars associated with pathogen are recognized by mannose receptors. The ingestion by mannose receptors is different in mechanism from other receptors ($F_{c\gamma}$ or complement) [18].

Phagosome

It is an organelle that gets formed by phagocytosis. This organelle, after being formed, moves toward the centrosome of the phagocyte and fuses with lysosomes to form a phagolysosome. Then, it gets degraded (oxygen-dependent- or oxygen-independent). Oxygen-dependent degradation depends on NADPH and reactive oxygen species. Oxygen-independent degradation depends on granule release having enzyme (lysozyme), lactoferrin, defensins, etc. Lactoferrin facilitates the sequestering of iron and provides unfavorable conditions for the growth of bacteria. Leukocytes also produce hydrogen cyanide during the process and are able to kill bacteria, fungus, and other pathogens through the release of toxic substances [20–22]. Various mediators involved in the cellular phase of inflammation are summarized in Table 2.

2.3.3 Treatment modalities

The treatment modalities for inflammation can be divided into two types—the first is physical and therapeutic modalities and the second one is the medications. Choice of modality used depends on the patient's condition and needs.

TABLE 2 Various mediators involved in cellular phase.

S. no	Mediator	Type of mediator	Origin	Function
1	Lysosome granules	Enzyme	Granulocytes	These granules contain numerous enzymes and can be distinguished into two types specific and azurophilic. The type depends on its content and their ability to breakdown substances
2	Histamine	Monoamine	Mast cells	It is stored in granules and is released when it responds to certain stimuli. It is responsible for dilation of arterioles and increase in permeability of veins
3	Interferon-γ	Cytokine	T-cells and Natural K-cells	It is important for maintenance of chronic inflammation. It possesses antiviral and antitumor properties
4	Interleukin-6	Cytokine	Macrophages, smooth muscle cells, adipocytes	It is pro inflammatory mediator secreted by adipocytes in obesity. IL-6 is secreted by macrophages too. It is secreted in response to pathogen associated molecular pattern (PAMP)
5	Interleukin-8	Chemokine	Macrophages	The neutrophils which exert weak effect on monocytesas well as eosinophils are activated by IL-8
6	Leukotriene B_4	Eicosanoid	Leukocytes and carcinoma cells	Mediation of leukocyte adhesion and help them in binding to endothelium. In case of neutrophils, it acts as a chemoattractant and initiates the formation of reactive oxygen species

TABLE 2 Various mediators involved in cellular phase—cont'd

S. no	Mediator	Type of mediator	Origin	Function
7	Leukotriene C_4, leukotriene D_4	Eicosanoid	Mast cells, eosinophils and macrophages	These facilitate the stimulation of mucus, increase the vascular permeability. It also promotes inflammation caused by eosinophils in eye, skin and lungs
8	5 HETE	Eicosanoid	Leukocytes	It is a precursor of 5-oxoeicosatetraeinoic acid. It possess low potency in stimulating neutrophils, eosinophils, chemotaxis and formation of reactive oxygen species
9	Prostaglandins	Eicosanoid	Mast cell	It is a group of lipids that is responsible for fever, pain and vasodilation
10	Interferon-α and Interleukin/-1	Cytokines	Macrophages	Both of these affect many cells by inducing inflammatory reactions like chemotaxis, fever. These cytokines result in loss of appetite and increase in cardiac rate

1. Physical and therapeutic modalities

It is used by the physiotherapists for their patients in order to achieve the therapeutic goals [23]. The various methods used in the treatment are enlisted below:

(i) *Electrical stimulation*

Lack of proper input of nerve in a muscle may be because of any peripheral nerve injury or a stroke, which results in the stiffness and atrophy of muscles. In that case, electrical stimulation by placing the electrodes on the skin helps to prevent the atrophy and contraction by providing a form of exercise. Transcutaneous electrical nerve stimulation (TENS) is a form of electrical stimulation that employs low current and does not lead to the contraction and stiffness of muscles. For TENS, a device that uses a battery will produce a current. The current is applied using electrodes that are placed on the skin. The advantage of this technique is that it is not painful though it produces a tingling sensation.

It can be applied many times in a day from 20 min to several hours. The duration will depend on the severity of pain. The disadvantage of this technique is that it may cause arrhythmias. So, people with cardiac disorder or those using pacemaker should not use it and it should not be used nearby the eyes.

(ii) *Traction*

This technique is used in rehabilitation centers and hospitals especially if the bones in the cervical region have degenerated. It can be used in homes too. It is most effective if people are sitting rather than lying down. Traction can be combined with physical therapies like stretching exercises. The precaution is that it should be used in the presence of a family member to avoid any injury.

(iii) *Massage*

Massage helps to get rid of pain and decreases swelling, and helps to loosen the tightened tissue. It is used in kneading injurious tissues of the body using hands so as to alleviate pain, improvement in circulation, and decrease muscular tension. Petrissage, effleurage, and trigger point massage are some of the techniques used for the purpose of massage. Massage should never be used in treating inflammation caused by thrombophlebitis.

(iv) *Thermal energy*

Therapeutic heat (thermotherapy) and cold (cryotherapy) constitute the conductive modalities. These techniques utilize thermal energy to produce local or generalized heating or cooling effects on superficial tissues. It can achieve maximum penetration of up to 1 cm or less [24].

(a) **Thermotherapy**: It involves warm whirlpools, hydrocollator packs, fluidotherapy, and paraffin baths. The physiological effect of heat includes the increase in elasticity of connective tissue, increase in metabolic rate, increase in blood flow, and reduced ischemia [24]. It also helps in the stimulation of fibroblast proliferation, increased proliferation of endothelial cells, and increase in the phagocytic activity of inflammatory cells [25–27]. It is contraindicated in malignancy, patients with tuberculosis, and in acute injury/inflammation.

There are a few additional considerations that need to be followed:

(i) A patient must be asked to differentiate among hot/cold stimuli in order to check the sensory integrity.

(ii) The pads should be wrapped up in 6–8 layers to protect the skin from burning.

(b) **Cryotherapy**: It involves ice massage, cold whirlpool, cold spray, and cold compression [24]. There will be vasoconstriction and decrease in the blood flow within 15–20 min. Also, the metabolic rate would also slow down. The technique would decrease the velocity of nerve conduction. Slow metabolism releases some inflammatory mediators and decreases edema. As a result of this, the oxygen demand of tissues will be decreased and their chances of injury from ischemia would also decrease [28,29].

Cold increase the threshold stimuli of muscle spindles and decrease the excitation of nerve endings. This results in increase in pain threshold and muscle spasm would also decrease [30,31]. Special precaution should be taken in the case of drug infection, damaged skin, hypertension, person with impaired sensation, etc.

(v) *Ultrasound*

This technique needs sound energy. Pressure waves will be created by the vibration of particles through a medium. The flow may either be delivered as a continuous mode or as a pulsed mode. Ultrasound has a capacity to increase pressure in tissues with depth because they can travel very well in the homogenous tissue (fat tissue) [32,33]. Earlier, it was used for its heating effects but it has the tendency to heat at the cell level. It has been proven that it alters all the phases of tissue repair. It also helps in the increase of phagocytic activity of macrophages [34]. It facilitates the release of chemical mediators from cells that attracts fibroblasts to the injury site and stimulates the production of collagen that ultimately strengthens the scar tissue [35]. Ultrasound also aids in relief from pain. This technique is of two types:

(a) **Pulsed ultrasound**: It accelerates the healing of fractures because of the increase of androgenic and osteogenic activities [36]. But, it is contraindicated in pregnancy, hemorrhagic conditions, and tuberculosis.

(b) **Continuous ultrasound**: It is mostly used when heat effects are desired but nonheating effects also occur [37]. It is contraindicated in malignancy, impaired memory and circulation, skin disease, for instance, eczema, psoriasis, etc.

(vi) *LASER*

The term LASER stand for "Light amplification for the stimulated emission of radiation." This technique involves electromagnetic radiation and photonic movement through space. A low power layer seems to have significant effect on soft tissues, pain management, and healing of fractures. It produces very small or no thermal effect. Laser stimulates cellular degranulation resulting in the release of growth factors, activation of phagocytosis at site of injury, and activation of fibroblasts. Laser absorbed by hemoglobin releases nitric oxide and leads to cell proliferation of endothelium. This results in the increase of microcirculation [38].

(vii) *Iontophoresis*

It is a technique involving electrical stimulation and is used for delivering medicament from the skin to the inflamed tissues. Most commonly, this method is applicable for steroids like dexamethasone for the treatment of inflammation. Steroids help to alleviate pain and provide relief to the swollen tissues.

2. **Medications**

Therapeutic drugs used to control the pain, inflammation and muscular spasm include—anesthetic drugs, analgesic drugs, NSAIDs, adrenocorticosteroids, and muscle relaxants.

(a) *Local anesthetics*

This category of drugs, e.g., lidocaine, procaine, and benzocaine, helps in the elimination of the short-term sensation of pain by blocking sensory transmission through peripheral nerves.

(b) *Analgesic drugs*

Aspirin can be used to alleviate pain and inflammation as well. But, it possesses anticlotting properties, due to which it cannot be used during the acute healing phase. Acetaminophen too can be used as analgesic and antipyretic agent. But, it does not possess antiinflammatory characteristics.

(c) *Nonsteroidal antiinflammatory drugs (NSAIDs)*

This category helps ion dilation of blood vessels and inhibition of production of prostaglandins. Prostaglandins increase blood flow, permeability of capillaries, and inflammation-induced edema. Also, they decrease sensitization of pain receptors toward the effect of pain-producing substances, for instance, bradykinin. Ibuprofen, naproxen sodium, and piroxicam are some of the commonly used NSAIDs used in the treatment of inflammation.

(d) *Adrenocorticoids*

These drugs can be applied topically, taken orally or injected onto the specific area, e.g., prednisone, cortisone, and hydrocortisone. But, long-term use of these drugs can damage the structures, depress adrenal glands, and may lead to osteoporosis.

(e) *Muscle relaxants*

Involuntary muscular tension, if not relaxed, may lead to intensive pain. This may result in buildup of certain metabolites that mediate pain. A vicious cycle is created leading to more pain, more spasm. Muscle relaxants help to break this pain-spasm cycle by reduction in muscle excitation and improvising motor function, e.g., Flexeril and Dantrium.

3 Herbal antiinflammatory agents

Herbal medicines are synthesized by experience and practicing indigenous medicinal systems from centuries. Although the medical system has done tremendous progress during the past few decades for the treatment of many diseases but the treatment of some serious diseases, for instance, inflammation, is still questionable. There are some drugs like NSAIDs, muscle relaxants, etc. but they are associated with numerous side effects. So our medicinal system requires certain drugs that possess greater efficacy and safety even at small doses. Herbal medicines are one of the great alternatives of synthetic derivatives. They are more acceptable with fewer side effects. These compounds are found to be a part of living flora and possess greater compatibility with the human body. So, it is high time to explore these herbal bioactives for their usage in the treatment of disease and their compatibility with other prescription medications.

Below are some of the herbal antiinflammatory agents:

1. Omega-3-fatty acids

It is called fish oil in United Kingdom. Cod liver oil is an example of omega-3-fatty acids and it can be used in the treatment of various muscular and skeletal diseases. This investigation was carried out by Curtis et al. in the 18th century [39,40]. But, cod liver oil, when exposed to air, undergoes rancidity of polyunsaturated oil. So, extraction techniques were improvised, using a nitrogen blanket as a protective compound and methods increasing oxygen-free encapsulation. The oxidation of oil can be prevented during the manufacturing process.

According to research, omega-3 fatty acids are one of the most effective anti-inflammatory agents [41–44]. Fish oil supplements are recommended by the American Heart Association to prevent various anti-inflammatory diseases. The countries with high consumption of fish have low incidence of depression and other neurological diseases. Many clinical studies have been carried out to show the effectiveness of fish oil in the treatment of arthritis as compared to the traditional antiinflammatory agents. The active constituents of fish oil, i.e., eicosapentaenoic acid (EPA) and docosahexaenoic acid (DNA), help to convert COX to PGE_3.

PGE_3 is a natural antiinflammatory agent and it inhibits the conversion of arachidonic acid to PGE_2 (high inflammatory substance). PGE_3 also leads to the inhibition of the synthesis of inflammatory cytokines TNF-α and IL-1b. A study was carried out on synovial cartilage to observe the effect of omega-3-EFA. It demonstrated that degenerative enzymes like aggrecanase and matrix metalloproteinase as well as TNF-α, IL-1, and COX-2 were reduced as a result of which inflammation was reduced.

According to a recent study on 250 patients suffering from cervical and lumbar disc disease NSAIDs were substituted with fish oil and thus proven to be used as an effective antiinflammatory agent. About 1.5–5 g/day of EPA and DHA is the recommended dose and it must be taken with meals. Steatorrhea and belching are some of the side effects of supplements, if it is not taken with meals. Fish oil is not recommended to be taken by patients using anticoagulant medicines.

2. White willow bark

The bark of the white willow has been widely used as an antiinflammatory and antipyretic agent since ancient times in Egyptian, Roman, and Indian civilizations. Increased use of aspirin may result in gastric bleeding. So, it was replaced with the herbal bioactive obtained from white willow bark. White willow bark nonselectively inhibits COX-1 and COX-2, which are used to block the prostaglandins [45]. Random placebo-controlled studies showed efficacious results in comparison to aspirin. White willow bark contains salicin. It is converted to salicylic acid in the liver. This salicylic acid possesses few side effects other than aspirin. But, it is comparatively costlier than aspirin and its use is limited to adults only. It is contraindicated in patients with peptic ulcers, diabetes, and renal disorders. The recommended daily dose is 240 mg/day [46–53].

3. *Curcuma longa* (Turmeric)

It is a most important indigenous plant that is widely used in India [54]. The most important active constituent of *C. longa* with antiinflammatory properties is curcumin [55]. Many clinical trials had been conducted to prove the antiinflammatory action of curcumin and the results suggested that it can effectively improvise the inflammation in rheumatoid arthritis and reduce the stiffness of joints and morning sickness as well, when compared to phenylbutazone that acts as a positive control [56].

In another clinical investigation, curcumin was found to be effective against gastric ulcers. Remission after 12 weeks was observed in the subjects [57]. Curcumin was found to be effective in inflammatory bowel syndrome too [58]. In the case of kidney transplant surgery, curcumin acts as a reducing agent so as to delay graft rejection [59]. Curcumin ameliorates ulcerative colitis [60] and psoriasis [61] by selectively prohibiting phosphorylase kinase [61].

4. Zingiber officinale (Ginger)

Depending upon the amount consumed, the oral administration of Z. officinale showed some inconsistent effects. A study was carried out in mice, which were administered some squeezed ginger extract once or twice. This leads to elevation of TNF-α in peritoneal cells. But, if this extract is administered for a long term, it increases the corticosterone level in serum and decreases the pro-inflammatory markers [62]. Another study was carried out for a period of 2 months in type-2 diabetes patients having low-grade inflammation. After 2 months, the level of TNF-α and high sensitivity C-reactive protein (hs-CRP) in the serum decreased to a definite level [63].

In the patients suffering from osteoarthritis, ginger has improved the pain to a level identical to diclofenac sodium, 100 mg. But the former shows no side effects [63]. Ginger powder ameliorates musculoskeletal disease and rheumatism by the inhibition of cyclooxygenase and lipoxygenase pathways in synovial fluid [64].

5. Rosmarinus officinalis (Rosemary)

A trial was carried out to assess the antiinflammatory potential of rosemary in patients suffering from osteoarthritis and rheumatoid arthritis for a period of 4 weeks. Hs-CRP, which is an index to evaluate the presence of inflammation, was found to be reduced in the patients. The antiinflammatory activity of R. officinalis in molecular scope has also been confirmed using a trial. The trial demonstrated that rosemarinic acid disturbs the activation of complement system by the inhibition of C_{3b} attachment; the minimum dose required for this effect was 34 µM [65].

In another study, rosemary was found to be more efficacious in treating gastric ulcers other than omeprazole. This is because of reduction in the mediators like TNF-α and IL-1 [66]. A very high dose (500 mg/kg) of rosemary extract has decreased the level of testosterone and spermatogenesis in rats that render them infertile [67]. Rosemary act as a topical antiinflammatory agent for wound healing in mice [67].

6. Borago officinalis

This plant possesses 25% of gamma linoleic acid (GLA). The elevation of prostaglandin E (PGE) level leads to increase in cyclic adenosine monophosphate (cAMP) as well. GLA can strongly suppress the level of TNF-α [68]. These mechanisms make borage oil a strong antiinflammatory agent against rheumatoid arthritis. On the other hand, this herb is contraindicated in pregnancy as it increases the chances of miscarriage [68]. Two random clinical trials were carried out to assess the antiinflammatory potential of borago. The first study was carried out using 1.4 g/day of dosage of borage seed oil. The comparison was carried out with placebo and the therapy continued for 6 months. At the end of this, the oil has ameliorated the disease to 36.8% in the treatment group.

The second study was carried out using a dose of 2.8 g/day. The study was carried out for 6 months. Rheumatoid arthritis was ameliorated to 64% in the treatment group in comparison to the control group where the disease was ameliorated to 2% [69]. For assessing the effectivity of this herb in treating atopic dermatitis, 12 clinical trials were conducted. Five of those trials have successfully proven the effectiveness of the herbs whereas, two of them improved some of the patients. In the rest of five trials, no observation has been made [70].

7. Oenothera biennis (Evening primrose)

The active constituents of this herb are aliphatic alcohols (e.g., tetracosanol), ferulic acid, and gamma linoleic acid (GLA). These constituents provide protection against inflammatory markers [71]. The oil also contains β-sitosterol and campesterol. They help to modulate nitric oxide. Because this herb modulates TNF-α, TXB_2, and IL-1β as well, and leads to the suppression of the COX-2 gene expression, primrose oil possess greater antiinflammatory action than borage oil [72]. A clinical trial was conducted to evaluate the antiinflammatory activity of primrose oil in combination with hemp seed oil. The evaluation was carried out over multiple sclerosis patients. They were allowed to take primrose oil/hemp oil and placebo randomly. IFN-Υ and IL-17 were significantly reduced in the treatment group. Alleviation of relapse rate of multiple sclerosis was observed in the patients of treatment group [73].

In another random clinical trial on rheumatoid arthritis, subjective improvement and decrease in the usage of NSAIDs was also observed [74].

8. Harpagophytum procumbens (Devil's claw)

The herb belongs to the family Pedaliaceae [75]. Harpagoside is the active constituent of this plant that is responsible for imparting antiinflammatory properties to this herb [76]. The mechanism that forms the basis of the antiinflammatory property is the inhibition of nitrous oxide, cytokines (TNF-α, IL-1β, IL-6), and PGE_2 as well. It also prevents the metabolism of arachidonic acid and biosynthesis of eicosanoids. This leads to inhibition of COX-2 and thereby reduces inflammation [77–79]. In a preclinical study, the herb did not show to be efficacious in the improvement of edema in the feet of rats (induced by carrageenan) [80]. But in a random clinical trial, the effectivity of herb in the remission of osteoarthritis was assessed [81]. The main side effect of this herb is that it causes gastrointestinal problems. So, it is contraindicated in patients having gastric ulcers, diabetes, and gall stones [75].

9. *Boswellia serrata*

The *Boswellia* tree produces an oleogum resin named *B. serrata* [82]. The herb was evaluated for its antiinflammatory properties in patients suffering from osteoarthritis. It was observed that frequency of swelling and pain in joints was alleviated dramatically and also joint flexibility and walking was also augmented at the end of the treatment. On the other hand, ESR, early morning stiffness, and requirement of administration of NSAIDs was also reduced.

A pilot study was carried out in patients of polyarthritis; it was recorded that there was no significant remission in the manifestations of patients during these 12 weeks of therapy using the extract of *B. serrata*. *B. serrata* has ameliorated an inflammatory bowel disease namely collagenous colitis in the therapy group in comparison to the placebo [83]. If *B. serrata* is given in combination with *C. longa* and *Glycyrrhiza glabra* it has shown effective results in improvising asthmatic symptoms in patients. Boswellic acid is the main active constituent of this gum, which inhibits the C_3 convertase enzyme and suppresses the complement system [84,85]. This herb possesses both topical and systemic inflammation characteristics [86].

10. *Rosa canina* (Dog rose)

It is a member of the Rosaceae family. The herb was evaluated for its antiinflammatory characteristics in patients of osteoarthritis and rheumatoid arthritis. In the patients who were suffering from osteoarthritis, it was observed that the pain was alleviated, the consumption of medicine was rescued, and there was significant reduction in the level of CRP after the treatment [87,88]. The antiinflammatory effect is due to the seed of this herb. In contrast to this, the dose of 10 g of rosehip powder per day for a period of 1 month does not show antiinflammatory action on patients with RA. Galactolipid is the main constituent of this herb, which has the tendency to inhibit nitrous oxide and is responsible for the antiinflammatory property of *Rosa canina* [89,90].

11. *Urtica dioica*

It belongs to the family Urticaceae. A pilot study was conducted using 50 mg diclofenac per day on the patients of acute arthritis along with 50 mg of *Urtica dioica*. Remarkable attenuation of the CRP level was observed. *U. dioica* in combination with NSAIDs had shown remarkable synergistic effects [91]. In an RCT, *U. dioica* applied topically on a thumb in osteoarthritis patients; the RCT revealed outstanding alleviation of pain and stiffness [92].

U. dioica if used in combination along with rosehip and willow bark can suppress IL-1β and COX-2. In allergic rhinitis, the extract has proven to be an excellent antiinflammatory agent by antagonizing a H_1 receptor and reduction of PGD_2 production. The herb exerts inhibitory effect on the mast cell tryptase [93].

12. *Uncaria tomentosa* (Cat's claw)

It belongs to the family Rubiaceae. An experimental study was conducted in over 45 patients of osteoarthritis. The patients were divided into two groups—placebo and active. Remission to some degree was noted after a period of 4 weeks. This was due to inhibition of TNF-α and reduction of PGE_2 production [94]. A double-blind placebo-controlled study of 24 weeks was performed for the evaluation of *U. tomentosa* extract in rheumatoid arthritis patients. The extract was administered with sulfasalazine. There was alleviated pain, tenderness, and swelling of the joints in the treatment group other than placebo [95]. The mechanism that lies behind the antiinflammatory effect of cat's claw is the downregulation of TNF-α, IL-1α, and 1β. An *in vivo* study showed little inactivation of COX-1 and COX-2 [96,97].

13. *Salvia officinalis* (Sage)

It belongs to the Lamiaceae family. Carnosic acid and carnosol are responsible for the antiinflammatory action of sage [98]. These active constituents inhibit the PGE_2 synthase-1 enzyme, which further inhibits the production of PGE_2 [99]. It is worth mentioning that Halicioglu et al. have reported generalized tonic-clonic seizures in a newborn and a child who exposed themselves to sage oil [100].

14. *Ribes nigrum* (Black currant)

This oil is rich in n-6PUFA, α-linoleic acid, and ϒ-linoleic acid [101]. A clinical trial of 6 weeks was conducted on rheumatoid arthritis patients, the results of which show reduction in inflammatory mediators (IL-1β and TNF-α) and attenuation of morning stiffness in the case of the experimental group [102]. The symptoms of disease reduced after a period of 24 weeks in the case of rheumatoid arthritis patients. There was not much difference observed in the case of placebo and treatment groups [103]. According to a study, the herb is capable of reducing the HSP70 and HSP90 heat shock proteins along with the expression of COX-2 in rats [104].

15. *Persea americana* (Avocado)

It belongs to the family Lauraceae. A randomized control study for a period of 3 months was carried out on osteoarthritis patients with a combination of NSAID; after a period of 45 days, it was noticed that the requirement of NSAID came to an end, but no change was observed in the pain score [105]. Then, three clinical trials were conducted for osteoarthritis patients to assess the effectivity of *P. americana*. Two of them revealed that the pain and disability were reduced and also, Lequesne's functional index (LFI), was also reduced but in the last trial no changes have been observed [106]. The follow-up of hip for 3 years in osteoarthritis patients demonstrated that there was no improvement in joint space width (JSW) but the JSW exacerbation was prevented up to 20% [107]. Extracts of avocadoes and soyabeans were administered topically and orally, in vulvar lichen sclerosus (VLS). The treatment period was of 24 weeks. After the treatment period, the signs and symptoms of the disease were significantly diminished [108].

16. *Elaeagnus angustifolia*

It belongs to the family Elaeagnaceae [109]. An RCT study over 28 patients in the treatment of oral lichen planus (OLP) revealed that pain and size of lesion was attenuated up to 50%–75% in the case group [109]. Another random clinical trial was conducted on 90 female osteoarthritis patients. The results revealed that proinflammatory mediators—TNF-α and matrix metalloprotein-1 (MMP-1) —were significantly attenuated whereas an antiinflammatory cytokine level of IL-10 was alleviated in the active therapy group [110]. The inhibition of COX-1 and COX-2 were responsible for the antiinflammatory action of *E. angustifolia*. The evidence also suggested that there is no correlation between corticosterone level and antiinflammatory action [111].

17. *Vaccinium myrtillus* (Bilberry)

It belongs to the family Vaccinium. A clinical trial with 400 g of bilberry was carried out over 27 patients, who were suffering from metabolic disorder. The outcome of the study showed that the levels of hs-CRP, IL-6, and IL-12 had diminished [112]. Another study was carried over 13 ulcerative colitis patients; the bilberry extract resulted in 63.4% remission along with fecal protection level [113].

18. *Olea europaea* (Olive)

It belongs to the family Oleaceae. Extra virgin olive oil has proven its positive effect by modulation of postprandial plasma lipopolysaccharide, TXB_2 and LTB_4 in the case of coronary heart disease demonstrated through healthy and metabolic syndrome volunteers [114,115]. Olive oil has found to be more useful than sunflower oil in wound healing and alleviation of hospitalization in case of second-degree burns [116].

19. Green tea

Green tea is known for its anticancer and cardiovascular properties since long. But, its antiinflammatory action for the treatment of arthritis has been discovered in a recent study. Polyphenolic compounds (catechins and epigallocatechin-3-galate) are found abundantly in green tea. Epigallocatechin-3-gallate inhibits the release of proteoglycan induced by IL-1 [117]. In vitro models in humans demonstrated that it causes the suppression of IL-16 and also the inhibition of aggrecanases, which are responsible for the degradation of cartilage. Research on green tea demonstrated an antiinflammatory and chondroprotective effect as well. According to the "Asian Paradox" it is being theorized that increased consumption of green tea may lead to significant cancer preventive, neuroprotective, and cardioprotective properties [118]. The dosage of green tea is 300–400 mg. Because of the caffeine content, green tea may cause gastric irritation in some cases.

20. *Capsaicin* (Chilli pepper)

It is a shrub that is cultivated in some regions of America but now it is cultivated throughout the world. The active constituent of the small fruit is capsaicin that is responsible for the pungency of the fruit. Capsaicin degenerates capsaicin-sensitive nerve endings (nociceptive nerve endings), which leads to the increase in the nociceptive threshold. Capsaicin activates vanilloid 1, which is a transient and main receptor. It causes the inhibition of NF-kB, which is responsible for its antiinflammatory activity. Capsaicin often causes a sense of burning whenever it comes in contact with human tissues, also in the digestive tract. It is often used in combination with other antiarthritic preparations [119,120].

4 In vivo and clinical studies in herbal formulations

For hundreds or even thousands of years several traditional herbs were used on humans to avoid and cure diseases [121]. Herbal drug products are preferred due to their lack of toxicity, low irritant content, and widespread consumer adoption [122]. Especially in the context of drug development from medicinal plants, it has a great benefit since ethnopharmacological evidence on traditional use is sometimes well recorded and might offer suggestions on therapeutically beneficial chemicals [123]. It is crucial to highlight that extracting plant components is the first significant stage in testing biological activity, with numerous advantages and disadvantages compared to isolating pure, active substances [124]. While herbal formulations were commonly used in the analyzed community, despite widespread confidence in the harmless existence of botanical extracts, the prevalence of reported side effects confirms that they should be considered a possible cause of adverse skin events [125]. Hence, dermatologists should be mindful of the factors that affect topical medication effectiveness and safety as high-volume prescribers [126]. Obviously, the topical route of administration is a useful way to accomplish dermal delivery of a drug to the diseased skin region [127]. It has several benefits: a straightforward approach to the site of action and local delivery of the active pharmaceutical ingredient (API) [127].

Herbal products, which are obtained from or produced naturally by the living organisms, are of preferred for their non- or less toxicity and are as effective as the conventional modern medications. Herbal formulation for percutaneous absorption is complicated as the penetration rate of the API depends on several factors including molecular size, water solubility, and hydrophile/lipophile balance [122]. It was proposed that the maximum molecular weight of 500 Da rule should be applied for compounds developed for topical drug delivery to ensure skin penetration [128]. The regular dosage of herbal medications in the form of crude extracts is usually concentrated and is not given at an accurate dose. This poses the risk of overdose and toxicity. Traditional herbal medications for skin application are commonly prepared by mixing the extracted powder with water, honey, vinegar, or wine, in which preparations are messy, poorly adhesive to the skin, unsanitary, and cannot be stored for a long time [122].

Nowadays, the drug formulations for topical administration have improved tremendously to suit the criteria needed for a more convenient and effective applications. Ointments, creams, patches, and gels are the common form of modern natural product preparations for dermal applications. These forms of formulations are however hardly penetrating the skin due to their size and hydrophobicity, thus leading to issues of poor bioavailability, distribution and stability of the herbal medicines.

As described previously in this chapter, there are techniques to enhance drug penetration through the skin, which mainly involved physical disturbance of the skin structure prior to drug delivery, such as by low-frequency ultrasound, electroporation, laser ablation, and microneedle arrays [129]. As these techniques damaging the natural barrier function of the skin before the drug can be transported deeper into the stratum corneum layers, one must consider the risks of complications such as permanent skin injury and secondary infection these techniques might cause. These have led to the exploration of nanotechnology to improve the current herbal-drug formulations for topical

administration through the skin. The use of nanosized carriers to be incorporated with the herbal product allows different ways of delivering the bioactive molecules into the deep skin layers. The nanocarriers (NC) can be designed to suit the need for dermal and transdermal drug delivery by making the particle small and having specific hydrophobicity/hydrophilicity for improved skin penetration. The NC could also allow specific targeting of cell populations, as well as acting as a depot for a sustained drug release.

Formulating for Efficacy (FFE) is a software program that assists formulators in selecting the appropriate excipient(s) for an active ingredient(s) in a formulation. The formulator's objective is to choose certain formulation components at the optimal concentrations to maximize active ingredient(s) distribution to the skin [130]. Numerous phytoconstituents, including flavonoids, triterpenoids, alkaloids, steroids, and phenols, have been shown to have antiinflammatory properties [131]. The topical use of pharmaceutical particles has been widely investigated with a view to dermal, follicular, or transdermal drug delivery (TDD) [129]. Transdermal topical medication delivery provides a noninvasive medication method [132]. TDDs is a noninvasive, painless technique of administering medication that takes precedence over other traditional delivery methods in this case [133]. However, this approach has several drawbacks, including skin reactions, skin discoloration, allergies, disturbance of the skin's barrier layers, and blood level changes [133]. Preclinical models, such as excised human skin, reconstructed skin, and animal models, all contribute to our understanding of the various forms of drug distribution into the skin [129]. The stratum corneum is thought to be responsible for the skin barrier function, which provides a significant difficulty in clinical practice when it comes to cutaneous administration of medicines [134]. Noninvasive imaging techniques such as high-frequency ultrasound scans, optical coherence tomography, laser-scan-microscopy, and in vivo microscopy are now available for human volunteers and have opened up a refined picture of in vivo anatomies in photoacoustic microscopy [129].

The herbal medications, which are not prepared following a standardized regulations, are prone to have poor quality, lack of standardization between batches, and risk of adulteration of plant materials [135]. The requirement to have a proper guideline to support the claimed quality and activity of herbal products is crucial to standardized and validate its therapeutic activity. According to the WHO guidelines [136], the development of herbal products must be done through nonclinical and clinical studies (Fig. 7). The nonclinical studies are to support the clinical investigation to determine the toxicity, efficacy, and pharmacokinetics of the drug. The toxicity studies involve both *in vitro* and *in vivo* investigations. The in vivo toxicity studies mainly use rodents for assessment of maximum tolerated

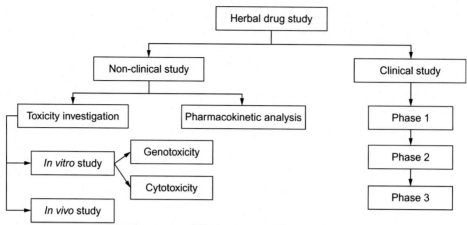

FIG. 7 Herbal drug investigation through clinical and nonclinical approaches.

dose, single-dose acute toxicity, and repeated dose toxicological effects. As for the pharmacokinetic studies, the analyses involve the determination of drug absorption after oral dosing or drug mobilization from the injection site, distribution of the API, as well as determination of the drug metabolism. For clinical considerations of herbal products, Good Clinical Practice should be followed during all clinical trial stages to ensure the quality and ethical standards are fulfilled. Biostatisticians should also be consulted in all the trial stages to ensure the sample size is adequate to meet the primary endpoint/objective. Preclinical models on the other hand, such as excised human skin, reconstructed skin, and animal models contribute to our understanding of various forms of drug distribution into the skin. Fig. 8 summarizes all the applications, challenges, and methods for natural products' delivery on human skin.

5 Nanocarriers

Nanotechnology involves the application of nanometer size range materials in various fields of science and technology. The application of nanotechnology in medicine, commonly termed as nanomedicine, is not only used in treatment modalities but also for diagnosis and monitoring purposes. Nanocarriers (NC) such as dendrimers, nanoparticles, and polymeric or lipid-based carriers are designed to form particulates at the nanometer size range and having specific physicochemical properties upon encapsulation or attachment with bioactive compounds. In general, the aims of NC in topical administration are to enhance drug-delivery efficacy by increasing the bioavailability, to reduce repeated administration and toxicity by ensuring sufficient retention within the skin and to enhance cell targeting by local administration to the skin surface.

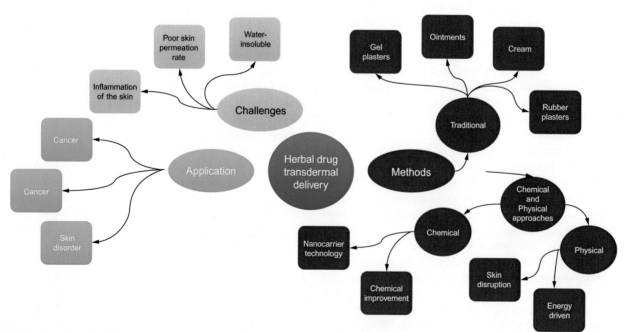

FIG. 8 Natural product delivery on the human skin: applications, challenges, and methods.

TABLE 3 The summary of nanocarriers and their preparation method for incorporation of antiinflammatory active herbal agents.

Nanocarrier	Herbal agent	Method/ technique	Formulations	Reference
Liposomes	Catechin	Solvent evaporation and sonication	(+)-Catechin, 4% w/v egg phosphatidylcholine, 1% cholesterol and additives including deoxycholic acid, dicetyl phosphate and polyethylene glycol with MW of 200 and 1000	[139]
Elastic vesicles (deformable liposomes)	Glycyrrhetinic acid	Film and high pressure homogenizer	Soybean phosphocholine, ($\pm$)-α-tocopherol, sodium deoxycholate, cholesterol, glycyrrhetinic acid	[140]
Glycerosomes	Paeoniflorin	Reverse-phase evaporation	Phospholipid (lipoid S 80), cholesterol, paeoniflorin, glycerol in water	[141]
Solid lipid nanoparticle, microemulsions	Triptolide	Emulsification-sonication	SLN containing 5% tristearin glyceride, 1.20% soybean lecithin, triptolide and 3.60% polyethylene glycol (400) monostearate; Microemulsion containing 40% isopropyl myristate, triptolide (oil phase), 50% Tween-80, 1,2-propylene glycol (5:1, v/v) and water	[142]
Nanostructured lipid Carriers	Quercetin	Emulsion evaporation-solidification	Quercetin, glyceryl monostearate, stearic acid, medium chain triglyceride, soya lecithin, TPGS	[143]
Lipospheres	Thymoquinone	Stirring and vortexing	Egg lecithin, propylene glycol, tricaprin, Tween 80, Cremophor RH 40, thymoquinone	[144]
Ethosomes	Ammonium glycyrrhizinate	Solvent evaporation	1%–3% w/v Phospholipon 90, 30%–45% (v/v) ethanol, ammonium glycyrrhizinate, and water to 100% (w/v)	[145]
Ethosomes	Matrine	Ethanol injection-sonication	1–3 g/L of lecithin, 30%–45% (v/v) ethanol, 0.25 g/L of cholesterol, matrine, or methylnicotinate and water	[146]
Nanoemulsions	Glycyrrhetic acid	Phase inversion temperature	3.1% w/w ceteareth-20, 6.9% w/w mixture of glyceryl stearate, ceteareth-12, cetearyl alcohol and cetyl palmitate, 3.5% w/w caprylic capric acid of saturated fatty alcohols C12-C18, 3.5% w/w dicaprylic carbonate. 0.5% w/w glycyrrhetic acid and 82.5% w/w water	[147]
PLGA-nanocarrier	Dictamnine	Antisolvent flash precipitation using bioreactor	Dictamnine, PLGA (85/15 L-lactide/glycolide copolymer), poly-vinylpyrrolidone	[148]

There are many advantages the NC could offer. As the herbal extracts consist of many constituents that work simultaneously and synergistically for the therapeutic efficacy, the use of NC would allow dosing of phytoconstituents in a bulk amount [137]. NC also enable smaller dose administrations since lesser amount of the herbal constituents are needed to reach the therapeutic target. This could also lead to less repeated administration and thus reducing patient compliance. The NC for topical administration purposes are developed to have various criteria to suit the need of dermal and transdermal penetration for local and systemic therapeutic effects, respectively [138]. The formulations of the herbal bioactives with NC have resulted in

various forms of nanoformulations, which include the application of solid lipid nanoparticles, nanoemulsions, liposomes, ethosomes, and other vesicular systems. Here in this chapter, a few selected types of NC are reviewed and simplified (Table 3) for their incorporation with antiinflammatory phytoconstituents and the in vivo and/or clinical studies done to determine the efficacy of the nanoformulations.

5.1 Liposomes

Liposomes are the spherical bilayer vesicles made of phospholipids that enclose an aqueous core. Liposomes can encapsulate both hydrophilic and hydrophobic compounds due to the different phases in their structure. Liposomes can interact with epidermal lipids and keratinocytes for improvement of drug retention in the skin [149]. Due to their inherent structural similarity with the natural phospholipids, liposomes are considered biocompatible and are commonly used as drug carriers.

Fang et al. [139] developed elastic liposomes for encapsulation of tea catechins via the solvent evaporation and sonication method. The catechins, which include epigallocatechin-3-gallate as the major component of the polyphenols in green tea, were proven to have antiinflammatory effects [150]. As the liposomes were incorporated with deoxycholic acid and diacetyl phosphate as the ionic surfactants, the permeation of NC was increased by five- to sevenfold. It was postulated that the liposomes permeate through the intercellular spaces of the stratum corneum layers.

The recent findings reported that the conventional liposomes were unable to penetrate deeply the skin and tend to remain confined in the upper layers of the stratum corneum [151]. Liposomes were also considered unstable as they tend to leak during the passing through the skin due to adherence to the inside wall of the skin, causing the collapse of the phospholipid-associated structures [152]. The issues associated with liposomal structure has led to the modulation of the liposomes into an improved version of the vesicular carriers known as deformable liposomes. Deformable liposomes which are also known as transfersome are the first generation of elastic vesicles made of phospholipids and an edge activator. Edge activators such as Tween 80, Span 80, and sodium cholate is responsible for destabilizing the lipid bilayers and causing the deformability of the liposomes, thus improving their penetration of the intact skin under the nonocclusion condition [153].

Deformable liposomes were used in the formulation of glycyrrhetinic acid for the treatment of dermatitis and eczema [140]. Glycyrrhetinic acid or glycyrrhetic acid (GA) is the hydrolytic product of glycyrrhizic acid, an antiinflammatory agent extracted from the root of *Glycyrrhiza glabra*, which is also the major active constituent of the licorice plant. The formulation of GA elastic vesicles with 10% ethanol produced particle size at the average of 87.3 ± 1.5 nm, which was smaller than the elastic vesicles without ethanol (106.4 ± 5.9 nm) and conventional liposomes (149.6 ± 9.9 nm). The GA elastic vehicles increased the skin deposition of GA upon nonocclusive application to the mice ears in vivo, as well as showing significant antiinflammatory activity by reducing the skin swelling of the induced chronic-contact dermatitis of the mice ears. The findings showed that the elastic vesicles were capable of enhancing the skin permeation of GA, thus suggesting the deformable liposomes are a promising carrier for transdermal drug delivery.

Another type of vesicular particles created to enhance the permeability of liposomes is known as glycerosomes. Apart from phospholipid and water, glycerosomes contain a high concentration of glycerol (10%–30% v/v), which modifies the fluidity of the liposomal bilayer [154]. Glycerosomes can be obtained using common techniques used to prepare conventional liposomes by having the one or more additives in the liposomal formulation such as the cholesterol.

Zhang et al. [141] developed paeoniflorin (PF)-loaded glycerosomes (PF-GL) to improve the transdermal delivery of PF for the potential treatment of rheumatoid arthritis (RA). The PF-GL were added with essential oil from *Speranskia tuberculate* (STO) as the transdermal enhancer to promote glycerosome penetration into the skin. PF is a monoterpene glucoside isolated from the root of *Paeonia lactiflora* Pall and has been used to treat several inflammatory diseases including RA. A in vivo study using rat knee joint model showed significantly higher accumulation (3.1-fold) of the PF in the synovium upon topical administration of the PF-GL with STO in comparison to the group treated with PF-GL without STO. The improved drug absorption in the synovium indicated that the glycerosomes formulation with STO has potential as the transdermal delivery vehicle for RA treatment.

5.2 Solid lipid nanoparticles (SLN)

The basic structure of having a solid lipophilic matrix at the particle core enables the SLN to entrap hydrophobic materials that solidify at room and body temperatures. SLN are usually dispersed in a liquid medium containing surfactants to stabilize the SLN formulations. The SLN are better suited for inflamed or damaged skin application due to their nontoxic and nonirritative lipid base components. The occlusive effect of SLN causing formation of film on the skin surface could reduce the transepidermal water loss in atopic eczema, as well as enhancing drug penetration through the stratum corneum due to the high hydration level in the skin.

Mei et al. [142] formulated SLN with triptolide (TP), a purified product from the extract of *Tripterygium wilfondil* Hook F, which is a plant used in traditional Chinese medicine. In the study, the formulation of SLN was compared with TP microemulsion by assessing their differences in the capacity of transdermal delivery and antiinflammatory activity. It was found that both SLN and microemulsions enhanced skin permeability of TP to 3.45 and 7.02 times higher than the TP control solution, respectively. The carrageenan-induced rat paw edema model showed superior activity by the SLN than the microemulsion in reducing the paw swelling, while the Frenud's adjuvant (CFA)-induced paw edema showed the opposite results. It was proposed that the SLN could have better stratum corneum penetration effect than the microemulsion if the surfactant concentration was increased.

5.3 Nanostructured lipid carriers (NLC)

The disadvantages of SLN such as low drug load, drug expulsion during storage, and high water content in the dispersion have led to the emergence of NLC [155]. As the second generation of lipid carriers, the NLC could increase the payload for active compounds and avoid compound expulsion during storage by having a mixture of different lipid molecules of solid and liquid lipids (oils) in the matrix. The amorphous state of the lipid matrix in NLC could also avoid the formation of lipid crystals as occurred in SLN, thus increasing the drug-loading capacity of the NLC.

NLC was used to be incorporated with quercetin (QT), a natural flavonoid most commonly studied for various pharmacological activities due to its antioxidation behavior against the reactive oxygen species-related diseases including skin damage caused by UV exposures. The QT-loaded NLC (QT-NLC) were formulated using the technique of emulsion evaporation-solidification at low temperatures [143]. The NLC produced were at the average size of 215 nm with high QT entrapment efficiency of 89.95%. The assessment of *in vitro* topical delivery revealed increased skin permeation and retention of QT in the epidermal and dermal layers. The QT-NLC were made into gels for ease of topical administration on the rat model of xylene-induced ear edema. The in vivo study revealed an increased rate of edema inhibition by the QT-NLC gels, which indicated the advantages of the NLC for topical delivery.

5.4 Lipospheres

Lipospheres are lipid-based nanocarriers containing a solid hydrophobic lipid core stabilized by a layer of phospholipid molecules (coat lipid) embedded on their surface. The internal core is the solid fat matrix where the bioactive compounds are dissolved or dispersed, as in Ref. [156]. Lipospheres are similar to the SLN and liposomes for its solid lipid core and having phospholipid layers as the outer coat, respectively. The combination of features from two different kinds of nanocarriers allows the lipospheres to be an ideal vehicle to improve transdermal drug delivery.

Thymoquinone (TQ) is a hydrophobic benzoquinone extracted from the black seeds of the *Nigella sativa* plant. TQ is known for its various pharmacological properties, which include antiinflammatory, antihyperglycemic, antihistamic, and anticancer properties. Due to the poor aqueous solubility and sensitivity toward light and pH variability, TQ was formulated into lipospheres for its application in topical psoriasis treatment [144]. The preparation of the lipospheres involved reconstitution of the liposphere preconcentrate in water prior to its application to reduce the water-/pH-induced degradation of TQ. The lipospheres were skin compatible and enhanced the skin penetration of TQ. The antipsoriatic activity of TQ determined from the imiquimod-induced psoriatic plaque model on BALB/c mice showed an improvement in phenotypic and histopathological features of the psoriatic skin thus suggesting the potential of TQ lipospheres in psoriasis management.

5.5 Ethosomes

Ethosomes are the lipid vesicles made of phospholipids, ethanol, and water. Ethosomes were originally designed as an alternative to liposomes, which explains the structural similarity between ethosomes and liposomes, except for the use of ethanol instead of cholesterol in ethosomes [151]. The high concentration of ethanol in the ethosome formulations is responsible in enhancing the skin permeation of the particles to release the drug load in the deeper layer of skin and thus into the systemic circulation. Ethosomes are soft, malleable, and highly deformable, making them easy to permeate intact through the skin. The ability of ethosomes to penetrate deep into the skin layers might be due to the ethanol binding to the polar group of lecithin molecules in the skin, therefore reducing the lipid melting point, increasing the fluidity of the lipids, and enhancing the permeability of the cell membrane [149].

Ammonium glycyrrhizinate (AG) is the ammonium salt of the glycyrrhizic acid, a derivative of glycyrrhetic acid. AG is known for its antiinflammatory activity and therefore was incorporated into ethosomes for topical application [145]. The AG-ethosomes were prepared by the solvent evaporation method to produce suspensions with particle size ranging from 100 to 350 nm, depending on the amount of ethanol and lecithin in the formulation. The ethosomal suspensions containing 45% (v/v) ethanol and 2% (w/v) lecithin showed skin tolerability in human volunteers up to 48 h of application. The AG-ethosomal formulations showed significant reduction of skin erythema compared to the treatment of free AG, possibly owing to the sustained AG release from the ethosomes, hence prolonging the therapeutic activity of the active compound.

Another ethosomal formulation of an antiinflammatory agent involved the incorporation of matrine, the major active component derived from the shrub plant, *Sophora flavescens* [146]. The matrine ethosomes prepared by the ethanol injection-method produced particles at 50–200 nm size range and matrine entrapment efficiency of 40%–90%. The study also reported a pattern of decreased ethosomal particle size with the increase of ethanol concentration, while a pattern of increase in particle size when higher phospholipid concentration was used. The antiinflammatory activity of matrine ethosomes was determined using an induced erythema model on in vivo rat skin. The results revealed significantly rapid reduction of the erythema by the matrine ethosomes in comparison to the matrine enanoethosome formulations. The ethosomes are proved to be an ideal nanocarrier due to their good skin tolerability and enhancement of the percutaneous permeations.

5.6 Nanoemulsions

Nanoemulsions are composed of two nonmiscible liquids, commonly oil and water that mix to form either oil-in-water (O/W) or water-in-oil (W/O) emulsions. These systems contain nanosized droplets that are stabilized by surfactant and cosurfactant via the formation of interfacial layers around the droplets, causing them to repel each other to maintain their individual particle structures within the same phase.

GA was formulated into nanoemulsions using a type of low-energy emulsification technique known as the phase inversion temperature method [147]. The method was able to produce nanoemulsion droplets in the size range of 180–240 nm. In a study of percutaneous absorption through excised human skin (stratum corneum and epidermis), the nanoemulsion was found to increase the GA transdermal permeability in comparison to the control solution of O/W emulsions. The antiinflammatory activity of the GA nanoemulsions was also proven by the inhibition of UVB-induced erythema performed on healthy human volunteers.

5.7 Polymeric nanoparticles

Nanoparticles constructed from polymers can be used as reservoirs for lipophilic herbal agents to improve drug delivery through the skin. Biodegradable and biocompatible polymeric nanoparticles are commonly used for the entrapment or attachment of active ingredients and can be of natural sources or synthetically made. Poly(lactide-*co*-glycolide) (PLGA) is one example of biodegradable, synthetic polymer that has been ubiquitously used to form nanoparticles for various biomedical purposes. Lin et al. [148] used PLGA-based nanocarriers for the incorporation of dictamnine, a component extracted from the root bark of *Dictamnus dasycarpus* Turcz for the treatment of atopic dermatitis (AD). Dictamnine has been used in Chinese medicine for many years for the treatment of inflammatory skin diseases such as eczema, urticaria, and pruritus vulvae [157]. The PLGA-dictamnine was prepared by an antisolvent precipitation technique using a bioreactor. The ultrarapid process managed to produce fine PLGA nanoparticle with sizes of approximately 186 nm. The oxazolone-induced atopic dermatitis model in mice revealed alleviation of the AD symptoms by the PLGA-dictamnine treatment, presumably due to the increased drug release and epidermal penetration compared to those of naked dictamnine. The PLGA-based nanoparticles, hence, were proven capable of penetrating the dermal tissues for enhanced drug delivery of dictamnine.

The summary of various nanocarriers and their preparation method for the incorporation of antiinflammatory active herbal agents is summarized in Table 3

6 Gels

Gels are semisolid structures composed of small- or large-molecule dispersions with the inclusion of a gelling agent/polymer in aqueous or hydroalcoholic liquid vehicles [158]. Gels have been used in many areas including the food, cosmetics, and pharmaceutical industries. Gels are one of the favorite delivery systems because of their easy preparation and ability to provide direct contact between the therapeutic agent and the site of absorption. The main ingredient of gels is the gelling agents, which form colloidal mixture in the liquid phase. The preparation of gels for therapeutic purposes may contain one or more medicinal substances, along with additional solvents such as alcohol, glycerine, and propylene glycol, preservatives such as propyl paraben and methyl paraben, as well as chelating agents.

Gels can be classified according to several different conditions but the most common is based on the colloidal phase and the type of solvent used. On the basis of the colloidal phase, the gels are classified either as a single-phase (organic gels) or a two-phase system (inorganic gels). The single-phase gels are composed of large organic molecules dissolved in a liquid phase to form a semisynthetic polymer, synthetic polymer, or natural gums. The two-phase gels have three-dimensional structures throughout the gel mass due to their large particle size in the dispersed phase. The gel mass (magma) generally has floccules of small particles, which contribute to the structure instability of the gel [159].

6.1 Organogels, hydrogels, xerogels, and aerogels

On the basis of solvent, gels can be classified into organogels (nonaqueous solvent), hydrogels (aqueous solvent), and aerogels/xerogels. Organogels are a semisolid system comprising an organic liquid phase that is immobilized by a three-dimensional network of intertwined self-assembled structures known as gelator fibers [160]. The organogels can be made of water-insoluble oleaginous (containing or producing oil) materials. Despite containing high liquid, the organogels behave and appeared like solids. Organogels can be further classified into either low-molecular organogelators or polymeric gelators depending on the nature of the gelling molecules.

Hydrogels are composed of hydrophilic homopolymers or copolymers that form three-dimensional cross-linked water-insoluble structures capable of swelling in the aqueous environment while maintaining their structural integrity [161]. Due to its ability of retaining high water

TABLE 4 The summary of novel gels and their preparation method for incorporation of antiinflammatory active herbal agents.

Herbal extract	Nanocarriers	Method/technique	Formulations	Reference
Capsaicin	Liposomes in Carbopol 1% w/w gel	Thin film hydration	Capsaicin, soya phosphatidylcholine, cholesterol	[162]
	Niosomes in Carbopol 1% w/w gel	Thin film hydration	Capsaicin, Span 80, cholesterol	
	Emulsomes in 1% w/w gel	Film hydration	Capsaicin, soya phosphatidylcholine, cholesterol, tristearin	
Psoralen	Liposomes in 15% w/w hydroxy propyl methyl cellulose gel	Thin film hydration	Psoralen, cationic liposomes = 3ß-[N-(N', N'-dimethylaminoethane)-carbamoyl] cholesterol hydrochloride, cholesterol; Anionic liposomes = egg lecithin, cholesterol, tetramyristoyl cardiolipin	[163]
Celastrol	Niosome gel	Thin film hydration method and probe sonication	Celastrol, Span 20: Span 60: cholesterol = 3:1:1 w/w	[164]
Curcumin	Nanoemulsion gel	Low-energy emulsification	Curcumin, oil phase (propylene glycol dicaprylocaprate, diethylene glycol monoethyl ether), Smix (Tween 20, polyethylene glycol (15)-hydroxy stearate), polyacrylic acid (carbopol 934) hydrogel	[165]
Tea tree oil and adapalene	Nanoemulsion gel	Spontaneous emulsification	0.1% adapalene, 6% tea tree oil, 10% dimethyl sulfoxide, Tween 80: Span 80 (75:25)	[166]
Triptolide	Solid lipid nanoparticle hydrogel	Emulsification-sonication	SLN containing triptolide, tristearin glyceride, stearic acid, lecithin or poloxamer 188, PEG400MS soybean lecithin, 0.5% glycerol, 1.5% Carbomer 940, double distilled water	[167]

content and soft consistency, hydrogels have been used for various medical applications including as drug-delivery vehicle in the formulation of microparticles and nanoparticles.

Xerogels are a solid form of gel with low solvent concentration. Xerogels are commonly formed by the solvent evaporation method, which results in high porosity and high surface area gel with small pore sizes. The xerogels tend to crack due to the extreme shrinkage during the drying process but are still able to retain their original shape. Aerogels are formed when the liquid phase of a gel is replaced with gas, resulting in a solid gel network retained having minimal or no shrinkage. In short, the drying process used on the gel determines the formation of either xerogels or aerogels.

6.2 Advanced gel-delivery systems

The advancement in gel delivery systems has brought forward the use of novel gel systems to improve drug delivery for local or systemic actions. These novel gels allow the controlled and sustained release of drugs, better tissue targeting, and providing more protection and stability to the API. The novel gels are also designed to react on stimuli for a more controlled release of the active compounds. Table 4 summarizes different types of novel gels used to incorporate antiinflammatory active herbal agents for topical drug delivery.

Nanogels are one of the advanced forms of gels created with many advantages including high biocompatibility, biodegradability and drug loading, as well as having the rapid swelling/contracting behavior. Nanogels are also termed as hydrogel nanoparticles, in which nanoparticulate system, the hydrogel or organogel matrices are uniformly dispersed. Nanoparticles can be placed inside the gel or positioned as the exosystems, for instance in the case of liposome mixtures or nanosuspensions' incorporation in gels [168].

Capsaicin is an active compound isolated from chili peppers that has the potential to treat psoriasis. Gupta et al. [162] incorporated capsaicin in the vesicular systems of liposomes, niosomes, and emulsomes in gels for localized and topical delivery of the antiinflammatory agent. The results of an in vivo drug localization study in the dorsal skin of rats showed capsaicin retention in the stratum corneum of 7.75, 4.8, and 2.9-fold for the emulsomal, liposomal, and niosomal gel systems respectively, as compared to plain gel. As the emulsomes had the highest entrapment efficiency, good physical stability, and able to continuously release the active compound in a sustained manner, it was concluded that the emulsomes-incorporated gels were the most effective among the three vesicular systems for the local delivery of the antipsoriatic agents through the topical route.

Another liposomal incorporation in gels was formulated with psoralen, a natural compound found in the seeds of *Psoralea corylifolia*. Psoralen is commonly combined with ultraviolet light A (UVA) radiation (PUVA) in the phototherapy treatment of psoriasis, eczema, vitiligo, and other skin problems. Doppalapudi et al. [163] developed topical PUVA with psoralen liposomal nanocarriers in the form of two different charged liposomes. The psoralen cationic and anionic gels showed high amelioration of psoriasis symptoms in mice when compared to the psoralen control solution. The improved efficacy of liposomal gels was associated with high drug penetration and skin deposition, which helped to alleviate the severity of the imiquimod (IMQ)-induced psoriasis-like skin inflammation.

Niosomes are the vesicles with bilayer membranes that mainly composed of nonionic surfactants and have better stability than liposomes. An extract from Chinese herbal medicine known as celastrol has been incorporated in a niosome gel for the improvement of its therapeutic effects against psoriasis [164]. Celastrol is a pentacyclic triterpenoid extracted from *Tripterygium wilfordii* Hook f. and has been used traditionally to treat rheumatoid arthritis and psoriasis. A celastrol-incorporated niosome gel was able to reduce the erythema on the mouse skin in the in vivo IMQ-induced psoriasis model. The niosome hydrogel was able to increase the water solubility of celastrol thus improving its antipsoriasis activity.

Emulgel or emulsion gel is a novel, topical, drug-delivery device that has the potential to be a boost for dermal treatment and cosmetology. Emulgels are the combination of emulsion and gel technologies and are formed either as oil-in-water or water-in-oil emulsions that are gelled by adding the gel-forming agent [169]. The advantages of emulgels include better drug entrapment than the conventional gels, less greasy features, longer shelf life than emulsions, and lower production cost than vesicular gels [170].

Nanoemulgel is the combination of nanoemulsions and emulgels. Algahtani et al. [165] formulated curcumin nanoemulsion, which later converted into nanoemulgel using Carbopol 934 as the gel-forming agent. The nanoemulgel formulations exhibited a faster healing of the psoriasis-like symptoms in mice compared to the curcumin gel and betamethasone-17-valerate gel (control), suggesting improved curcumin penetration by the nanoemulgels in psoriatic skin. Najafi-Taher et al. [166] formulated tea tree oil-based nanoemulsions that were incorporated with adapalene, a naphthoic acid used for the topical treatment of acne vulgaris. The nanoemulsion was subsequently incorporated with 1% Carbopol 934 to convert the formulation into the gel form. The in vivo skin irritation study revealed no irritation and erythema from the use of the adapalene-loaded tea tree oil nanoemulsion gel, indicating its potential to be used in acne vulgaris treatment.

Solid lipid nanoparticles were also incorporated into the hydrogel. Mei et al. [167] formulated the SLN hydrogels with triptolide and found that the nanoparticulate structure of SLN was maintained upon conversion to gels, thus avoiding the SLN aggregation in the system, as well as having a longer shelf life. The soybean lecithin and lipids in the SLN formulations also helped in reducing the adverse side effects of triptolide. From the carrageenan-induced paw edema test, the SLN-hydrogel was able to reduce the rat paw inflammation twofold higher than that of conventional triptolide hydrogel. The antiinflammatory activity was attributed to the increased cumulative absorption of triptolide upon topical application of the SLN hydrogels.

The summary of different novel gels and their preparation method for the incorporation of antiinflammatory active herbal agents is given in Table 4.

7 Films

Nowadays, medicated films have received much interest as a topical application therapy due to their ease of application, capacity to target a specific area with an appropriate dose, and capacity to terminate therapy at any time by removing the device [171]. The basic backbone for film preparation is the polymeric film forming device (natural and synthetic) that may be employed alone or together [171]. There are some characteristics for films, which must be taken into considerations such as, water solubility, water vapor permeability (WVP), and moisture content [172]. Film-forming solution (FFS) is a recent substance used to supply several drugs transdermally. In general, FFS consists of drugs and film polymer(s) that are dissolved into a vehicle and essential excipients [173]. Table 5 shows some of the

TABLE 5 Examples of using herbal extract in formulation of film against inflammation.

Herbal extract	Formulation of film	Characteristics	Reference
Apocynum cannabinum	Apocynin (0.05 g) film using casein (CAS) as a film-forming protein, benzalkonium chloride (0.01%) as a preservative, CAS (0.5 g), and glycerol (0.8 g)	Application of apocynin films on rat paw before or after an induction of carrageenan paw, which showed a significant decrease in paw swelling and elevation of the edema inhibition	[171]
Piper nigrum	Piperine-rich herbal mixture plus film-forming solution (PHM-E FFS) at final concentration 3% w/w	PHM-E FFS showed antiinflammatory activity with low viscosity and the Newtonian behavior. Also, it exhibited moderate-to-high potency for inhibition of inflammatory signs in the rats	[173]
Curcuma longa	Curcumin or diferuloylmethane (1,7-bis-[4-hydroxy-3-methoxyphenyl]-1,6-heptadiene-3,5-dione): Using mucoadhesive films	No side effects have been documented and healing in all cases was unpredictable	[174]
Shikonin (Prepared from plant)	Biopolymeric film containing bioactive naphthoquinone	Reduced lesion morphological sign intensity in the patient population investigated, and due to faster pain alleviation, inflammatory damaging focal epithelialization in the oral mucosa	[175]
Azadirachta indica	Biocomposite film (incorporate collagen film)	Good antiinflammatory activity	[176]

examples of film formulation from herbal extracts for inflammation.

The mechanical parameters of the films were determined using the following equations using a computerized tensile strength tester [177].

The following formula was used to compute the percentage elongation at break, E_b, of the tested films:

$$E_b = \frac{L_e - L_o}{L_o} \times 100$$

where L_o is its original length and L_e is the film's length after elongation.

Hook's law was used to determine the film's modulus of elasticity (ME):

$$B = \text{ME} \left(\frac{L_e - L_o}{L_o} \right) \qquad (1)$$

The tensile strength, B, of the films under test was determined using the following equation:

$$B = \frac{F}{A} \qquad (2)$$

where F is the maximum force exposed to the film, and A is its cross-sectional area.

8   Ointments/creams

Essential oils are odorous, poisonous compounds, present in the flowers, fruits, leaves, and roots of many plants. For over 2000 years, the production of these odorous compounds from plants has been an effective task [178]. The leaves, flowers, and stems of *Ocimum basilicum* have various medicinal features, and one of the most important is antiinflammatory feature and constituents such as methylchavicol (estragol) linalool, eugenol, and 1,8-cineole [179]. Peppermint oil obtained from *Mentha piperita* also showed an antiinflammatory effect on its oil from steam distillation from the stems effect. The oil is extracted from stems, and leaves by steam distillation and its major constituents include 1,8-cineole, menthofurane, menthone, menthol, pulegone, and menthyl acetate [179]. Fennel oil is made by steam distilling the crushed seeds of *Foeniculum vulgare*, a member of the Apiaceae or Umbelliferae family. This plant exhibits antiinflammatory properties. Its major components are trans-anethole (phenolic ester), fenchone (ketone), α-pinene (monoterpene), and methyl chavicol (phenol) [179]. *Cuminum cyminum* from the same family can be used as an antiinflammatory. Its main components include cuminaldehyde, γ-terpinene, β-pinene, *p*-mentadienal, and *p*-cymene [179]. To evaluate the various properties, numerous cream batches have been produced and physicochemically characterized. Most of the produced creams may look dark brown mainly because of the presence of phyto-constituents incorporated as extracts.

The USP describes creams as "a semisolid emulsion that comprises more than 20% of aqueous phase and/or less than 50% of oleaginous phase for external application to the skin" [180]. Some advantages of plant-based ointments are described below.

Pharmaceutical ointments are quickly applied on the skin and form an occlusive barrier at the site of application, eliminating moisture removal from the skin. This is particularly beneficial when it comes to restoring the physical features of the skin (e.g., due to inflammation).

Pharmaceutical ointments have lubricating/emollient effects, which can be used to minimize trauma to an infected site during spread.

The hydrophobicity and retention of pharmaceutical ointments are advantageous when applied to mucosa, such as an inflamed hemorrhoid or the eyelids, where fluid flow/inflammation will usually help to dilute other formulations (e.g., oil-in-water creams); however, it should be cautioned that applying ointments on wet surfaces may be challenging due to the hydrophobic properties of the majority of ointments.

Owing to the opaque nature of pastes (as a result of their high solid content), this formulation is suitable for use as a sunblock.

Pharmaceutical ointments, in general, remain at the site of delivery, allowing for a longer period of opioid release than is possible for many other topical dosage formulations. Pharmaceutical pastes' improved viscosity ensures that a dense layer of the drug type is added to the site of operation, which exhibits exceptional persistence. This property is especially advantageous when protection is needed on an inflamed spot, as is the case with eczema and psoriasis.

The chemical stability of hydrolyzed medicinal agents can be significantly improved by the application of pharmaceutical ointments and pastes.

Pharmaceutical pastes are often porous due to their high solid content, allowing moisture to escape from the applied spot. Additionally, pastes can serve as an absorbent of moisture and chemicals contained within exudates.

Nevertheless, the disadvantage concerns that the ointments are generally greasy and difficult to remove (and are therefore often cosmetically unacceptable) [180]. Most of the plant-based creams utilize in vivo animal models for evaluation on the efficacy. For this, the backs of animal like rats are properly shaved 24 h prior to administration of the sample. The cream is given to animals' skin patches and the application site is evaluated at 24, 48, and 72 h for changes in any dermal responses. The irritation index is developed to determine the cream's irritant potential using the following the Draize rating criteria [181]:

Erythema and escher formation	
No erythema	0
Very slight erythema (barely perceptible)	1
Well-defined erythema	2
Moderate-to-severe erythema	3

Erythema and escher formation	
Severe erythema (beef redness) to escher formation	
Preventing grading of erythema	4
Edema formation	
No edema	0
Very slight edema (barely perceptible)	1
Slight edema (edges of area well defined by definite raising)	2
Moderate edema (raised approximately 1 mm)	3
Severe edema (raised more than 1 mm and extending beyond)	
Area of exposure	4

9 Patent's perspective

According to the granted patents' search (https://link.lens.org/iL034O78Kck, accessed on June 1, 2021), the number of patents granted over the last 5 years has been steadily increasing since 2016 (from 50 in 2016 to 110 in 2020), indicating a high demand for topical antiinflammatory formulations based on herbal bioactives. In terms of distribution, the majority of patents were granted in the United States, followed by European Patents and Australia, with the United States accounting for 77.6% of all world patents. As per the numbers, Amarin Pharmaceuticals le Ltd was granted 25 patents, with Soni Paresh as the lead inventor (24 document counts). Most granted patents are for herbal combinations with bioactive compositions for treating eczema, analgesics-based snake venoms, antimicrobial, mucosal tissue, inflammatory disorders, psoriasis, seborrheic keratosis, and other inflammatory skin ailments. *Curcuma longa* L. is a well-known patented herb that contains bioactive phenolic diketones such as curcumin, demethoxycurcumin, and bisdemethoxycurcumin in microemulsion and nanoemulsion formulations [182,183]. Traditional Chinese Medicine herbs such as Sheng Di Huang, Da Huang, and Jin Yin Hua have been advocated as topical treatments for eczema and/or other skin and scalp conditions [184]. Due to the medical benefits of plant-based therapeutic agents, there will be a strong demand for topical-based antiinflammatory formulations on herbal bioactives in the future.

10 Conclusions and future direction

In a nutshell, antiinflammatory activities of several phytoconstituents have been demonstrated. Some of these include flavonoids, triterpenoids, and alkaloids. Although it is widely perceived that natural products are safe, there is also evidence suggesting that they are not safe to use once taken. Despite broad belief in the safety of botanical extracts and widespread usage of herbal formulations in the community, it goes without saying that the topical route of administration is an effective technique to deliver drugs to the skin region through the dermal layer of the skin for inflammation. The rapid emergence and evolution of nanomedicine has shown how novel drug-delivery systems can address the pharmacological limitations of traditional herbal medicines. The exciting potential of topical nanoformulations is that they can deliver potent herbal constituents in a targeted manner. Modern formulations using *in silico*, predictive formulation development tools, and computational methods are preferred and could be the frontier in future research for topical delivery of antiinflammatory agents due to benefits such as a clear approach to the region of action and local distribution of a plant's active medicinal ingredient.

References

[1] Antiinflammatory actions of cat's claw: the role of NF-κB, Aliment. Pharmacol. Ther. 12 (12) (1998) 1279–1289, https://doi.org/10.1046/j.1365-2036.1998.00424.x.

[2] M.A. Abu-Al-Basal, Healing potential of Rosmarinus officinalis L. on full-thickness excision cutaneous wounds in alloxan-induced-diabetic BALB/c mice, J. Ethnopharmacol. 131 (2) (2010) 443–450, https://doi.org/10.1016/j.jep.2010.07.007.

[3] A. Aderem, D.M. Underhill, Mechanisms of phagocytosis in macrophages, Annu. Rev. Immunol. 17 (1) (1999) 593–623, https://doi.org/10.1146/annurev.immunol.17.1.593.

[4] C.R. Afonso, R.S. Hirano, A.L. Gaspar, E.G.L. Chagas, R.A. Carvalho, F.V. Silva, G.R. Leonardi, P.S. Lopes, C.F. Silva, C.M.P. Yoshida, Biodegradable antioxidant chitosan films useful as an anti-aging skin mask, Int. J. Biol. Macromol. 132 (2019) 1262–1273, https://doi.org/10.1016/j.ijbiomac.2019.04.052.

[5] Ajazuddin, A. Alexander, A. Khichariya, S. Gupta, R.J. Patel, T.K. Giri, D.K. Tripathi, Recent expansions in an emergent novel drug delivery technology: Emulgel, J. Control. Release 171 (2) (2013) 122–132, https://doi.org/10.1016/j.jconrel.2013.06.030.

[6] N. Akhtar, V. Singh, M. Yusuf, R.A. Khan, Non-invasive drug delivery technology: development and current status of transdermal drug delivery devices, techniques and biomedical applications, Biomed. Eng./Biomedizinische Technik 65 (3) (2020) 243–272, https://doi.org/10.1515/bmt-2019-0019.

[7] S. Viji Chandran, T.S. Amritha, M. Pandimadevi, A preliminary in vitro study on the bovine collagen film incorporated with Azadirachta indica plant extract as a potential wound dressing material, Int. J. PharmTech Res. 8 (6) (2015) 248–257. http://www.sphinxsai.com/2015/ph_vol8_no6/2/(248-257)V8N6PT.pdf.

[8] L. Allen, H.C. Ansel, Ansel's Pharmaceutical Dosage Forms and Drug Delivery Systems, 2013.

[9] G.P. Amaral, N.R. de Carvalho, R.P. Barcelos, F. Dobrachinski, R. de Lima Portella, M.H. da Silva, T.H. Lugokenski, G.R.M. Dias, S.C.A. da Luz, A.A. Boligon, M.L. Athayde, M.A. Villetti, F.A. Antunes Soares, R. Fachinetto, Protective action of ethanolic extract of Rosmarinus officinalis L. in gastric ulcer prevention induced by ethanol in rats, Food Chem. Toxicol. 55 (2013) 48–55, https://doi.org/10.1016/j.fct.2012.12.038.

[10] H.P.T. Ammon, Modulation of the immune system by Boswellia serrata extracts and boswellic acids, Phytomedicine 17 (11) (2010) 862–867, https://doi.org/10.1016/j.phymed.2010.03.003.

[11] A. Anil, S.K. Gujjari, M.P. Venkatesh, Evaluation of a curcumin-containing mucoadhesive film for periodontal postsurgical pain control, J. Indian Soc. Periodontol. 23 (5) (2019) 461–468, https://doi.org/10.4103/jisp.jisp_700_18.

[12] S.H. Ansari, F. Islam, M. Sameem, Influence of nanotechnology on herbal drugs: a review, J. Adv. Pharm. Technol. Res. 3 (3) (2012) 142–146, https://doi.org/10.4103/2231-4040.101006.

[13] H.M. Anter, I.I.A. Hashim, W. Awadin, M.M. Meshali, Novel antiinflammatory film as a delivery system for the external medication with bioactive phytochemical "Apocynin", Drug Des. Devel. Ther. 12 (2018) 2981–3001, https://doi.org/10.2147/DDDT.S176850.

[14] R. Asasutjarit, P. Sookdee, S. Veeranondha, A. Fuongfuchat, A. Itharat, Application of film-forming solution as a transdermal delivery system of piperine-rich herbal mixture extract for anti-inflammation, Heliyon 6 (6) (2020), e04139, https://doi.org/10.1016/j.heliyon.2020.e04139.

[15] A.G. Atanasov, B. Waltenberger, E.M. Pferschy-Wenzig, T. Linder, C. Wawrosch, P. Uhrin, V. Temml, L. Wang, S. Schwaiger, E.H. Heiss, J.M. Rollinger, D. Schuster, J.M. Breuss, V. Bochkov, M.D. Mihovilovic, B. Kopp, R. Bauer, V.M. Dirsch, H. Stuppner, Discovery and resupply of pharmacologically active plant-derived natural products: a review, Biotechnol. Adv. 33 (8) (2015) 1582–1614, https://doi.org/10.1016/j.biotechadv.2015.08.001.

[16] W.A. Banks, Characteristics of compounds that cross the blood-brain barrier, BMC Neurol. 9 (1) (2009), https://doi.org/10.1186/1471-2377-9-S1-S3.

[17] W.A. Banks, Physiology and pathology of the blood brain barrier: implications for microbial pathogenesis drug delivery and neurodegenerative disorders, J. Neurovirol. 5 (6) (1994) 538–555.

[18] J. Bauer, S. Kuehnl, J.M. Rollinger, O. Scherer, H. Northoff, H. Stuppner, O. Werz, A. Koeberle, Carnosol and carnosic acids from Salvia officinalis inhibit microsomal prostaglandin E2 synthase-1, J. Pharmacol. Exp. Ther. 342 (1) (2012) 169–176, https://doi.org/10.1124/jpet.112.193847.

[19] J.J.F. Belch, D. Ansell, R. Madhok, A. O'Dowd, R.D. Sturrock, Effects of altering dietary essential fatty acids on requirements for non-steroidal anti-inflammatory drugs in patients with rheumatoid arthritis: a double blind placebo controlled study, Ann. Rheum. Dis. 47 (2) (1988) 96–104, https://doi.org/10.1136/ard.47.2.96.

[20] J.E. Bernstein, D.R. Bickers, M.V. Dahl, J.Y. Roshal, Treatment of chronic postherpatic neuralgia with topical capsaicin. A preliminary study, J. Am. Acad. Dermatol. 17 (1987) 93–98.

[21] L. Biedermann, J. Mwinyi, M. Scharl, P. Frei, J. Zeitz, G.A. Kullak-Ublick, S.R. Vavricka, M. Fried, A. Weber, H.U. Humpf, S. Peschke, A. Jetter, G. Krammer, G. Rogler, Bilberry ingestion improves disease activity in mild to moderate ulcerative colitis—an open pilot study, J. Crohn's Colitis 7 (4) (2013) 271–279, https://doi.org/10.1016/j.crohns.2012.07.010.

[22] A. Bishayee, R.J. Thoppil, A. Mandal, A.S. Darvesh, V. Ohanyan, J.G. Meszaros, E. Háznagy-Radnai, J. Hohmann, D. Bhatia, Black currant phytoconstituents exert chemoprevention of diethylnitrosamine-initiated hepatocarcinogenesis by suppression of the inflammatory response, Mol. Carcinog. 52 (4) (2013) 304–317, https://doi.org/10.1002/mc.21860.

[23] F. Blotman, E. Mahen, A. Wulwik, H. Carpard, A. Lopez, Efficacy and safety of avocado/soyabean unsaponifiables in the treatment of symptomatic osteoarthritis of knee and hip. A prospective

multicentre, three months, randomized, double blind, placebo-controlled trial, Rev. Rheum. 64 (12) (1997) 825–834.

[24] P. Bogani, C. Galli, M. Villa, F. Visioli, Postprandial anti-inflammatory and antioxidant effects of extra virgin olive oil, Atherosclerosis 190 (1) (2007) 181–186, https://doi.org/10.1016/j.atherosclerosis.2006.01.011.

[25] A. Borghi, M. Corazza, S. Minghetti, G. Toni, A. Virgili, Avocado and soybean extracts as active principles in the treatment of mild-to-moderate vulvar lichen sclerosus: results of efficacy and tolerability, J. Eur. Acad. Dermatol. Venereol. 29 (6) (2015) 1225–1230, https://doi.org/10.1111/jdv.12617.

[26] J.L. Borowitz, P.G. Gunasekar, G.E. Isom, Hydrogen cyanide generation by µ-opiate receptor activation: possible neuromodulatory role of endogenous cyanide, Brain Res. 768 (1–2) (1997) 294–300, https://doi.org/10.1016/S0006-8993(97)00659-8.

[27] J.D. Bos, M.M.H.M. Meinardi, The 500 Dalton rule for the skin penetration of chemical compounds and drugs, Exp. Dermatol. 9 (3) (2000) 165–169, https://doi.org/10.1034/j.1600-0625.2000.009003165.x.

[28] R. Bundy, A.F. Walker, R.W. Middleton, J. Booth, Turmeric extract may improve irritable bowel syndrome symptomology in otherwise healthy adults: a pilot study, J. Altern. Complement. Med. 10 (6) (2004) 1015–1018, https://doi.org/10.1089/acm.2004.10.1015.

[29] T.J. Burke, 5 Questions-and answers-about MIRE treatment, Adv. Skin Wound Care 16 (7) (2003) 369–371, https://doi.org/10.1097/00129334-200312000-00016.

[30] A. Camargo, O.A. Rangel-Zuñiga, C. Haro, E.R. Meza-Miranda, P. Peña-Orihuela, M.E. Meneses, C. Marin, E.M. Yubero-Serrano, P. Perez-Martinez, J. Delgado-Lista, J.M. Fernandez-Real, M.D. Luque De Castro, F.J. Tinahones, J. Lopez-Miranda, F. Perez-Jimenez, Olive oil phenolic compounds decrease the postprandial inflammatory response by reducing postprandial plasma lipopolysaccharide levels, Food Chem. 162 (2014) 161–171, https://doi.org/10.1016/j.foodchem.2014.04.047.

[31] M.J. Caterina, D. Julius, The vanilloid receptor: a molecular gateway to the pain pathway, Annu. Rev. Neurosci. 24 (2001) 487–517, https://doi.org/10.1146/annurev.neuro.24.1.487.

[32] G. Chen-yu, Y. Chun-fen, L. Qi-lu, T. Qi, X. Yan-wei, L. Wei-na, Z. Guang-xi, Development of a Quercetin-loaded nanostructured lipid carrier formulation for topical delivery, Int. J. Pharm. 430 (1–2) (2012) 292–298, https://doi.org/10.1016/j.ijpharm.2012.03.042.

[33] Y.C. Cheng, T.S. Li, H.L. Su, P.C. Lee, H.M.D. Wang, Transdermal delivery systems of natural products applied to skin therapy and care, Molecules (Basel, Switzerland) 25 (21) (2020), https://doi.org/10.3390/molecules25215051.

[34] S. Chrubasik, E. Eisenberg, E. Balan, T. Weinberger, R. Luzzati, C. Conradt, Treatment of low back pain exacerbations with willow bark extract: a randomized double-blind study, Am. J. Med. 109 (1) (2000) 9–14, https://doi.org/10.1016/S0002-9343(00)00442-3.

[35] S. Chrubasik, O. Künzel, A. Model, C. Conradt, A. Black, Treatment of low back pain with a herbal or synthetic anti-rheumatic: a randomized controlled study. Willow bark extract for low back pain, Rheumatology 40 (12) (2001) 1388–1393.

[36] S. Chrubasik, W. Enderlein, R. Bauer, W. Grabner, Evidence for antirheumatic effectiveness of Herba Urticae dioicae in acute arthritis: a pilot study, Phytomedicine 4 (2) (1997) 105–108, https://doi.org/10.1016/S0944-7113(97)80052-9.

[37] J.M. Chung, K.H. Lee, H. Yuichi, W.D. Willis, Effects of capsaicin applied to a peripheral nerve on the responses of primate spinothalamic tract cells, Brain Res. 329 (1–2) (1985) 27–38, https://doi.org/10.1016/0006-8993(85)90509-8.

[38] M. Corazza, A. Borghi, M. Lauriola, A. Virgili, Use of topical herbal remedies and cosmetics: a questionnaire-based investigation in dermatology out-patients, J. Eur. Acad. Dermatol. Venereol. 23 (11) (2009) 1298–1303, https://doi.org/10.1111/j.1468-3083.2009.03314.x.

[39] J.A. Crowell, B.K. Kusserow, W.L. Nyborg, Functional changes in WBC after microsonation ultrasound, Med. Biol. 3 (2) (1997) 185–190.

[40] C.L. Curtis, C.E. Hughes, C.R. Flannery, C.B. Little, J.L. Harwood, B. Caterson, n-3 Fatty acids specifically modulate catabolic factors involved in articular cartilage degradation, J. Biol. Chem. 275 (2) (2000) 721–724, https://doi.org/10.1074/jbc.275.2.721.

[41] C.L. Curtis, S.G. Rees, C.B. Little, C.R. Flannery, C.E. Hughes, C. Wilson, C.M. Dent, I.G. Otterness, J.L. Harwood, B. Caterson, Pathologic indicators of degradation and inflammation in human osteoarthritic cartilage are abrogated by exposure to n-3 fatty acids, Arthritis Rheum. 46 (6) (2002) 1544–1553, https://doi.org/10.1002/art.10305.

[42] M.L. Daviglus, J. Stamler, A.J. Orencia, A.R. Dyer, K. Liu, P. Greenland, M.K. Walsh, D. Morris, R.B. Shekelle, Fish consumption and the 30-year risk of fatal myocardial infarction, N. Engl. J. Med. 336 (15) (1997) 1046–1053, https://doi.org/10.1056/NEJM199704103361502.

[43] A.G. De Boer, P.J. Gaillard, Drug targeting to the brain, Annu. Rev. Pharmacol. Toxicol. 47 (2007) 323–355, https://doi.org/10.1146/annurev.pharmtox.47.120505.105237.

[44] P.G. De Deyne, M. Kirsch-Volders, In vitro effects of therapeutic ultrasound on the nucleus of human fibroblasts, Phys. Ther. 75 (7) (1995) 629–634, https://doi.org/10.1093/ptj/75.7.629.

[45] A.J. Domb, Lipospheres for controlled delivery of substances, in: Microencapsulation, 1993, pp. 217–316.

[46] K.B.M. Tijburg, T. Mattern, J.D. Folts, U.M. Weisgerber, M.B. Katan, Tea flavonoids and cardiovascular diseases: a review, Crit. Rev. Food Sci. Nutr. 37 (8) (1997) 771–785, https://doi.org/10.1080/10408399709527802.

[47] D. Draper, S. Sunderland, Examination of the law of grotthis-drapes: does ultrasound penetrate subcutaneous fat in humans, J. Athl. Train. 28 (3) (1993) 248–250.

[48] D.O. Draper, J.C. Castel, D. Castel, Rate of temperature increase in human muscle during 1 MHz and 3 MHz continuous ultrasound, J. Orthop. Sports Phys. Ther. 22 (4) (1995) 142–150, https://doi.org/10.2519/jospt.1995.22.4.142.

[49] V.N. Drozdov, V.A. Kim, E.V. Tkachenko, G.G. Varvanina, Influence of a specific ginger combination on gastropathy conditions in patients with osteoarthritis of the knee or hip, J. Altern. Complement. Med. 18 (6) (2012) 583–588, https://doi.org/10.1089/acm.2011.0202.

[50] D.A. El-Setouhy, N.S.A. El-Malak, Formulation of a novel tianeptine sodium orodispersible film, AAPS PharmSciTech 11 (3) (2010) 1018–1025, https://doi.org/10.1208/s12249-010-9464-2.

[51] M.M.A. Elsayed, O.Y. Abdallah, V.F. Naggar, N.M. Khalafallah, Deformable liposomes and ethosomes: mechanism of enhanced skin delivery, Int. J. Pharm. 322 (1–2) (2006) 60–66, https://doi.org/10.1016/j.ijpharm.2006.05.027.

[52] E. Ernst, Avocado-soybean unsaponifiables (ASU) for osteoar-thritis—a systematic review, Clin. Rheumatol. 22 (4–5) (2003) 285–288, https://doi.org/10.1007/s10067-003-0731-4.

[53] T.S. Reese, M.J. Karnovsky, Fine structural localization of a blood-brain barrier to exogenous peroxidase, J. Cell Biol. 34 (1) (1967) 207–217, https://doi.org/10.1083/jcb.34.1.207.

[54] S. Farahbakhsh, S. Arbabian, F. Emami, B.R. Moghadam, H. Ghoshooni, A. Noroozzadeh, H. Sahraei, L. Golmanesh, C. Jalili, H. Zrdooz, Inhibition of cyclooxygenase type 1 and 2 enzyme by aqueous extract of Elaeagnus Angustifolia in mice, Basic Clin. Neurosci. 2 (2) (2011) 31–37. http://bcn.tums.ac.ir/browse.php?a_id=88&slc_lang=en&sid=1&ftxt=1.

[55] B.L. Fiebich, S. Chrubasik, Effects of an ethanolic Salix extract on the release of selected inflammatory mediators in vitro, Phytome-dicine 11 (2–3) (2004) 135–138, https://doi.org/10.1078/0944-7113-00338.

[56] B.L. Fiebich, B.L. Fiebich, M. Heinrich, K.O. Hiller, N. Kammerer, Inhibition of TNF-α synthesis in LPS-stimulated primary human monocytes by Harpagophytum extract SteiHap 69, Phytomedicine 8 (1) (2001) 28–30, https://doi.org/10.1078/0944-7113-00002.

[57] G.A. FitzGerald, Coxibs and cardiovascular disease, N. Engl. J. Med. 351 (17) (2004) 1709–1711, https://doi.org/10.1056/NEJMp048288.

[58] R.H. Foster, G. Hardy, R.G. Alany, Borage oil in the treatment of atopic dermatitis, Nutrition 26 (7–8) (2010) 708–718, https://doi.org/10.1016/j.nut.2009.10.014.

[59] L.T. Fox, M. Gerber, J. Du Plessis, J.H. Hamman, Transdermal drug delivery enhancement by compounds of natural origin, Molecules 16 (12) (2011) 10507–10540, https://doi.org/10.3390/molecules161210507.

[60] R. Furst, I. Zundorf, Plant derived anti-inflammatory compounds: hopes and disappointments regarding the translation of preclinical knowledge into clinical progress, Mediat. Inflamm. (2014).

[61] J.J. Gagnier, M. van Tulder, B. Berman, C. Bombardier, Herbal med-icine for low back pain, Cochrane Database Syst. Rev. (Online) 2 (2006), CD004504.

[62] S. Ganguly, A.K. Dash, A novel in situ gel for sustained drug delivery and targeting, Int. J. Pharm. 276 (1–2) (2004) 83–92, https://doi.org/10.1016/j.ijpharm.2004.02.014.

[63] S. Ghosh, M.J. May, E.B. Kopp, NF-κB and rel proteins: evolution-arily conserved mediators of immune responses, Annu. Rev. Immunol. 16 (1998) 225–260, https://doi.org/10.1146/annurev.immunol.16.1.225.

[64] O.P. Gulati, Pycnogenolinvenous disorders: a review, Eur. Bull. Drug Res. 7 (1999) 8–13.

[65] R. Gupta, M. Gupta, S. Mangal, U. Agrawal, S.P. Vyas, Capsaicin-loaded vesicular systems designed for enhancing localized delivery for psoriasis therapy, Artif. Cells Nanomed. Bio-technol. 44 (3) (2016) 825–834, https://doi.org/10.3109/21691401.2014.984301.

[66] V. Gyurkovska, K. Alipieva, A. Maciuk, P. Dimitrova, N. Ivanovska, C. Haas, T. Bley, M. Georgiev, Anti-inflammatory activity of Devil's claw in vitro systems and their active constituents, Food Chem. 125 (1) (2011) 171–178, https://doi.org/10.1016/j.foodchem.2010.08.056.

[67] O. Halicioglu, G. Astarcioglu, I. Yaprak, H. Aydinlioglu, Toxicity of salvia officinalis in a newborn and a child: an alarming report, Pediatr. Neurol. 45 (4) (2011) 259–260, https://doi.org/10.1016/j.pediatrneurol.2011.05.012.

[68] H. Hanai, T. Iida, K. Takeuchi, F. Watanabe, Y. Maruyama, A. Andoh, T. Tsujikawa, Y. Fujiyama, K. Mitsuyama, M. Sata, M. Yamada, Y. Iwaoka, K. Kanke, H. Hiraishi, K. Hirayama, H. Arai, S. Yoshii, M. Uchijima, T. Nagata, Y. Koide, Curcumin maintenance therapy for Ulcerative colitis: randomized, multicenter, double-blind, placebo-controlled trial, Clin. Gastroenterol. Hepatol. 4 (12) (2006) 1502–1506, https://doi.org/10.1016/j.cgh.2006.08.008.

[69] S. Hannoodee, D.N. Nasuruddin, Acute Inflammation Response, StatPearls Publishing, Treasure Island, FL, 2022.

[70] T.M. Haqqi, D.D. Anthony, S. Gupta, N. Ahmad, M.S. Lee, G.K. Kumar, H. Mukhtar, Prevention of collagen-induced arthritis in mice by a polyphenolic fraction from green tea, Proc. Natl. Acad. Sci. U. S. A. 96 (8) (1999) 4524–4529, https://doi.org/10.1073/pnas.96.8.4524.

[71] M.C.Y. Heng, M.K. Song, J. Harker, M.K. Heng, Drug-induced sup-pression of phosphorylase kinase activity correlates with resolution of psoriasis as assessed by clinical, histological and immunohisto-chemical parameters, Br. J. Dermatol. 143 (5) (2000) 937–949, https://doi.org/10.1046/j.1365-2133.2000.03767.x.

[72] P. Henneke, D.T. Golenbock, Phagocytosis, innate immunity, and host-pathogen specificity, J. Exp. Med. 199 (1) (2004) 1–4, https://doi.org/10.1084/jem.20031256.

[73] S.S.W. Ho, R.L. Illgen, R.W. Meyer, P.J. Torok, M.D. Cooper, B. Reider, Comparison of various icing times in decreasing bone metabolism and blood flow in the knee, Am. J. Sports Med. 23 (1) (1995) 74–76, https://doi.org/10.1177/036354659502300112.

[74] T.R. Hoare, D.S. Kohane, Hydrogels in drug delivery: progress and challenges, Polymer 49 (8) (2008) 1993–2007, https://doi.org/10.1016/j.polymer.2008.01.027.

[75] K. Hostanska, G. Daum, R. Saller, Cytostatic and apoptosis inducing activity of boswellic acids towards malignant cell lines in-vitro, Anticancer Res. 22 (2002) 2853–2864.

[76] T.H.W. Huang, V.H. Tran, R.K. Duke, S. Tan, S. Chrubasik, B.D. Roufogalis, C.C. Duke, Harpagoside suppresses lipopolysaccharide-induced iNOS and COX-2 expression through inhibition of NF-κB activation, J. Ethnopharmacol. 104 (1–2) (2006) 149–155, https://doi.org/10.1016/j.jep.2005.08.055.

[77] M.A. Hughes, C. Tang, G.W. Cherry, Effect of intermittent radiant warming on proliferation of human dermal endothelial cells in vitro, J. Wound Care 12 (4) (2003) 135–137, https://doi.org/10.12968/jowc.2003.12.4.26487.

[78] S. Indulekha, P. Arunkumar, D. Bahadur, R. Srivastava, Thermore-sponsive polymeric gel as an on-demand transdermal drug delivery system for pain management, Mater. Sci. Eng. C 62 (2016) 113–122, https://doi.org/10.1016/j.msec.2016.01.021.

[79] F. Joo, Endothelial cells of the brain and other organ systems: some similarities and differences, Prog. Neurobiol. (1996) 255–273, https://doi.org/10.1016/0301-0082(95)00046-1.

[80] A. Jain, V. Pooladanda, U. Bulbake, S. Doppalapudi, T.A. Rafeeqi, C. Godugu, W. Khan, Liposphere mediated topical delivery of thy-moquinone in the treatment of psoriasis, Nanomedicine 13 (7) (2017) 2251–2262, https://doi.org/10.1016/j.nano.2017.06.009.

[81] M. Jan, T. Stelmaszynska, The Respiratory Bust and Its Physio-logical Significance, 1988.

[82] Y. Javadzadeh, L. Azharshekoufeh Bahari, Therapeutic nanostructures for dermal and transdermal drug delivery, in: Nano- and Microscale Drug Delivery Systems: Design and Fabrication, Elsevier, 2017, pp. 131–146, https://doi.org/10.1016/B978-0-323-52727-9.00008-X.

[83] R. Jebbawi, S. Fruchon, C.-O. Turrin, M. Blanzat, R. Poupot, Supramolecular and macromolecular matrix nanocarriers for drug delivery in inflammation-associated skin diseases, Pharmaceutics 12 (12) (2020) 1224, https://doi.org/10.3390/pharmaceutics12121224.

[84] J.S. Jurenka, Anti-inflammatory properties of curcumin, a major constituent of Curcuma longa: a review of preclinical and clinical research, Altern. Med. Rev. 14 (2) (2009) 141–153.

[85] A. Kapil, N. Moza, Anticomplementary activity of Boswellic acids—an inhibitor of C3-convertase of the classical complement pathway, Int. J. Immunopharmacol. 14 (7) (1992) 1139–1143, https://doi.org/10.1016/0192-0561(92)90048-P.

[86] R.E. Kast, Borage oil reduction of rheumatoid arthritis activity may be mediated by increased cAMP that suppresses tumor necrosis factor-alpha, Int. Immunopharmacol. 1 (12) (2001) 2197–2199, https://doi.org/10.1016/S1567-5769(01)00146-1.

[87] R. Kaur, A. Sharma, V. Puri, I. Singh, Preparation and characterization of biocomposite films of carrageenan/locust bean gum/montmorrillonite for transdermal delivery of curcumin, BioImpacts 9 (1) (2019) 37–43, https://doi.org/10.15171/bi.2019.05.

[88] A. Kharazmi, Laboratory and pre-clinical studies on anti-inflammatory and anti-oxidant properties of rose hip powder- identification and characterization of active component GOPO®, Osteoarthr. Cartil. 16 (1) (2008).

[89] S. Khogta, J. Patel, K. Barve, V. Londhe, Herbal nano-formulations for topical delivery, J. Herbal Med. 20 (2020), 100300, https://doi.org/10.1016/j.hermed.2019.100300.

[90] N. Kimmatkar, V. Thawani, L. Hingorani, R. Khiyani, Efficacy and tolerability of Boswellia serrata extract in treatment of osteoarthritis of knee—a randomized double blind placebo controlled trial, Phytomedicine 10 (1) (2003) 3–7, https://doi.org/10.1078/094471103321648593.

[91] S.S. Kitchen, C.J. Partridge, A review of therapeutic ultrasound, Physiotherapy 76 (10) (1990) 593–600.

[92] R.J. Ko, Adulterants in Asian patent medicines [2], N. Engl. J. Med. 339 (12) (1998) 847, https://doi.org/10.1056/NEJM199809173391214.

[93] M. Kolehmainen, O. Mykkänen, P.V. Kirjavainen, T. Leppänen, E. Moilanen, M. Adriaens, D.E. Laaksonen, M. Hallikainen, R. -Puupponen-Pimiä, L. Pulkkinen, H. Mykkänen, H. Gylling, K. Poutanen, R. Törrönen, Bilberries reduce low-grade inflammation in individuals with features of metabolic syndrome, Mol. Nutr. Food Res. 56 (10) (2012) 1501–1510, https://doi.org/10.1002/mnfr.201200195.

[94] S.M.-D. la Paz, M.A. Fernandez-Arche, M. Angel-Martin, M.D. Garcia-Gimenez, The sterols isolated from evening primrose oil modulate the release of pro-inflammatory mediators, Phytomedicine 19 (12) (2012) 1072–1076.

[95] P.C. Leung, E.C.H. Ko, W.S. Siu, E.S.Y. Pang, C.B.S. Lau, Selected topical agents used in traditional Chinese medicine in the treatment of minor injuries—a review, Front. Pharmacol. 7 (2016), https://doi.org/10.3389/fphar.2016.00016.

[96] L.J. Leventhal, E.G. Boyce, R.B. Zurier, Treatment of rheumatoid arthritis with blackcurrant seed oil, Rheumatology 33 (9) (1994) 847–852, https://doi.org/10.1093/rheumatology/33.9.847.

[97] S. Li, Y. Qiu, S. Zhang, Y. Gao, Enhanced transdermal delivery of 18β-glycyrrhetic acid via elastic vesicles: In vitro and in vivo evaluation, Drug Dev. Ind. Pharm. 38 (7) (2012) 855–865, https://doi.org/10.3109/03639045.2011.630395.

[98] C.Y. Lin, Y.T. Hsieh, L.Y. Chan, T.Y. Yang, T. Maeda, T.M. Chang, H.C. Huang, Dictamnine delivered by PLGA nanocarriers ameliorated inflammation in an oxazolone-induced dermatitis mouse model, J. Control. Release 329 (2021) 731–742, https://doi.org/10.1016/j.jconrel.2020.10.007.

[99] D.M. Lindsay, J. Dearness, C.C. McGinley, Electrotherapy usage trends in private physiotherapy practice in Alberta, Physiother. Can. 47 (1) (1995) 30–34.

[100] W.J. Liu, Traditional Herbal Medicine Research Methods: Identification, Analysis, Bioassay, and Pharmaceutical and Clinical Studies, 2011.

[101] D. Loew, J. Möllerfeld, A. Schrödter, S. Puttkammer, M. Kaszkin, Investigations on the pharmacokinetic properties of Harpagophytum extracts and their effects on eicosanoid biosynthesis in vitro and ex vivo, Clin. Pharmacol. Ther. 69 (5) (2001) 356–364, https://doi.org/10.1067/mcp.2001.115445.

[102] A. Madisch, S. Miehlke, O. Eichele, Boswellia serrata extract for treatment of collagenous colitis. A double-blind randomized placebo-controlled multicentre trial, Int. J. Physiother. Phytopharmacol. 15 (2008) 6–7.

[103] E. Maheu, C. Cadet, M. Marty, D. Moyse, I. Kerloch, P. Coste, M. Dougados, B. Maziéres, T.D. Spector, H. Halhol, J.M. Grouin, M. Lequesne, Randomised, controlled trial of avocado-soybean unsaponifiable (Piascledine) effect on structure modification in hip osteoarthritis: the ERADIAS study, Ann. Rheum. Dis. 73 (2) (2014) 376–384, https://doi.org/10.1136/annrheumdis-2012-202485.

[104] S. Mahluji, A. Ostadrahimi, M. Mobasseri, V.E. Attari, L. Payahoo, Anti-inflammatory effects of Zingiber officinale in type 2 diabetic patients, Adv. Pharm. Bull. 3 (2) (2013) 273–276, https://doi.org/10.5681/apb.2013.044.

[105] M.L. Manca, M. Zaru, M. Manconi, F. Lai, D. Valenti, C. Sinico, A.M. Fadda, Glycerosomes: a new tool for effective dermal and transdermal drug delivery, Int. J. Pharm. 455 (1–2) (2013) 66–74, https://doi.org/10.1016/j.ijpharm.2013.07.060.

[106] S.K. Manna, A. Mukhopadhyay, B.B. Aggarwal, Resveratrol suppresses TNF-induced activation of nuclear transcription factors NF-κB, activator protein-1, and apoptosis: potential role of reactive oxygen intermediates and lipid peroxidation, J. Immunol. 164 (12) (2000) 6509–6519, https://doi.org/10.4049/jimmunol.164.12.6509.

[107] M.A. Maranduca, D. Branisteanu, D.N. Serban, D.C. Branisteanu, G. Stoleriu, N. Manolache, I.L. Serban, Synthesis and physiological implications of melanic pigments (review), Oncol. Lett. 17 (5) (2019) 4183–4187, https://doi.org/10.3892/ol.2019.10071.

[108] C. Marstrand, L. Warholm, Kharazmi, K. Winther, The anti-inflammatory capacity of rose hip is strongly dependent on the seeds—a comparison of animal and human studies, Osteoarthr. Cartil. 21 (2013).

[109] G. McGregor, B. Fiebich, A. Wartenberg, S. Brien, G. Lewith, T. Wegener, Devil's claw (Harpagophytum procumbens): an anti-inflammatory herb with therapeutic potential, Phytochem. Rev. 4 (1) (2005) 47–53, https://doi.org/10.1007/s11101-004-2374-8.

[110] M. Sandoval-Chacon, J.H. Thompson, X.J. Weng, Anti-inflammatory actions of cat's claw: the role of NF-kB, Pharmacol. Ther. Aliment. 12 (1998) 1279–1289.

[111] A. Vogt, C. Wischke, A.T. Neffe, N. Ma, U. Alexiev, A. Lendlein, Nanocarriers for drug delivery into and through the skin—do

existing technologies match clinical challenges? J. Control. Release 242 (2) (2016) 3–15, https://doi.org/10.1016/j.jconrel.2016.07.027.

[112] S. Meng, L. Sun, L. Wang, Z. Lin, Z. Liu, L. Xi, Z. Wang, Y. Zheng, Loading of water-insoluble celastrol into niosome hydrogels for improved topical permeation and anti-psoriasis activity, Colloids Surf. B: Biointerfaces 182 (2019), 110352, https://doi.org/10.1016/j.colsurfb.2019.110352.

[113] M.A. Merrick, K.L. Knight, C.D. Ingersoll, J.A. Potteiger, The effects of ice and compression wraps on intramuscular temperatures at various depths, J. Athl. Train. 28 (3) (1993) 236–245.

[114] S. Montserrat-De La Paz, M.A. Fernández-Arche, M. Ángel-Martín, M.D. García-Giménez, Phytochemical characterization of potential nutraceutical ingredients from Evening Primrose oil (Oenothera biennis L.), Phytochem. Lett. 8 (1) (2014) 158–162, https://doi.org/10.1016/j.phytol.2013.08.008.

[115] E. Mur, F. Hartig, G. Eibl, M. Schirmer, Randomized double blind trial of an extract from the pentacyclic alkaloid-chemotype of uncaria tomentosa for the treatment of rheumatoid arthritis, J. Rheumatol. 29 (4) (2002) 678–681.

[116] K. Murphy, Janeway's immunobiology, in: Garland Science, 1956, ISBN: 9780815342434.

[117] R.H. Müller, M. Radtke, S.A. Wissing, Solid lipid nanoparticles (SLN) and nanostructured lipid carriers (NLC) in cosmetic and dermatological preparations, Adv. Drug Deliv. Rev. 54 (2002) S131–S155, https://doi.org/10.1016/S0169-409X(02)00118-7.

[118] A. Vintiloiu, J.C. Leroux, Organogels and their use in drug delivery—a review, J. Control. Release 125 (3) (2008) 179–192, https://doi.org/10.1016/j.jconrel.2007.09.014.

[119] M. Najmi, Z.V. Shariatpanahi, M. Tolouei, Z. Amiri, Effect of oral olive oil on healing of 10-20% total body surface area burn wounds in hospitalized patients, Burns 41 (3) (2015) 493–496, https://doi.org/10.1016/j.burns.2014.08.010.

[120] Z. Nikniaz, A. Ostadrahimi, R. Mahdavi, A. Ebrahimi, a., & Nikniaz, L., Effects of Elaeagnus angustifolia L. supplementation on serum levels of inflammatory cytokines and matrix metalloproteinases in females with knee osteoarthritis, Complement. Ther. Med. 22 (5) (2014) 864–869, https://doi.org/10.1016/j.ctim.2014.07.004.

[121] S. Nipanikar, S. Chitlange, D. Nagore, Evaluation of anti-inflammatory and antimicrobial activity of AHPL/AYCAP/0413 capsule, Pharm. Res. 9 (3) (2017) 273, https://doi.org/10.4103/0974-8490.210328.

[122] T. Nishiyama, T. Mae, H. Kishida, M. Tsukagawa, Y. Mimaki, M. Kuroda, Y. Sashida, K. Takahashi, T. Kawada, T. Nakagawa, M. Kitahara, Curcuminoids and sesquiterpenoids in turmeric (Curcuma longa L.) suppress an increase in blood glucose level in type 2 diabetic KK-Aγ mice, J. Agric. Food Chem. 53 (4) (2005) 959–963, https://doi.org/10.1021/jf0483873.

[123] C.D.R. Nunes, M.B. Arantes, S.M. de Faria Pereira, L.L. da Cruz, M. de Souza Passos, L.P. de Moraes, I.J.C. Vieira, D.B. de Oliveira, Plants as sources of anti-inflammatory agents, Molecules 25 (16) (2020), https://doi.org/10.3390/molecules25163726.

[124] T. Ohishi, S. Goto, P. Monira, M. Isemura, Y. Nakamura, Anti-inflammatory action of green tea, Antiinflamm. Antiallergy Agents Med. Chem. 15 (2) (2016) 74–90, https://doi.org/10.2174/1871523015666160915154443.

[125] WHO, Operational guidance: Information needed to support clinical trials of herbal products, 2005. World Health Organization on behalf of the Special Programme for Research and Training in Tropical Diseases.

[126] A. Otto, J. Du Plessis, J.W. Wiechers, Formulation effects of topical emulsions on transdermal and dermal delivery, Int. J. Cosmet. Sci. 31 (1) (2009) 1–19, https://doi.org/10.1111/j.1468-2494.2008.00467.x.

[127] R. Pahwa, A. Goyal, P. Bansal, Chronic inflammation, Stat. Pearls 1 (2022).

[128] D. Paolino, G. Lucania, D. Mardente, F. Alhaique, M. Fresta, Ethosomes for skin delivery of ammonium glycyrrhizinate: in vitro percutaneous permeation through human skin and in vivo anti-inflammatory activity on human volunteers, J. Control. Release 106 (1–2) (2005) 99–110, https://doi.org/10.1016/j.jconrel.2005.04.007.

[129] W.M. Pardridge, Drug and gene targeting to the brain with molecular Trojan horses, Nat. Rev. Drug Discov. 1 (2) (2002) 131–139, https://doi.org/10.1038/nrd725.

[130] I. Pather, T.Z. Woldemariam, Novel Formulations and Uses for Curcuma Extracts, A.P. Office, 2018.

[131] I. Pather, T.Z. Woldemariam, et al., Method of Producing a Safe, Whole-Extract of Curcuma for Oral and Topical Use, 2019.

[132] K.R. Patil, U.B. Mahajan, B.S. Unger, S.N. Goyal, S. Belemkar, S.J. Surana, S. Ojha, C.R. Patil, Animal models of inflammation for screening of anti-inflammatory drugs: implications for the discovery and development of phytopharmaceuticals, Int. J. Mol. Sci. 20 (18) (2019), https://doi.org/10.3390/ijms20184367.

[133] Q. Peng, Z. Wei, B.H.S. Lau, Pycnogenol inhibits tumor necrosis factor_alpha_induced nuclear factor kappa B activation and adhesion molecule expression in human vascular endothelial cells, Cell. Mole. Life Sci. 57 (5) (2000) 834–841, https://doi.org/10.1007/s000180050045.

[134] J. Piscoya, Z. Rodriguez, S.A. Bustamante, N.N. Okuhama, M.J.S. Miller, M. Sandoval, Efficacy and safety of freeze-dried cat's claw in osteoarthritis of the knee: mechanisms of action of the species Uncaria guianensis, Inflamm. Res. 50 (9) (2001) 442–448, https://doi.org/10.1007/PL00000268.

[135] D. Poeckel, C. Greiner, M. Verhoff, O. Rau, L. Tausch, C. Hörnig, D. Steinhilber, D. Schubert-Zsilavecz, O. Werz, Carnosic acid and carnosol potently inhibit human 5-lipoxygenase and suppress pro-inflammatory responses of stimulated human polymorphonuclear leukocytes, Biochem. Pharmacol. 76 (1) (2008) 91–97, https://doi.org/10.1016/j.bcp.2008.04.013.

[136] W.E. Prentie, Therapeutic Modalities in Rehabilitation, 2011.

[137] C. Prucksunand, B. Indrasukhsri, M. Leethochawalit, K. Hungspreugs, Phase II clinical trial on effect of the long turmeric (Curcuma longa Linn) on healing of peptic ulcer, Southeast Asian J. Trop. Med. Public Health 32 (1) (2001) 208–215. https://seameotropmednetwork.org/publication_current_issue.html.

[138] C. Puglia, L. Rizza, M. Drechsler, F. Bonina, Nanoemulsions as vehicles for topical administration of glycyrrhetic acid: characterization and in vitro and in vivo evaluation, Drug Deliv. 17 (3) (2010) 123–129, https://doi.org/10.3109/10717540903581679.

[139] J.Y. Fang, T.L. Hwang, Y.L. Huang, C.L. Fang, Enhancement of the transdermal delivery of catechins by liposomes incorporating anionic surfactants and ethanol, Int. J. Pharm. 310 (1–2) (2006) 131–138, https://doi.org/10.1016/j.ijpharm.2005.12.004.

[140] C. Rubin, M. Bolander, J.P. Ryaby, M. Hadjiargyrou, The use of low-intensity ultrasound to accelerate the healing of fractures, J. Bone Joint Surg. A 83 (2) (2001) 259–270, https://doi.org/10.2106/00004623-200102000-00015.

[141] K. Zhang, Y. Zhang, Z. Li, N. Li, N. Feng, Essential oil-mediated glycerosomes increase transdermal paeoniflorin delivery:

[142] Z. Mei, H. Chen, T. Weng, Y. Yang, X. Yang, Solid lipid nanoparticle and microemulsion for topical delivery of triptolide, Eur. J. Pharm. Biopharm. 56 (2) (2003) 189–196, https://doi.org/10.1016/S0939-6411(03)00067-5.

[143] S. Schmieder, P. Patel, K. Krishnamurthy, Research techniques made simple: drug delivery techniques, part 1: concepts in transepidermal penetration and absorption, J. Investig. Dermatol. 135 (11) (2015) 1, https://doi.org/10.1038/jid.2015.343.

[144] A.R. Setty, L.H. Sigal, Herbal medications commonly used in the practice of rheumatology: mechanisms of action, efficacy, and side effects, Semin. Arthritis Rheum. 34 (6) (2005) 773–784, https://doi.org/10.1016/j.semarthrit.2005.01.011.

[145] P.P. Shah, P.R. Desai, A.R. Patel, M.S. Singh, Skin permeating nanogel for the cutaneous co-delivery of two anti-inflammatory drugs, Biomaterials 33 (5) (2012) 1607–1617, https://doi.org/10.1016/j.biomaterials.2011.11.011.

[146] A. Sharma, V. Puri, P. Kumar, I. Singh, Biopolymeric, nanopatterned, fibrous carriers for wound healing applications, Curr. Pharm. Des. 26 (38) (2020) 4894–4908, https://doi.org/10.2174/1381612826666200701152217.

[147] D. Shoskes, C. Lapierre, M. Cruz-Corerra, N. Muruve, R. Rosario, B. Fromkin, M. Braun, J. Copley, Beneficial effects of the bioflavonoids curcumin and quercetin on early function in cadaveric renal transplantation: a randomized placebo controlled trial, Transplantation 80 (11) (2005) 1556–1559, https://doi.org/10.1097/01.tp.0000183290.64309.21.

[148] N. Shraibom, Herbal Combinations for Treating Eczema, 2020.

[149] C. Randall, H. Randall, F. Dobbs, C. Hutton, H. Sanders, Randomized controlled trial of nettle sting for treatment of base-of-thumb pain, J. R. Soc. Med. 93 (6) (2000) 305–309, https://doi.org/10.1177/014107680009300607.

[150] E. Rein, A. Kharazmi, K. Winther, A herbal remedy, Hyben Vital (stand. powder of a subspecies of Rosa canina fruits), reduces pain and improves general wellbeing in patients with osteoarthritis—a double-blind, placebo-controlled, randomised trial, Phytomedicine 11 (5) (2004) 383–391, https://doi.org/10.1016/j.phymed.2004.01.001.

[151] S.R.I.N. Reis, L.M.M. Valente, A.L. Sampaio, A.C. Siani, M. Gandini, E.L. Azeredo, L.A. D'Avila, J.L. Mazzei, M.D.G.M. Henriques, C.F. Kubelka, Immunomodulating and antiviral activities of Uncaria tomentosa on human monocytes infected with dengue virus-2, Int. Immunopharmacol. 8 (3) (2008) 468–476, https://doi.org/10.1016/j.intimp.2007.11.010.

[152] S. Rezapour-Firouzi, S.R. Arefhosseini, F. Mehdi, E.M. Mehrangiz, B. Baradaran, E. Sadeghihokmabad, S. Mostafaei, S.M.B. Fazljou, M.A. Torbati, S. Sanaie, F. Zamani, Immunomodulatory and therapeutic effects of hot-nature diet and co-supplemented hemp seed, evening primrose oils intervention in multiple sclerosis patients, Complement. Ther. Med. 21 (5) (2013) 473–480, https://doi.org/10.1016/j.ctim.2013.06.006.

[153] B. Roschek, R.C. Fink, M. McMichael, R.S. Alberte, Nettle extract (Urtica dioica) affects key receptors and enzymes associated with allergic rhinitis, Phytother. Res. 23 (7) (2009) 920–926, https://doi.org/10.1002/ptr.2763.

[154] A.L.M. Ruela, A.G. Perissinato, M.E.D.S. Lino, P.S. Mudrik, G.R. Pereira, Evaluation of skin absorption of drugs from topical and transdermal formulations, Braz. J. Pharm. Sci. 52 (3) (2016) 527–544, https://doi.org/10.1590/s1984-82502016000300018.

[155] B. Schmid, I. Kötter, L. Heide, Pharmacokinetics of salicin after oral administration of a standardised willow bark extract, Eur. J. Clin. Pharmacol. 57 (5) (2001) 387–391, https://doi.org/10.1007/s002280100325.

[156] J.P. Schwager, N. Richard, S. Woffram, Anti-inflammatory and chondro-protective effects of rosehip powder and its constituent galactolipids Gopo, Osteoarthr. Cartil. 16 (4) (2008).

[157] S. Singh, A. Khajuria, S.C. Taneja, R.K. Johri, J. Singh, G.N. Qazi, Boswellic acids: a leukotriene inhibitor also effective through topical application in inflammatory disorders, Phytomedicine 15 (6–7) (2008) 400–407, https://doi.org/10.1016/j.phymed.2007.11.019.

[158] K.L. Soeken, S.A. Miller, E. Ernst, Herbal medicines for the treatment of rheumatoid arthritis: a systematic review, Rheumatology 42 (5) (2003) 652–659, https://doi.org/10.1093/rheumatology/keg183.

[159] T. Someya, M. Amagai, Toward a new generation of smart skins, Nat. Biotechnol. (2019) 382–388, https://doi.org/10.1038/s41587-019-0079-1.

[160] K.C. Srivastava, T. Mustafa, Ginger (Zingiber officinale) in rheumatism and musculoskeletal disorders, Med. Hypotheses 39 (4) (1992) 342–348, https://doi.org/10.1016/0306-9877(92)90059-L.

[161] T. Stelmaszynska, Formation of HCN by human phagocytosing neutrophils—1. Chlorination of Staphylococcus epidermidis as a source of HCN, Int. J. Biochem. 17 (3) (1985) 373–379, https://doi.org/10.1016/0020-711X(85)90213-7.

[162] B.J. Taheri, F. Ambari, Z. Maleki, S. Boostani, A. Zarghi, F. Buralibaba, Efficacy of Elaeagnus angustifolia topical gel in the treatment of symptomatic oral lichen planus, J. Dent. Res. Dent. Clin. Dent. Prospects 4 (1) (2010) 29–32.

[163] S. Doppalapudi, A. Jain, D.K. Chopra, W. Khan, Psoralen loaded liposomal nanocarriers for improved skin penetration and efficacy of topical PUVA in psoriasis, Eur. J. Pharm. Sci. 96 (2017) 515–529, https://doi.org/10.1016/j.ejps.2016.10.025.

[164] E. Touitou, N. Dayan, L. Bergelson, B. Godin, M. Eliaz, Ethosomes—novel vesicular carriers for enhanced delivery: characterization and skin penetration properties, J. Control. Release 65 (3) (2000) 403–418, https://doi.org/10.1016/S0168-3659(99)00222-9.

[165] M.S. Algahtani, M.Z. Ahmad, J. Ahmad, Nanoemulsion loaded polymeric hydrogel for topical delivery of curcumin in psoriasis, J. Drug Deliv. Sci. Technol. 59 (2020), https://doi.org/10.1016/j.jddst.2020.101847.

[166] R. Najafi-Taher, B. Ghaemi, A. Amani, Delivery of adapalene using a novel topical gel based on tea tree oil nano-emulsion: permeation, antibacterial and safety assessments, Eur. J. Pharm. Sci. 120 (2018) 142–151, https://doi.org/10.1016/j.ejps.2018.04.029.

[167] Z. Mei, Q. Wu, S. Hu, X. Li, X. Yang, Triptolide loaded solid lipid nanoparticle hydrogel for topical application, Drug Dev. Ind. Pharm. 31 (2) (2005) 161–168, https://doi.org/10.1081/DDC-200047791.

[168] D. Stewart, The Chemistry of Essential Oils Made Simple: God's Love Manifest in Molecules, 2005.

[169] O. Uchechi, J.D. Ogbonna, A.A. Attama, Nanoparticles for dermal and transdermal drug delivery, App. Nanotechnol. Drug Deliv. 4 (2014) 193–227.

[170] H. Ueda, K. Ippoushi, A. Takeuchi, Repeated oral administration of a squeezed ginger (Zingiber officinale) extract augmented the serum corticosterone level and had anti-inflammatory properties, Biosci. Biotechnol. Biochem. 74 (11) (2010) 2248–2252, https://doi.org/10.1271/bbb.100456.

[171] J. Watson, M.L. Byars, P. Mcgill, A.W. Kelman, Cytokine and prostaglandin production by monocytes of volunteers and rheumatoid arthritis patients treated with dietary supplements of blackcurrant seed oil, Rheumatology 32 (12) (1993) 1055–1058, https://doi.org/10.1093/rheumatology/32.12.1055.

[172] M. Weston, C. Taber, L. Casagranda, M. Cornwall, Changes in local blood volume during cold gel pack application to traumatized ankles, J. Orthop. Sports Phys. Ther. 19 (4) (1994) 197–199, https://doi.org/10.2519/jospt.1994.19.4.197.

[173] L.W. Whitehouse, M. Znamirowska, C.J. Paul, Devil's claw (Harpagophytum procumbens): no evidence for anti-inflammatory activity in the treatment of arthritic disease, Can. Med. Assoc. J. 129 (3) (1983) 249–251.

[174] J.W. Wiechers, C.L. Kelly, T.G. Blease, J.C. Dederen, Formulating for efficacy1, Int. J. Cosmet. Sci. 26 (4) (2004) 173–182, https://doi.org/10.1111/j.1467-2494.2004.00211.x.

[175] H. Wolburg, S. Noell, A. Mack, K. Wolburg-Buchholz, P. Fallier-Becker, Brain endothelial cells and the glio-vascular complex, Cell Tissue Res. 335 (1) (2009) 75–96, https://doi.org/10.1007/s00441-008-0658-9.

[176] D. Wu, M. Meydani, L.S. Leka, Z. Nightingale, G.J. Handelman, J.B. Blumberg, S.N. Meydani, Effect of dietary supplementation with black currant seed oil or the immune response of healthy elderly subjects, Am. J. Clin. Nutr. 70 (4) (1999) 536–543, https://doi.org/10.1093/ajcn/70.4.536.

[177] Z. Xia, A. Sato, M.A. Hughes, G.W. Cherry, Stimulation of fibroblast growth in vitro by intermittent radiant warming, Wound Repair Regen. 8 (2) (2000) 138–144, https://doi.org/10.1046/j.1524-475X.2000.00138.x.

[178] J. Xie, S. Huang, H. Huang, X. Deng, P. Yue, J. Lin, M. Yang, L. Han, D.K. Zhang, Advances in the application of natural products and the novel drug delivery systems for psoriasis, Front. Pharmacol. 12 (2021), https://doi.org/10.3389/fphar.2021.644952.

[179] W. Xiu-qin, Operational guidance: information needed to support clinical trials of herbal products, Chinese J. Clin. Pharmacol. Ther. (2007).

[180] B. Yang, H.B. Lee, S. Kim, Y.C. Park, K. Kim, H. Kim, Decoction of Dictamnus Dasycarpus Turcz. Root bark ameliorates skin lesions and inhibits inflammatory reactions in mice with contact dermatitis, Pharmacogn. Mag. 13 (51) (2017) 483–487, https://doi.org/10.4103/0973-1296.211034.

[181] E.B. Zagorodnyaya, G.I. Oskol'Skii, A.Y. Basharov, E.L. Lushnikova, L.M. Nepomnyashchikh, A.S. Zagorodnii, Biopolymeric film containing bioactive naphthoquinone (Shikonin) in combined therapy of inflammatory destructive lesions in the buccal mucosa, Bull. Exp. Biol. Med. 156 (2) (2013) 232–235, https://doi.org/10.1007/s10517-013-2318-7.

[182] A. Sahu, N. Rawal, M.K. Pangburn, Inhibition of complement by covalent attachment of rosmarinic acid to activated C3b, Biochem. Pharmacol. 57 (12) (1999) 1439–1446, https://doi.org/10.1016/S0006-2952(99)00044-1.

[183] Z. Zhaowu, W. Xiaoli, Z. Yangde, L. Nianfeng, Preparation of matrine ethosome, its percutaneous permeation in vitro and anti-inflammatory activity in vivo in rats, J. Liposome Res. 19 (2) (2009) 155–162, https://doi.org/10.1080/08982100902722381.

[184] B.V. Zlokovic, The blood-brain barrier in health and chronic neurodegenerative disorders, Neuron 57 (2) (2008) 178–201, https://doi.org/10.1016/j.neuron.2008.01.003.

Chapter 18

Therapeutic potential of plant-derived flavonoids against inflammation

Reyaz Hassan Mir[a,b,*], Roohi Mohi-ud-din[c,*], Prince Ahad Mir[d], Mudasir Maqbool[e], Nazia Banday[f], Saeema Farooq[f], Syed Naeim Raza[g], and Pooja A. Chawla[h]

[a]*Pharmaceutical Chemistry Division, Chandigarh College of Pharmacy, Landran, Punjab, India,* [b]*Pharmaceutical Chemistry Division, Department of Pharmaceutical Sciences, University of Kashmir, Srinagar, Jammu and Kashmir, India,* [c]*Sher-I-Kashmir Institute of Medical Sciences, Srinagar, Jammu and Kashmir, India,* [d]*Amritsar Pharmacy College, Amritsar, Punjab, India,* [e]*Pharmacy Practice Division, Department of Pharmaceutical Sciences, University of Kashmir, Srinagar, Jammu and Kashmir, India,* [f]*Pharmacognosy & Phytochemistry Division, Department of Pharmaceutical Sciences, University of Kashmir, Srinagar, Jammu and Kashmir, India,* [g]*Pharmaceutics Division, Department of Pharmaceutical Sciences, University of Kashmir, Srinagar, Jammu and Kashmir, India,* [h]*Department of Pharmaceutical Chemistry and Analysis, ISF College of Pharmacy, Moga, Punjab, India*

1 Natural products introduction

Natural products are the chemical ingredients synthesized by living organisms via semisynthetic or synthetic methods. Since ancient times natural sources are being utilized by human beings as a primary source for food, shelter, and curative remedies and since the last few decades tremendous research has been carried out on natural herbs for the search and development of novel therapeutic agents beneficial for human health without or with least side effects. Commonly, the term natural product is considered the other name for secondary metabolites [1,2]. These secondary metabolites are the organic ingredients that exert various pharmacological effects on human health, but do not contribute directly in various process like reproduction, growth, development, etc. [3,4]. Nutraceuticals, cosmetics, and pharmaceuticals are the main industries in which natural ingredients are purposely used as the main constituents [5,6]. These are basically small molecules with some structural changes and are less than 3000 Da in molecular weight [7–9].

The relative study of natural products inspires scientists to isolate, identify, and characterize active compounds from natural plants and further use them to develop pharmacologically active molecules. However, natural ingredients are extremely cumbersome to isolate and very challenging to synthesize [10,11]. Natural products are frequently regarded as an initial point for drug discovery in chemical synthesis, from which synthetic derivatives can be synthesized with upgraded efficiency, safety, and purity [12–15].

2 Flavonoids

Flavonoids are a large group of polyphenolic phytoconstituents and are represented as 2-phenyl-benzo-γ-pyrone derivatives [16,17]. Flavonoids are chiefly available in dietary substances like vegetables, tea, fruits, and legumes [18]. Flavonoids possess a wide variety of health stimulating benefits and are an essential ingredient in numerous pharmaceuticals, nutraceuticals, cosmetics, and medicinal therapies, due to their enzymatic function modification tendency, and also possess various biological activities like antiinflammatory, antioxidant, anticarcinogenic and antimutagenic potency against neurodegenerative disease. Flavonoids also potently block various enzymes like cyclo-oxygenase, xanthine oxidase, phosphoinositide 3-kinase, and lipoxygenase [19]. In the natural state, Generally, flavonoids are mined from plants and are available in various parts. In plants, flavonoids play an important role in the coloring and aroma of fruits and flowers which, in turn, helps in attracting pollinators [20,21]. They also shield plants from various abiotic and biotic stresses and also from harmful UV radiations [22,23]. Flavonoids are mainly digested in the intestines and their metabolites are directed toward the liver, where they are further digested. These digested metabolites are carried to targeted cells, either disintegrated into aglycones due to microflora, or expelled via feces or urine. Flavonoids that are not digested by the intestines are directed toward the colon, where they get debased by the colonic microflora and then reabsorbed [24–26]. Flavonoids are also known as bioflavonoids due to their various pharmacological effects. They potently scavenge reactive

---

*Authors contributed equally.

Recent Developments in Anti-Inflammatory Therapy. https://doi.org/10.1016/B978-0-323-99988-5.00019-X

oxygen species, particularly hydroxyl, superoxides, and lipid radicals [27–29] and, due to this property flavonoids possess antibacterial, antiinflammatory, antiviral, antioxidant, anticancer, and immunomodulatory potency [30,31].

2.1 Classification

Flavonoids structurally possess two benzene moieties (A and B) which are connected with an oxygen-containing heterocyclic ring C. On the basis of the B-ring configuration, linkage between rings B and C, and glycosylation and hydroxylation designs in three rings, flavonoids can be categorized into various subcategories which includes flavonols, flavones, flavanones, anthocyanidins, and isoflavones [32,33].

Flavonols: Flavonols are flavonoids that possess a ketonic group in their ring structure. They constitute a multiplex category of polyphenolic compounds ranging from monomeric flavan-3-ols (e.g., epicatechin, catechin, and gallocatechin) to polymeric procyanidins called condensed tannins [34]. Flavonols are predominantly found in fruits and related products, like fruit jams or juices. They are also available in cereals, cocoa, apples, red wine, kiwi, and tea. In vegetative products and legumes excluding lentils and broad beans, flavonols are found in very low quantities [35].

Various findings have reported that flavonols encourage nitric oxide concentration in smoker's blood and antithesis few smoking-allied injuries in blood vessels. Scientists revealed that 176–185 mg of flavonols prominently intensifies nitric oxide circulation and flow-facilitated expansion. Similarly, prolonged uptake of a flavonol-rich diet results in a persistent rise in endothelial functions and avoids future heart-related infections [27]. Catechins are a vital representative of this category and are also regarded as building blocks for tannins. These constituents are available in the skin and seed of unripened fruits. The various subtypes of catechins include catechin 3-gallate, epigallocatechin, gallocatechin 3-gallate, epicatechin 3-gallate, epicatechin, gallocatechin, catechin 3-gallate, and catechins and are mainly available in chocolates, apples, apricots, red wine, red raspberry, black and green tea, blackberry, and peach [36]. Catechins inhibit protein oxidation due to the free radical engulfing ability. In addition, it retains the capability to decrease covalent variation of protein triggered by ROS or its by-products [37].

Flavones: Flavones are structurally analogous to flavonols that contain an additional hydroxyl group at position 3. Luteolin and apigenin are the most common flavones available. Luteolin is predominantly available in fruits and vegetables like celery, parsley, broccoli, onion leaves, carrots, chrysanthemum flowers, cabbages, apple skins, and peppers [38], whereas, apigenin is available in parsley, onions, oranges, tea, wheat sprouts, and chamomile. Apigenin is a chief constituent of chamomile, and possess antiphlogistic, antispasmodic, and antibacterial potency. Various studies have demonstrated that apigenin exhibits significant anticarcinogenic, antiinflammatory, and antioxidant potency [39]. Apigenin revealed antitumor potency by blocking ornithine decarboxylase, an enzyme crucial in tumor formation [40].

Luteolin-rich plants are widely used in Chinese traditional medicines for the treatment of inflammatory infections, hypertension, and as anticancer agents. Luteolin exhibited various pharmacological benefits like antiinflammation antiallergy, and anticarcinogenic [41]. Furthermore, luteolin is scanned for antioxidant potency and it has been demonstrated that luteolin prominently blocks ROS-triggered DNA and protein and lipid injury. Luteolin revealed its potency via defending or prolonging internal antioxidants like glutathione-S-transferase, glutathione reductase, and superoxide dismutase [42].

Flavanones: Flavanones are another vital subcategory of flavonoids commonly found in citrus fruits like grapes, oranges, and lemons. Eriodictyol, naringenin, and hesperitin are some common examples of flavanones. These constituents impart a bitter taste to the peel and juice of citrus fruits. Flavanones possess numerous pharmacological benefits like antiinflammatory, hypolipidimic, hypocholestremic, and antioxidant potency due to their radical engulfing ability [43–45]. Flavanones are also known as dihydroflavones due to saturation at carbon 2 and 3 in ring C; and this saturation differentiates two subcategories of flavonoids [46]. Flavanones demonstrate potent antitumor potency by decreasing DNA injury, cancer growth, and multiplication [47]. Flavanones, especially naringenin, revealed antimutagenic potency due to their ability to protect DNA from injury triggered by UV radiations and free radicals [48].

Isoflavonoids: Isoflavones are a typical and an essential subcategory of flavonoids. Structurally, isoflavones contain a 3-phenylchromen frame, a derivative of 2-phenylchromen frame synthesized by an aryl-relocation mechanism. Isoflavones chiefly occur in legumes, especially in soy, chickpeas, sunflower seeds, clover sprouts, black beans, and lima beans [49]. Daidzein and genistein are the chief isoflavones found in dietary products, which occur in four associated chemical structures, namely aglycones, 6'-O-malonylglucosides, 6'-O-acetylglucosides, and 7-O-glucosides [50]. In the course of plants and microscopic organism interaction, isoflavones play a crucial role in the synthesis of phytoalexins, an antimicrobial compound. Isoflavones like daidzein and genistein are widely considered as phyto-estrogens due to their estrogenic potency [51]. Isoflavones have demonstrated beneficial effects in alleviating menopausal symptoms, cardiovascular infections and also inhibit carcinogenesis. In addition, isoflavones are very beneficial in reducing the lipid profile [52].

Anthocyanidins: Anthocyanidins are a cluster of phytoconstituents that act as natural coloring agents that impart color to the various parts of a plant like fruits and flowers [53]. This particular flavonoid category is abundantly available in cocoa, honey, vegetables, fruits, teas, cereals, olive oil, and nuts. They are also available in berries like strawberries, black currant, elderberries, blueberries, and their extract along with red wine [54]. The coloring nature of anthocyanidins prominently relies on the pH and on acylation or methylation of hydroxyl groups in rings A and B [46]. Peonidin, cyanidin, delphinidin, petunidin, malvidin, and pelargonidin are the most common anthocyanidins available in vegetables and fruits. These constituents differ only in the position and number of methoxyl and hydroxyl groups as substituents [53]. Anthocyanidins play a crucial role in cholesterol disintegration, heart-related infections, and acute sight, along with cytotoxic and antioxidant potency [55]. Anthocyanidins target cells responsible for the growth of atherosclerosis. Scientifically, it was proved that anthocyanidins possess defensive potency against TNF-α-triggered MCP-1 (chemokine monocyte chemotactic protein 1) [56].

Neoflavonoids: Neoflavonoids are a group of polyphenolic agents with a 4-phenylchromen backbone without a hydroxyl moiety at the second position instead of a 2-phenylchromen-4-one backbone in flavonoids [57]. Neoflavonoids are subcategorized into two groups based on the backbone structure. These include neoflavones with a 4-phenylcoumarin (or 4-aryl-coumarin) backbone and neoflavenes with a 4-phenylchromen backbone. Calophyllolide was the first neoflavone isolated in 1951 from the seeds of *Calophyllum inophyllum* [58] and Dalbergichromene is a neoflavene isolated from the stem bark of *Dalbergia sissoo* [59].

Chalcones: Chalcones are another subcategory of flavonoids. They are also known as open chain flavonoids due to the lack of "ring C" in the basic skeleton. Chalconaringenin, arbutin, phloridzin, and phloretin are some common examples of this category. Chalcones are abundantly available in certain wheat products, pears, bearberries, tomatoes, and strawberries. Chalcones and their related products have gained huge response due to various biological and nutritional effects [60]. Researchers have demonstrated that chalcones possess anticancer, antiinflammatory, antioxidant, antitubercular, and antimicrobial benefits [61].

3 Introduction to inflammation

Inflammation is a defensive reaction to trauma, illness, damage to tissue, or harmful stimuli. Inflammation caused by microbial infections is normally a critical and challenging protective reaction. Tissue damage or injury that does not occur without any presence of microorganisms, a situation known as sterile inflammation, can also induce inflammation [62–64]. In the majority of cases, inflammation is an immunological response that is autocontrolled and organized for the resolution of infections or for the repair of damaged wounds and tissues. However, inflammation may generate a dysfunctional response or it may be accompanied with a physiologic stability imbalance without directly related inflammatory stimuli. When the trigger components are not included; an inflammatory illness can be triggered and chronic systemic damage causing inflammatory disturbances can occur [64–66]. Inflammation entails the recruitment by certain signals caused by inflammatory triggers of innate immune cells that have phagocytic characteristics. Proinflammatory cytokines as well as chemokines are secreted by these intrinsic cells, which attract lymphocytes and boost an immune system adaptive response. Reactive nitrogen species, reactive oxygen species, and other proteases are generated during an inflammatory immune response, which can promote proliferation, tissue damage, or fibrosis, all of which can lead to chronic inflammation [64,67]. Inflammation has been observed to be closely associated with various noninfectious disorders. Various serious ailments, like diabetes, cancer, autoimmune, cardiovascular problems, and neurological diseases (Fig. 1), arise from tissue lesions and genome changes generated by continual low-grade inflammation of the tissue or organ around it. Existing treatments for the majority of these chronic disorders sometimes cause more weakness than the condition itself, which guarantees that therapeutic options for patients are safer, less toxic, and more economical. Reducing chronic inflammation is a good method in the fight against various human disorders [68]. Substantial consumption of red meat, meat products, heavy or trans-fat diets built on processed constituents, or alcohol are all proinflammatory processes [64,69]. A balanced diet of vegetables, fruits, and whole grains, with nonprocessed, sugar-free meals, as well as an active and healthy lifestyle, appears to be connected to a lower incidence of inflammatory problems [64,70,71].

Numerous bioactive fruit and vegetable components, such as carotenoids, vitamins, flavonoids, minerals, and fibers, have been demonstrated to function independently as well as synergistically to provide consumers with a high level of nutritive value and medical benefits. In this regard, flavonoids have risen in popularity in recent years, thanks to a slew of large studies examining their potential human health benefits [64,72,73]. Flavonoids are a type of natural substance that is present in vegetables, fruits, as well as some drinks. Flavonoids are secondary plant metabolites having a polyphenolic core. These also have a variety of positive enzymatic and antioxidant qualities that are linked to diseases like Alzheimer's (AD), cancer, and atherosclerosis, among others [19,23,74–79]. These have been related to a variety of health-promoting qualities and are used in pharmacology, nutraceuticals, therapeutics, and cosmetics, due to its high antiinflammatory, antioxidant, anticancer,

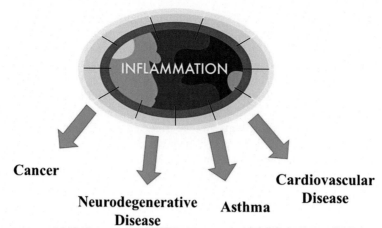

FIG. 1   Association of inflammation with various diseases.

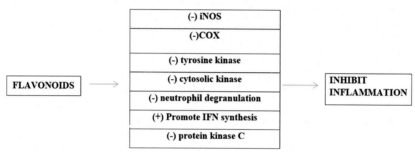

FIG. 2   Effect of flavonoids on inflammation [80].

and antimutagenic characteristics, as well as its capacity to regulate key cell enzyme activities (Fig. 2) [19,81–83]. Flavonoid compounds are plant extracts that can be found in many parts of plants. Vegetables employ flavonoids to help them grow and protect themselves against plaque formation. They are phenolic compounds with a low molecular weight that are abundantly found in plants. In higher plants, they are one of the most distinctive types of chemicals. In most angiosperm families, several flavonoids may be easily identified as floral pigments. They can be found in all parts of plants, not just flowers [19,84–86]. The functional mechanisms of flavonoids are still not completely known. Plant-derived compounds, on the other hand, are documented to exhibit a broad spectrum of pharmacological actions for a long time. The current trends in flavonoid research and development are the collection, detection, characterization, and activities of flavonoids, as well as their uses for health benefits. The industry is also predicting potential uses and manufacturing using molecular docking and bioinformatics data.

3.1   Protein kinases and transcription factor inhibition

PK (Protein kinases) have long been known to play a role in signal transmission during inflammation. Several flavonoids can regulate numerous core kinases involved in

multiple signaling pathways using this approach [64,87]. Flavonoids have been reported to inhibit kinases viz. tyrosine kinases, phosphatidylinositol kinase, phosphoinositol kinase, protein kinase C, and cyclin-dependent kinase 4 [64,88,89]. Inflammation also activates a number of kinases, which are fundamental for the transmission of signals involving lipid and protein phosphorylation (e.g., protein tyrosine kinase, protein kinase C, and phosphatidylinositol kinase). Roles of the suppression of the flavonoid protein C in lymphocyte modulation and release of antigen-based basophil histamine have been widely examined [90,91]. Flavonoids may regulate protein kinases via inhibiting transcription factors like NF-κB [64,92]. This factor controls several inflammatory cytokines, chemokines, and molecules of cell adhesion. IκB operates as an antagonistic molecule of NF-κB, but during inflammation IκB undergoes phosphorylation and is eliminated during the course of inflammation. Therefore, NF-κB from the cytoplasm is transported to the nucleus, causing activation of several proinflammatory genes. Flavonoids have been reported to regulate NF-κB as well as IκB activities, which have a profound effect on cell activation. Flavonoids may also modulate CD4 + T Helper 2 (Th2) cytokines like transducer and activator of signal for transcription 6 (STAT-6) and GATA-3 [64,93–96]. The primary transcription factor induced during inflammatory processes is NF-κB. In normal settings, a protein inhibitor κB (i.e., IκBα) retains the transcription factor subunits (p50 and p65) in an inactive cytoplasm. If TNF-α stimulates the activation of the IκB kinase, a series of complicated signaling cascades occurs that turn phosphorylates IκBα into the dissociation of the NF-κB inhibitor [97,98]. In addition, NF-κB gets translocated to the nucleus wherein it attaches to particular binding sites and areas with the DNA and encourages several proinflammatory genes for various biochemical media and enzymes to be transcribed. In spite of the a lot of research that shows the favorable effects of flavonoids on NF-κB activation, relatively few focused on its activities and structural characteristics [98,99].

3.2 Inhibition of phosphodiesterases

PDEs (phosphodiesterases) are enzymes that can be found in a range of tissues and organs in mammals. The secondary messengers' cyclic guanosine monophosphate (cGMP) as well as cyclic adenosine monophosphate (cAMP), which modulate cyclic nucleotide levels, are hydrolyzed and inactivated by them. Low cyclic nucleotide concentrations or short-term duration in tissues or organs have been associated with asthma, erectile dysfunction in men, diabetes, and Alzheimer's disease, to name a few [100,101]. Phosphodiesterases like cAMP phosphodiesterase are inhibited by flavonoids. cAMP is a second messenger molecule that regulates a wide range of cell activities during inflammation. Increasing cAMP levels is linked to antiinflammatory effects. Phosphodiesterases are enzymes that catalyze the hydrolysis of cAMP in order to maintain appropriate cAMP levels. Flavonoids' phosphodiesterase inhibitory actions can prevent cAMP breakdown and prolong cAMP propagation [64,102,103]. The suppression of phosphodiesterases in chronic and allergic inflammations is of special therapeutic value. Flavonoids have been connected to this inhibitory function in a number of traditional medical remedies, and phosphodiesterase suppression is an essential activity linked to a variety of medicinal plants. In investigations, flavone aglycones with five or more methoxy substitutions were found to be potent cAMP phosphodiesterase inhibitors; however, C-glycosyl flavones and flavone-*O*-glycosides were found to be less effective than aglycones [90,104,105].

3.3 Antioxidant activity

Free radicals, such as nitrogen-derived radicals and oxygen-derived radicals, are produced when tissue is damaged, and they have an unfavorable effect on cell activity [64,106]. Free radicals are highly reactive and damaging to DNA, lipids, and proteins, due to the presence of unpaired electrons. It is also documented that both lipid peroxidation in cell membranes as well as oxidative damage to nucleic acids

and proteins are caused by free radicals. A high production of free radicals, a lack of transition metal ion sequestration, and a lack of free radical scavenging activity all contribute to oxidative stress [64,107]. Due to their inhibitory activity on free radical formation and scavenging capacity for reactive oxygen and nitrogen species, flavonoids have antioxidant capabilities. Flavonoids are antioxidants because of their molecular structure, distinct replacement sequences within the structure, plus phenolic hydrogen atoms, which enables their functioning as hydrogen-donating moieties [64,108,109]. Scavenging reactive oxygen species; lowering reactive oxygen species creation (by inhibiting enzymes or chelating trace elements engaged in free radical production); and finally, upregulation or protection of antioxidant defenses are some of the antioxidant potentials [110–112]. The majority of the mechanisms outlined above are involved in flavonoid activity. The relationship between radical scavenging activity as well as enzyme functions could be the cause of some of the effects they mediate. Glutathione *S*-transferase, microsomal monooxygenase, NADH oxidase, mitochondrial succinoxidase, and other ROS-producing enzymes are all inhibited by flavonoids. Antioxidant action is influenced by the presence, position, structure, and total quantity of sugar moieties in flavonoids (flavonoid glycosides). Aglycones are more powerful antioxidants than their glycoside counterparts. Multiple studies have found that as the number of glycosidic moieties in flavonol glycosides from tea, their antioxidant potential decreased. Despite the fact that glycosides are typically weaker antioxidants than aglycones, a glucose moiety can sometimes increase absorption [112–114].

3.4 Impact on arachidonic acid metabolism

The phospholipase A2 enzyme (PLA2) produces arachidonic acid from phospholipids from plasma membranes during the course of the inflammation process. After arachidonic acid is digested by various oxygenases viz. cyclooxygenase (COX) and lipoxygenase (LOX), inflammatory mediators like thromboxanes, prostaglandins, as well as leukotrienes are generated [64,115]. Flavonoids also have the ability to block enzymes implicated in the metabolism of arachidonic acid, lowering the production of inflammatory cytokines produced by this route. In addition, flavonoids can prevent the synthesis of prostaglandins, thromboxanes, and leukotrienes by preventing the formation of PLA2, COX, as well as LOX enzymes [64,116–119]. As inflammatory mediators, cyclooxygenase and lipoxygenase play a crucial role. They play a role in the secretion of arachidonic acid, which serves as a key component of the inflammatory process. Neutrophils with lipoxygenase produce arachidonic acid chemotactic molecules. These also cause the secretion of cytokines. Certain phenolic substances have demonstrated that both cyclooxygenase and 5-lipoxygenase pathways are inhibited [120–123]. This restriction lowers arachidonic acid release. The specific process by which these enzymes are inhibited is not established. In particular, quercetin blocks simultaneously cyclooxygenase and lipoxygenase, hence decreasing the synthesis of these inflammatory metabolites [123–126].

3.5 Effects in immune cells

Flavonoids influence cell activation, maturation, signaling, cytokine production, and secretory mechanisms in a variety of immune cells due to their diverse properties and activities. For example, inhibiting maturation markers like CD80 and CD86, which are necessary for CD4 + T cell activation and are higher when DCs mature, has been shown to impede DC maturation. This would lead to an inhibitory effect in cytokine release and a proliferative CD4 + T cell response [64,127–129]. By modulating iron metabolism, flavonoids have an effect on DCs' inflammatory response. Various studies have suggested that some flavonoids can suppress the production of prostaglandins and histamine by mast cells, neutrophils, and other immune cells, as well as the production of proinflammatory mediators or chemokines by neutrophils, mast cells, as well as other immune cells [64,130–133]. Flavonoids can bind to cytokine targets, such as the "IL-17RA" part of the IL-17 receptor, suppressing signaling, according to the research. They can also stop inflammatory receptors like the high-affinity IgE receptor and others from signaling downstream [64,134,135]. Flavonoids may reduce monocyte adhesion, or diminish activation as well as proliferative responsiveness of some immune cells involved in chronic

inflammation [64,136,137]. IL-4, IL-5, as well as IL-13 are among the cytokines implicated in the beginning and regulation of the allergic response, as well as the generation of IgE. Such cytokines are involved in the distinguishing as well as activation processes of the Th2 type CD4+ cells, IgE B lymphocyte differentiation, chemotaxis, mucus hypersecretion, and bronchoconstrictions [138–140]. The inhibition of granulocytic cell chemoattractant components by some flavonoids has been shown to reduce the stimulation of the eosinophilic inflammatory responsiveness [140–142].

4 Role of flavonoids in various inflammation-associated diseases

4.1 Cancer

Flavonoids may help in regulating the action of growth factors responsible for the development of tumors [143]. Quercetin, when studied in prostate cancer cell lines of humans, was observed to cause programmed cell death [144]. Apigenin, a flavonoid, has also been observed to inhibit the activity of certain enzymes [145]. Rutin, when given to rats at a concentration of 100 mg/kg (pancreatitis model) for a month, considerably decreased the concentration of certain marker enzymes (Table 1) [158]. In diabetic kidney disorder, naringenin was observed to restrain the spread of glomerular meningeal cells [159]. A natural flavonoid, luteoloside found in *Gentiana macrophylla*, has been studied for its antitumor activity in in vitro as well as in vivo methods. An in vitro study conducted on hepatocellular carcinoma cells has shown that luteoloside exerted

TABLE 1 Antiinflammatory effects of flavonoids in various inflammation associated diseases.

Disease	Compound	Response	Reference
Cancer	Quercetin	Inhibition of cancer cell replication	[146,147]
	Isoflavone	Suppression of lung, breast, ovarian, endometrial, and colorectal cancers	
Neurodegenerative diseases	Apigenin	Memory enhancement and improvement in learning as well	[148–154]
	Nobiletin	Improvement of mice memory	
	Baicalein	Intraperitoneal route at a concentration of 10 mg/kg in 1 x FAD model was known to prevent memory loss	
	Fisetin	In several models for Alzheimer's disorder was seen to avert the loss of intellectual learning	
	Rutin	Avert the loss of memory	
Asthma	Quercetin	Exhibits antiinflammatory property via murine model of airways allergic inflammation	[134,155]
	Luteolin	Suppresses histamine and prostaglandin release from mast cells	
	Genistein	Inhibition proinflammatory cytokines in mast cells as well as GATA-3, STAT-6	

TABLE 1 Antiinflammatory effects of flavonoids in various inflammation associated diseases—cont'd

Disease	Compound	Response	Reference
CVD	Quercetin	Decrease in oxidative stress and cardio-protective properties	[156,157]
	Luteolin	Enhancement of systolic/diastolic function in rat hearts after ischemia	
	Puerarin	Decline in inflammatory responses and NF-κB activation	
	Anthocyanidin	Suppresses adhesion of monocytes to endothelial cells	

an inhibitory action on cancerous cells. An in vivo study conducted on BALB/c mice has also shown the inhibitory action of luteoloside in metastasis [160]. A flavonoid found in green tea, i.e., EGCG, is known to cause growth inhibition in skin cancer cells [161]. A novel synthetic flavonoid, LFG-500, has been studied in vivo using mice induced with lung cancer. It has been observed that LGF-500 considerably inhibited the metastasis of cancerous cells [162]

It has been proved by numerous in vitro and in vivo models that flavonoids possibly possess a defensive action toward the growth and development of several kinds of tumors [163–165].

Some flavonoids from *Trichosanthes kirilowii*, viz., acacetin, genkwanin, and isorhamnetin have happened to inhibit the growth and development of breast cancer [166]. Quercetin has been seen to exert its action on telomeric sequences wherein it causes disruption in telomeric end elongation that, in turn, affects the replication of cancerous cells [146]. Leaves of *Diospyros kaki,* used for making tea in Asian countries, possess the flavonoids that have been observed to cause growth inhibition of cancer cells in mice liver [167]. A 5 year study conducted on 1063 women (75 years old and above) has revealed that women with higher flavonoid consumption had lower chances of cancer development [168]. Among the various flavonoids, viz., flavones, isoflavones, flavanones, flavanols, and anthocyanidins, it has been seen that the greater consumption of flavanols and flavonols is correlated with the reduction in colorectal cancer cases [169]. It also considerably caused reduction in colorectal and breast cancers [147].

4.2 Neurodegenerative diseases

In various studies 7,8-dihydroxyflavone (a flavone) has been examined in the 5 x FAD model. It has been observed that in mice (aged 1 year old) when 7,8-dihydroxyflavone was injected at a concentration of 5 mg/kg intraperitoneally, there was a positive change in performance in the Y-maze test [170]. Using the same model, i.e., 5 x FAD model when 7,8-DHF was given through an intraperitoneal route at a

concentration of 5 mg/kg every day for a month it was observed to improve the memory power [171].

Apigenin, a flavone was used in the model 2 x FAD, in which 40 mg/kg was administered to mice orally for 3 months. It was seen that there was memory enhancement and improvement in learning as well [148]. Nobiletin, a citrus flavone was used in the model 1 x FAD, in which 10 mg/kg daily was administered intraperitoneally for about 4 months. It was observed that memory was enhanced [172]. In a 3 x FAD model, nobiletin was given every day at concentrations 10 and 30 mg/kg intraperitoneally for 12 weeks. It was noted to improve the memory of mice [149]. Also, in several assays it was observed that nobiletin when administered in mice intraperitoneally at concentration 10 and 50 mg/kg helped in the improvement of mice memory [173].

Baicalein, a flavone when given through the intraperitoneal route at a concentration of 10 mg/kg in a 1 x FAD model was known to prevent memory loss [150]. Fisetin, a flavonol in several models for Alzheimer's disorder, was seen to avert the loss of intellectual learning. It was efficient when given orally at a concentration of 25 mg/kg daily as well as intraperitoneally at a dose of 20 mg/kg [151–153]. Quercetin has been studied in various models of Alzheimer's disorder. It was given at a concentration of 25 mg/kg everyday either orally or intraperitoneally. It was observed that the nanoencapsulated particles of quercetin were twice as efficient as quercetin (free) in memory enhancement and learning improvement in mice [174–176].

Rutin, a combination of quercetin and rutinose, was studied in rats. It was injected intraperitoneally at a concentration of 100 mg/kg every day for a month and was noted to avert the loss of memory [154]. Green tea has increased concentration of flavanols, which includes epigallocatechin gallate (EGCG) that has been studied in several models of AD. It has been observed that the EGCG, when taken for a prolonged period, enhanced the cognitive functions [177,178]. Hesperidin and puerarin, when administered daily at a concentration of 100 and 30 mg/kg, correspondingly in animals were proven to be beneficial in several models of AD [179]. Baicalein, a flavone, when studied in various models of Parkinson's disorder was observed to reduce the DA neuron loss and also enhanced behavioral functions [180–182].

7,8-DHF, when given orally at a concentration of 12–16mg/kg daily to rats, was seen to reduce DA neuron loss and also enhance behavioral functions [183]. In mice using the MPTP model, 7,8-DHF, when given at a concentration of 5mg/kg every day, intraperitoneally, was seen to improve motor functions and also prevented the loss of DA neurons [184]. Also, in monkeys, when administered orally at a concentration of 30mg/kg daily, 7,8-DHF was known to prevent loss of DA neurons [185].

Quercetin, when administered orally at 100 and 200mg/kg daily in mice, caused improvement in the motor functions [186]. Rutin, when administered intraperitoneally at a dose of 10 and 30mg/kg daily, was observed to enhance motor activity [187]. Fisetin, when administered at a concentration of 10–25mg/kg daily, was seen to increase dopamine levels in mice [188]. Kaempferol, a flavonol administered orally at doses 25, 50, and 100mg/kg daily, was also seen to improve dopamine levels in mice [189]. Catechin at doses 10 and 30mg/kg daily when used intraperitoneally in rats [190], EGCG given orally at a concentration of 25mg/kg daily in mice [191], and epicatechin when given to rats at a concentration of 100mg/kg daily orally [192] were known to improve behavioral functions. Naringenin, when administered orally at varying concentrations of 25, 50, and 100mg/kg daily, improved the levels of dopamine [193]. Hesperetin, when given orally at a concentration of 50mg/kg daily, improved behavioral functions and also prevented DA neuron loss [194]. Isoflavones, puerarin and genistein, have been studied in PD animal models. Both the compounds were known to improve neuronal functions [179,195]. Chrysin, a flavone, when administered orally at 50mg/kg daily, was known to improve the behavioral activity in rats when studied on Huntington's disease model [196]. 7,8-DHF, when given orally at a concentration of 5mg/kg daily in a mice model of HD helped to present the progression of motor and cognitive deficits [197]. Fisetin has also been seen to prevent Huntington's disease [198].

In a study, it has been observed that quercetin at a concentration of 25mg/kg daily when taken orally caused reduction in motor deficits [199]. In alternative experiment, it was given intraperitoneally at a concentration of 50mg/kg that also helped to enhance motor activity [200]. Rutin was studied for its action in the 3-NP rat model at a concentration of 25 and 50mg/kg administered daily. It was observed that it helped to avert the impairments induced due to 3-NP in motor functions [201]. Kaempferol injected daily at a concentration of 25mg/kg in the 3-NP model for rats lowered the motor damage [202]. Hesperidin, at a concentration of 100mg/kg daily given orally to the same model (3-NP rat model), also lessened motor damage [203].

Genistein, an isoflavone administered daily at a concentration of 10 and 20mg/kg intraperitoneally, was also observed to exert protective action in the 3-NP rat model [204].

The intake of berries containing anthocyanins in diet daily at a concentration of about 100mg/kg was known to prevent damage to motor functions [205]. In a SOD1-G93A mice model, a method for studying amyotrophic lateral sclerosis (ALS), 7,8-DHF at a concentration of 5mg/kg intraperitoneally on alternate days helped to prevent the age-related reduction of motor activity [206].

Fisetin at a concentration of 9mg/kg taken orally also facilitated to avert the progress of motor deficiencies and also improved the life span [207].

4.3 Role of flavonoids in asthma

Asthma is a chronic complex respiratory disorder. It is represented by the obstruction of air passages, their inflammation, and the hyperactivity of bronchia. It involves complex pathophysiology, and various immune responses. For example, allergens induce allergic asthma and Th2 cell-related immune responses play a key role in its mediation. Th2 cells produce cytokines, which are important in B cells for IgE class switching; also they help in the involvement of mast cells and eosinophils [208]. In these types of asthma cases, flavonoids, like flavones, isoflavones, flavonols, and anthocyanidins, display promising results in asthma. Oligomeric proanthocyanidins (OPCs), which is a flavonoid polymer, decreased the inflammation of the airways and reduced the infiltration by inflammatory cells. These results were observed in studies conducted in a murine model of asthma. Also Th2 cytokines, and IgE, an allergic specific immunoglobulin, were reduced by OPCs. In addition to these, pulmonary CD11c+ DCs maturation was inhibited by OPCs. It was brought about by minimizing the costimulatory molecule CD86's expression as a result of which, in CD4+T cells, promotion in their proliferative responses gets affected [127]. In the commencement and progression of asthma, mast cells play an important role. Mast cells are capable of releasing mediators that develop cooperation between different types of cells vital in this disorder [209]. In the previous studies conducted so far, which involved human mast cells developed in culture, it was found that luteolin-like flavones were responsible for decreasing the prostaglandin D2 and histamine from these cells [210]. In contrast to this, recent studies showed that tetramethoxyluteolin (methlut), a structural analog of luteolin and also a new flavone, was more potent in the reduction of histamine release and other mediators involved in asthma. Luteolin and this new flavone suppressed the discharge of mediators such as TNF, histamine, and β-hexosaminidase. In addition to this, in mast cells derived from human cord blood the discharge of CCL2 was reduced; as a consequence, the inflammatory cells are not recruited. The intracellular calcium blockade and obstruction of NF-κB at the gene and protein levels would be the possible mechanisms for the mast cell suppression shown by luteolin and its analog [133]. On the other hand, flavonols, the other flavonoid type, suppress the discharge of cytokines from mast cells or basophils. In addition to this, flavonols also possess antiinflammatory activity [131,132,155]. Onions, broccoli, or apples contain quercetin, which is a flavonol. In a murine model of airways allergic inflammation quercetin showed antiinflammatory activity upon oral administration in a microemulsion form. The levels of the cytokines IL-5 and IL-4 was decreased by quercetin; also, there was reduction in the involvement of eosinophils to the bronchoalveolar fluid [155]. In the same model, other flavonols such as kaempferol upon oral administration caused a decrease in the intrusion of eosinophils in the air passage and in the lungs. Kaempferol blocked the degranulation of eosinophils. The mechanism of action in the abovementioned studies lies in the NF-κB blockade. [131].

In another model of asthma using guinea pigs, antiinflammatory activity was depicted by isoflavones. For example, in the guinea pig asthmatic model genistein, an isoflavone, caused a reduction in airway hyperresponsiveness and acute bronchoconstriction, which was induced by the allergen ovalbumin (OVA). Genistein inhibits protein tyrosine kinases, thereby stabilizing the mast cells and this is thought to be a probable mechanism of its action. [211]. Red berries, apples, or plums contain cyanidin, which is a type of anthocyanidin. It was found to decrease inflammation induced by Th17 cells; also, it caused a reduction in hyperresponsiveness in the studies conducted in various mouse models in which severe asthma was induced [135].

The above results suggest that flavonoids have a promising role in the management of asthma.

4.4 Role of flavonoids in CVD

The cardioprotective effect of flavonoids on the initiation and development of CVD have been described in studies conducted in vitro and in vivo. In one such study, a reassuring cardioprotective effect was shown by luteolin in a rat model with myocardial ischemia reperfusion (I/R) injury [212]. As per this study, the serum levels of IL-18, IL-1β, and TNF-α in rats was reduced by luteolin and also it was found that NLRP3, ASC, TLR4, MyD88, and NF-κB were downregulated. The other species, *Abelmoschus manihot*, provides a good source of flavonoids and the total flavonoids extracted from it showed the cardioprotective activity by reducing myocardial ischemia reperfusion (I/R) injury in a rat model. These flavonoids act by inhibiting the NLRP3 inflammasome [213]. In fruits, procyanidin flavonoids are commonly found; these type of flavonoids show their protective effects on vessels by inhibiting activation of the NLRP3 inflammasome [214]. There was decrease in inflammation and atherosclerosis on quercetin intake as depicted in experiments using various animal models [215,216]. Similarly, in different animal models Baicalin,

a flavone, which is found in various herbs particularly in rhizomes, showed a cardioprotective effect. It was particularly effective against myocardial ischemic injury and atherosclerosis. In one of the experiments, cardiac hypertrophy was induced by a pressure overload and baicalin showed a cardioprotective effect. The conditions like cardiac dysfunction and myocardial hypertrophy were improved by this flavonoid; also, it decreased apoptosis and fibrosis in heart tissue [217].

5 Conclusions

The various inflammatory disorders including CVD, cancer, or allergies are mainly due to dysregulation in inflammatory processes. The influence that diet has over inflammatory disorders has been well established from the past one decade, and in this context, the importance of flavonoids as a key component of a healthy diet has gained tremendous consideration because of its antiinflammatory associated properties. Recently published data from various in vitro studies have added new insights that various subclasses of flavonoids can regulate in different stages of inflammation. Besides, the use of novel experimental animal models has provided numerous information toward the understanding of the prospective health benefits of flavonoids. These important advances have provided us a knowledge that a healthy diet rich in flavonoids has an impact in the complexity of chronic inflammatory disorders. However, a much deeper understanding of the antioxidant and antiinflammatory effects of flavonoids in various chronic disorders further needs to be investigated at the clinical level.

References

[1] A.D. Kinghorn, Y.-W. Chin, S.M. Swanson, Discovery of natural product anticancer agents from biodiverse organisms, Curr. Opin. Drug Discov. Devel. 12 (2) (2009) 189.

[2] N.A. Lone, et al., Bioactivity guided isolation and characterization of anti-hepatotoxic markers from *Berberis pachyacantha Koehne*, Pharm. Res. Mod. Chinese Med. 4 (2022) 100144.

[3] J. Krause, G. Tobin, Discovery, development, and regulation of natural products, in: Using Old Solutions to New Problems-Natural Drug Discovery in the 21st Century, 2013, pp. 1–35 (Chapter 1).

[4] R.H. Mir, et al., A comprehensive review on journey of pyrrole scaffold against multiple therapeutic targets, Anticancer Agents Med. Chem. 22 (19) (2022) 3291–3303.

[5] A. Baiano, Potential use of bioactive compounds from waste in the pharmaceutical industry, in: Utilisation of Bioactive Compounds from Agricultural and Food Waste, CRC Press, 2017, pp. 383–401.

[6] P.A. Mir, et al., Anticancer potential of thymoquinone: a novel bioactive natural compound from *Nigella sativa* L., Anticancer Agents Med. Chem. 22 (20) (2022) 3401–3415.

[7] D.A. Dias, et al., Current and future perspectives on the structural identification of small molecules in biological systems, Metabolites 6 (4) (2016) 46.

[8] A.J. Shah, et al., Clinical Biomarkers and Novel Drug Targets to Cut Gordian Knots of Alzheimer's Disease, 2022.

[9] R.H. Mir, et al., Isoflavones of soy: chemistry and health benefits, in: Edible Plants in Health and Diseases, Springer, 2022, pp. 303–324.

[10] R. Cooper, G. Nicola, Natural Products Chemistry: Sources, Separations and Structures, CRC Press, 2014.

[11] R.H. Mir, et al., Resveratrol: A Potential Drug Candidate With Multispectrum Therapeutic Application, vol. 73, 2022, pp. 99–137.

[12] G. Appendino, A. Minassi, O. Taglialatela-Scafati, Recreational drug discovery: natural products as lead structures for the synthesis of smart drugs, Nat. Prod. Rep. 31 (7) (2014) 880–904.

[13] N. Chintoju, et al., Importance of natural products in the modern history, Res. Rev. J. Hosp. Clin. Pharm. 1 (1) (2015) 5–10.

[14] R. Mohi-Ud-Din, et al., The regulation of endoplasmic reticulum stress in cancer: special focuses on luteolin patents, Molecules 27 (8) (2022) 2471.

[15] R.H. Mir, et al., Curcumin as a privileged scaffold molecule for various biological targets in drug development, Stud. Nat. Prod. Chem. 73 (2022) 405–434.

[16] I. Erlund, Review of the flavonoids quercetin, hesperetin, and naringenin. Dietary sources, bioactivities, bioavailability, and epidemiology, Nutr. Res. 24 (10) (2004) 851–874.

[17] R. Mohi-Ud-Din, et al., Recent insights into therapeutic potential of plant-derived flavonoids against cancer, Anticancer Agents Med. Chem. 22 (20) (2022) 3343–3369.

[18] X. Li, et al., Chemical composition and antioxidant and anti-inflammatory potential of peels and flesh from 10 different pear varieties (Pyrus spp.), Food Chem. 152 (2014) 531–538.

[19] A. Panche, A. Diwan, S. Chandra, Flavonoids: an overview, J. Nutr. Sci. (2016) 5.

[20] R. Griesbach, Biochemistry and genetics of flower color, Plant Breed Rev. 25 (2005) 89–114.

[21] G. Ahmad, et al., Assessment of anti-inflammatory activity of 3-acetylmyricadiol in LPSStimulated Raw 264.7 macrophages, Comb Chem. High Throughput Screen 25 (1) (2022) 204–210.

[22] A. Takahashi, T. Ohnishi, The significance of the study about the biological effects of solar ultraviolet radiation using the exposed facility on the international space station, Biol. Sci. Space 18 (4) (2004) 255–260.

[23] A.J. Shah, et al., Depression: an insight into heterocyclic and cyclic hydrocarbon compounds inspired from natural sources, Curr. Neuropharmacol. 19 (11) (2021) 2020–2037.

[24] S.H. Thilakarathna, H. Rupasinghe, Flavonoid bioavailability and attempts for bioavailability enhancement, Nutrients 5 (9) (2013) 3367–3387.

[25] R. Mohi-ud-Din, et al., Plant-derived natural compounds for the treatment of amyotrophic lateral sclerosis: an update, Curr. Neuropharmacol. 20 (1) (2022) 179–193.

[26] A. Bhagat, et al., Oreganum Vulgare: in-vitro assessment of cytotoxicity, molecular dock-ing studies, antioxidant and anti-inflammatory activity in LPS Stimulat-ed RAW 264.7 cells, Med. Chem. 16 (2020) 1–11.

[27] K.M. Brodowska, Natural flavonoids: classification, potential role, and application of flavonoid analogues, Eur. J. Biol. Res. 7 (2) (2017) 108–123.

[28] R. Mohi-Ud-Din, et al., Berberine in the treatment of neurodegenerative diseases and nanotechnology enabled targeted delivery, Comb. Chem. High Throughput Screen. 25 (4) (2022) 616–633.

[29] R.H. Mir, et al., Natural anti-inflammatory compounds as drug candidates in Alzheimer's disease, Curr. Med. Chem. 28 (23) (2021) 4799–4825.

[30] S.-H. Wang, Y.-L. Hu, T.-X. Liu, Plant distribution and pharmacological activity of flavonoids, Tradit. Med. Res 4 (2019) 269–287.

[31] N.B. Sabreen, M.M. Bhat, M.J.F.I.N.P.C.V. Hussain, Coumarin Derivatives as Potential Anti-inflammatory Agents for Drug Development, vol. 8, 2021, pp. 213–238.

[32] T.-Y. Wang, Q. Li, K.-S. Bi, Bioactive flavonoids in medicinal plants: structure, activity and biological fate, Asian J. Pharm. Sci. 13 (1) (2018) 12–23.

[33] M. Kumar, et al., Molecular and biochemical evidence on the protective effects of quercetin in isoproterenol-induced acute myocardial injury in rats, J. Biochem. Mol. Toxicol. 31 (1) (2017) 1–8.

[34] D. Pascual-Teresa, D.A. Moreno, C. García-Viguera, Flavanols and anthocyanins in cardiovascular health: a review of current evidence, Int. J. Mol. Sci. 11 (4) (2010) 1679–1703.

[35] K.R. Määttä-Riihinen, et al., Catechins and procyanidins in berries of Vaccinium species and their antioxidant activity, J. Agric. Food Chem. 53 (22) (2005) 8485–8491.

[36] A. Gramza, J. Korczak, R. Amarowicz, Tea polyphenols-their antioxidant properties and biological activity-a review, Polish J. Food Nutr. Sci. 14 (3) (2005) 219.

[37] J.A. Vinson, et al., Phenol antioxidant quantity and quality in foods: fruits, J. Agric. Food Chem. 49 (11) (2001) 5315–5321.

[38] Y. Lin, et al., Luteolin, a flavonoid with potential for cancer prevention and therapy, Curr. Cancer Drug Targets 8 (7) (2008) 634–646.

[39] D. Patel, S. Shukla, S. Gupta, Apigenin and cancer chemoprevention: progress, potential and promise, Int. J. Oncol. 30 (1) (2007) 233–245.

[40] M. Horinaka, et al., The dietary flavonoid apigenin sensitizes malignant tumor cells to tumor necrosis factor–related apoptosis-inducing ligand, Mol. Cancer Ther. 5 (4) (2006) 945–951.

[41] G. Galati, P.J. O'brien, Potential toxicity of flavonoids and other dietary phenolics: significance for their chemopreventive and anticancer properties, Free Radic. Biol. Med. 37 (3) (2004) 287–303.

[42] T. Lapidot, M.D. Walker, J. Kanner, Antioxidant and prooxidant effects of phenolics on pancreatic β-cells in vitro, J. Agric. Food Chem. 50 (25) (2002) 7220–7225.

[43] M. Denaro, A. Smeriglio, D. Trombetta, Antioxidant and anti-inflammatory activity of citrus flavanones mix and its stability after in vitro simulated digestion, Antioxidants 10 (2) (2021) 140.

[44] X. Montané, et al., Current perspectives of the applications of polyphenols and flavonoids in cancer therapy, Molecules 25 (15) (2020) 3342.

[45] M.K. Khan, O. Dangles, A comprehensive review on flavanones, the major citrus polyphenols, J. Food Compos. Anal. 33 (1) (2014) 85–104.

[46] T. Iwashina, Flavonoid properties of five families newly incorporated into the order Caryophyllales, Bull. Natl. Mus. Nat. Sci. 39 (2013) 25–51.

[47] A. Trzeciakiewicz, et al., Molecular mechanism of hesperetin-7-O-glucuronide, the main circulating metabolite of hesperidin, involved in osteoblast differentiation, J. Agric. Food Chem. 58 (1) (2010) 668–675.

[48] K. Gao, et al., The citrus flavonoid naringenin stimulates DNA repair in prostate cancer cells, J. Nutr. Biochem. 17 (2) (2006) 89–95.

[49] F. Marin, J. Perez-Alvarez, C. Soler-Rivas, Isoflavones as functional food components, in: Studies in Natural Products Chemistry, Elsevier, 2005, pp. 1177–1207.

[50] T. Clavel, et al., Isoflavones and functional foods alter the dominant intestinal microbiota in postmenopausal women, J. Nutr. 135 (12) (2005) 2786–2792.

[51] K. Szkudelska, L. Nogowski, Genistein—a dietary compound inducing hormonal and metabolic changes, J. Steroid Biochem. Mol. Biol. 105 (1-5) (2007) 37–45.

[52] J. Yeung, T.-F. Yu, Effects of isoflavones (soy phyto-estrogens) on serum lipids: a meta-analysis of randomized controlled trials, Nutr. J. 2 (1) (2003) 1–8.

[53] S. de Pascual-Teresa, C. Santos-Buelga, J.C. Rivas-Gonzalo, Quantitative analysis of flavan-3-ols in Spanish foodstuffs and beverages, J. Agric. Food Chem. 48 (11) (2000) 5331–5337.

[54] B.I. Nwiloh, A.A. Uwakwe, J.O. Akaninwor, Phytochemical screening and GC-FID analysis of ethanolic extract of root bark of Salacia nitida L. *Benth*, J. Med. Plants Stud. 4 (6) (2016) 283–287.

[55] D. Bagchi, et al., Anti-angiogenic, antioxidant, and anti-carcinogenic properties of a novel anthocyanin-rich berry extract formula, Biochem. Mosc. 69 (1) (2004) 75–80.

[56] M. Garcia-Alonso, et al., Red wine anthocyanins are rapidly absorbed in humans and affect monocyte chemoattractant protein 1 levels and antioxidant capacity of plasma, J. Nutr. Biochem. 20 (7) (2009) 521–529.

[57] S.-F. Wu, et al., Anti-inflammatory and cytotoxic neoflavonoids and benzofurans from Pterocarpus santalinus, J. Nat. Prod. 74 (5) (2011) 989–996.

[58] M. Garazd, Y.L. Garazd, V. Khilya, Neoflavones. 1. Natural distribution and spectral and biological properties, Chem. Nat. Compd. 39 (1) (2003) 54–121.

[59] P. Devi, Phytochemical and pharmacological profiling of Dalbergia sissoo Roxb. *Stem*, J. Pharmacogn. Phytochem. 6 (6) (2017) 2483–2486.

[60] Z. Nowakowska, A review of anti-infective and anti-inflammatory chalcones, Eur. J. Med. Chem. 42 (2) (2007) 125–137.

[61] S. Tekale, et al., Biological role of chalcones in medicinal chemistry, in: Vector-Borne Diseases-Recent Developments in Epidemiology and Control, IntechOpen, 2020.

[62] F. Behnia, S. Sheller, R. Menon, Mechanistic differences leading to infectious and sterile inflammation, Am. J. Reprod. Immunol. 75 (5) (2016) 505–518.

[63] G.Y. Chen, G. Nuñez, Sterile inflammation: sensing and reacting to damage, Nat. Rev. Immunol. 10 (12) (2010) 826–837.

[64] S.J. Maleki, J.F. Crespo, B. Cabanillas, Anti-inflammatory effects of flavonoids, Food Chem. 299 (2019), 125124.

[65] C. Franceschi, J. Campisi, Chronic inflammation (inflammaging) and its potential contribution to age-associated diseases, J. Gerontol. A Biomed. Sci. Med. Sci. 69 (Suppl_1) (2014) S4–S9.

[66] M.E. Kotas, R. Medzhitov, Homeostasis, inflammation, and disease susceptibility, Cell 160 (5) (2015) 816–827.

[67] H. Shen, D. Kreisel, D.R. Goldstein, Processes of sterile inflammation, J. Immunol. 191 (6) (2013) 2857–2863.

[68] R. Ginwala, et al., Potential role of flavonoids in treating chronic inflammatory diseases with a special focus on the anti-inflammatory activity of apigenin, Antioxidants 8 (2) (2019) 35.

[69] V. Bouvard, et al., Carcinogenicity of consumption of red and processed meat, Lancet Oncol. 16 (16) (2015) 1599–1600.

[70] L. Schwingshackl, B. Bogensberger, G. Hoffmann, Diet quality as assessed by the healthy eating index, alternate healthy eating index, dietary approaches to stop hypertension score, and health outcomes: an updated systematic review and meta-analysis of cohort studies, J. Acad. Nutr. Diet. 118 (1) (2018) 74–100. e11.

[71] S.G. van Breda, T.M. de Kok, Smart combinations of bioactive compounds in fruits and vegetables may guide new strategies for personalized prevention of chronic diseases, Mol. Nutr. Food Res. 62 (1) (2018) 1700597.

[72] R.H. Liu, Health-promoting components of fruits and vegetables in the diet, Adv. Nutr. 4 (3) (2013) 384S–392S.

[73] J.L. Slavin, B. Lloyd, Health benefits of fruits and vegetables, Adv. Nutr. 3 (4) (2012) 506–516.

[74] M. Burak, Y. Imen, Flavonoids and their antioxidant properties, Turkiye Klin Tip Bil Derg 19 (1999) 296–304.

[75] A. Castañeda-Ovando, et al., Chemical studies of anthocyanins: a review, Food Chem. 113 (4) (2009) 859–871.

[76] Y.K. Lee, et al., (−)-Epigallocatechin-3-gallate prevents lipopolysaccharide-induced elevation of beta-amyloid generation and memory deficiency, Brain Res. 1250 (2009) 164–174.

[77] R.H. Mir, et al., Natural anti-inflammatory compounds as drug candidates in Alzheimer's disease, Curr. Med. Chem. 28 (23) (2021) 4799–4825.

[78] R. Mohi-Ud-Din, et al., Plant-derived natural compounds for the treatment of amyotrophic lateral sclerosis: an update, Curr. Neuropharmacol. 20 (1) (2022) 179–193.

[79] Z. Sobhani, et al., Medicinal species of the genus Berberis: a review of their traditional and ethnomedicinal uses, phytochemistry and pharmacology, Adv. Exp. Med. Biol. 1308 (2021) 547–577.

[80] H.K. Sandhar, et al., A review of phytochemistry and pharmacology of flavonoids, Int. Pharm. Sci. 1 (1) (2011) 25–41.

[81] D. Metodiewa, A. Kochman, S. Karolczak, Evidence for antiradical and antioxidant properties of four biologically active N, N-diethylaminoethyl ethers of flavaone oximes: a comparison with natural polyphenolic flavonoid rutin action, IUBMB Life 41 (5) (1997) 1067–1075.

[82] E.H. Walker, et al., Structural determinants of phosphoinositide 3-kinase inhibition by wortmannin, LY294002, quercetin, myricetin, and staurosporine, Mol. Cell 6 (4) (2000) 909–919.

[83] P.A. Mir, et al., Anti-inflammatory and anti-helminthic potential of methanolic and aqueous extract of polygonum alpinum rhizomes, J. Drug Deliv. Ther. 9 (3) (2019) 455–459.

[84] B.H. Havsteen, The biochemistry and medical significance of the flavonoids, Pharmacol. Ther. 96 (2-3) (2002) 67–202.

[85] P. Dewick, Front matter and index, in: Medicinal Natural Products: A Biosynthetic Approach, second ed., John Wiley & Sons, Ltd, Chichester, 2001.

[86] R.H. Mir, M.H. Masoodi, Anti-inflammatory plant polyphenolics and cellular action mechanisms, Curr. Bioact. Compd. 16 (6) (2020) 809–817.

[87] D.-X. Hou, T. Kumamoto, Flavonoids as protein kinase inhibitors for cancer chemoprevention: direct binding and molecular modeling, Antioxid. Redox Signal. 13 (5) (2010) 691–719.

[88] G. Lolli, et al., Inhibition of protein kinase CK2 by flavonoids and tyrphostins. A structural insight, Biochemistry 51 (31) (2012) 6097–6107.

[89] T. Yokoyama, Y. Kosaka, M. Mizuguchi, Structural insight into the interactions between death-associated protein kinase 1 and natural flavonoids, J. Med. Chem. 58 (18) (2015) 7400–7408.

[90] P. Rathee, et al., Mechanism of action of flavonoids as anti-inflammatory agents: a review, Inflamm. Allergy Drug Targets (Formerly Curr. Drug Targets Inflamm. Allergy) (Discontinued) 8 (3) (2009) 229–235.

[91] P.C. Ferriola, V. Cody, E. Middleton Jr., Protein kinase C inhibition by plant flavonoids: kinetic mechanisms and structure-activity relationships, Biochem. Pharmacol. 38 (10) (1989) 1617–1624.

[92] H.-L. Peng, et al., Fisetin inhibits the generation of inflammatory mediators in interleukin-1β–induced human lung epithelial cells by suppressing the NF-κB and ERK1/2 pathways, Int. Immunopharmacol. 60 (2018) 202–210.

[93] Y. Lin, et al., The NF-κB activation pathways, emerging molecular targets for cancer prevention and therapy, Expert Opin. Ther. Targets 14 (1) (2010) 45–55.

[94] L. Chen, et al., Intracellular signaling pathways of inflammation modulated by dietary flavonoids: the most recent evidence, Crit. Rev. Food Sci. Nutr. 58 (17) (2018) 2908–2924.

[95] F. Gao, et al., Genistein attenuated allergic airway inflammation by modulating the transcription factors T-bet, GATA-3 and STAT-6 in a murine model of asthma, Pharmacology 89 (3-4) (2012) 229–236.

[96] C. Liu, et al., The flavonoid 7, 4′-dihydroxyflavone inhibits MUC5AC gene expression, production, and secretion via regulation of NF-κB, STAT6, and HDAC2, Phytother. Res. 29 (6) (2015) 925–932.

[97] K. Meijer, et al., Cell-based screening assay for anti-inflammatory activity of bioactive compounds, Food Chem. 166 (2015) 158–164.

[98] M. Catarino, et al., The antiinflammatory potential of flavonoids: mechanistic aspects, in: Studies in Natural Products Chemistry, Elsevier, 2016, pp. 65–99.

[99] M.A. Panaro, et al., Anti-inflammatory effects of resveratrol occur via inhibition of lipopolysaccharide-induced NF-κB activation in Caco-2 and SW480 human colon cancer cells, Br. J. Nutr. 108 (9) (2012) 1623–1632.

[100] R. Rahimi, et al., A review of the herbal phosphodiesterase inhibitors; future perspective of new drugs, Cytokine 49 (2) (2010) 123–129.

[101] C. Sabphon, et al., Phosphodiesterase inhibitory activity of the flavonoids and xanthones from Anaxagorea luzonensis, Nat. Prod. Commun. 10 (2) (2015). p. 1934578X1501000222.

[102] Y.-Q. Guo, et al., Prenylated flavonoids as potent phosphodiesterase-4 inhibitors from Morus alba: isolation, modification, and structure-activity relationship study, Eur. J. Med. Chem. 144 (2018) 758–766.

[103] B. Wahlang, et al., Role of cAMP and phosphodiesterase signaling in liver health and disease, Cell. Signal. 49 (2018) 105–115.

[104] A. Kusano, et al., Inhibition of adenosine 3′, 5′-cyclic monophosphate phosphodiesterase by flavonoids from licorice roots and 4-arylcoumarins, Chem. Pharm. Bull. 39 (4) (1991) 930–933.

[105] C. Dehmlow, N. Murawski, H. de Groot, Scavenging of reactive oxygen species and inhibition of arachidonic acid metabolism by silibinin in human cells, Life Sci. 58 (18) (1996) 1591–1600.

[106] M. Mittal, et al., Reactive oxygen species in inflammation and tissue injury, Antioxid. Redox Signal. 20 (7) (2014) 1126–1167.

[107] S.B. Nimse, D. Pal, Free radicals, natural antioxidants, and their reaction mechanisms, RSC Adv. 5 (35) (2015) 27986–28006.

[108] G.-L. Chen, et al., Antioxidant and anti-inflammatory properties of flavonoids from lotus plumule, Food Chem. 277 (2019) 706–712.

[109] X. Li, et al., Comparison of the antioxidant effects of quercitrin and isoquercitrin: Understanding the role of the 6″-OH group, Molecules 21 (9) (2016) 1246.

[110] B. Halliwell, J.M. Gutteridge, Free Radicals in Biology and Medicine, Oxford University Press, USA, 2015.

[111] A. Mishra, S. Kumar, A.K. Pandey, Scientific validation of the medicinal efficacy of Tinospora cordifolia, Sci. World J. 2013 (2013).

[112] S. Kumar, A.K. Pandey, Chemistry and biological activities of flavonoids: an overview, Sci. World J. 2013 (2013).

[113] E.J. Brown, et al., Structural dependence of flavonoid interactions with Cu^{2+} ions: implications for their antioxidant properties, Biochem. J. 330 (3) (1998) 1173–1178.

[114] A. Ratty, N. Das, Effects of flavonoids on nonenzymatic lipid peroxidation: structure-activity relationship, Biochem. Med. Metab. Biol. 39 (1) (1988) 69–79.

[115] N. Yahfoufi, et al., The immunomodulatory and anti-inflammatory role of polyphenols, Nutrients 10 (11) (2018) 1618.

[116] R. Kumar, et al., Exploring the binding mechanism of flavonoid quercetin to phospholipase A2 fluorescence spectroscopy and computational approach, Eur. J. Exp. Biol. 7 (2017) 33.

[117] M. Novo Belchor, et al., Evaluation of rhamnetin as an inhibitor of the pharmacological effect of secretory phospholipase A2, Molecules 22 (9) (2017) 1441.

[118] D. González Mosquera, et al., Flavonoids from Boldoa purpurascens inhibit proinflammatory cytokines (TNF-α and IL-6) and the expression of COX-2, Phytother. Res. 32 (9) (2018) 1750–1754.

[119] Z. Hanáková, et al., Anti-inflammatory activity of natural geranylated flavonoids: cyclooxygenase and lipoxygenase inhibitory properties and proteomic analysis, J. Nat. Prod. 80 (4) (2017) 999–1006.

[120] M. Ferrandiz, M. Alcaraz, Anti-inflammatory activity and inhibition of arachidonic acid metabolism by flavonoids, Agents Actions 32 (3) (1991) 283–288.

[121] M. Ferrandiz, A. Nair, M. Alcaraz, Inhibition of sheep platelet arachidonate metabolism by flavonoids from Spanish and Indian medicinal herbs, Pharmazie 45 (3) (1990) 206–208.

[122] M.J. Laughton, et al., Inhibition of mammalian 5-lipoxygenase and cyclo-oxygenase by flavonoids and phenolic dietary additives: relationship to antioxidant activity and to iron ion-reducing ability, Biochem. Pharmacol. 42 (9) (1991) 1673–1681.

[123] R.J. Nijveldt, et al., Flavonoids: a review of probable mechanisms of action and potential applications, Am. J. Clin. Nutr. 74 (4) (2001) 418–425.

[124] T. Yoshimoto, et al., Flavonoids: potent inhibitors of arachidonate 5-lipoxygenase, Biochem. Biophys. Res. Commun. 116 (2) (1983) 612–618.

[125] H. Kim, et al., Effects of naturally-occurring flavonoids and biflavonoids on epidermal cyclooxygenase and lipoxygenase from guinea-pigs, Prostaglandins Leukot. Essent. Fat. Acids 58 (1) (1998) 17–24.

[126] J. Robak, R. Gryglewski, Bioactivity of flavonoids, Pol. J. Pharmacol. 48 (6) (1996) 555–564.

[127] Y. Li, et al., Oligomeric proanthocyanidins attenuate airway inflammation in asthma by inhibiting dendritic cells maturation, Mol. Immunol. 91 (2017) 209–217.

[128] W. Lin, et al., Quercetin protects against atherosclerosis by inhibiting dendritic cell activation, Mol. Nutr. Food Res. 61 (9) (2017) 1700031.

[129] M. Masilamani, et al., Soybean isoflavones regulate dendritic cell function and suppress allergic sensitization to peanut, J. Allergy Clin. Immunol. 128 (6) (2011) 1242–1250. e1.

[130] V. Galleggiante, et al., Dendritic cells modulate iron homeostasis and inflammatory abilities following quercetin exposure, Curr. Pharm. Des. 23 (14) (2017) 2139–2146.

[131] J.-H. Gong, et al., Kaempferol suppresses eosionphil infiltration and airway inflammation in airway epithelial cells and in mice with allergic asthma, J. Nutr. 142 (1) (2012) 47–56.

[132] Z. Weng, et al., Quercetin is more effective than cromolyn in blocking human mast cell cytokine release and inhibits contact dermatitis and photosensitivity in humans, PLoS One 7 (3) (2012), e33805.

[133] Z. Weng, et al., The novel flavone tetramethoxyluteolin is a potent inhibitor of human mast cells, J. Allergy Clin. Immunol. 135 (4) (2015) 1044–1052. e5.

[134] D.H. Kim, et al., Genistein inhibits pro-inflammatory cytokines in human mast cell activation through the inhibition of the ERK pathway, Int. J. Mol. Med. 34 (6) (2014) 1669–1674.

[135] C. Liu, et al., The flavonoid cyanidin blocks binding of the cytokine interleukin-17A to the IL-17RA subunit to alleviate inflammation in vivo, Sci. Signal. 10 (467) (2017).

[136] C. Del Bo', et al., Different effects of anthocyanins and phenolic acids from wild blueberry (Vaccinium angustifolium) on monocytes adhesion to endothelial cells in a TNF-α stimulated proinflammatory environment, Mol. Nutr. Food Res. 60 (11) (2016) 2355–2366.

[137] H.-W. Zhang, et al., Flavonoids inhibit cell proliferation and induce apoptosis and autophagy through downregulation of PI3Kγ mediated PI3K/AKT/mTOR/p70S6K/ULK signaling pathway in human breast cancer cells, Sci. Rep. 8 (1) (2018) 1–13.

[138] G.A. Ramirez, et al., Eosinophils from physiology to disease: a comprehensive review, Biomed. Res. Int. 2018 (2018).

[139] D. Karo-Atar, et al., Therapeutic targeting of the interleukin-4/interleukin-13 signaling pathway: in allergy and beyond, BioDrugs 32 (3) (2018) 201–220.

[140] G. Martínez, M.R. Mijares, J.B. De Sanctis, Effects of flavonoids and its derivatives on immune cell responses, Recent Patents Inflamm. Allergy Drug Discov. 13 (2) (2019) 84–104.

[141] D.N. Che, et al., Fisetin inhibits IL-31 production in stimulated human mast cells: possibilities of fisetin being exploited to treat histamine-independent pruritus, Life Sci. 201 (2018) 121–129.

[142] M. Sakai-Kashiwabara, S. Abe, K. Asano, Suppressive activity of quercetin on the production of eosinophil chemoattractants from eosinophils in vitro, In Vivo 28 (4) (2014) 515–522.

[143] J.B. White, et al., Some natural flavonoids are competitive inhibitors of Caspase-1, -3 and -7 despite their cellular toxicity, Food Chem. 131 (4) (2012) 1453–1459.

[144] M.R. Vijayababu, et al., Effects of quercetin on insulin-like growth factors (IGFs) and their binding protein-3 (IGFBP-3) secretion and induction of apoptosis in human prostate cancer cells, J. Carcinog. 5 (2006) 10.

[145] L.Y. Wang, J. Kuang, J. Li, Apigenin regulates lipopolysaccharides-induced activation of inflammasome, Zhonghua Yi Xue Za Zhi 91 (34) (2011) 2435–2439.

[146] A. Tawani, A. Kumar, Structural insight into the interaction of flavonoids with human telomeric sequence, Sci. Rep. 5 (1) (2015) 1–13.

[147] G. Grosso, et al., A comprehensive meta-analysis on dietary flavonoid and lignan intake and cancer risk: level of evidence and limitations, Mol. Nutr. Food Res. 61 (4) (2017) 1600930.

[148] L. Zhao, et al., Neuroprotective, anti-amyloidogenic and neurotrophic effects of apigenin in an Alzheimer's disease mouse model, Molecules 18 (8) (2013) 9949–9965.

[149] A. Nakajima, et al., Nobiletin, a citrus flavonoid, improves cognitive impairment and reduces soluble Aβ levels in a triple transgenic mouse model of Alzheimer's disease (3XTg-AD), Behav. Brain Res. 289 (2015) 69–77.

[150] S.-Q. Zhang, et al., Baicalein reduces β-amyloid and promotes non-amyloidogenic amyloid precursor protein processing in an Alzheimer's disease transgenic mouse model, J. Neurosci. Res. 91 (9) (2013) 1239–1246.

[151] A. Currais, et al., Modulation of p25 and inflammatory pathways by fisetin maintains cognitive function in Alzheimer's disease transgenic mice, Aging Cell 13 (2) (2014) 379–390.

[152] A. Currais, et al., Fisetin reduces the impact of aging on behavior and physiology in the rapidly aging SAMP8 mouse, J. Gerontol. A Biol. Sci. Med. Sci. 73 (3) (2018) 299–307.

[153] A. Ahmad, et al., Neuroprotective effect of fisetin against amyloid-beta-induced cognitive/synaptic dysfunction, neuroinflammation, and neurodegeneration in adult mice, Mol. Neurobiol. 54 (3) (2017) 2269–2285.

[154] S. Moghbelinejad, et al., Rutin activates the MAPK pathway and BDNF gene expression on beta-amyloid induced neurotoxicity in rats, Toxicol. Lett. 224 (1) (2014) 108–113.

[155] A.P. Rogerio, et al., Anti-inflammatory effect of quercetin-loaded microemulsion in the airways allergic inflammatory model in mice, Pharmacol. Res. 61 (4) (2010) 288–297.

[156] M. Bartekova, et al., Cardioprotective effects of acute and chronic treatment with flavonoid quercetin against ischemia/reperfusion injury in isolated rat hearts: focus on the role of age in the efficiency of treatment, J. Mol. Cell. Cardiol. 120 (2018) 20–21.

[157] J. Roslan, et al., Quercetin ameliorates oxidative stress, inflammation and apoptosis in the heart of streptozotocin-nicotinamide-induced adult male diabetic rats, Biomed. Pharmacother. 86 (2017) 570–582.

[158] R. Aruna, A. Geetha, P. Suguna, Rutin modulates ASC expression in NLRP3 inflammasome: a study in alcohol and cerulein-induced rat model of pancreatitis, Mol. Cell. Biochem. 396 (1-2) (2014) 269–280.

[159] F. Chen, et al., Naringin ameliorates the high glucose-induced rat mesangial cell inflammatory reaction by modulating the NLRP3 Inflammasome, BMC Complement. Altern. Med. 18 (1) (2018) 192.

[160] S.-H. Fan, et al., Luteoloside suppresses proliferation and metastasis of hepatocellular carcinoma cells by inhibition of NLRP3 inflammasome, PLoS One 9 (2) (2014), e89961.

[161] L.Z. Ellis, et al., Green tea polyphenol epigallocatechin-3-gallate suppresses melanoma growth by inhibiting inflammasome and IL-1β secretion, Biochem. Biophys. Res. Commun. 414 (3) (2011) 551–556.

[162] D. Yang, et al., LFG-500, a novel synthetic flavonoid, suppresses epithelial-mesenchymal transition in human lung adenocarcinoma cells by inhibiting NLRP3 in inflammatory microenvironment, Cancer Lett. 400 (2017) 137–148.

[163] V.C. George, G. Dellaire, H.P.V. Rupasinghe, Plant flavonoids in cancer chemoprevention: role in genome stability, J. Nutr. Biochem. 45 (2017) 1–14.

[164] K. Jilani, S. Manasa, Raspberry Pi based color speaker, Int. J. Electron. Commun. Eng. 1 (2014) 8–12.

[165] S. Srivastava, et al., Quercetin, a natural flavonoid interacts with DNA, arrests cell cycle and causes tumor regression by activating mitochondrial pathway of apoptosis, Sci. Rep. 6 (1) (2016) 1–13.

[166] H. Zhang, et al., Surface metallization of ABS plastics for nickel plating by molecules grafted method, Surf. Coat. Technol. 340 (2018) 8–16.

[167] L. Chen, et al., Antitumor and immunomodulatory activities of total flavonoids extract from persimmon leaves in H22 liver tumor-bearing mice, Sci. Rep. 8 (1) (2018) 10523.

[168] K.L. Ivey, et al., Flavonoid intake and all-cause mortality, Am. J. Clin. Nutr. 101 (5) (2015) 1012–1020.

[169] C. Dae-Il, L. Seung-Yong, An experimental study on the static behavior of steel composite rahmen with partial horizontally prestressed, J. Korean Soc. Adv. Compos. Struct. 8 (3) (2017) 7–12.

[170] L. Devi, M. Ohno, 7,8-dihydroxyflavone, a small-molecule TrkB agonist, reverses memory deficits and BACE1 elevation in a mouse model of Alzheimer's disease, Neuropsychopharmacology 37 (2) (2012) 434–444.

[171] Z. Zhang, et al., 7,8-Dihydroxyflavone prevents synaptic loss and memory deficits in a mouse model of Alzheimer's disease, Neuropsychopharmacology 39 (3) (2014) 638–650.

[172] H. Onozuka, et al., Nobiletin, a citrus flavonoid, improves memory impairment and Abeta pathology in a transgenic mouse model of Alzheimer's disease, J. Pharmacol. Exp. Ther. 326 (3) (2008) 739–744.

[173] A. Nakajima, et al., Nobiletin, a citrus flavonoid, ameliorates cognitive impairment, oxidative burden, and hyperphosphorylation of tau in senescence-accelerated mouse, Behav. Brain Res. 250 (2013) 351–360.

[174] E. Zaplatic, et al., Molecular mechanisms underlying protective role of quercetin in attenuating Alzheimer's disease, Life Sci. 224 (2019) 109–119.

[175] L.C.G.E.I. Moreno, et al., Effect of the oral administration of nanoencapsulated quercetin on a mouse model of Alzheimer's disease, Int. J. Pharm. 517 (1) (2017) 50–57.

[176] A.M. Sabogal-Guáqueta, et al., The flavonoid quercetin ameliorates Alzheimer's disease pathology and protects cognitive and emotional function in aged triple transgenic Alzheimer's disease model mice, Neuropharmacology 93 (2015) 134–145.

[177] J.M. Walker, et al., Beneficial effects of dietary EGCG and voluntary exercise on behavior in an Alzheimer's disease mouse model, J. Alzheimers Dis. 44 (2) (2015) 561–572.

[178] Y. Guo, et al., (-)-Epigallocatechin-3-gallate ameliorates memory impairment and rescues the abnormal synaptic protein levels in the frontal cortex and hippocampus in a mouse model of Alzheimer's disease, Neuroreport 28 (10) (2017) 590–597.

[179] S. Zhang, et al., Effects of three flavonoids from an ancient traditional Chinese medicine Radix puerariae on geriatric diseases, Brain Circ. 4 (4) (2018) 174–184.

[180] K.C. Hung, et al., Baicalein attenuates α-synuclein aggregation, inflammasome activation and autophagy in the MPP(+)-treated nigrostriatal dopaminergic system in vivo, J. Ethnopharmacol. 194 (2016) 522–529.

[181] Y. Cheng, et al., Neuroprotective effect of baicalein against MPTP neurotoxicity: behavioral, biochemical and immunohistochemical profile, Neurosci. Lett. 441 (1) (2008) 16–20.

[182] X. Zhang, et al., Therapeutic effects of baicalein on rotenone-induced Parkinson's disease through protecting mitochondrial function and biogenesis, Sci. Rep. 7 (1) (2017) 9968.

[183] D. Luo, et al., 7,8-dihydroxyflavone protects 6-OHDA and MPTP induced dopaminergic neurons degeneration through activation of TrkB in rodents, Neurosci. Lett. 620 (2016) 43–49.

[184] X.-H. Li, et al., 7,8-Dihydroxyflavone ameliorates motor deficits via suppressing α-synuclein expression and oxidative stress in the MPTP-induced mouse model of Parkinson's disease, CNS Neurosci. Ther. 22 (7) (2016) 617–624.

[185] J. He, et al., Neuroprotective effects of 7, 8-dihydroxyflavone on midbrain dopaminergic neurons in MPP(+)-treated monkeys, Sci. Rep. 6 (2016) 34339.

[186] C. Lv, et al., Effect of quercetin in the 1-methyl-4-phenyl-1, 2, 3, 6-tetrahydropyridine-Induced mouse model of Parkinson's disease, Evid. Based Complement. Alternat. Med. 2012 (2012), 928643.

[187] M.M. Khan, et al., Rutin protects dopaminergic neurons from oxidative stress in an animal model of Parkinson's disease, Neurotox. Res. 22 (1) (2012) 1–15.

[188] P. Maher, Protective effects of fisetin and other berry flavonoids in Parkinson's disease, Food Funct. 8 (9) (2017) 3033–3042.

[189] S. Li, X.P. Pu, Neuroprotective effect of kaempferol against a 1-methyl-4-phenyl-1,2,3,6-tetrahydropyridine-induced mouse model of Parkinson's disease, Biol. Pharm. Bull. 34 (8) (2011) 1291–1296.

[190] M.D. Teixeira, et al., Catechin attenuates behavioral neurotoxicity induced by 6-OHDA in rats, Pharmacol. Biochem. Behav. 110 (2013) 1–7.

[191] Q. Xu, et al., Epigallocatechin gallate Has a neurorescue effect in a mouse model of Parkinson disease, J. Nutr. 147 (10) (2017) 1926–1931.

[192] M. Rubio-Osornio, et al., Epicatechin reduces striatal MPP⁺-induced damage in rats through slight increases in SOD-Cu, Zn activity, Oxid. Med. Cell. Longev. 2015 (2015), 276039.

[193] S. Mani, et al., Naringenin decreases α-synuclein expression and neuroinflammation in MPTP-induced Parkinson's disease model in mice, Neurotox. Res. 33 (3) (2018) 656–670.

[194] Z. Kiasalari, et al., Protective effect of oral hesperetin against unilateral striatal 6-hydroxydopamine damage in the rat, Neurochem. Res. 41 (5) (2016) 1065–1072.

[195] M. Kujawska, J. Jodynis-Liebert, Polyphenols in Parkinson's disease: a systematic review of in vivo studies, Nutrients 10 (5) (2018) 642.

[196] S. Thangarajan, S. Ramachandran, P. Krishnamurthy, Chrysin exerts neuroprotective effects against 3-Nitropropionic acid induced behavioral despair—mitochondrial dysfunction and striatal apoptosis via upregulating Bcl-2 gene and downregulating Bax—Bad genes in male wistar rats, Biomed. Pharmacother. 84 (2016) 514–525.

[197] G. García-Díaz Barriga, et al., 7,8-dihydroxyflavone ameliorates cognitive and motor deficits in a Huntington's disease mouse model through specific activation of the PLCγ1 pathway, Hum. Mol. Genet. 26 (16) (2017) 3144–3160.

[198] P. Maher, et al., ERK activation by the polyphenols fisetin and resveratrol provides neuroprotection in multiple models of Huntington's disease, Hum. Mol. Genet. 20 (2) (2010) 261–270.

[199] R. Sandhir, A. Mehrotra, Quercetin supplementation is effective in improving mitochondrial dysfunctions induced by 3-nitropropionic acid: Implications in Huntington's disease, Biochim. Biophys. Acta (BBA) - Mol. Basis Dis. 1832 (3) (2013) 421–430.

[200] J. Chakraborty, et al., Quercetin improves behavioral deficiencies, restores astrocytes and microglia, and reduces serotonin metabolism in 3-nitropropionic acid-induced rat model of Huntington's Disease, CNS Neurosci. Ther. 20 (1) (2014) 10–19.

[201] S.N. Suganya, T. Sumathi, Effect of rutin against a mitochondrial toxin, 3-nitropropionicacid induced biochemical, behavioral and histological alterations-a pilot study on Huntington's disease model in rats, Metab. Brain Dis. 32 (2) (2017) 471–481.

[202] R. Lagoa, et al., Kaempferol protects against rat striatal degeneration induced by 3-nitropropionic acid, J. Neurochem. 111 (2) (2009) 473–487.

[203] E.T. Menze, et al., Potential neuroprotective effects of hesperidin on 3-nitropropionic acid-induced neurotoxicity in rats, Neurotoxicology 33 (5) (2012) 1265–1275.

[204] E.T. Menze, et al., Genistein improves sensorimotor gating: mechanisms related to its neuroprotective effects on the striatum, Neuropharmacology 105 (2016) 35–46.

[205] F. Kreilaus, et al., Therapeutic effects of anthocyanins and environmental enrichment in R6/1 Huntington's disease mice, J. Huntingtons Dis. 5 (3) (2016) 285–296.

[206] O.T. Korkmaz, et al., 7,8-Dihydroxyflavone improves motor performance and enhances lower motor neuronal survival in a mouse model of amyotrophic lateral sclerosis, Neurosci. Lett. 566 (2014) 286–291.

[207] T.H. Wang, et al., Fisetin exerts antioxidant and neuroprotective effects in multiple mutant hSOD1 models of amyotrophic lateral sclerosis by activating ERK, Neuroscience 379 (2018) 152–166.

[208] M. Schatz, L. Rosenwasser, The allergic asthma phenotype, J. Allergy Clin. Immunol. Pract. 2 (6) (2014) 645–648.

[209] D.E.A. Komi, L. Bjermer, Mast cell-mediated orchestration of the immune responses in human allergic asthma: current insights, Clin. Rev. Allergy Immunol. 56 (2) (2019) 234–247.

[210] M. Kimata, et al., Effects of luteolin, quercetin and baicalein on immunoglobulin E-mediated mediator release from human cultured mast cells, Clin. Exp. Allergy 30 (4) (2000) 501–508.

[211] W. Duan, et al., Antiinflammatory effects of genistein, a tyrosine kinase inhibitor, on a guinea pig model of asthma, Am. J. Respir. Crit. Care Med. 167 (2) (2003) 185–192.

[212] X. Zhang, et al., The protective effect of Luteolin on myocardial ischemia/reperfusion (I/R) injury through TLR4/NF-κB/NLRP3 inflammasome pathway, Biomed. Pharmacother. 91 (2017) 1042–1052.

[213] D. Lv, et al., The cardioprotective effect of total flavonoids on myocardial ischemia/reperfusion in rats, Biomed. Pharmacother. 88 (2017) 277–284.

[214] H. Yang, et al., Procyanidin B2 inhibits NLRP3 inflammasome activation in human vascular endothelial cells, Biochem. Pharmacol. 92 (4) (2014) 599–606.

[215] J. Guillermo Gormaz, S. Quintremil, R. Rodrigo, Cardiovascular disease: a target for the pharmacological effects of quercetin, Curr. Top. Med. Chem. 15 (17) (2015) 1735–1742.

[216] X. Lin, et al., Quercetin protects against heat stroke-induced myocardial injury in male rats: antioxidative and antiinflammatory mechanisms, Chem. Biol. Interact. 265 (2017) 47–54.

[217] Y. Zhang, et al., Baicalin attenuates cardiac dysfunction and myocardial remodeling in a chronic pressure-overload mice model, Cell. Physiol. Biochem. 41 (3) (2017) 849–864.

Chapter 19

Heterocycles in managing inflammatory diseases

Bhupender Nehra[a], Pooja A. Chawla[b], Parteek Prasher[c], and Devidas S. Bhagat[d]

[a]*Department of Pharmaceutical Sciences, Guru Jambheshwar University of Science & Technology, Hisar, Haryana, India,* [b]*Department of Pharmaceutical Chemistry and Analysis, ISF College of Pharmacy, Moga, Punjab, India,* [c]*Department of Chemistry, University of Petroleum & Energy Studies, Dehradun, Uttarakhand, India,* [d]*Department of Forensic Chemistry and Toxicology, Government Institute of Forensic Science, Aurangabad, Maharashtra, India*

1 Introduction

The word "heterocycle" comprises two terms, i.e., prefix "hetero" directs toward the presence of noncarbon atoms such as nitrogen (N), oxygen (O), sulfur (S), etc., and suffix "cycle" indicates the existence of one or more rings (five- or six-membered rings) in the structure of the molecule [1]. In the design and development of various potent pharmacological compounds, heterocycles are the most promising and widely employed structural nucleus. Compounds with heterocyclic rings play an important role in drug discovery and development of effective therapeutic candidates, making heterocyclic compounds one of the most important fields of medicinal chemistry study [2]. Researchers have also noticed that heterocyclic scaffolds have attracted their interest as a possible core moiety for delivering lead compounds in a variety of domains of medicinal chemistry. The heterocycles may be five-membered heterocycles (pyrazole, imidazole, isoxazole, pyrazoline, thiazole, triazole, tetrazole, pyrrole, furan, and thiophene, for example), six-membered heterocycles (pyridine, piperidine, dioxane, and pyrimidine, for example), and fused heterocycles (such as pyridine, piperidine, dioxane (indole, quinoline, and benzimidazole, etc.) [1,2].

From several past years, most of these five- and six-membered heterocyclic scaffolds act like the core structure of numerous drug compounds and have elicited wide range of pharmacological activity (shown in Figs. 1 and 2) [1,2]. Apart from five- and six-membered heterocyclic moieties, many fused heterocycles also exhibited promising pharmacological potential in the eradication of a variety of diseases (shown in Fig. 3). These single heterocyclic and fused heterocyclic scaffolds have attracted the keen interest from researchers and are widely explored to provide lead molecules in the diverse area of medicinal chemistry.

Nowadays, the heterocyclic nucleus find use in miscellaneous applications in pharmaceutical as well as agrochemical areas. Numerous heterocycles containing molecules are widely used in the discovery of potent drug compounds by acting as a core scaffold in pharmaceutical, agrochemical as well as textile industries [3]. Heterocycles have also emerged as being essential in the metabolism of all living cells. Furthermore, a substantial part of the genome is also composed of heterocycle-based nucleobases including purines and pyrimidines. Various antibiotics such as penicillin, cephalosporins, macrolides, etc. and natural occurring alkaloids including morphine, reserpine, and vinblastine and many more are available in the market having heterocyclic scaffolds in their structures [3,4]. Also, various clinical trial candidates and marketed drugs bearing heterocyclic moieties are available such as indomethacin (indole-based), miconazole (imidazole-based), celecoxib (pyrazole-based), nitrofurantoin (furan-based), ranitidine (furan-based), cloxacillin (isoxazole-based), tolmetin (pyrrole-based), mebendazole (benzimidazole-based), ethosuximide (pyrrolidine-based), clonidine (imidazoline-based), pyrantel (thiophene-based), cefotaxime (1,3 thiazole-based), and many more. Moreover, drug molecules consisted of a heterocyclic scaffold as the core nucleus displayed diverse biological implications including antiinflammatory, antitubercular, anti-HIV, antimicrobial, anticancer, anticonvulsant, antifungal, antioxidant, antidiabetic, antihypertensive, antitumor, insecticidal, and herbicidal agents, etc. [5–13] (shown in Fig. 4).

2 Mechanism of actions involved for heterocyclic scaffold-based marketed drugs in the treatment of inflammation

For decades, researchers have found heterocyclic moieties to be the most appealing and promising core scaffold due to their wide range of therapeutic implications in the pharmaceutical field. To treat inflammation, a variety of marketed and approved medicines with a heterocyclic core

Recent Developments in Anti-Inflammatory Therapy. https://doi.org/10.1016/B978-0-323-99988-5.00010-3

FIG. 1 Five-membered heterocycles used in pharmacologically active molecules.

furan
1H-pyrazole
thiophene
1H-pyrrole
dioxolane
pyrazolidine
pyrazoline
thiazole
imidazole
isothiazole
triazole
tetrazole
isoxazole
oxazole
oxadiazole

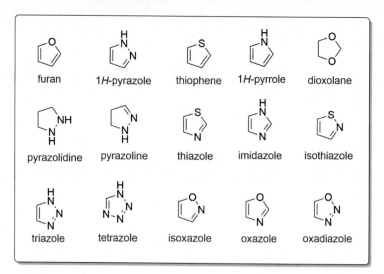

FIG. 2 Six-membered heterocycles used in pharmacologically active molecules.

pyridine
pyran
pyrimidine
thiopyran
2H-1,2-thiazine
piperidine
oxane
dioxane
piperazine
2H-1,2-oxazine

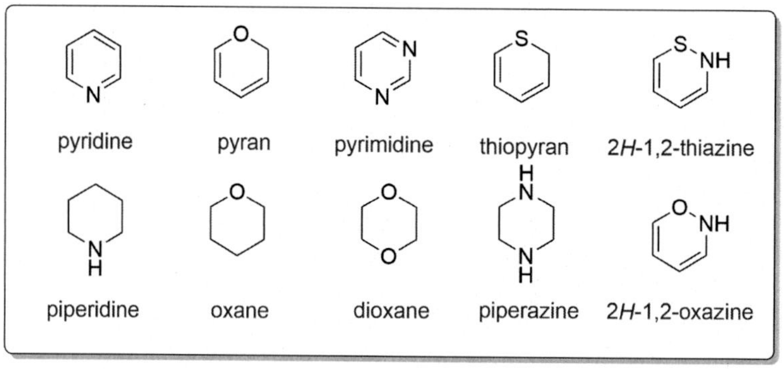

FIG. 3 Fused heterocycles used in pharmacologically active molecules.

1H-indole
1H-indazole
benzimidazole
purine
benzofuran
quinoline
quinoxaline
2H-chromene
benzothiazole
isatin

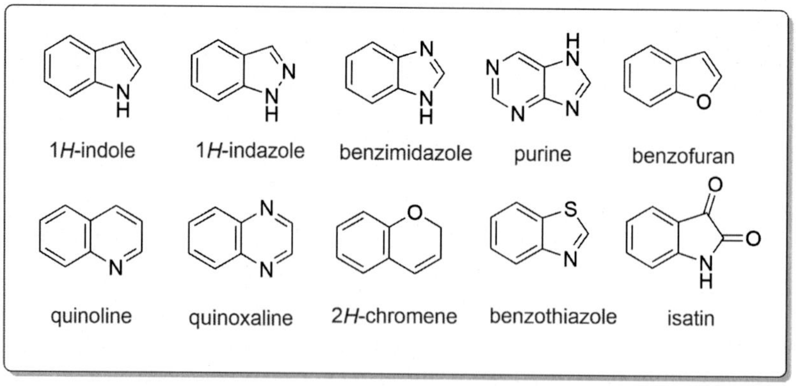

FIG. 4 Various pharmacological activity exhibited by numerous heterocyclic scaffolds.

Anti-Convulsant
Anti-Inflammatory
Anti-Malarial
Anti-Cancer
Anti-diabetic
Anti-Oxidant
Antibacterial & Antifungal
Five-membered, Six-membered and fused heterocycles

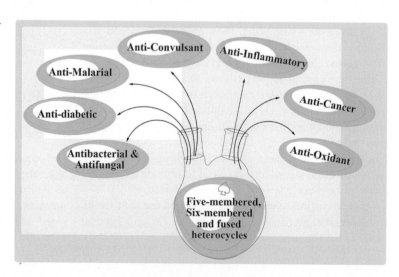

nucleus are employed [14]. Nonsteroidal antiinflammatory medications (NSAIDs) are the most common licensed pharmaceuticals on the market with a heterocyclic core nucleus for the treatment of inflammation, pain, and fever. Nonsteroidal antiinflammatory medicines work by preventing the stimulation of cyclo-oxygenase isoenzymes, which leads to a reduction in the generation of pro-inflammatory prostaglandins at the injury site [14,15]. The cyclo-oxygenase enzyme catalyzes the manufacture of prostaglandins and thromboxane from arachidonic acid, which is created by the inflammatory stimulation of membrane phospholipids. The cyclo-oxygenase-1 (COX-1) and cyclo-oxygenase-2 (COX-2) isoenzymes are important for causing inflammation in the body. COX-1 is a constitutive isoform that is involved in a variety of physiological functions in the body, including platelet aggregation, renal blood flow modulation, and gastric mucosal layer protection. COX-1 suppression is also linked to gastrointestinal (GI) discomfort due to the decreased synthesis of stomach-protective prostaglandins, as well as renal toxicity. COX-2 is an inducible isoform that is induced by a variety of stimuli (growth factors, hormones, oncogenes, and mitogens) and causes inflammation and cancer in the body [15,16]. Both isoenzymes of cyclooxygenase catalyze the conversion of arachidonic acid to endoperoxides, which leads to the formation of inflammatory chemical mediators like prostaglandins, prostacyclin, and thromboxane [16].

NSAIDs with low COX-1 or COX-2 isoform inhibitory capacity may also act as antipyretics and analgesics, with the COX-3 isoform being targeted to relieve pain and inflammation in the central nervous system (brain and spinal cord), heart, and aorta [16,17]. Aside from these pathways, many NSAIDs do not inhibit cyclo-oxygenase isoforms (COX-1/COX-2 or COX-3) and instead bind to alternative enzymes like prostaglandin synthase, prostacyclin synthase, thromboxane synthase, and 5-lipoxygenase, which are responsible for the production of prostaglandins, prostacyclin, and thromboxane (Fig. 5) [18,19].

3 Heterocyclic scaffold-based marketed drugs in the treatment of inflammation

Nonselective or classical NSAIDs are able to inhibit both cyclo-oxygenase isoenzymes (COX-1 and COX-2). Thereby, nonselective or classical NSAIDs present with or without a heterocyclic core scaffold such as antipyrine/phenzone, ketoprofen, indomethacin, aspirin, carprofen, diclofenac, aceclofenac, acemetacin, ibuprofen, naproxen, ketorolac, mefenamic acid, piroxicam, tenoxicam, phenylbutazone, oxyphenylbutazone, ramifenazone, famprofazone, morazone, flurbiprofen, flunixin, tepoxalin, etc. (shown in Figs. 6 and 7) are used to treat short-term fever,

inflammation and pain but may also display gastrointestinal ulceration and renal toxicity due to nonselective inhibition of the COX-1 isoenzyme [20–25].

To prevent the adverse effects of COX-1 inhibition, selective or nonclassical NSAIDs that exclusively inhibit the cyclo-oxygenase-2 (COX-2) isoform have been developed. COX-2 inhibitors, such as nimesulide, meloxicam, nabumetone, etodolac, tolmetin, and others, are primarily accessible on the market and have the ability to inhibit COX-2 isoforms while having just a minor or partial inhibitory capability for COX-1 isoforms [26–28] (as depicted in Fig. 8).

Furthermore, selective COX-2 inhibitors such as celecoxib, rofecoxib, parecoxib, etoricoxib, valdecoxib, lumiracoxib, dexibuprofen, and others (shown in Fig. 9) are available on the market, which do not have the adverse effects associated with nonselective COX inhibitors [29,30].

Also, certain NSAIDs, such as paracetamol, metamizole, propyfenazone, aminopyrine, and nefopam, may work as antipyretics and analgesics by targeting the COX-3 isoform to alleviate pain and inflammation related with the central nervous system (brain and spinal cord), heart, and aorta (shown in Fig. 10) [31,32].

4 Heterocyclic scaffold-based antiinflammatory compounds under clinical development

Heterocyclic scaffolds are a common motif that can be used to make a variety of pharmacologically active compounds and are a noteworthy pharmacophore for medicinal research [33]. A large number of intriguing reports in the literature have piqued researchers' interest in investigating the medicinal significance of heterocyclic moieties in the design and development of innovative medication candidates [34]. Aside from the heterocycle-based commercialized medications that are already being used for incardination of various diseases, there are some heterocyclic scaffolds containing lead candidates that are currently being developed in clinical trials, as detailed below.

E-6087 is a derivative of Enficoxib, also known as E-6132, it is a pyrazoline heterocyclic nucleus containing compounds, which are structurally analogs as that of selective cyclooxygenase-2 (COX-2) inhibitors. It acts via selective inhibition of the COX-2 isoform and is enduring phase-I clinical trials process as a nonsteroidal antiinflammatory agent (NSAID) used in the treatment of osteoarthritis and pain [35,36]. SC560 is a selective COX-2 isoenzyme inhibitor used for the treatment of various kinds of inflammatory disorders [37]. SC558 is a pyrazole derivative, which binds in a much more effective way toward the COX-1 isoform, as compared to the COX-2

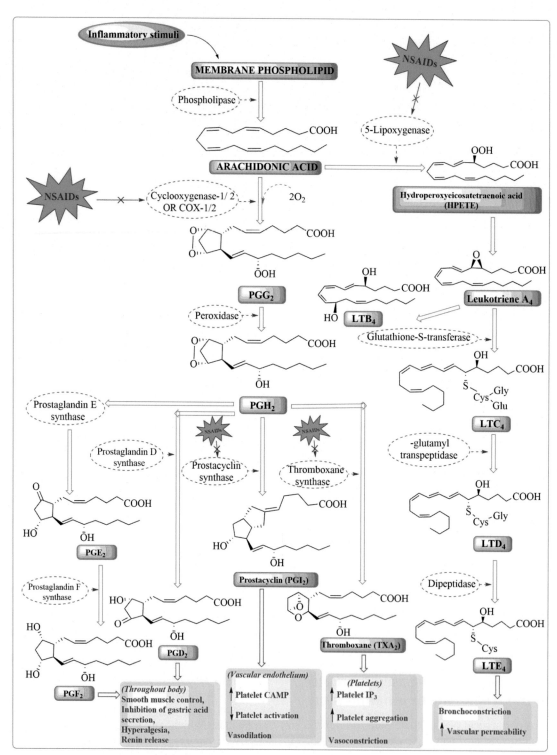

FIG. 5 Biosynthesis of various inflammatory chemical mediators and role of NSAIDs.

isoenzyme. So, SC558 is a selective COX-1 isoenzyme inhibitor used for the eradication of inflammation including PM10-induced endothelial disorders [38]. SC558 has also displayed a potent role as an antihepatitis C (HCV) and antiproliferative agent [39].

Further, SC581 is another pyrazole heterocyclic scaffold-based compound, which acts via selectively inhibiting COX-2 isoform to treat various kinds of inflammatory diseases including edema, osteoarthritis, and pain [40]. Moreover, DuP697 is a thiophene heterocyclic core

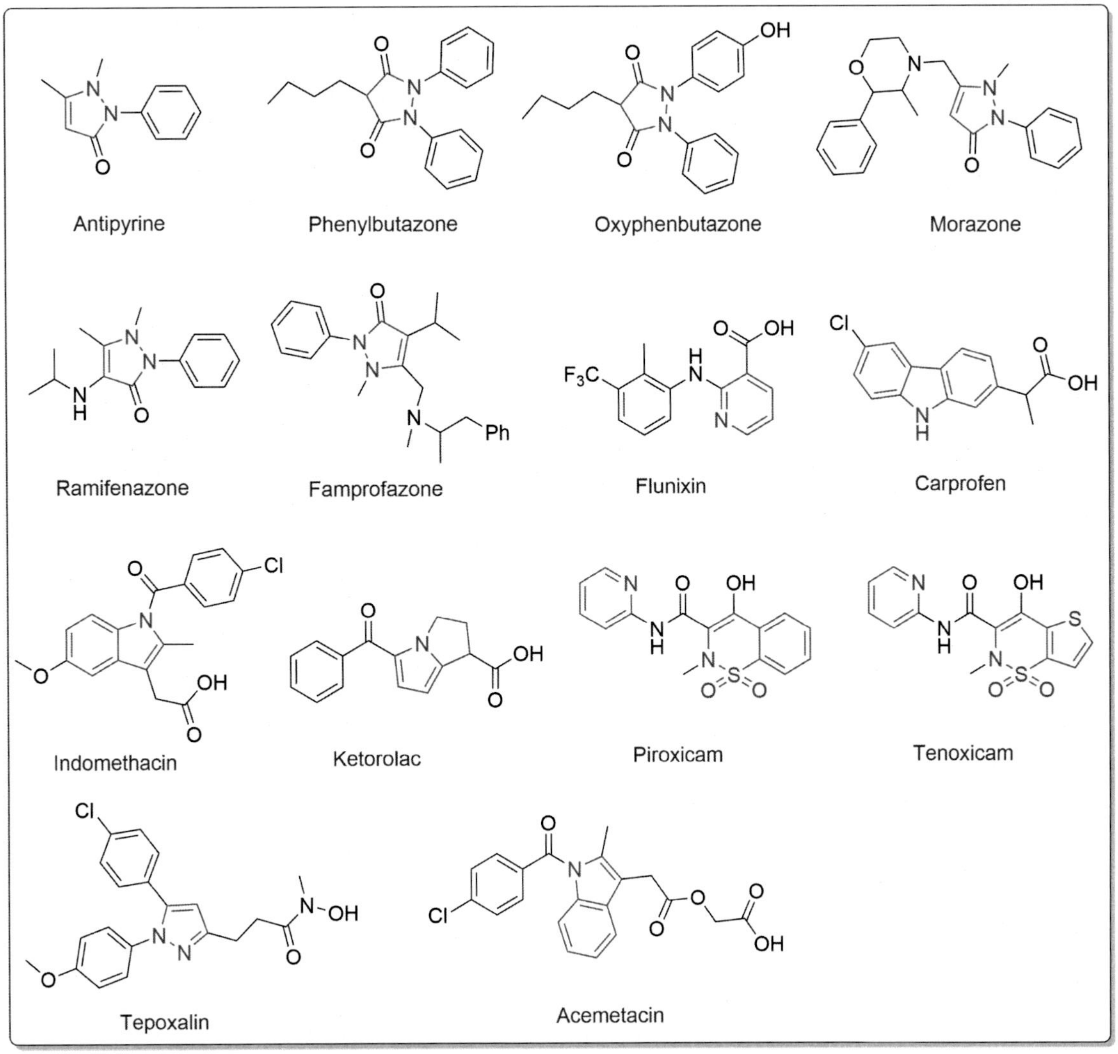

FIG. 6 Structures of nonselective or classical NSAIDs with a heterocyclic core scaffold.

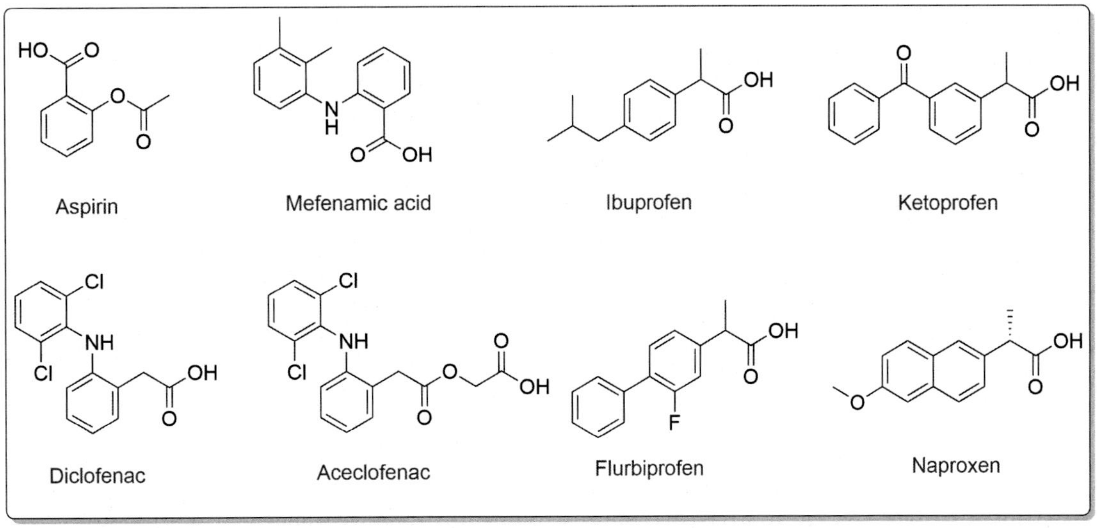

FIG. 7 Structures of nonselective or classical NSAIDs without a heterocyclic core scaffold.

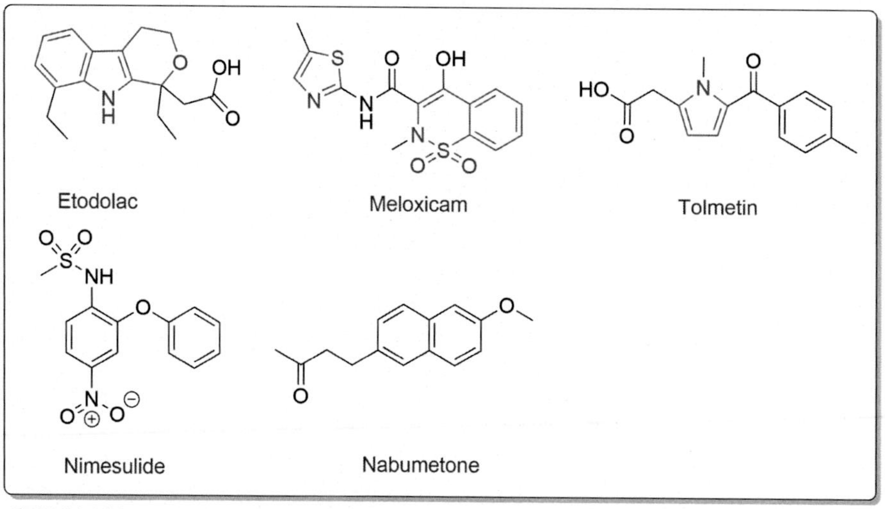

FIG. 8 Preferentially COX-2 inhibitors with or without a heterocyclic core scaffold.

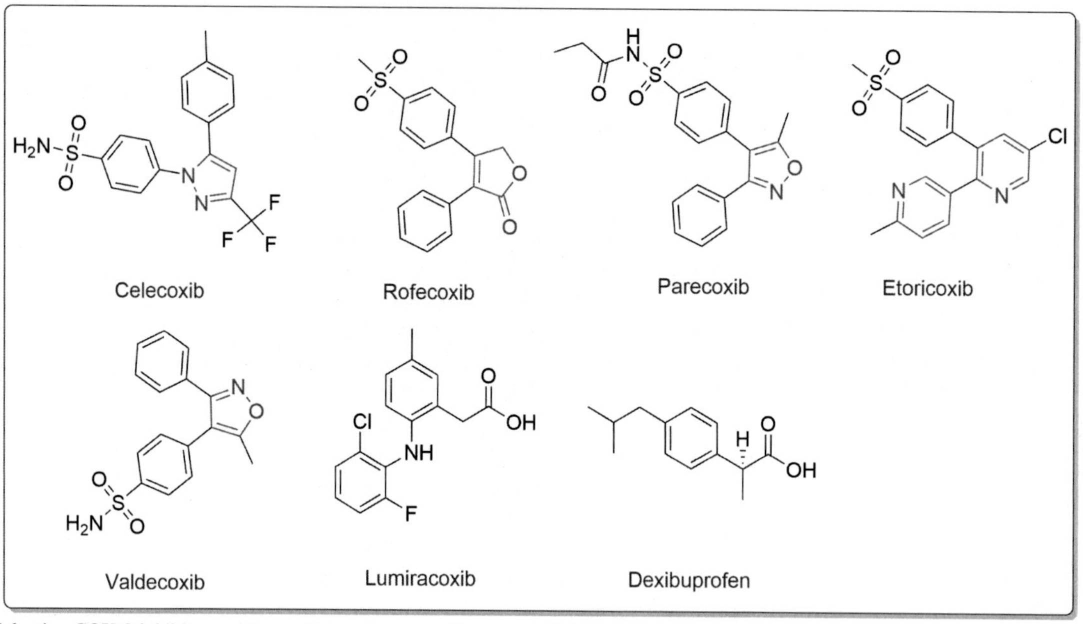

FIG. 9 Selective COX-2 inhibitors with or without a heterocyclic core scaffold.

FIG. 10 Structures of poor COX-1 or COX-2 inhibitors with or without a heterocyclic core scaffold.

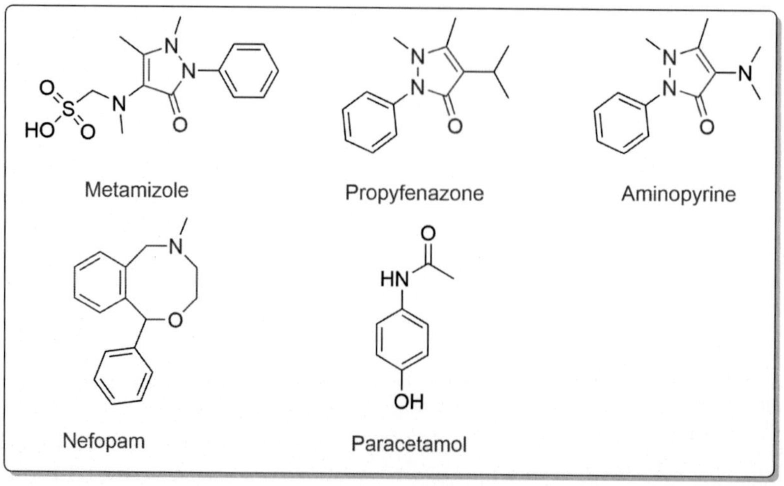

moiety containing a derivative, which acts via selective inhibition of the COX-2 isoenzyme to eradicate numerous types of inflammatory dysfunctions [41]. In the continuous efforts to eliminate toxicity associated with COX-1 inhibition, NS-398 and BF-389 binds toward COX-2 isoenzyme selectively, not at the COX-1 isoenzyme and hence, acts via selective inhibition of the COX-2 isoform [42,43] (shown in Fig. 11).

5 Recent advancements in heterocyclic derivatives as potent antiinflammatory agents

Several heterocyclic moieties have seen significant advances in the design and development of lead molecules in medicinal chemistry over the past several decades. As a result, a large number of research reports have been published and made available to assess the pharmacological potential of heterocyclic scaffolds including chemicals. Furthermore, the antiinflammatory potential of heterocyclic compounds has been described in various previous reviews. Heterocyclic rings were examined by Sondhi et al. [44] as a possible scaffold for designing and developing heterocyclic compounds with significant antiinflammatory action. Aside from the antiinflammatory properties, there are numerous evaluations that describe the potential of heterocyclic derivatives in the treatment of various disorders. The therapeutic importance of heterocyclic derivatives in numerous disease areas was highlighted in a review by Dua et al. [45]. The current improvements and prospective pharmacological responses of several heterocyclic compounds were reviewed by Saini et al. [46]. Despite these studies, there

are a plethora of research reports available that are likely to explain the design and development of various heterocyclic compounds with significant antiinflammatory activity.

6 Various heterocyclic scaffolds to display significant antiinflammatory activity

6.1 Pyrazoline derivatives as antiinflammatory agents (shown in Fig. 12)

The incorporation of heteroatoms such as N, O, or S, primarily in the A- and D-rings of steroidal structures, has been shown to have a wide range of biological functions, as well as reduced toxicity and increased bioavailability, according to certain research. Cai et al. (2019) discussed the design, synthesis, and antiinflammatory assessment of novel D-ring substituted steroidal pyrazoline derivatives in light of these facts. In comparison to the reference medicine dexamethasone ($IC_{50} = 0.62$M), compound **1g** was determined to be the most active contender, with an IC_{50} value of 0.86M against LPS-treated RAW 264.7 cells [47]. Eid et al. also revealed the design, synthesis, and antiinflammatory evaluation of many novel pyrazoline derivatives (2018). In comparison to the standard medicine indomethacin (relative potency = 100), **2f** was the most promising molecule among all series, with a relative potency of 104% at 4h [48]. Chen et al. (2017) also showed how to design, synthesize, and test a library of novel phenyl-pyrazoline-coumarin hybrid compounds for antiinflammatory properties. Compound **3m**, in particular, had the most effective antiinflammatory activity, inhibiting TNF and IL-6 by 40.38% and 41.17%,

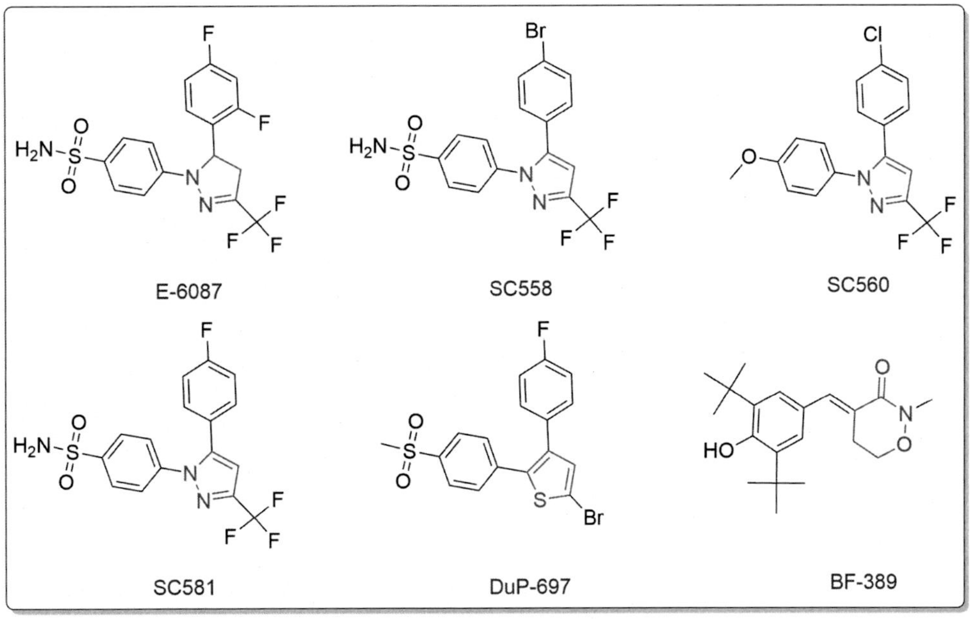

FIG. 11 Heterocycles containing antiinflammatory candidates under clinical development.

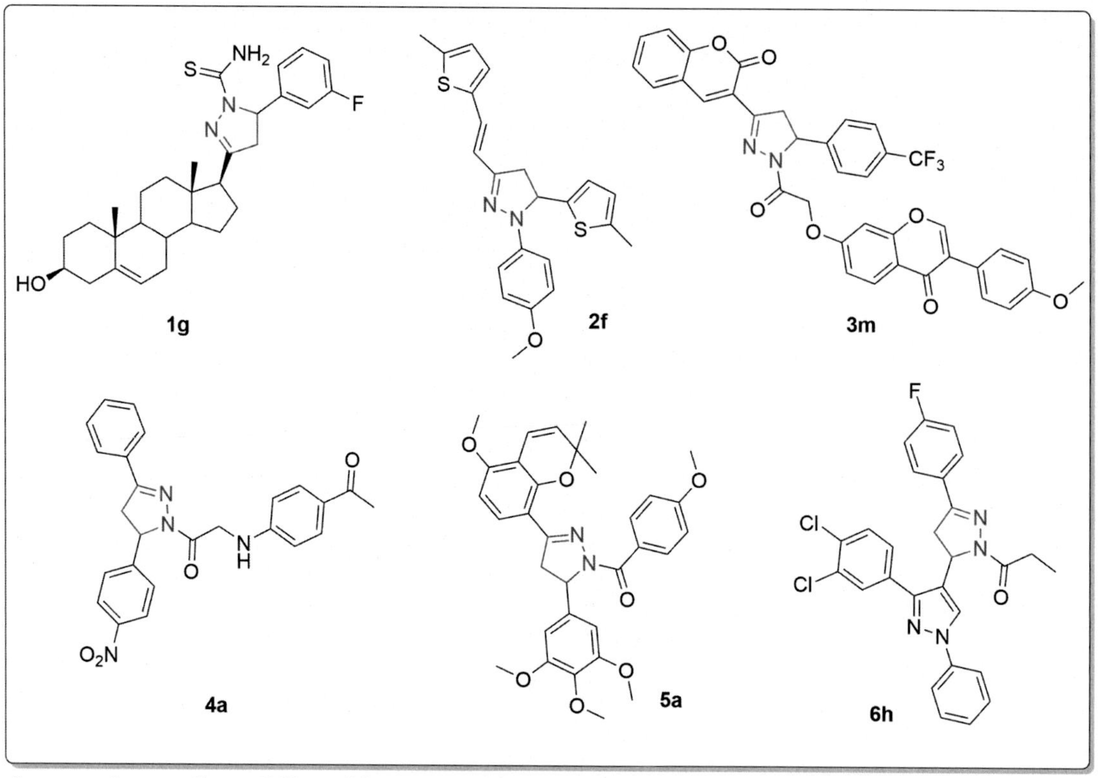

FIG. 12 Structures of a pyrazoline scaffold containing potent antiinflammatory compounds.

respectively, at a concentration of 10M [49]. Abdel-Sayed et al. also reported on the design, synthesis, characterization, and antiinflammatory evaluation of novel 1,3,5-trisubstituted pyrazoline derivatives, as well as a molecular docking research (2016). Compound **4a** inhibited COX-2 in vitro significantly, with an IC$_{50}$ value of 10M [50]. Jiqiang He et al. (2015) also developed and synthesized a library of 28 pyrazoline derivatives, which they tested for antiinflammatory efficacy. In comparison to indomethacin (inhibitory rate = 60.60%), compound **5a** suppressed LPS-induced NO generation at a concentration of 10M with an inhibitory rate of 80% [51]. Viveka et al. (2015) published a paper in the same year detailing the design, synthesis, and antiinflammatory, analgesic, and antibacterial assessment of a series of novel pyrazole-attached substituted pyrazoline hybrid compounds. The N-acylated derivative **6h** showed the most promising edema inhibitory activity among this group (75.56%) [52].

6.2 Indole derivatives as antiinflammatory agents
(shown in Fig. 13)

Song et al. (2019) reported the design, synthesis, and antiinflammatory evaluation of novel indole-dithiocarbamate derivatives. Among all, compound **7o** was found to be most active candidate with an IC$_{50}$ value in the nanomolar level and exhibited remarkable inhibition against IL-6 as well as TNF-α production [53]. Furthermore, design, synthesis, characterization, and antiinflammatory evaluation with dual

inhibition of COX and 5-LOX along with a molecular docking study of novel indole-2-amide derivatives was reported by Huang et al. (2019). Hereby, compound **8b** displayed the most potent *in vitro* COX-2 inhibition with an IC$_{50}$ value of 23.21 nM and a selectivity index (COX-1/COX-2) of 17.45 [54]. Furthermore, Birmann et al. (2018) demonstrated the design, synthesis, and antiinflammatory evaluation of a new selenium compound 3-(4-chlorophenylselanyl)-1-methyl-1H-indole (**9a**). Particularly, compound 3-(4-chlorophenylselanyl)-1-methyl-1H-indole (**9a**) exhibited a good CMI value that provides potent antiinflammatory activity [55]. Moreover, the design, synthesis, and antiinflammatory evaluation of N-acyl-substituted indole-clubbed benzimidazoles and naphthoimidazole hybrid derivatives was disclosed by Abraham et al. [56]. Results of an *in vitro* HRBC (human red blood cells) membrane stabilization test for antiinflammatory evaluation revealed that **10a** was most promising compound with significant antiinflammatory activity. Also, Pedada et al. [57] designed and synthesized indole-containing isoxazole derivatives and evaluated them for antiinflammatory and anticancer activity. Among these all, compound **11o** showed remarkable sPLA2 inhibitory activity with an IC$_{50}$ value of $10.23 \pm 0.91 \mu M$, which was more potent than standard ursolic acid (IC$_{50} = 12.59 \pm 1.03 \mu M$) [57]. In the same year, Liu et al. [58] reported the design, synthesis, and antiinflammatory evaluation of a series of new indole-2-carboxamide derivatives. From this series, derivative **12g** exhibited most

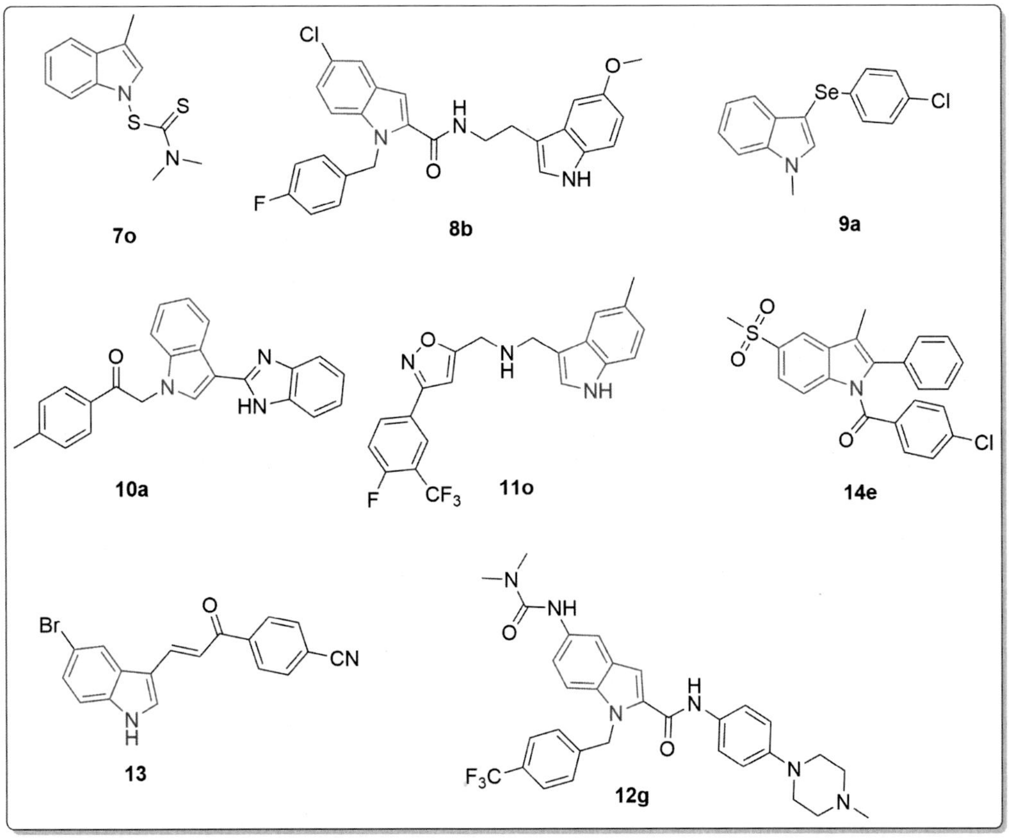

FIG. 13 Structures of an indole scaffold containing potent antiinflammatory compounds.

promising antiinflammatory activity against IL-6 and TNF-α production with IC_{50} values of $1.24 \pm 0.43 \mu M$ and $2.67 \pm 0.76 \mu M$, respectively [58]. Moreover, Ozdemir et al. [59] reported the design, synthesis, and antiinflammatory evaluation of novel indole-based chalcone derivatives. Among all, compound **13** was found to be most active candidate against both COX-1 and COX-2 with IC_{50} values of $8.1 \pm 0.2 \mu g/mL$ and $9.5 \pm 0.8 \mu g/mL$, respectively [59]. In the same year, the design, synthesis, and characterization along with antiinflammatory and analgesic evaluation of new 3-methyl-2-phenyl-1-substituted-indole derivatives was reported by Abdellatif et al. [60]. Hereby, compound 14e displayed most potent in vitro selective COX-2 inhibition with an IC_{50} value of $1.65 \pm 1.02 \mu M$ and a selectivity index (COX-1/COX-2) of 25.67 [60].

6.3 Pyrazole derivatives as antiinflammatory agents (shown in Fig. 14)

Taher et al. (2019) reported the design, synthesis, antiinflammatory as well as analgesic evaluation with a docking simulation study of novel pyrazole derivatives. Among all, compound **15** found to be the most active candidate having good affinity of -13.400kcal/mol toward COX-2 binding pocket [61]. In the same year, the design, synthesis, charac-

terization, and antiinflammatory evaluation of new pyrazole derivatives was reported by Hassan et al. (2019). Hereby, compound **16a** displayed the most potent in vitro COX-2 inhibition with an IC_{50} value of $19.87 \pm 0.57 \text{nM}$ [62]. Abdellatif et al. (2019) demonstrated the design, synthesis and antiinflammatory and antidiabetic PPAR-γ agonistic evaluation of thiazolidine-appended pyrazole hybrid compounds. Particularly, compound **17c** exhibited the most potent selective COX-2 inhibition with an IC_{50} value of $0.63 \mu M$ and a selectivity index (COX-1/COX-2) of 9.15 [63]. Furthermore, the design, microwave-assisted synthesis along with antibacterial and antiinflammatory evaluation of coumarin-pyrazole hybrid derivatives was disclosed by Chavan et al. (2018). The results of an in vivo antiinflammatory evaluation revealed that **18f** was most promising compound with 67.27% inhibition of heat-induced protein denaturation [23]. Furthermore, Nossier et al. (2017) designed and synthesized a new pyrazole endowed with different nitrogenous heterocyclic scaffolds and evaluated them for antiinflammatory activity. Among these all, compound **19b** showed remarkable with % inhibition of edema of 89.57%, as compared to the standard drug indomethacin (% inhibition = 72.99%) [64]. In the same year, Abd El Razik et al. (2017) reported the design, synthesis, and antiinflammatory evaluation of a series of new

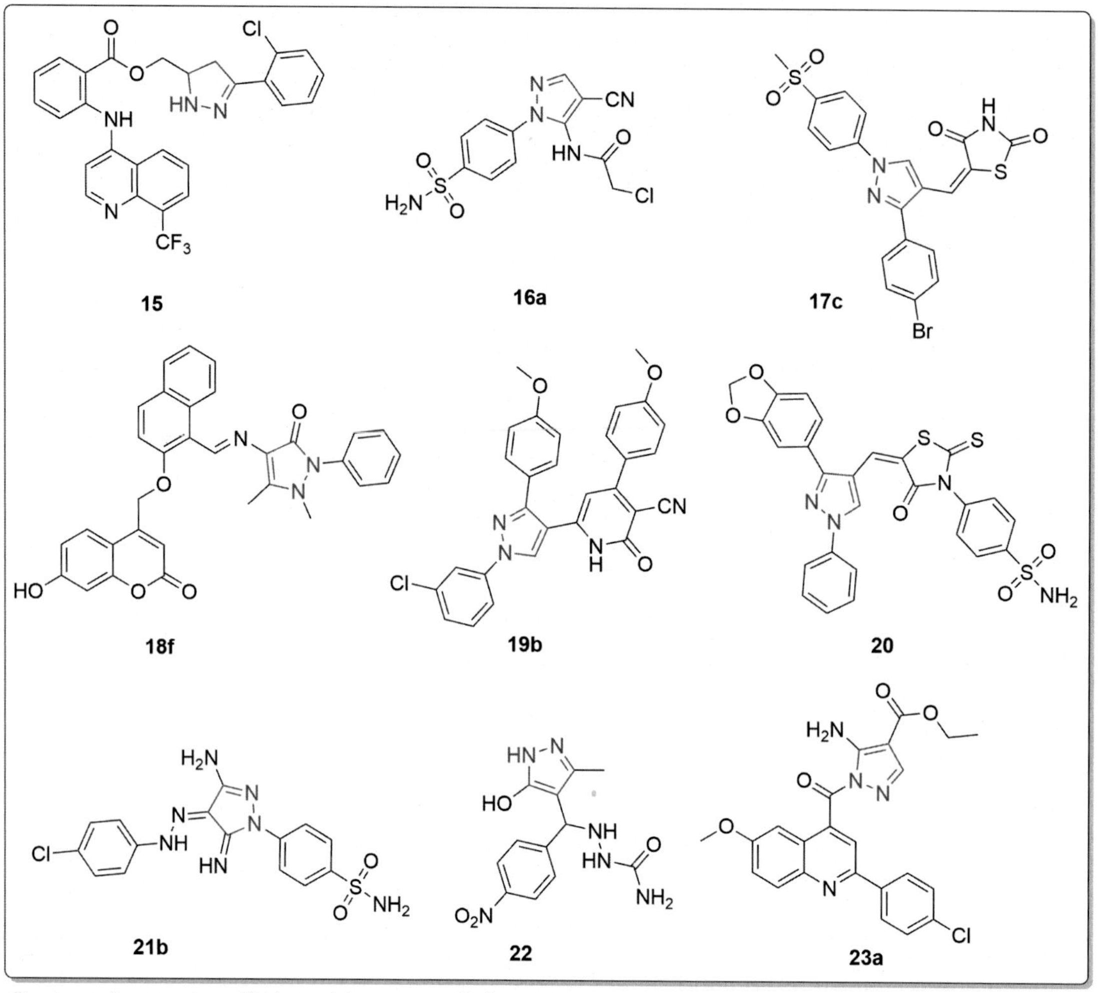

FIG. 14 Structures of a pyrazole scaffold containing potent antiinflammatory compounds.

benzodioxole-pyrazole hybrid derivatives. From this series, derivative **20** exhibited the most promising selective COX-2 inhibition with an IC$_{50}$ value of 0.33 μM and a selectivity index (COX-1/COX-2) of 12.06 [65]. Also, Abdelgawad et al. (2017) reported the design, synthesis, and antiinflammatory evaluation along with a docking study of novel pyrazole-clubbed hydrazone derivatives. Among all, compound **21b** was found to be most active candidate against COX-2 isoform with an IC$_{50}$ value of 0.58 μM, which was more potent than standard drug celecoxib (IC$_{50}$ = 0.87 μM) [66]. Moreover, the design, synthesis, and characterization along with antiinflammatory and antimicrobial evaluation of new pyrazole derivatives was reported by Kumar et al. (2015). Among all, compound **22** displayed the most potent antiinflammatory activity with 82.1%, that was more than standard drug diclofenac sodium (% activity = 75%) [22]. In the same year, El-Feky et al. (2015) described the design, synthesis, and antiinflammatory evaluation along with a docking study of novel pyrazole-appended quinoline derivatives. Among all, compound **23a** was found to be most active candidate against the

COX-2 isoform with an IC$_{50}$ value of 0.26 μM, which was more promising than the reference drug celecoxib (IC$_{50}$ = 0.28 μM) [67].

6.4 Thiazole derivatives as antiinflammatory agents (shown in Fig. 15)

Han et al. (2021) reported the design, synthesis, and antiinflammatory evaluation as sEH inhibitory activity of novel 2-aminobenzo[d]thiazole derivatives. Among all, compound **24d** was found to be most active candidate with potent sEH inhibitory activity having an IC$_{50}$ value of 0.082 μM [68]. Furthermore, the design, synthesis, characterization, and antiinflammatory evaluation with dual inhibition of COX-2 and 5-LOX of new thiazole derivatives was reported by Jacob et al. (2020). Hereby, compound **25l** displayed the most potent in vitro COX-1, COX-2, and 5-LOX inhibition with IC$_{50}$ values of 5.55, 0.09, and 0.38 μM, respectively [69]. Also, the design, synthesis, characterization, and antiinflammatory, antimicrobial

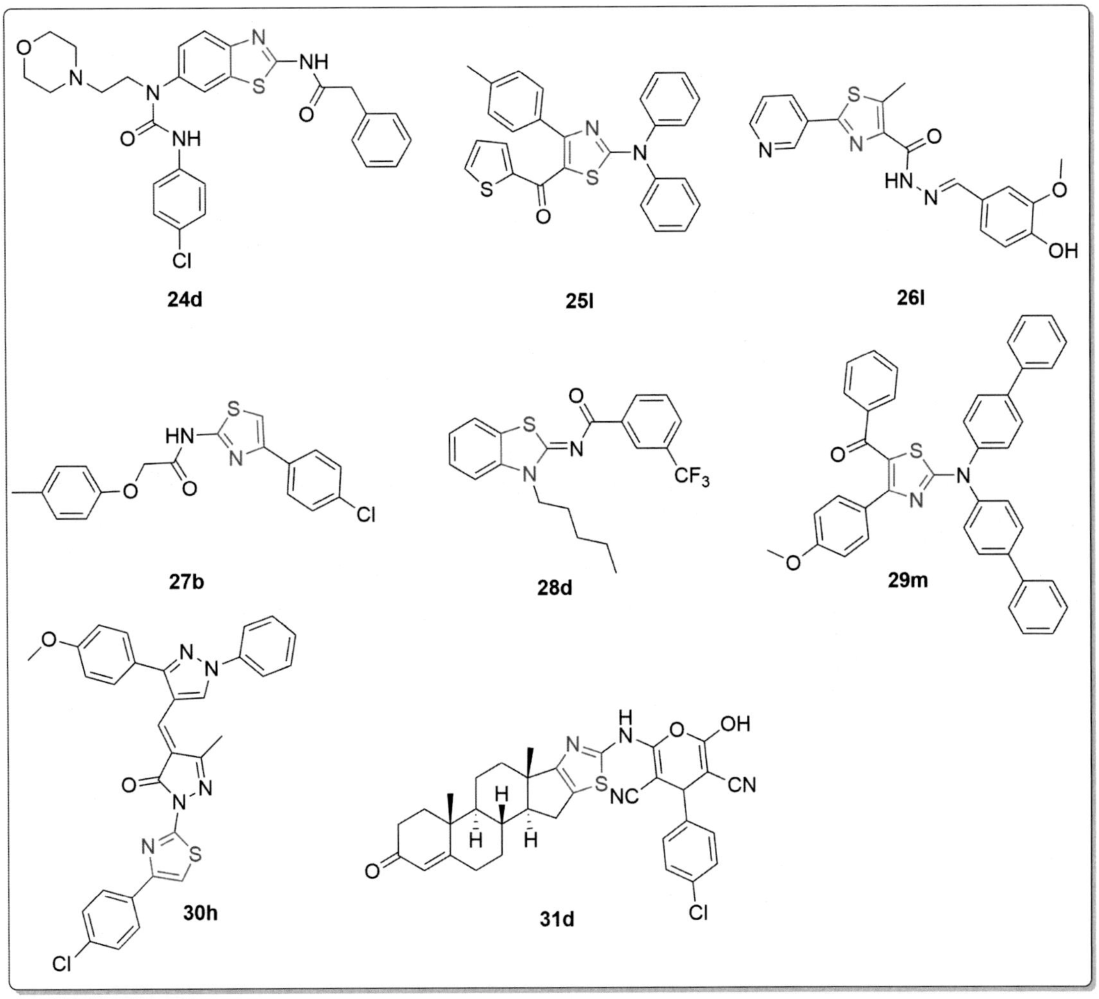

FIG. 15 Structures of a thiazole scaffold containing potent antiinflammatory compounds.

evaluation with a molecular docking study of novel pyridine- and thiazole-clubbed hydrazide derivatives was reported by Kamat et al. (2020). Among these, compound **26l** displayed the most potent inhibition of protein denaturation with an IC_{50} value of 46.29 μg/mL [70]. Khamees et al. (2020) reported the design, synthesis, and antiinflammatory evaluation of novel phenoxy thiazole acetamide derivatives. Among all, compound **27b** was found to be the most active candidate in COX-2 inhibition with an IC_{50} value of 3.13 μM, which was more than the standard drug diclofenac sodium ($IC_{50} = 8.2$ μM) [71]. Furthermore, the design, synthesis, characterization, and antiinflammatory evaluation as well as a cannabinoid-II receptor agonistic study of novel thiazole and benzothiazole derivatives was reported by Ghonim et al. (2019). Hereby, compound **28d** displayed the most potent cannabinoid-II receptor agonistic activity with an EC_{50} value of 128.82 nM [72]. Also, Sinha et al. (2018) demonstrated the design, synthesis, and antiinflammatory evaluation as

the 5-LOX inhibitory potential of new substituted 2-aminothiazole derivatives. Particularly, **29m** exhibited potent 5-LOX inhibitory activity with an IC_{50} value of 0.9 ± 0.1 μM [73]. Then, the design, synthesis, and antiinflammatory evaluation along with a docking study of pyrazole-clubbed thiazole hybrid derivatives was disclosed by Kamble et al. (2016). The results of an in vitro antiinflammatory evaluation revealed that **30h** was the most promising compound with % COX-2 inhibition of 78.91%, which found to be more than indomethacin (% COX-II inhibition = 32.89%) [74]. Moreover, Mohareb et al. (2015) designed and synthesized thiazole, thiophene, pyridine, and pyran derivatives derived from androstenedione and evaluated them for antiinflammatory and antiulcer activity. Among these all, compound **31d** showed maximum protection from carrageenan-induced paw edema at a dose of 40 mg/kg with 89%, as compared to standard drug indomethacin (% protection = 96%) [75].

6.5 Thiophene derivatives as antiinflammatory agents (shown in Fig. 16)

The design, synthesis, and in vivo antiinflammatory, COX-1/COX-2, and 5-LOX inhibitory evaluation of novel 2,3,4-trisubstituted thiophene derivatives were reported by Qandeel et al. (2020). Among all, compound **32b** was found to be the most active candidate with potent COX-2 inhibitory activity having an IC_{50} value of 5.45 μM [76]. In the same year, the design, synthesis, characterization, and antiinflammatory and antitubercular evaluation of novel pyrazole-endowed thiophene derivatives was reported by Nayak et al. (2020). Among these, compound **33b** displayed the most potent inhibition of protein denaturation with an IC_{50} value of 34.1 μg/mL [77]. Further, El-Shoukrofy et al. (2019) reported the design, synthesis, and in vivo antiinflammatory, COX-1/COX-2 and 5-LOX inhibitory evaluation along with a docking study of new pyrazole-endowed thiophene, thienopyrimidine, and thienotriazolopyrimidine derivatives. Among all, compound **34** was found to be the most active candidate in COX-2 inhibition with an IC_{50} value of 0.048 μM, which was comparable to that of the standard drug celecoxib (IC_{50} = 0.045 μM) [78]. Furthermore, the design, synthesis, characterization, and antiinflammatory evaluation as well as a docking study of novel thiophene-clubbed pyrazole derivatives was reported by Prabhudeva et al. [79]. Hereby, compound **35l** displayed most potent $sPLA_2$ inhibitory activity with an IC_{50} value of 10.106 ± 0.095 μM [79]. Furthermore, Mahajan et al. [80] demonstrated the design, synthesis, and antiinflammatory evaluation of new thiophene-appended quinoline based β-diketones and derivatives. Particularly, **36a** exhibited potent antiinflammatory activity with an EC_{50} value of 11.00 ± 1.26 μM, which was comparable to that of standard drug diclofenac sodium ($EC_{50} = 11.70 \pm 0.98$ μM) [80]. In the same year, the design, synthesis, and antiinflammatory as well as antiulcer evaluation of thiophene, thieno[2,3-d] pyrimidine, 1,2,4-triazole, pyran, and pyridine derivatives was disclosed by El-Sayed et al. (2016). Among all these, compound **37c** showed maximum protection from carrageenin-induced paw edema at a dose of 40 mg/kg with 99%, which was more than that of the standard drug indomethacin (% protection = 96%) [81]. Moreover, Helal et al. [82] designed and synthesized novel thiophene derivatives and evaluated them for antiinflammatory activity. Among all these, compound **38** showed maximum protection from carrageenin-induced paw edema at 4 h with 58.46%, which was more than that of the standard drug indomethacin (% protection = 47.73%) [82].

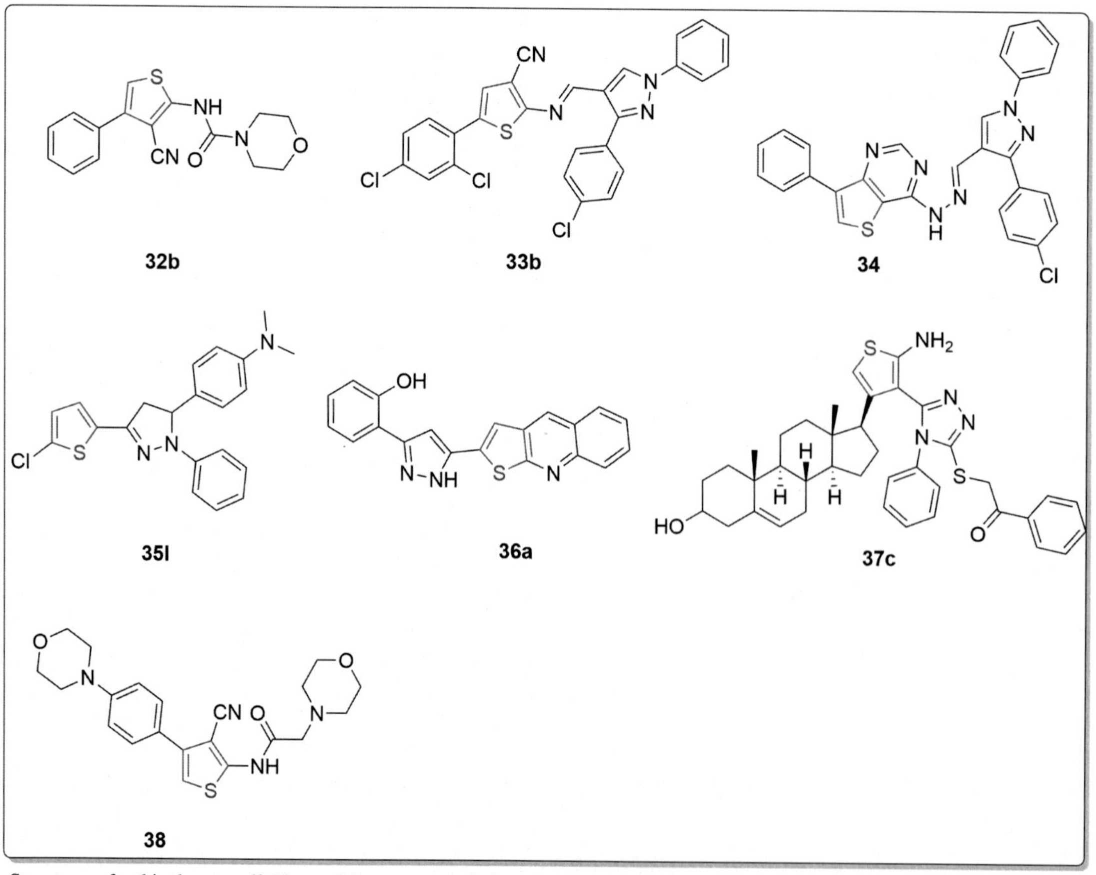

FIG. 16 Structures of a thiophene scaffold containing potent antiinflammatory compounds.

6.6 Triazole derivatives as antiinflammatory agents (shown in Fig. 17)

Boshra et al. (2019) reported the design, synthesis, and antiinflammatory evaluation along with a docking study of novel 2′-hydroxychalcone-triazole hybrid derivatives. Among all, compound **39f** was found to be most active candidate with potent COX-2 inhibitory activity, having an IC_{50} value of 0.041 μM and a selectivity index of 319.51 [83]. Furthermore, the design, synthesis, characterization, p38α MAP kinase inhibition, antiinflammatory evaluation and docking simulation study of novel quinoxaline-endowed triazole derivatives was reported by Tariq et al. (2018). Among these, compound **40f** displayed the most potent antiinflammatory activity with potent edema inhibition of 84.15% [84]. In the continuation of research work, design, synthesis, characterization, p38α MAP kinase inhibition, antiinflammatory evaluation, and docking simulation study of new 1,2,4-triazole-clubbed benzothiazole/benzoxazole derivatives was reported by Tariq et al. (2018). Compound **41b** displayed the most potent antiinflammatory activity with potent edema inhibition of 84.43% [85]. Furthermore, Zhang et al. (2017) reported the design, synthesis, and antiinflammatory evaluation along with a docking study of new perimidine-endowed triazole derivatives. Among all, compound **42n** was found to be most active candidate with 49.26% inhibition at 50 mg/kg drug concentration, which was more potent than that of standard drug ibuprofen (% inhibition = 28.13%) [86]. Furthermore, the design, synthesis, characterization, and antiinflammatory evaluation of novel 1,2,4-triazole derivatives was reported by Paprocka et al. [87]. The result revealed that most compounds displayed remarkable antiinflammatory activity [87].

6.7 Tetrazole derivatives as antiinflammatory agents (shown in Fig. 18)

Labib et al. [88] reported the design, synthesis, and antiinflammatory evaluation including COX-2, PGE2, TNF-α,

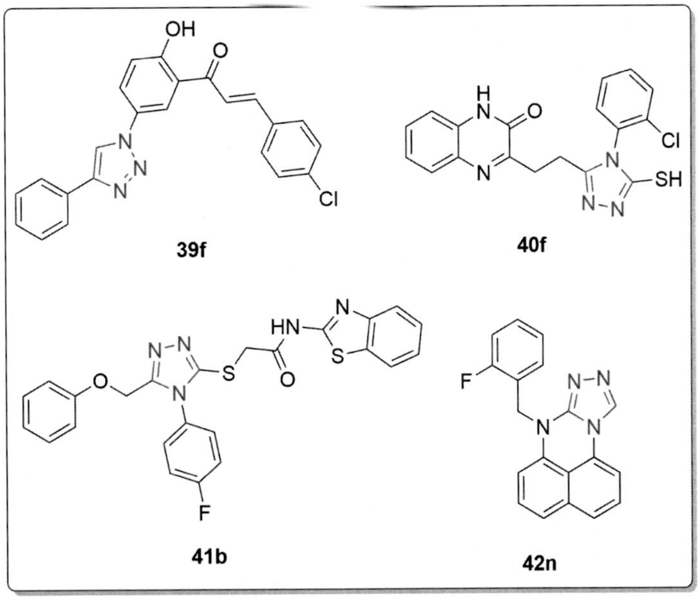

FIG. 17 Structures of a triazole scaffold containing potent antiinflammatory compounds.

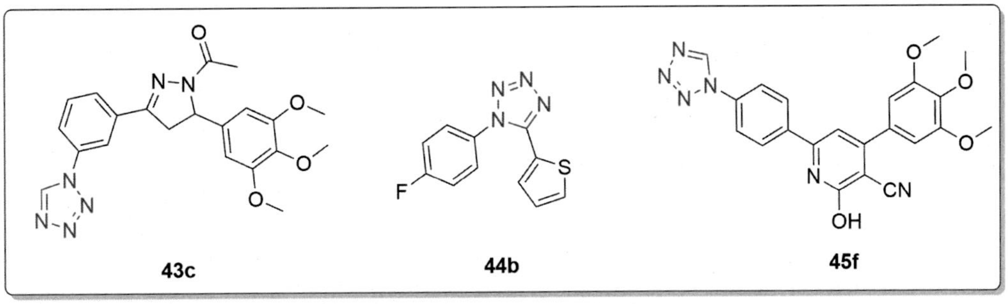

FIG. 18 Structures of a tetrazole scaffold containing potent antiinflammatory compounds.

and IL-6 inhibitory activity of novel tetrazole derivatives. Among all, compound **43c** was found to be the most active candidate with potent COX-2 inhibitory activity, having an IC_{50} value of $0.039 \pm 0.0003\,\mu M$ and selectivity index of 317.95, which was more potent than that of the standard drug celecoxib ($IC_{50} = 0.045 \pm 0.0035\,\mu M$) and indomethacin ($IC_{50} = 0.080 \pm 0.0057\,\mu M$) [88]. Furthermore, the design, synthesis, characterization, antiinflammatory evaluation, and docking simulation study of novel tetrazole-endowed heterocycle hybrid compounds was reported by Sribalan et al. [89]. Among these, compound **44b** displayed most potent antiinflammatory activity with potent edema inhibition of 74.44%, which was comparable to that of the standard drug diclofenac sodium (% inhibition = 79.03%) [89]. Moreover, the design, synthesis, characterization, antiinflammatory as well as ulcerogenic liability evaluation and a docking simulation study of new tetrazole and cyanamide derivatives was reported by Lamie et al. [90]. Among all, compound **45f** was found to be most active candidate against the COX-2 isoform with an IC_{50} value of $0.14\,\mu M$ and a selectivity index of 0.14, which was more potent than that of the standard drug celecoxib ($IC_{50} = 0.16\,\mu M$), diclofenac ($IC_{50} = 0.8\,\mu M$), and indomethacin ($IC_{50} = 0.49\,\mu M$) [90].

6.8 Benzoxazole derivatives as antiinflammatory agents (shown in Fig. 19)

Yatam et al. [91] reported the design, synthesis, and antiinflammatory as well as antioxidant evaluation of novel 2 (((5-aryl-1,2,4-oxadiazol-3-yl)methyl)thio)benzo[d]oxazole derivatives. Among all, compound **46j** was found to be most active candidate with potent COX-2 inhibitory activity having an IC_{50} value of $4.83\,\mu M$ [91]. Furthermore, the design, synthesis, characterization, antiinflammatory evaluation, and a docking simulation study of novel benzo[d]oxazole derivatives were reported by Shakya et al. [92]. Among these, compound **47i** displayed the most potent antiinflammatory activity with potent edema inhibition of 45.1%, as compared to the standard drug diclofenac sodium (% inhibition = 69.5%) and ibuprofen (% inhibition = 64.7%) [92].

6.9 Imidazole derivatives as antiinflammatory agents (shown in Fig. 20)

Nascimento et al. [93] reported the design, synthesis, and antiinflammatory evaluation of novel, substituted fluorophenyl imidazole (**48a**). Results revealed that substituted

FIG. 19 Structures of a benzoxazole scaffold containing potent antiinflammatory compounds.

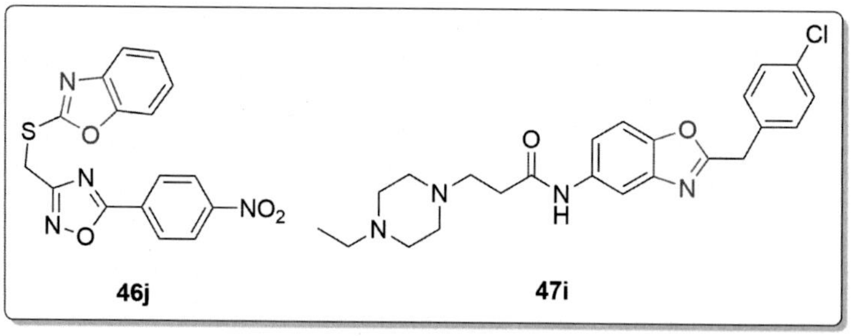

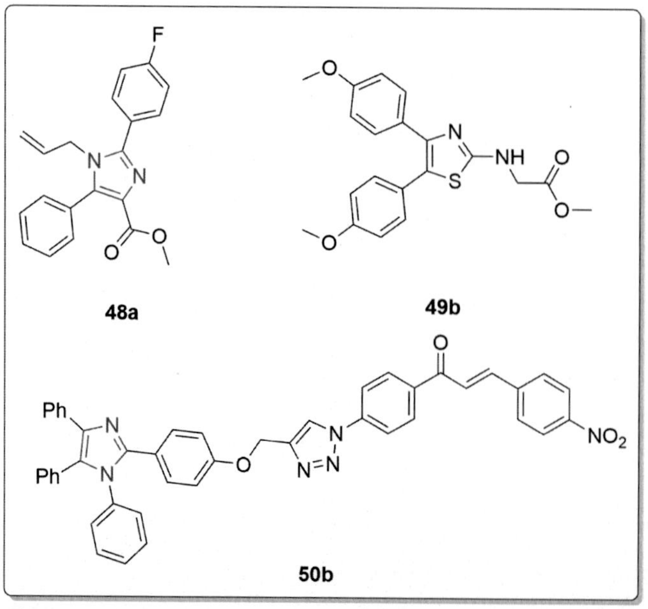

FIG. 20 Structures of imidazole scaffold containing potent antiinflammatory compounds.

fluorophenyl imidazole (**48a**) showed remarkable antiinflammatory potential via inhibiting intracellular pathways including p38, MAPK, and NF-κB [93]. Furthermore, the design, synthesis, characterization, and docking studies for antiinflammatory evaluation of novel 1,2,3-triazole ring embedded 4-(1,4,5-triphenyl-1H-imidazol-2-yl) phenol derivatives were described by Kumar et al. [94]. Among these, compound **49b** exhibited an excellent docking score of 208.357 and 168.763 with COX-1 and COX-2 active sites, respectively [94]. In the same year, Abdelazeem et al. [95] reported the design, synthesis, and antiinflammatory as well as analgesic evaluation of novel diarylthiazole and diarylimidazole derivatives. Among all, compound **50b** was found to be most potent candidate against COX-1 with an IC_{50} value of 0.32 μM and a selectivity index of 28.84 for both COX isoforms [95].

7 Conclusions

Heterocyclic molecules play a significant role in the design and development of promising drug candidates and hence, are widely investigated by the researchers to afford lead compounds in various fields of medicinal chemistry. These versatile heterocyclic structures provide an exclusive three-dimensional arrangement that permits numerous substitution patterns to deliver potent, desired pharmacological responses including antiinflammatory, antimicrobial, analgesic, anticancer, antitrypanosomal, antiepileptic, antidiabetic, MAO-inhibitory, antiviral, etc. On the other hand, inflammation remains one of the major challenging disorders endowed with initial symptoms such as pain, swelling, redness, and heat. Nowadays, drug resistance to the available drug regimen represents a massive challenge for researchers to design and develop novel, prominent drug molecules with tremendous potency and least adverse effects including a variety of allergies and inflammation. Also, limited marketed drugs having a heterocyclic core scaffold, i.e., mainly nonsteroidal antiinflammatory drugs (NSAIDs) are in use to relieve acute as well as chronic inflammatory syndromes. Hence, identification, design, and development of novel antiinflammatory agents is an emerging need to eliminate various kinds of inflammations. Hereby, considering the abovementioned facts, in this chapter we have reviewed the recently developed heterocyclic derivatives as prominent molecules displaying potential to eradicate inflammation along with much emphasis on SAR studies to establish the relationship between biological activity and target site interactions.

References

[1] P. Arora, V. Arora, H. Lamba, D. Wadhwa, Importance of heterocyclic chemistry: a review, Int. J. Pharmaceut. Sci. Drug Res. 9 (2012) 2947–2954, https://doi.org/10.13040/IJPSR.0975-8232.3.

[2] P. Gupta, Synthesis of bioactive imidazoles: a review, Chem. Sci. J. (2015), https://doi.org/10.4172/2150-3494.100091.

[3] P.V. Thanikachalam, R.K. Maurya, V. Garg, V. Monga, An insight into the medicinal perspective of synthetic analogs of indole: a review, Eur. J. Med. Chem. 180 (2019) 562–612, https://doi.org/10.1016/j.ejmech.2019.07.019.

[4] F.D. Hart, P.L. Boardman, Indomethacin a new non-steroid antiinflammatory agent, Br. Med. J. 2 (5363) (1963) 965–970, https://doi.org/10.1136/bmj.2.5363.965.

[5] A. Huttner, E.M. Verhaegh, S. Harbarth, A.E. Muller, U. Theuretzbacher, J.W. Mouton, Nitrofurantoin revisited: A systematic review and meta-analysis of controlled trials, J. Antimicrob. Chemother. 70 (9) (2015) 2456–2464, https://doi.org/10.1093/jac/dkv147.

[6] P. Chawla, S. Kalra, R. Kumar, R. Singh, S.K. Saraf, Novel 2-(substituted phenyl Imino)-5-benzylidene-4-thiazolidinones as possible non-ulcerogenic tri-action drug candidates: synthesis, characterization, biological evaluation And docking studies, Med. Chem. Res. 28 (3) (2019) 340–359, https://doi.org/10.1007/s00044-018-02288-z.

[7] M. Matias, S. Silvestre, A. Falcao, G. Alves, Recent highlights on molecular hybrids potentially useful in central nervous system disorders, Mini-Rev. Med. Chem. 17 (6) (2017) 486–517, https://doi.org/10.2174/1389557517666161111110121.

[8] G. Mishra, N. Sachan, P. Chawla, Synthesis and evaluation of thiazolidinedione-coumarin adducts as antidiabetic, antiinflammatory and antioxidant agents, Lett. Org. Chem. 12 (6) (2015) 429–445, https://doi.org/10.2174/1570178612666150424235603.

[9] M. Amir, S.A. Javed, H. Kumar, Synthesis of some 1,3,4-oxadiazole derivatives as potential antiinflammatory agents, ChemInform 38 (39) (2007), https://doi.org/10.1002/chin.200739109.

[10] T. Chandra, N. Garg, S. Lata, K.K. Saxena, A. Kumar, Synthesis of substituted acridinyl pyrazoline derivatives and their evaluation for anti-inflammatory activity, Eur. J. Med. Chem. 45 (5) (2010) 1772–1776, https://doi.org/10.1016/j.ejmech.2010.01.009.

[11] H. Sharma, P.A. Chawla, R. Bhatia, 1,3,5-Pyrazoline derivatives in CNS disorders: Synthesis, biological evaluation and structural insights through molecular docking, CNS Neurol. Disord. Drug Targets 19 (6) (2020) 448–465, https://doi.org/10.2174/1871527319999200818182249.

[12] M. Akhter, A. Husain, B. Azad, M. Ajmal, Aroylpropionic acid based 2,5-disubstituted-1,3,4-oxadiazoles: synthesis and their antiinflammatory and analgesic activities, Eur. J. Med. Chem. 44 (6) (2009) 2372–2378, https://doi.org/10.1016/j.ejmech.2008.09.005.

[13] B. Jayashankar, K.M. Lokanath Rai, N. Baskaran, H.S. Sathish, Synthesis and pharmacological evaluation of 1,3,4-oxadiazole bearing bis(heterocycle) derivatives as anti-inflammatory and analgesic agents, Eur. J. Med. Chem. 44 (10) (2009) 3898–3902, https://doi.org/10.1016/j.ejmech.2009.04.006.

[14] P.N. Kalaria, S.C. Karad, D.K. Raval, A review on diverse heterocyclic compounds as the privileged scaffolds in antimalarial drug discovery, Eur. J. Med. Chem. 158 (2018) 917–936, https://doi.org/10.1016/j.ejmech.2018.08.040.

[15] H. Nakamura, Cyclooxygenase (COX)-2 selective inhibitors: aspirin, a dual COX-1/COX-2 inhibitor, to COX-2 selective inhibitors, Folia Pharmacol. Japon. 118 (3) (2001) 219–230, https://doi.org/10.1254/fpj.118.219.

[16] K. Takeuchi, Y. Hayashi, A. Tanaka, Functional mechanism for up-regulation of COX-2 induced by COX-1 inhibition in rat stomachs:

importance of gastric hypermotility, Gastroenterology A174 (2003), https://doi.org/10.1016/s0016-5085(03)80864-8.

[17] B.J. Anderson, Paracetamol (acetaminophen): mechanisms of action, Paediatr. Anaesth. 18 (10) (2008) 915–921, https://doi.org/10.1111/j.1460-9592.2008.02764.x.

[18] J. Martel-Pelletier, D. Lajeunesse, P. Reboul, J.P. Pelletier, Therapeutic role of dual inhibitors of 5-LOX and COX, selective and non-selective non-steroidal anti-inflammatory drugs, Ann. Rheum. Dis. 62 (6) (2003) 501–509, https://doi.org/10.1136/ard.62.6.501.

[19] A. Gaddi, A.F.G. Cicero, E.J. Pedro, Clinical perspectives of anti-inflammatory therapy in the elderly: The lipoxigenase (LOX)/cycloxigenase (COX) inhibition concept, Arch. Gerontol. Geriatr. 38 (3) (2004) 201–212, https://doi.org/10.1016/j.archger.2003.10.001.

[20] R. Bhutani, D.P. Pathak, A. Husain, G. Kapoor, R. Kant, A review on recent development of pyrazoline as a pharmacologically active molecule, Int. J. Pharmaceut. Sci. Res. 6 (10) (2015) 4113.

[21] S. Kumar, S. Bawa, S. Drabu, R. Kumar, H. Gupta, Biological activities of pyrazoline derivatives—a recent development, Recent Pat. Antiinfect. Drug Discov. 4 (3) (2009) 154–163, https://doi.org/10.2174/157489109789318569.

[22] R. Surendra Kumar, I.A. Arif, A. Ahamed, A. Idhayadhulla, Anti-inflammatory and antimicrobial activities of novel pyrazole analogues, Saudi J. Biol. Sci. 23 (5) (2016) 614–620, https://doi.org/10.1016/j.sjbs.2015.07.005.

[23] R.R. Chavan, K.M. Hosamani, Microwave-assisted synthesis, computational studies and antibacterial/ anti-inflammatory activities of compounds based on coumarin-pyrazole hybrid, R. Soc. Open Sci. 5 (5) (2018), 172435, https://doi.org/10.1098/rsos.172435.

[24] Rahman, M., & Sidhiqui, A. (n.d.). Pyrazoline derivatives: a worthy insight into the recent advances and potential pharmacological activities. Int. J. Pharmaceut. Sci. Drug Res., 2010(3), 165–175.

[25] E.S. Ramadan, E.M. Sharshira, R.I. El Sokkary, N. Morsy, Synthesis and antimicrobial evaluation of some heterocyclic compounds from 3-aryl-1-phenyl-1H-pyrazole-4-carbaldehydes, Zeitsch. Für Naturforsc. B 73 (6) (2018) 389–397, https://doi.org/10.1515/znb-2018-0009.

[26] A. Bennett, G. Villa, Nimesulide: An NSAID that preferentially inhibits COX-2, and has various unique pharmacological activities, Expert Opin. Pharmacother. 1 (2) (2000) 277–286, https://doi.org/10.1517/14656566.1.2.277.

[27] N.H. Amin, M.T. El-Saadi, A.A. Hefny, A.H. Abdelazeem, H.A. Elshemy, K.R. Abdellatif, Anti-inflammatory indomethacin analogs endowed with preferential COX-2 inhibitory activity, Future Med. Chem. 10 (21) (2018) 2521–2535, https://doi.org/10.4155/fmc-2018-0224.

[28] M. Del Tacca, R. Colucci, M. Fornai, C. Blandizzi, Efficacy and tolerability of meloxicam, a COX-2 preferential nonsteroidal anti-inflammatory drug, Clin. Drug Investig. 22 (12) (2002) 799–818, https://doi.org/10.2165/00044011-200222120-00001.

[29] P.M. Sivakumar, M. Doble, Quantitative structure-activity relationships for commercially available inhibitors of COX-2, Med. Chem. 4 (2) (2008) 110–115, https://doi.org/10.2174/157340608783789112.

[30] C. Marot, P. Chavatte, D. Lesieur, Comparative molecular field analysis of selective cyclooxygenase-2 (COX-2) inhibitors, Quant. Structure-Activity Relation. 19 (2) (2000) 127–134, https://doi.org/10.1002/1521-3838(200004)19:2<127::AID-QSAR127>3.0.CO;2-P.

[31] R. Botting, S.S. Ayoub, COX-3 and the mechanism of action of paracetamol/acetaminophen, Prostaglandins Leukot. Essent. Fatty Acids

72 (2) (2005) 85–87. Churchill Livingstone https://doi.org/10.1016/j.plefa.2004.10.005.

[32] S.S. Ayoub, Paracetamol (acetaminophen): a familiar drug with an unexplained mechanism of action, Temperature 1–21 (2021), https://doi.org/10.1080/23328940.2021.1886392.

[33] C. Congiu, M.T. Cocco, V. Onnis, Design, synthesis, and in vitro antitumor activity of new 1,4-diarylimidazole-2-ones and their 2-thione analogues, Bioorg. Med. Chem. Lett. 18 (3) (2008) 989–993, https://doi.org/10.1016/j.bmcl.2007.12.023.

[34] M.A. Iñiguez, C. Punzón, C. Cacheiro-Llaguno, M.D. Díaz-Muñoz, J. Duque, R. Cuberes, I. Alvarez, E.M. Andrés, J. Buxens, H. Buschmann, J.M. Vela, M. Fresno, Cyclooxygenase-independent inhibitory effects on T cell activation of novel 4,5-dihydro-3 trifluoromethyl pyrazole cyclooxygenase-2 inhibitors, Int. Immunopharmacol. 10 (10) (2010) 1295–1304, https://doi.org/10.1016/j.intimp.2010.07.013.

[35] R.F. Reinoso, R. Farrán, T. Moragon, A. Garcı́a-Soret, L. Martı́nez, Development and validation of two chromatographic methods for the quantification of E-6087 and one of its metabolites, E-6132, in rat plasma, J. Pharm. Biomed. Anal. 24 (5–6) (2001) 897–911, https://doi.org/10.1016/s0731-7085(00)00558-6.

[36] R.F. Reinoso, R. Farrán, T. Moragón, A. García-Soret, L. Martínez, Pharmacokinetics of E-6087, a new anti-inflammatory agent, in rats and dogs, Biopharm. Drug Dispos. 22 (6) (2001) 231–242, https://doi.org/10.1002/bdd.258.

[37] S.-M. Yeom, M.-S. Kim, E. Lingenfelter, J. Broadwell, A methocarbamol combination to prevent toxicity of non-steroidal anti inflammatory drugs, Korean J. Clin. Lab. Sci. (2017) 88–98, https://doi.org/10.15324/kjcls.2017.49.2.88.

[38] V. Limongelli, M. Bonomi, L. Marinelli, F.L. Gervasio, A. Cavalli, E. Novellino, M. Parrinello, Molecular basis of cyclooxygenase enzymes (COXs) selective inhibition, Proc. Natl. Acad. Sci. 107 (12) (2010) 5411–5416, https://doi.org/10.1073/pnas.0913377107.

[39] K.V.V.M. Sai Ram, G. Rambabu, J.A.R.P. Sarma, G.R. Desiraju, Ligand coordinate analysis of SC-558 from the active site to the surface of COX-2: A molecular dynamics study, J. Chem. Inf. Model. 46 (4) (2006) 1784–1794, https://doi.org/10.1021/ci050142i.

[40] M.J. Alam, O. Alam, S.A. Khan, M.J. Naim, M. Islamuddin, G.S. Deora, Synthesis, anti-inflammatory, analgesic, COX1/2-inhibitory activity, and molecular docking studies of hybrid pyrazole analogues, Drug Des. Devel. Ther. 10 (2016) 3529–3543, https://doi.org/10.2147/DDDT.S118297.

[41] D.G. Munroe, C.Y. Lau, Turning down the heat: new routes to inhibition of inflammatory signaling by prostaglandin H2 synthases, Chem. Biol. 2 (6) (1995) 343–350, https://doi.org/10.1016/1074-5521(95)90212-0.

[42] M. Perkins, A. Dray, Novel pharmacological strategies for analgesia, Ann. Rheum. Dis. 55 (10) (1996) 715–722, https://doi.org/10.1136/ard.55.10.715.

[43] S. Wong, S.J. Lee, M.R. Frierson, J. Proch, T.A. Miskowski, B.S. Rigby, S.J. Schmolka, R.W. Naismith, D.C. Kreutzer, R. Lindquist, Antiarthritic profile of BF-389—a novel anti-inflammatory agent with low ulcerogenic liability, Agents Actions 37 (1–2) (1992) 90–98, https://doi.org/10.1007/BF01987895.

[44] S.M. Sondhi, M. Dinodia, J. Singh, R. Rani, Heterocyclic compounds as anti-inflammatory agents, Curr. Bioactive Comp. 3 (2) (2007) 91–108, https://doi.org/10.2174/157340707780809554.

[45] R. Dua, S. Shrivastava, S. Sonwane, S. Srivastava, Pharmacological significance of synthetic heterocycles scaffold: a review, Adv. Biol. Res. 5 (3) (2011) 120–144.

[46] Saini, M., Kumar, A., Dwivedi, J., Singh, R., & Review. (n.d.). Biological significances of heterocyclic compounds. Int. J. Pharmaceut. Sci. Drug Res., 2013(3), 66–77.

[47] X. Cai, S. Zhao, D. Cai, J. Zheng, Z. Zhu, D. Wei, Z. Zheng, H. Zhu, Y. Chen, Synthesis and evaluation of novel D-ring substituted steroidal pyrazolines as potential anti-inflammatory agents, Steroids 146 (2019) 70–78, https://doi.org/10.1016/j.steroids.2019.03.012.

[48] N.M. Eid, R.F. George, Facile synthesis of some pyrazoline-based compounds with promising anti-inflammatory activity, Future Med. Chem. 10 (2) (2018) 183–199, https://doi.org/10.4155/fmc-2017-0144.

[49] L.Z. Chen, W.W. Sun, L. Bo, J.Q. Wang, C. Xiu, W.J. Tang, J.B. Shi, H.P. Zhou, X.H. Liu, New arylpyrazoline-coumarins: Synthesis and anti-inflammatory activity, Eur. J. Med. Chem. 138 (2017) 170–181, https://doi.org/10.1016/j.ejmech.2017.06.044.

[50] M.A. Abdel-Sayed, S.M. Bayomi, M.A. El-Sherbeny, N.I. Abdel-Aziz, K.E.H. Eltahir, G.S.G. Shehatou, A.A.M. Abdel-Aziz, Synthesis, anti-inflammatory, analgesic, COX-1/2 inhibition activities and molecular docking study of pyrazoline derivatives, Bioorg. Med. Chem. 24 (9) (2016) 2032–2042, https://doi.org/10.1016/j.bmc.2016.03.032.

[51] J. He, L. Ma, Z. Wei, J. Zhu, F. Peng, M. Shao, L. Lei, L. He, M. Tang, L. He, Y. Wu, L. Chen, Synthesis and biological evaluation of novel pyrazoline derivatives as potent anti-inflammatory agents, Bioorg. Med. Chem. Lett. 25 (11) (2015) 2429–2433, https://doi.org/10.1016/j.bmcl.2015.03.087.

[52] S. Viveka, S. Dinesha, P., Nagaraja, G. K., Ballav, S., & Kerkar, S., Design and synthesis of some new pyrazolyl-pyrazolines as potential anti-inflammatory, analgesic and antibacterial agents, Eur. J. Med. Chem. 101 (2015) 442–451, https://doi.org/10.1016/j.ejmech.2015.07.002.

[53] Z. Song, Y. Zhou, W. Zhang, L. Zhan, Y. Yu, Y. Chen, W. Jia, Z. Liu, J. Qian, Y. Zhang, C. Li, G. Liang, Base promoted synthesis of novel indole-dithiocarbamate compounds as potential anti-inflammatory therapeutic agents for treatment of acute lung injury, Eur. J. Med. Chem. 171 (2019) 54–65, https://doi.org/10.1016/j.ejmech.2019.03.022.

[54] Y. Huang, B. Zhang, J. Li, H. Liu, Y. Zhang, Z. Yang, W. Liu, Design, synthesis, biological evaluation and docking study of novel indole-2-amide as anti-inflammatory agents with dual inhibition of COX and 5-LOX, Eur. J. Med. Chem. 180 (2019) 41–50, https://doi.org/10.1016/j.ejmech.2019.07.004.

[55] P.T. Birmann, F.S.S. Sousa, D.H. de Oliveira, M. Domingues, B.M. Vieira, E.J. Lenardão, L. Savegnago, 3-(4-Chlorophenylselanyl)-1-methyl-1H-indole, a new selenium compound elicits an antinociceptive and anti-inflammatory effect in mice, Eur. J. Pharmacol. 827 (2018) 71–79, https://doi.org/10.1016/j.ejphar.2018.03.005.

[56] R. Abraham, P. Prakash, K. Mahendran, M. Ramanathan, A novel series of N-acyl substituted indole-linked benzimidazoles and naphthoimidazoles as potential anti inflammatory, anti biofilm and anti microbial agents, Microb. Pathog. 114 (2018) 409–413, https://doi.org/10.1016/j.micpath.2017.12.021.

[57] S.R. Pedada, N.S. Yarla, P.J. Tambade, B.L. Dhananjaya, A. Bishayee, K.M. Arunasree, G.H. Philip, G. Dharmapuri, G. Aliev, S. Putta, G. Rangaiah, Synthesis of new secretory

[58] Z. Liu, L. Tang, H. Zhu, T. Xu, C. Qiu, S. Zheng, Y. Gu, J. Feng, Y. Zhang, G. Liang, Design, synthesis, and structure-activity relationship study of novel indole-2-carboxamide derivatives as anti-inflammatory agents for the treatment of sepsis, J. Med. Chem. 59 (10) (2016) 4637–4650, https://doi.org/10.1021/acs.jmedchem.5b02006.

[59] A. Özdemir, M.D. Altıntop, G. Turan-Zitouni, G.A. Çiftçi, İ. Ertorun, Ö. Alataş, Z.A. Kaplancıklı, Synthesis and evaluation of new indole-based chalcones as potential antiinflammatory agents, Eur. J. Med. Chem. 89 (2015) 304–309, https://doi.org/10.1016/j.ejmech.2014.10.056.

[60] K.R.A. Abdellatif, P.F. Lamie, H.A. Omar, 3-Methyl-2-phenyl-1-substituted-indole derivatives as indomethacin analogs: design, synthesis and biological evaluation as potential anti-inflammatory and analgesic agents, J. Enzyme Inhib. Med. Chem. 31 (2) (2016) 318–324, https://doi.org/10.3109/14756366.2015.1022174.

[61] A.T. Taher, M.T. Mostafa Sarg, N.R. El-Sayed Ali, N. Hilmy Elnagdi, Design, synthesis, modeling studies and biological screening of novel pyrazole derivatives as potential analgesic and anti-inflammatory agents, Bioorg. Chem. 89 (2019), 103023, https://doi.org/10.1016/j.bioorg.2019.103023.

[62] G.S. Hassan, D.E. Abdel Rahman, E.A. Abdelmajeed, R.H. Refaey, M. Alaraby Salem, Y.M. Nissan, New pyrazole derivatives: synthesis, anti-inflammatory activity, cycloxygenase inhibition assay and evaluation of mPGES, Eur. J. Med. Chem. 171 (2019) 332–342, https://doi.org/10.1016/j.ejmech.2019.03.052.

[63] K.R.A. Abdellatif, W.A.A. Fadaly, G.M. Kamel, Y.A.M.M. Elshaier, M.A. El-Magd, Design, synthesis, modeling studies and biological evaluation of thiazolidine derivatives containing pyrazole core as potential anti-diabetic PPAR-γ agonists and anti-inflammatory COX-2 selective inhibitors, Bioorg. Chem. 82 (2019) 86–99, https://doi.org/10.1016/j.bioorg.2018.09.034.

[64] E.S. Nossier, H.H. Fahmy, N.M. Khalifa, W.I. El-Eraky, M.A. Baset, D.J. McPhee, Design and synthesis of novel pyrazole-substituted different nitrogenous heterocyclic ring systems as potential anti-inflammatory agents, Molecules 22 (4) (2017), https://doi.org/10.3390/molecules22040512.

[65] H.A. Abd El Razik, M.H. Badr, A.H. Atta, S.M. Mouneir, M.M. Abu-Serie, Benzodioxole-pyrazole hybrids as anti-inflammatory and analgesic agents with COX-1,2/5-LOX inhibition and antioxidant potential, Arch. Pharm. 350 (5) (2017) 1700026, https://doi.org/10.1002/ardp.201700026.

[66] M.A. Abdelgawad, M.B. Labib, M. Abdel-Latif, Pyrazole-hydrazone derivatives as anti-inflammatory agents: Design, synthesis, biological evaluation, COX-1,2/5-LOX inhibition and docking study, Bioorg. Chem. 74 (2017) 212–220, https://doi.org/10.1016/j.bioorg.2017.08.014.

[67] S.A.H. El-Feky, Z.K. Abd El-Samii, N.A. Osman, J. Lashine, M.A. Kamel, H.K. Thabet, Synthesis, molecular docking and anti-inflammatory screening of novel quinoline incorporated pyrazole derivatives using the Pfitzinger reaction II, Bioorg. Chem. 58 (2015) 104–116, https://doi.org/10.1016/j.bioorg.2014.12.003.

[68] Y. Han, D. Huang, S. Xu, L. Li, Y. Tian, S. Li, C. Chen, Y. Li, Y. Sun, Y. Hou, Y. Sun, M. Qin, P. Gong, Z. Gao, Y. Zhao, Ligand-based optimization to identify novel 2-aminobenzo[d]thiazole derivatives as

potent sEH inhibitors with anti-inflammatory effects, Eur. J. Med. Chem. 212 (2021), 113028, https://doi.org/10.1016/j.ejmech.2020.113028.

[69] P.J. Jacob, S.L. Manju, Identification and development of thiazole leads as COX-2/5-LOX inhibitors through in-vitro and in-vivo biological evaluation for anti-inflammatory activity, Bioorg. Chem. 100 (2020), 103882, https://doi.org/10.1016/j.bioorg.2020.103882.

[70] V. Kamat, R. Santosh, B. Poojary, S.P. Nayak, B.K. Kumar, M. Sankaranarayanan, Faheem, S. Khanapure, D.A. Barretto, S.K. Vootla, Pyridine- and thiazole-based hydrazides with promising anti-inflammatory and antimicrobial activities along with their in silico studies, ACS Omega 5 (39) (2020) 25228–25239, https://doi.org/10.1021/acsomega.0c03386.

[71] H.A. Khamees, Y.H.E. Mohammed, S. Ananda, F.H. Al-Ostoot, Y. Sangappa, S. Alghamdi, S.A. Khanum, M. Madegowda, Effect of o-difluoro and p-methyl substituents on the structure, optical properties and anti-inflammatory activity of phenoxy thiazole acetamide derivatives: theoretical and experimental studies, J. Mol. Struct. 1199 (2020), https://doi.org/10.1016/j.molstruc.2019.127024.

[72] A.E. Ghonim, A. Ligresti, A. Rabbito, A.M. Mahmoud, V. Di Marzo, N.A. Osman, A.H. Abadi, Structure-activity relationships of thiazole and benzothiazole derivatives as selective cannabinoid CB2 agonists with in vivo anti-inflammatory properties, Eur. J. Med. Chem. 180 (2019) 154–170, https://doi.org/10.1016/j.ejmech.2019.07.002.

[73] S. Sinha, M. Doble, S.L. Manju, Design, synthesis and identification of novel substituted 2-amino thiazole analogues as potential anti-inflammatory agents targeting 5-lipoxygenase, Eur. J. Med. Chem. 158 (2018) 34–50, https://doi.org/10.1016/j.ejmech.2018.08.098.

[74] R.D. Kamble, R.J. Meshram, S.V. Hese, R.A. More, S.S. Kamble, R. N. Gacche, B.S. Dawane, Synthesis and in silico investigation of thiazoles bearing pyrazoles derivatives as anti-inflammatory agents, Comput. Biol. Chem. 61 (2016) 86–96, https://doi.org/10.1016/j.compbiolchem.2016.01.007.

[75] R.M. Mohareb, M.Y. Zaki, N.S. Abbas, Synthesis, anti-inflammatory and anti-ulcer evaluations of thiazole, thiophene, pyridine and pyran derivatives derived from androstenedione, Steroids 98 (2015) 80–91, https://doi.org/10.1016/j.steroids.2015.03.001.

[76] N.A. Qandeel, A.K. El-Damasy, M.H. Sharawy, S.M. Bayomi, N.S. El-Gohary, Synthesis, in vivo anti-inflammatory, COX-1/COX-2 and 5-LOX inhibitory activities of new 2,3,4-trisubstituted thiophene derivatives, Bioorg. Chem. 102 (2020), 103890, https://doi.org/10.1016/j.bioorg.2020.103890.

[77] S.G. Nayak, B. Poojary, V. Kamat, Novel pyrazole-clubbed thiophene derivatives via Gewald synthesis as antibacterial and anti-inflammatory agents, Arch. Pharm. 353 (12) (2020) 2000103, https://doi.org/10.1002/ardp.202000103.

[78] M.S. El-Shoukrofy, H.A. Abd El Razik, O.M. AboulWafa, A.E. Bayad, I.M. El-Ashmawy, Pyrazoles containing thiophene, thienopyrimidine and thienotriazolopyrimidine as COX-2 selective inhibitors: Design, synthesis, in vivo anti-inflammatory activity, docking and in silico chemo-informatic studies, Bioorg. Chem. 85 (2019) 541–557, https://doi.org/10.1016/j.bioorg.2019.02.036.

[79] M.G. Prabhudeva, S. Bharath, A.D. Kumar, S. Naveen, N.K. Lokanath, B.N. Mylarappa, K.A. Kumar, Design and environmentally benign synthesis of novel thiophene appended pyrazole analogues as anti-inflammatory and radical scavenging agents: crystallographic, in silico modeling, docking and SAR characterization, Bioorg. Chem. 73 (2017) 109–120, https://doi.org/10.1016/j.bioorg.2017.06.004.

[80] P. Mahajan, M. Nikam, A. Asrondkar, A. Bobade, C. Gill, Synthesis, antioxidant, and anti-inflammatory evaluation of novel thiophene-

fused quinoline based β-diketones and derivatives, J. Heterocyclic Chem. 54 (2) (2017) 1415–1422, https://doi.org/10.1002/jhet.2722.

[81] N.N.E. El-Sayed, M.A. Abdelaziz, W.W. Wardakhan, R.M. Mohareb, The Knoevenagel reaction of cyanoacetylhydrazine with pregnenolone: Synthesis of thiophene, thieno[2,3-d]pyrimidine, 1,2,4-triazole, pyran and pyridine derivatives with anti-inflammatory and anti-ulcer activities, Steroids 107 (2016) 98–111, https://doi.org/10.1016/j.steroids.2015.12.023.

[82] M.H. Helal, M.A. Salem, M.A. Gouda, N.S. Ahmed, A.A. El-Sherif, Design, synthesis, characterization, quantum-chemical calculations and anti-inflammatory activity of novel series of thiophene derivatives, Spectrochim. Acta—Part A: Mol. Biomol. Spectrosc. 147 (2015) 73–83, https://doi.org/10.1016/j.saa.2015.03.070.

[83] A.N. Boshra, H.H.M. Abdu-Allah, A.F. Mohammed, A.M. Hayallah, Click chemistry synthesis, biological evaluation and docking study of some novel 2′-hydroxychalcone-triazole hybrids as potent anti-inflammatory agents, Bioorg. Chem. 95 (2020), 103505, https://doi.org/10.1016/j.bioorg.2019.103505.

[84] S. Tariq, O. Alam, M. Amir, Synthesis, anti-inflammatory, p38α MAP kinase inhibitory activities and molecular docking studies of quinoxaline derivatives containing triazole moiety, Bioorg. Chem. 76 (2018) 343–358, https://doi.org/10.1016/j.bioorg.2017.12.003.

[85] S. Tariq, P. Kamboj, O. Alam, M. Amir, 1,2,4-Triazole-based benzothiazole/benzoxazole derivatives: Design, synthesis, p38α MAP kinase inhibition, anti-inflammatory activity and molecular docking studies, Bioorg. Chem. 81 (2018) 630–641, https://doi.org/10.1016/j.bioorg.2018.09.015.

[86] H.J. Zhang, X.Z. Wang, Q. Cao, G.H. Gong, Z.S. Quan, Design, synthesis, anti-inflammatory activity, and molecular docking studies of perimidine derivatives containing triazole, Bioorg. Med. Chem. Lett. 27 (18) (2017) 4409–4414, https://doi.org/10.1016/j.bmcl.2017.08.014.

[87] R. Paprocka, M. Wiese, A. Eljaszewicz, A. Helmin-Basa, A. Gzella, B. Modzelewska-Banachiewicz, J. Michalkiewicz, Synthesis and anti-inflammatory activity of new 1,2,4-triazole derivatives, Bioorg. Med. Chem. Lett. 25 (13) (2015) 2664–2667, https://doi.org/10.1016/j.bmcl.2015.04.079.

[88] M.B. Labib, A.M. Fayez, E.-S. El-Nahass, M. Awadallah, P.A. Halim, Novel tetrazole-based selective COX-2 inhibitors: design, synthesis, anti-inflammatory activity, evaluation of PGE2, TNF-α, IL-6 and histopathological study, Bioorg. Chem. 104 (2020), 104308, https://doi.org/10.1016/j.bioorg.2020.104308.

[89] R. Sribalan, G. Banuppriya, M. Kirubavathi, V. Padmini, Synthesis, biological evaluation and in silico studies of tetrazole-heterocycle hybrids, J. Mol. Struct. 1175 (2019) 577–586, https://doi.org/10.1016/j.molstruc.2018.07.114.

[90] P.F. Lamie, J.N. Philoppes, A.A. Azouz, N.M. Safwat, Novel tetrazole and cyanamide derivatives as inhibitors of cyclooxygenase-2 enzyme: design, synthesis, anti-inflammatory evaluation, ulcerogenic liability and docking study, J. Enzyme Inhib. Med. Chem. 32 (1) (2017) 805–820, https://doi.org/10.1080/14756366.2017.1326110.

[91] S. Yatam, S.S. Jadav, R. Gundla, K.P. Gundla, G.M. Reddy, M.J. Ahsan, J. Chimakurthy, Design, synthesis and biological evaluation of 2 (((5-aryl-1,2,4-oxadiazol-3-yl)methyl)thio)benzo[d]oxazoles: new antiinflammatory and antioxidant agents, ChemistrySelect 3 (37) (2018) 10305–10310, https://doi.org/10.1002/slct.201801558.

[92] A.K. Shakya, A. Kaur, B.O. Al-Najjar, R.R. Naik, Molecular modeling, synthesis, characterization and pharmacological evaluation of benzo[d]oxazole derivatives as non-steroidal anti-inflammatory

agents, Saudi Pharmaceut. J. 24 (5) (2016) 616–624, https://doi.org/10.1016/j.jsps.2015.03.018.

[93] M.V.P. dos Santos Nascimento, A.C. Mattar Munhoz, A.B.M. De Campos Facchin, E. Fratoni, T.A. Rossa, M. Mandolesi Sá, C.C. Campa, E. Ciraolo, E. Hirsch, E.M. Dalmarco, New pre-clinical evidence of anti-inflammatory effect and safety of a substituted fluorophenyl imidazole, Biomed. Pharmacother. 111 (2019) 1399–1407, https://doi.org/10.1016/j.biopha.2019.01.052.

[94] B. Sathish Kumar, P.V. Anantha Lakshmi, Synthesis and molecular docking studies of novel 1,2,3-triazole ring-containing 4-(1,4,5-triphenyl-1H-imidazol-2-yl)phenol derivatives as COX inhibitors, Res. Chem. Intermed. 44 (1) (2018) 455–467, https://doi.org/10.1007/s11164-017-3113-2.

[95] A.H. Abdelazeem, M.T. El-Saadi, A.G. Safi El-Din, H.A. Omar, S.M. El-Moghazy, Design, synthesis and analgesic/anti-inflammatory evaluation of novel diarylthiazole and diarylimidazole derivatives towards selective COX-1 inhibitors with better gastric profile, Bioorg. Med. Chem. 25 (2) (2017) 665–676, https://doi.org/10.1016/j.bmc.2016.11.037.

Chapter 20

In vivo models of understanding inflammation (in vivo methods for inflammation)

Poonam Negi[a], Shweta Agarwal[b], Prakrati Garg[c,d], Aaliya Ali[c,d], and Saurabh Kulshrestha[c,d]

[a]School of Pharmaceutical Sciences, Shoolini University, Solan, Himachal Pradesh, India, [b]Department of Pharmaceutics, L.R Institute of Pharmacy, Solan, Himachal Pradesh, India, [c]School of Applied Sciences and Biotechnology, Shoolini University, Solan, Himachal Pradesh, India, [d]Center for Omics and Biodiversity Research, Shoolini University, Solan, Himachal Pradesh, India

1 Introduction

Inflammation is the most common as well as a basic protective reaction of dwelling tissues to damage or to chemical exposure [1]. When there is a cell injury, the living machine responds to it and this response is inflammation. It is an all-time as well as essential shielding process against the damaging stimuli that includes infectious agents, physical, thermal, chemical agents, cancerous cells, ischemia, and antigen-antibody reactions with the aid of enhanced blood flow to the vicinity of injured tissue site [1,2]. It is a result of the spread of stimuli, together with immune reactions due to UV irradiation, physical damage, and microbial attack. The definitive key symptoms of the infections are warmth, ache, redness, and swelling. The inflammation cascades are responsible for the resulting illnesses, which constitute persistent bronchial asthma, psoriasis, multiple sclerosis, arthritis, and inflammatory bowel ailment [1]. Inflammation is likewise a first-rate threat to the affected person. It will increase the sickness and suffering of the patient because of the morbidity as well as the pain. The cyclooxygenase, arachidonic acid, and lipoxygenase-mediated activation of nearby inflammatory mediators including prostaglandins, thromboxane A2, leukotrienes, platelet-activating components, and prostacyclin have a critical role in the destruction of tissue and cause pain related to irritation [3,4]. Moreover, the inflammation is responsible for pus formation, which precludes the absorption of various antibiotics into the affected tissues resulting in tissue destruction [5]. Diseases related to inflammation are widely recognized as the key source of morbidity in the masses [6]. The inflammatory situation is related to the activated immune machine, consisting of activated biomolecules and immune cells.

Inflammation may be categorized as either acute, chronic, or miscellaneous [7–9]. Acute irritation can be a preliminary reaction of the body to damaging stimuli. Usually, the chronic irritation commences in 2–4 days after the start of the acute reaction and may remain for weeks to months and may be years because of the endurance of the beginning stimulus, involvement of the normal recovery technique, recurrent spells of acute inflammation, or low-grade soldering because of persevered production of immune response mediators. Chronic inflammation refers to granuloma formation. In the production of thromboxane, prostacyclin, and prostaglandins, cyclooxygenase (COX) is the primary enzyme. The enzymes might be involved in inflammation and responsible for pain as well as platelet aggregation [2]. There is appearance of acute inflammatory responses like warmth, redness, loss of function, and swelling. The enhanced flow of blood, nerve fiber sensitization, and increased vascular permeability are related to redness, pain, and swelling, respectively. The protecting consequences of the cascade related to inflammation and capability for tissue damage are typically balanced in a regular state. On the other hand, continual irritation is normally distinguished by enormous damage as well as restoration of wounded tissues from an inflammatory reaction [10]. If out of control, inflammation may become alarming in several diseased states like inflammatory bowel diseases, neoplastic variations, rheumatoid arthritis, psoriasis, a couple of sclerosis, and immune-inflammatory ailments [11]. Moreover, there is a link between chronic infection and various steps of tumorigenesis. It has also been identified as a threat for the incidence of various kinds of cancers [12]. The existence of low-grade continued inflammation is

Recent Developments in Anti-Inflammatory Therapy. https://doi.org/10.1016/B978-0-323-99988-5.00017-6

responsible for long-term sickness. The treatment of inflammatory sicknesses like inflammatory bowel diseases and rheumatoid arthritis (continual sickness) is still a matter of concern because of the lack of effective as well as safe medicine. Inflammation has been known to be a very common cause in most people for acute as well as persistent debilitating sicknesses and constitutes an important basis of morbidity in the current modern lifestyle. If not given proper attention, it may lead to the development of various illnesses like Alzheimer's disease, atherosclerosis, cancer, and rheumatoid arthritis, diabetes along with autoimmune, chronic pulmonary, and other cardiovascular problems. Inflammation includes a complicated community of several mediators, diffusion of cells, and implementation of numerous pathways [13]. Inflammation includes two primary processes, early inflammatory response later followed by restoration. Acute and persistent are two types of inflammation. Various unique animal models like ultraviolet erythema in guinea pigs, vascular permeability, paw edema in rats, croton-oil ear edema in rats and mice, adjuvant-induced arthritis, collagen-induced arthritis and papaya latex-Induced arthritis are made use of in the premedical study for the assessment of antiinflammatory potential. Animal models are used for the evaluation of inflammation, the pathogenesis of illnesses, and to check the capability of anti-inflammatory agents for medical use [1].

This chapter comprehensively discusses the animal models for the evaluation of inflammation and mechanisms of infection therein. The chapter encompasses the definition of inflammatory techniques and models used to observe the etiopathogenesis of inflammation in general, as well as their advantages and disadvantages for pharmacological assessment of antiinflammatory drug development from synthetic as well as natural sources.

2 The need for antiinflammatory agents

Inflammatory sicknesses, along with rheumatic diseases, are a crucial health issue globally, and in most of the human populace health is afflicted by these inflammation-associated problems. Numerous agents are available to deal with different types of inflammatory sicknesses; their extended use results in extreme detrimental effects. It is a traditional clinical practice to manage and treat inflammatory diseases with nonsteroidal or steroidal drugs. Nonsteroidal antiinflammatory drugs (NSAIDs) reduce the functions in the early steps of biosynthesis of prostaglandins by inhibiting cyclooxygenase (COX). To reduce undesired effects of inflammation the NSAIDs are the essential drugs [14]. The persistent use of NSAIDs is attached to renal, cardiovascular, and gastrointestinal toxicities [15]. Excess use of corticosteroids results in arrest of growth, hypertension, osteoporosis, and hyperglycemia [16], and on discontinuation relapse of symptoms and toxicity is a big problem

[14]. Thus, the development of safe and effective antiinflammatory drugs is very much warranted [17].

Antiinflammatory extracts derived from natural sources offer a rational and effective alternative for the management of inflammatory problems [15]. These products are safe to use, have good efficacy, are budget-friendly, and are biocompatible options for treating inflammation-related disorders [18]. Many nations like India, Sri Lanka, China, and Brazil have an interesting history of use of herbal products in therapeutics traditionally and also offer reliable protection of these herbal medicines. In the present times, the main focus in terms of experimental research is on pharmacological as well as molecular mechanisms as they are responsible for healing as well as health benefits. However, in the evolution of novel antiinflammatory leads, unification of conventional knowledge and indigenous assets will be of great use [6]. Many explorations on plant species, being used as folk remedy against inflammation, have increased the popularity of herbal preparations as antiinflammatory drugs. The efficacy of antiinflammatory phytoactives is due to their activity on pivotal regulatory molecules which includes cytokines, cyclooxygenase (COX), and inducible nitric oxide synthase (iNOS) [19,20].

3 The inflammatory cascade

There is involvement of many complex mediators in inflammation along with a localized rise in leukocytes at the site of inflammation. During inflammation, prostaglandins (the universal substance) modulate and direct tissue responses. The pathology of colonic adenoma, Alzheimer's disease, cancer, and cardiovascular disease involves the biosynthesis of prostaglandins. The short- and long-term inflammation happens in three stages; the first stage begins with an improved vascular permeability, leukocyte influx, accompanied by the formation of granuloma as well as tissue restoration [21]. There is release of different mediators because of adhesion molecules, chemokines, cytokines, arachidonic acid, and platelet-activating factors that initiate chemotaxis. Due to the host proteins like coagulation factors, kinins, and microbial products, there is activation of inflammatory mediators. The kinins, as well as complement proteins, originate from plasma. Furthermore, in the improvement of inflammatory diseases like arthritis, cancers, and asthma there is the involvement of cytokines, histamine, and prostaglandins originated from cells as well as arachidonic acid metabolites like 12-hydroxyeicosatetraenoic acid (12-HETE), leukotrienes (LTs), and prostaglandins (PGs) [22]. The activation of cell elements is a result of the phenomenon known as inflammation. Furthermore, there is the existence of diverse groups of biochemical mediators like kinases (MAP kinase, JNKs, p38 kinase), matrix metalloproteinases (MMPs), transcription elements, and cytokines (interleukin-1, e.g., TNF-α).

4 Key players of inflammation

4.1 Mediators derived from lipids

Arachidonic acid (AA) plays a main role as an eicosanoid precursor as well as a fundamental component of all body cells. Diverse phospholipase enzymes are brought into play, especially phospholipase A2 (PLA2). PLA2 is responsible for the liberation of AA from membrane phospholipids. Metabolism of AA takes place through multiple pathways with the aim to form a couple of oxygenated molecules called eicosanoids. There is the production of thromboxane (prostanoids) as well as prostaglandins (PGs) due to cyclooxygenase (COX). On the other hand, the lipoxins (LXs) and leukotrienes (LTs) are produced from lipoxygenases (LOX). Furthermore, cytochrome P450 enzymes form epoxyeicosatrienoic acids (EETs) [23]. Eicosanoids modify the diverse inflammatory and homeostatic system, which is connected to several diseases [24]. The pro-inflammatory interest of mediators derived from lipids has been elaborately documented. Constriction of the bronchii, secretion of mucus, vasodilation, and vascular permeability are all linked to PGs. Leukotrienes, on the other hand, are thought to be bronchoconstrictors as well as activators of vasodilation and permeability of the vasculature. Leukotriene B4 (LTB4) is linked to the activation of the neutrophils and the generation of superoxide. It also boosts the production of interleukin-6 (IL-6) and incites early gene transcription of additional cytokines. The 5-lipoxygenase (5-LOX) enzyme is required for leukotriene production, and leukotrienes (LTs) are important mediators in inflammatory and allergy responses. As a result, inhibiting 5-LOX is a viable therapy option for dermatitis and psoriasis. Another mediator causing constriction of the bronchi, activation of platelets, and chemotaxis is the platelet-activating factor (PAF), which is produced by a variety of inflammatory cells such as macrophages, neutrophils, eosinophils, and endothelial cells [13].

4.2 Pro-inflammatory cytokines

Cytokines affect immunological responses and inflammation in different ways. The family of cytokines includes interferons, interleukins, tumor necrosis factors, and colony stimulatory factors. In target cells, cytokines influence the expression of molecule adhesion, mobile growth, apoptosis, immunoglobulin synthesis, and chemotaxis [13]. When monocytes and macrophages are activated, pro-inflammatory cytokines such as tumor necrosis factor (TNF-α), interleukin-1 (IL-1β), and interleukin-6 (IL-6β) are released. TNF-α is associated with the spread of tumor cells and the pathophysiology of rheumatoid arthritis. IL-1 causes bone resorption by activating lymphocytes. TNF-α and IL-1β modify adhesion molecule expression and also

trap circulating leukocytes; and cytokines activate intracellular signaling cascades that lead to transcription [25].

4.3 Vasoactive mediators

Histamine is an extensively distributed and produced pro-inflammatory mediator found mostly in mast cells and in basophil leukocytes. Following tissue injury, the released histamine results in a transient increase in permeability. Histamine causes contractions of the endothelial cells and permits fluid and proteins to pass through the interendothelial junctions. Histamine increases vascular permeability, which causes edema and promotes gastric acid secretion. It causes endothelial cell enlargement and leukocyte adhesion at higher doses. As a result, histamine is the most important mediator that triggers initial vascular alterations during an inflammatory reaction. Serotonin is a neurotransmitter present in the intestine, the brain, and platelets, and it is the primary source of increased vascular permeability and muscle contraction. It also causes venous constriction and reduces capillary flow, resulting in stasis, at greater concentrations. Bradykinin causes cellular endothelial separation, resulting in gaps in postcapillary venules and increased permeability of the vasculature [13].

4.4 Hydrolytic enzymes

Activated pro-inflammatory cells secrete accumulated proteolytic enzymes during inflammation. The main elastic component of arteries and lungs, and proteins such as collagen, proteoglycans, and immunoglobulins undergo elastin hydrolysis and endothelial movement of activated pro-inflammatory mediators resulting from the liberation of human leukocyte elastase (HLE) from active polymorphonuclear leukocytes (PMNL) [13].

4.5 Reactive oxygen species (ROS)

Inflammation and oxidative stress are pathologically linked to a variety of disorders [26]. The function of reactive oxygen species (ROS) in cell defense systems is critical. The reactive oxygen species (ROS), liberated by inflammatory cells raises oxidative pressure, which activates intracellular signaling pathways and promotes pro-inflammatory gene expression. The endogenous and unfastened antioxidative mechanisms and radical scavengers are hampered by the increased production of radicals and peroxides, causing functionally important systems to deteriorate [13].

4.6 Transcription factors

Genes' transcription, which is involved in apoptosis, adhesion of cells, proliferation, mobile pressure response, response of the immune system, pathways of inflammation, and tissue remodeling is controlled by nuclear factor-kappa beta (NF-κB), which acts as the primary regulator of the immune and inflammatory responses [27]. It also controls the expression of inflammatory cytokines such as IL-1, IL-2, IL-6, IL-8, and TNF-α, as well as genes encoding COX-2, iNOS, mobile adhesion molecules, immune receptors, and growth factor receptors. Glucocorticoids, aspirin at high doses, and sulfasalazine all inhibit NF-κB activation. As a result, NF-κB is an exciting remedial target for the treatment of inflammatory diseases.

4.7 Complement system

The anaphylatoxins C3a and C5a, as well as the membrane assault complex, are formed when the complement cascade is activated. C5a is a powerful chemoattractant that promotes antibody creation and release of cytokines, PGs, and leukotrienes, as well as oxidative stress. Inflammatory cells such as neutrophils, eosinophils, monocytes, and T lymphocytes are also attracted to it. C5a is an example of a product that features influencing biological activity that starts the inflammatory cascade [13].

5 In vivo models of understanding inflammation

In vivo screening methods for assessing the effectiveness and potency of antiinflammatory drugs involve producing inflammation in investigational animals such as rats, mice, dogs, and monkeys of both sexes.

5.1 Vascular permeability

Vascular permeability rises during the stages of inflammation, allowing plasma additives such as antibodies to reach infected or wounded tissues. This is exploited for the calculation of the inhibitory effect of a drug against phlogistic substances-induced elevated vascular permeability. Prostaglandins, histamine, and leukotrienes are released in response to stimulation, causing arterioles and venules to dilate and permeability of the vasculature to rise. Consequently, excess proteins of the plasma, fluids, and edemas are created. The important dye, Evan's, blue can be used to identify the greater rate of permeability by infiltrating the injected locations [28].

5.1.1 Enhanced permeability of the vasculature by the Arthus reaction

Methodology

In this approach, four Wistar rats can be employed in each group. Administration of distilled water 1% w/v 1 mL/100 g orally in the control group, the test chemical in another group, and diclofenac 10 mL/kg by the intraperitoneal

way in the standard group is done. Rats are given 0.25 mL of a 0.6% v/v acetic acid solution intraperitoneally thereafter. Evan's blue (10% w/v) is injected into the tail vein at a rate of 10 mL/kg intravenously. After 30 min, ether is used as anesthesia to anesthetize the animals and then animals are sacrificed. To expose the viscera, the abdomen is dissected. The animals are held in place with a flap of their abdominal wall. The peritoneal fluid (exudates) is collected, filtered, and diluted with normal saline solution before centrifuging for 15 min at 3000 rpm. Using a spectrophotometer, the absorbance (A) of the supernatant is determined at 590 nm [29].

Evaluation

Reduced permeability is indicated by a decrease in dye concentration on assessing the absorbance values.

5.1.2 Acetic acid/compound 48/80-induced vascular permeability

The test is intended to assess the suppressive action of medications and compounds in the presence of phlogistic agents such as acetic acid and compound 48/80, which cause increased permeability of the vasculature. Compound 48/80 causes mast cell degranulation and is a powerful promoter of the release of histamine. Vascular permeability increases during the inflammatory phase to permit plasma constituents like antibodies and complements to reach infected or wounded tissues. When mast cells are stimulated, mediators like histamine, prostaglandins, and leukotrienes are liberated. The dilation of arterioles and venules improves vascular permeability. Proteins of plasma and fluids are extravasated, increasing the permeability of the vasculature and causing edema. The application of Evan's blue dye at the injection site identifies the accelerated vascular permeability [30].

5.1.3 UV-erythema in guinea pigs

Levels of prostaglandin E (PGE) in the skin of guinea pigs have been demonstrated to improve after 24 h of exposure to UV (ultraviolet light) between 280 and 320 nm. The evolution of PGE phases corresponded to the erythema's delayed appearance. The appearance of UV erythema on albino guinea pig skin was delayed by phenylbutazone and other NSAIDs (nonsteroidal antiinflammatory drugs). An initial sign of inflammation is redness followed by exudation of plasma and edema formation [31].

Methodology

Albino guinea pigs, both male and female, having a weight of approximately 350 g, can be employed in this approach. A total of 18 h before the experiment animals are shaved on sides and back using a suspension of barium chloride or depilatory cream. On the second day of the experiment, the compound to be tested is dissolved in the vehicle, and 30 min before UV exposure, half of the test compound is given to the animal by gastrogavage. Vehicle treatment is only given to the control group of animals. Animals are kept in leather shackles with holes of size 1.5 cm × 2.5 cm for the penetration of UV radiation to the affected zone. And finally, the rest of the test compound is added and after 2 and 4 h of exposure, erythema is recorded [1].

Evaluation

A double blind procedure is used to evaluate the degree of erythema. The scores below are used:

0—Absence of erythema
1—Weak erythema
2—Strong erythema
4—Very strong erythema

A total count of 0 in animals is said to be in the protected zone. Calculation of the duration of the effect and ED50 values is done by calculating scores above 2 and 4 [32].

5.1.4 Pleurisy tests

Induction of pleurisy in animals is done by various sources of irritants like dextran, enzymes, microbes, mast cell degranulation, histamine, prostaglandins, and antigen bradykinin, and by using irritants that are nonspecific like carrageenan and turpentine [33,34]. Exudative inflammation is a symptom of pleurisy [33]. Phlogistic substances such as dextran, carrageenan, enzymes, antigens, and compound 48/80 can also cause it in experimental animals. In the evaluation of acute inflammation, carrageenan-induced pleurisy is performed. This model is used to assess phenomena such as fluid leakage, leukocyte movement, and biochemical characteristics in exudates [33]. Quantity determination of exudates of the pleura, total protein content, and curbing of leukocyte movement is employed to demonstrate the acute antiinflammatory activity of test substances [35].

Methodology

One dose of 0.1 mL carrageenan is given intravenously to animals (mice) for the induction of pleurisy. After 4 h, the animals are killed by overdosing with ether and the pleural cavity is cleansed with 1.0 mL of sterile phosphate-buffered saline (PBS) having heparin (20 IU per mL). Exudate presence, level of nitric oxide (NO), adenosine deaminase activity, myeloperoxidase, and total differential leukocyte counts are all measured in pleural lavage samples. In a Neubauer's chamber, the total leukocyte count is determined. The C-reactive protein level in blood is also determined. In another series of experiments, animals are given Evan's blue dye solution (25 mg/kg, i.v.) 30 min prior to carrageenan administration to assess the extent of pleural exudation [36].

Estimation is done by interpolating from an Evan's blue dye standard curve in the range of 0.01–50 g/mL; the dye amount at 600 nm is determined by colorimetry with the help of an ELISA Plate Reader.

Evaluation

The average of every investigational group's values is calculated and compared to that of the control groups. The ED50 values for different doses are also calculated.

5.2 Edema

5.2.1 Croton-oil ear edema in rats and mice

Edema of the ear generated by croton oil or its irritating ingredient 12-O-tetradecanoylphorbol-13-acetate (TPA) is exploited to gauge the antiinflammatory effect of steroidal and nonsteroidal antiinflammatory medications. This model of skin inflammation is valuable for evaluating systemic and local antiinflammatory drugs because topical croton oil application promotes vasodilation, permeability of vasculature, influx of neutrophils, production of eicosanoids, and serotonin and histamine liberation [37]. This model can be used to test plant extracts as well as synthetic antiinflammatory drugs. Increased vascular permeability is primarily caused by PGI2 and LTB4, and COX and LOX inhibitory drugs are anticipated to reduce TPA-induced inflammation. Furthermore, TPA's pro-inflammatory effects are aided by protein kinase C activation, which turns on other enzymes such as mitogen-activated protein kinases (MAPKs) and phospholipase A2. COX, LOX, and PLA2 inhibitors, as well as corticoids, can reduce inflammation that occurs after TPA is applied topically [38]. The 5-lipoxygenase (5-LOX) and cyclooxygenase (COX) enzymes increase dilation and permeability of the vasculature, polymorphonuclear leukocyte movement, the deliverance of histamine and serotonin, and mild formation of inflammatory eicosanoids. In animal models of crotons, COX and 5-LOX inhibitors, leukotriene B4 (LTB4) antagonists, and corticosteroids demonstrated topical antiinflammatory activity [20].

Both rats and mice are utilized in this process; typically, rats of male gender (SD) weighing 80–60 g and male Swiss mice weighing 18 and 22 g are chosen and clustered in accordance to body weight. An amount of 15 μL containing an acetone solution of 75 g croton oil is spread on the inner surface of each animal's right ear in this method. Diethyl ether is used to anesthetize the animals at a rate of 0.02 mL in rats and 0.01 mL in mice [1].

Methodology

The control group receives an irritating solution while the left ear is left untreated, and indomethacin is utilized as a standard or reference. For inflammation reduction, different levels of dose of the test medication are administered to the inner surface of the mouse's right ear. After the test and standard drugs are applied, animals are sacrificed by dislocating the cervical vertebra. An approximately 8-mm diameter plug is taken out from each of the treated and untreated ears. The measure of edematous response is taken by calculating the weight difference between the two plugs [1].

Evaluation

The main focus of this procedure is to ascertain the antiinflammatory potential of steroid drugs. Calculation of percentage antiinflammatory activity is done by the formula [1],

$$\%\text{Antiinflammatory activity}$$
$$= (\text{wt.of the treated ear} - \text{wt.of untreated ear/wt.}$$
$$\text{of the control ear}) \times 100.$$

5.2.2 Ear edema induced by Oxazolone in mice

The most commonly utilized allergy-causing agent for the beginning of delayed-type hypersensitivity (DTH) is oxazolone, which causes an increase in CD8+ T-lymphocytes and skin sensitization. The topical use of oxazolone boosts arachidonate metabolites such prostaglandins and leukotrienes in tissues [39]. Chronic contact dermatitis is caused by applying oxazolone to an experimental animal's ear regularly. Persistent swelling of the ear, visible inflammatory cell penetration, and significant hyperplasia of the epidermis are all prominent symptoms. Oxazolone also induces an increase in interferon-α (IFN-α) levels and minor changes in IL-4 levels. Interferon activates a variety of inflammatory cells, promotes keratinocyte proliferation, and induces epidermal thickening [40]. This is a delayed contact hypersensitivity paradigm that aids in the quantitative assessment of medication regarding antiinflammatory activity at the topical and systemic levels.

Methodology

Mice are used in this method and 12 animals or any other such number can be used in each group. A 0.01-mL injection of 0.5% oxazolone in acetone is given to the right ear three times in a week for sensitization, whereas acetone alone is given in the control group of animals. Inside the right ear, another injection of 0.01 mL 2% oxazolone solution is given, this time with test or standard solutions. Each group of 10–15 mice is given either the irritant or the test medication or chemical solution. The left ear remains untreated, and inflammation develops after 24h. The animals are sacrificed under anesthesia, and an 8-mm diameter disc is pierced from both sides, allowed to dry and is then weighed. Weight discrepancy is a sign that edema is developing [1].

Evaluation

For each test and control group, the average of weight gain is calculated and statistically compared [41,42].

5.2.3 Paw edema in rats

Antiinflammatory medications' efficacy in reducing edema in the rat's hind paw following injection of a phlogistic agent such as brewer's yeast, formaldehyde, dextran, egg albumin, kaolin, Aerosil, and others is assessed by this method. The paw volume is noted before and after the application of irritant, and the treated animals' volume of paw is compared to that of the control group. Three separate phases of carrageenan-induced rat paw edemas have been identified. Phase one is triggered by mast cell degranulation and the release of histamine and serotonin (1h), phase two is triggered by the liberation of bradykinin and pain, and phase three is triggered by the creation of eicosanoid (3–4h). As a result, this model assesses to which mediator's inhibition is the test compound's antiinflammatory action related.

Methodology

The animals utilized are usually Sprague-Dawley rats of both male and female gender, weighing between 100 and 150g. The animals are starved overnight. The rats are given 5mL water through a stomach tube (control) or the test medication mixed in the same volume to ensure consistent hydration. The rats are challenged 30min later with a subcutaneous injection of 0.05mL of 1% solution of carrageenan into the plantar side of the left hind paw. At the level of the lateral malleolus, marking of the paw is done with ink and then immersed in mercury up to this point. Plethysmographic measurements of the paw volume are taken immediately after injection, 3 and 6h later, and finally 24h later. For plethysmography of the paw, various devices can be used, including mercury for paw immersion. More advanced apparatuses relying on the principle of converting the volume increase by immersion of paw into a proportional voltage with the help of a pressure transducer, and a sensitive method for measuring the paw volume by connecting a Mettler Delta Range toploading balance with a microcrystal are also commercially available.

Evaluation

For each animal, the augmentation in paw volume after 3 or 6h is computed as a percentage of the volume determined immediately after the irritant injection. Animals that have been effectively treated have substantially less edema. For each time interval, the difference in average values between treated and control animals is assessed and statistically analyzed. The differences at varied time intervals provide an insight into the antiinflammatory effect's persistence. For active medications, a dose-response curve is generated, and ED50 values are calculated [29,43].

5.2.4 Paw edema induced by Carrageenan in rats

In rats, acute swelling is generated by injecting a solution of carrageenan in saline, which causes acute swelling that peaks after 3–5h and diminishes after 24h [44]. This inflammation evaluation model can be used to assess inflammatory mediator production at locations of inflammation, nonsteroidal antiinflammatory medication's antiinflammatory characteristics, and the efficiency of claimed analgesic substances in reversing cutaneous sensitivity. Carrageenan-induced inflammation in the footpad, manifested as edema and hypersensitivity, is one of the methods used to produce and measure it.

The antiinflammatory action of a variety of substances is assessed using this method [45]. This is a unique model of acute inflammation with a higher level of repeatability. Carrageenan is a phlogistic agent that is nonantigenic and has no systemic effects [46]. The activation of the complement system and inflammatory mediators is attributed to sulfated sugars found in carrageenan. The early phase of inflammation is triggered by carrageenan's stimulation of phospholipase A2, whereas the cytotoxicity advances the inflammation. Carrageenan distends postcapillary venules, causing inflammatory fluid and cells to exude. Several pro-inflammatory mediators are released during this process. The early exudative inflammatory phase is represented by these events, and their suppression stops the inflammatory process [47]. The carrageenan model is associated with the triggering on of the cyclooxygenase pathway. An antiinflammatory effect is seen in this preclinical model using glucocorticoids and prostaglandin antagonists. A biphasic curve depicts the edema caused by carrageenan. The ordeal of injection and release of acute phase mediators, including serotonin and histamine, are largely responsible for the initial phase of carrageenan-induced inflammation. The primary participants in the development of phase two of carrageenan-induced inflammation, occurring 3h after carrageenan injection, are prostaglandins [48].

Methodology

Male or female SD rats weighing between 150 and 170g may be used in this method. Overnight, the animals are starved. The animals should be divided into groups based on the test substances used. The rats are tested by injecting 0.05mL of a 1% carrageenan solution into the plantar side of the left hind paw 30min later. At the lateral malleolus level, the paw is marked with ink and immersed in mercury up to the mark for measurement of volume [49].

Evaluation

At 3, 6, and 24h following the injection, a plethysmometer or a micrometer is used to measure the paw volume and the paw volume growth is calculated after 3 and 6h. At each period, the difference in average values between treated and control group animals is assessed to determine the percentage increase in paw volume. The ED50 values are calculated using a dose-response curve for the active medications. Animals in the treated group generally have markedly reduced edema than those in the control group [49].

Calculations

$$\%\text{Inhibition of edema} = A - B/A \times 100 \ [45]$$

where A is the volume of edema in the control group and B is the volume of edema in the treated group.

5.2.5 Arachidonic acid-induced ear edema in mice

One of the most significant advantages of this strategy is that it decreases the effect of interanimal variability in inflammatory stimulus reactivity and makes up for consistent bias in removing both of the animal's ears. The proportional weight increases are ascertained using a paired t-test of the two values. A total of 24h before applying arachidonic acid to the ear, the mice of one group will be treated with compound 48/80 subcutaneously [50].

Methodology

A solution of 2mg arachidonic acid in 10:1 tetrahydrofuran: methanol is administered topically to the inner surface of both ears of the animal. For first dose-dependency experiments, varying quantities of arachidonic acid in ethanol are used. In most cases, compounds that have been evaluated for their inhibitory capability are mixed into the arachidonic acid solution and administered solely to the ear on the left side. On each ear of the control animals, only the solvent is applied. Animals have to be sacrificed after 1h by the method of dislocation of the cervical vertebra.

Evaluation

Both left and right ears are weighed after cutting them off at the base of hairline and the swelling caused by arachidonic acid is assessed as an elevation in the weight of the right ears compared to the weight of the right ears of solvent-treated control animals, expressed as a percentage of the weight of the right ears of solvent-treated control animals. The increase in the weight of left ears above the weight of the left ears of the control animals in the presence of the test chemical will also be represented as a fraction of the weight of the solvent-treated left ears [50]

These values are given as percentage of the full (right ear) swelling, and so a percentage inhibition by the test compound can be assessed.

5.2.6   Ear edema induced by Xylene in mice

Drugs' acute inflammatory potential can be assessed in mice [51]. The mice are split randomly into different groups of eight animals each. The groups are vehicle control, ASA positive control, and test groups. The drugs are administered orally for 6 consecutive days. After 1 h of oral administration on day 7, 30 µL of xylene has to be spread on both the surfaces of the right ear to cause edema. The left ear will serve as a control. The animals are sacrificed by cervical dislocation 30 min after treating with xylene. The right and left ears of mice have to be taken out using a cork borer of diameter 8 mm and after this, the ears are weighed. The edema weight difference is measured for the right and left ears of the same mice. The comparison of the percentage of suppression with the control group is then done [52].

5.2.7   Paw edema induced by histamine/5-HT

The screening of different antiinflammatory drugs is done using histamine- and 5-HT-induced paw inflammation models. A major mediator of acute inflammation is histamine. Histamine and 5-HT increase vascular permeability and cause inflammation when combined with prostaglandins [53].

The leakage of fluid and proteins of the plasma into extracellular spaces is caused by the subplantar injection of histamine. It promotes the movement of lymph and, as a result, the formation of edema. H1 receptors are acted upon by histamine, causing the contraction and separation of endothelial cells at their boundaries which increases the permeability of the vasculature. Histamine also causes hyperalgesia and inflammation by releasing neuropeptides and prostaglandins. Interendothelial gaps are created by acute phase mediators like 5-HT, which enhance vascular permeability. These mediators are found in the granules of mast cells and are produced when they are stimulated. These mediators promote plasma extravagance by acting through receptors on surrounding capillaries [54].

5.2.8   Bradykinin-induced paw edema

Prostaglandins (PGs) have a role in this technique (PGs). Bradykinin stimulates phospholipase activity, which increases PG production. The ability of indomethacin to prevent paw edema induced by bradykinin supports the theory that PGs are involved in the development of paw edema, which is induced by bradykinin. When human endothelial cell cultures are incubated with bradykinin, metabolites of arachidonic acid are produced [55].

5.2.9   Paw edema induced by dextran

Enhancement in the permeability of the vasculature, kinin activation, and liberation of chemical substances such as histamine and serotonin are all involved in the dextran-induced paw edema, which results in osmotic edema with little neutrophils and proteins [56]. Dextran causes edema that develops quickly and is only temporary [57]. Following dextran injection, histamine and serotonin are released, resulting in interactions between these mediators and their receptors (H1, H2, and 5HT2).

5.2.10   Paw edema induced by lipopolysaccharide (LPS)

In the mouse paw, LPS has been accepted to cause increase in TNF-α, IL-1, and myeloperoxidase activity based on time. The screening of medicines that show action against TNF-mediated inflammation is aided by LPS-induced paw edema. LPS is injected subplantarly in the rat paw, causing an immediate inflammatory response which is localized, and edema of the injected paw [58].

5.2.11   Paw edema induced by formalin

This model is quite similar to human arthritis. It is considered a good experimental paradigm for evaluating the antiinflammatory effects of various drugs over time. Inflammation caused by formalin is biphasic. Histamine, 5-HT, prostaglandins, and bradykinin participate in the early neurogenic phase, while histamine, 5-HT, prostaglandins, and bradykinin take part in the later inflammatory phase. Opioids and other CNS-acting medications inhibit both stages equally. NSAIDs and corticosteroids, which operate through the peripheral nervous system, are the only medications that suppress the second phase [59].

5.3   Granuloma

5.3.1   Granuloma pouch technique

The administration of irritating chemicals into the subcutaneous (sc) air pouch causes granulation tissue to proliferate. Endothelial cells and fibroblasts make up the majority of the tissues. In addition, irritating chemical administration promotes macrophage and polymorphonuclear leukocyte infiltration. There is a chance that developing tissue will be exposed to carcinogenic and mutagenic chemicals in this model. It's preferable to inject the test chemicals inside an air pouch since this ensures that the compounds being tested are in close proximity with the target cells [30].

When an irritating material is introduced into a subcutaneous pocket of air, granulation tissue's proliferation is initiated which eventually entirely fills the interior of the pouch. Fibroblasts, endothelial cells, and macrophage and polymorphonuclear leukocyte infiltration make up this tissue. This rapidly developing tissue in the GPA is susceptible to carcinogenic and mutagenic substances. The ability to put the test chemicals in close proximity with the cells to be targeted by injecting them into the pocket of air is one of the system's key advantages. The substance can be administered orally as well as parenterally. It does not give quantifiable data on the test chemicals' cytotoxicity in vivo.

Methodology

The animals utilized are Sprague-Dawley rats weighing between 150 and 200 g for control and test groups. The backs of animals are shaved and cleaned. A pneumoderma is created in the center of the dorsal skin using a very tiny needle and 20 mL air injected under anesthesia [60].

Air is removed from the pouch 48 h later, and any adhesions that arise are broken 72 h later. As an irritant, 1 mL of 20% carrageenan suspension formulated in sesame oil might be made use of instead of croton oil. On commencement of the development of the pouch, the animals are given the test chemical or the standard every day, either orally or subcutaneously. The chemical to be tested is injected into the air sac simultaneously with the irritant to test local activity. The animals are sacrificed under anesthethesia after 3 or 4 days. Exudate is accumulated in glass cylinders once the bag is opened. The pouches are rinsed with 1 mL saline, the exudates are chilled on ice, and the volume is measured. After staining with Erythrosine B, the aggregate of leukocytes that moved into the pouch is determined, and the residual exudates are centrifuged at 3000 rpm for 10 min at 4°C, and the supernatant is kept at −20°C until used [1].

Evaluation

The mean value for control and test groups' exudates is determined. Statistical methods are used to make the comparison [60].

5.3.2 Cotton wool granuloma

Subcutaneous implantation of compressed cotton pellet-induced foreign body granulomas in rats is carried out in this method. Apart from fluid infiltration, histologically large cells and undifferentiated connective tissue can be seen after a few days. Weighing the dry pellets after removal can be used to determine the quantity of freshly produced connective tissue. If the cotton pellets are treated with carrageenan, more intense granuloma development is seen.

Methodology

Rats weighing 180–200 g can be utilized in the experiment. The test medicines are given by the oral route, once every day for 7 days, whereas the control group receives the vehicle. Under mild ether anesthesia and sterile procedure, two sterilized cotton wool pellets are inserted in the subcutaneous layer, one on either side of the animal's belly. On the seventh day, the rats are sacrificed. Wet weight is measured after dissecting the implanted pellets. Thymuses are also taken apart. The dry weight of both the pellet and the thymus is measured after 18 h of drying at 60°C.

Evaluation

The test medicines' percent granuloma inhibition, as well as the weights of the transudate and granuloma, are determined. The increase in body weight is also noted [43].

5.3.3 Glass rod granuloma

Glass rod granuloma exhibits signs of proliferative inflammation that has been present for a long time. Wet weight as well as dry weight, chemical composition and characteristics, may be assessed in newly created connective tissue.

Methodology

The ends of glass rods possessing a diameter of 6 mm are rounded off by flame melting and cut to a length of 40 mm. The rear skin of male Sprague-Dawley rats having approximately 130 g weight, is shaved and cleaned after they have been anesthetized with ether. With closed blunted forceps, a tunnel is created in the subcutaneous layer in the cranial direction from a caudal incision. A glass rod is inserted through the tube and eventually lands on the animal's back. Sutures are used to seal the incision wound. The animals are separated into cages. For 20–40 days, the rods are left in place. Drug treatment might be given for the entire duration or only during the final 10–20 days. The animals are finally sacrificed under carbondioxide anesthesia. The glass rods are produced in conjunction with the connective tissue that surrounds them, forming a tube. The glass rod is removed and the sac of granuloma is turned inside out, resulting in a simple section of connective tissue. The granuloma tissue's wet weight is reported. The granuloma tissue is finally dried and the weight of dry tissue is reported. Biochemical studies, like collagen and glycosaminoglycan assessment, are also possible.

Evaluation

This approach may be used to determine a number of factors. When compared to the reference compound, the weight of the granuloma is usually found to be lowered by the test compound [29].

5.3.4 Granuloma induced by cotton pellet

The pathogenic sequence of events of chronic inflammation is represented by this model. It is a commonly utilized paradigm for evaluating novel drugs' persistent antiinflammatory efficacy. Monocyte infiltration, fibroblast proliferation, angiogenesis, and exudation are all signs of it [61]. This model is used to gauge the transudation and proliferation-related aspects of chronic inflammation. A persistent inflammatory condition is marked by the development of granulomatous tissue. Granulation tissue is a highly vascularized reddish mass formed by augmentation of macrophages, neutrophils, and fibroblasts, as well as growth of tiny blood vessels. The amount of fluid absorbed by the pellet has a significant impact on the granuloma's moist (wet) weight. The development of transudate and granulomatous tissue is connected to the moist and dry weight of cotton pellets, respectively. Inflammation is inhibited by corticosteroids during the proliferative phase [62].

5.4 Arthritis

5.4.1 Collagen-induced arthritis (CIA)

Injections of type II collagenin (CII) in the dermis and an adjuvant are used to induce the procedure. Heterologous CII from chick, bovine, or rat origin is commonly utilized for induction. This is an MHC-dependent condition that is distinguished by joint inflammation accompanied with erosion, mediated by T and B cells in the body. However, the etiology and duration of the disease differ noticeably based on the genetic framework of the animal and the source of the CII utilized to induce disease [63].

Methodology

Animals used must be 8–10 weeks old at the time of immunization. By stirring at 4°C overnight, native type II collagen is mixed with 0.1N acetic acid at a concentration level of 2 mg/mL. Before adding it to incomplete Freund's adjuvant, thermally annihilated Mycobacterium tuberculosis is crushed in a mortar and pestle (IFA). A homogenizer is used at high speed to emulsify equal amounts of adjuvant and collagen solution for 2 min. Each animal gets a 0.1 mL injection of the resultant emulsion intradermally in the tail. With 100 g of denatured CII, other animal groups are vaccinated in the same way. On day 28, an intradermal injection of 100 g of antigen whose emulsification is done in

incomplete Freund's adjuvant is administered in the dorsal skin. As a first injection, the control animals receive an equivalent amount of 0.1N acetic acid emulsified with IFA having 250 g of Mycobacterium tuberculosis, followed by a booster dose of acetic acid in IFA only on day 28.

Evaluation

Each mouse is allocated an arthritic index based on the given criteria: 0, no symptoms of arthritis; (1) single-joint swelling and redness; (2) multiple-joint inflammation; and (3) severe swelling, joint erosion, and/or ankylosis. Every paw is given a score between 0 and 3, and the paws having arthritis are multiplied by their score, with the index equal to the total of all the paws (72.93).

5.4.2 Adjuvant-induced arthritis model in rats

The most frequently used animal model for arthritis is Freund's full adjuvant-induced arthritis in rats, which has clinical and laboratory characteristics that resemble the clinical aspects of rheumatoid arthritis in humans [4]. This model is responsive to antiinflammatory and immunosuppressive medications, making it suitable for research into the pathophysiology and pharmacological regulation of the progress of inflammation, and also the evaluation of analgesic therapeutic potential. The eicosanoid pathway, namely inhibitors of cyclooxygenases (COX 1 and COX 2)—NSAIDs—are focus of the rat adjuvant-induced arthritis model (nonsteroidal antiinflammatory drugs) [64].

Methodology

An intradermal injection of Freund's Complete Adjuvant (FCA) containing 1.0 mg dry thermally annihilated Mycobacterium tuberculosis per milliliter of sterile paraffin oil is injected into the foot pad of a male rat's left hind paw to cause arthritis. For injection, a 1 mL glass syringe with locking hubs and a 26G needle were utilized. Because the thick nature of the adjuvant makes injecting problematic, the rats are sedated with ether inhalation before and during the injection of adjuvant. A digital plethysmometer was used to check the swelling in each paw from the ankle regularly (up to 21 days) [7,65,66].

5.4.3 Papaya latex-induced arthritis

To investigate the antiinflammatory effect of slow acting antirheumatic medicines (SARMs), a papaya latex-induced model of experimental rheumatoid arthritis was established. Prostaglandins are recognized as having a role in papaya latex-induced inflammation [1].

Methodology

A solution of papaya latex of concentration 0.25% is prepared and 0.1 mL of it is injected into the rat hind paw (made in 0.05M sodium acetate buffer, pH 4.5, having 0.01% thymol). The impact peaks at 3h and lasts for over 5h. For NSAIDs like aspirin and ibuprofen, and steroidal antiinflammatory medications, the technique is sensitive [67,68].

5.4.4 Monosodium urate crystal-induced arthritis

Purine's unmetabolized product, uric acid, is deposited in the synovial joint, causing bradykinin activation, neutrophil granulocyte build-up, and an intermittent episode of acute arthritis or gout. To cause arthritis, sodium urate crystal suspensions (20mg) are injected intradermally into the knee joint of experimental animals. After the injection, the animals are seen to be in excruciating agony and prostration as if they were having an intense gout attack.

Methodology

A monosodium urate (MSU) crystal suspension, free from endotoxins, is injected in a volume of 0.2mL (4mg) in the right foot pad to cause inflammation. Days 0–3 are taken into account. Normal therapy and testing is started on day 0 half an hour before the MSU injection and is continued for 3 days.

Preparation of monosodium urate crystals

MSU crystals are prepared by dissolving 4g uric acid in 800mL water, heating with sodium hydroxide solution (9mL/0.5N), adjusting the pH to 8.9 at 60°C. This is then cooled for 12h in a cold room, washed and dried. The needle-shaped crystals are suspended in sterile saline (20mg/mL) after recovering them.

5.4.5 Grip strength of arthritic animals

In this approach, arthritis is induced by injecting silver nitrate into the tibiotarsal joint of rats or injecting talc in intra-articular regions of pigeons. With irritated paws, this reduces locomotor activity. NSAIDs, steroids, DMARDs, and antihistamines are all effective medications for which this test can be carried out. [69].

5.4.6 Complete Freund's adjuvant (CFA)-induced arthritis

In experimental mice, the CFA-induced arthritis model represents persistent inflammation with numerous systemic alterations as well as synovial hyperplasia [70]. Massive leukocyte infiltration, a rise in levels of chemokines and cytokines, such as IL-1 and TNF-α, the giving off of reactive oxygen species (ROS), cartilage and bone damage, as well as edema and deformation, are its symptoms. CFA injection in the rat's footpad results in the expansion of periarticular tissues like ligaments and joint capsules. Edema caused by CFA rises progressively during the early stages of inflammation and then stabilizes after 2 weeks. The reduction in paw inflammation caused by CFA is a measure of the test drug's antiinflammatory efficacy. Measurement of injected (ipsilateral) and noninjected (contralateral) paw edema, as well as antioxidant approximation, visual arthritis scoring system, nitrite content assessment, hematological and biochemical estimations, and radiological and histopathological evaluations, all aid in determining the likely mechanisms of the antiinflammatory and analgesic activities of test compounds [71].

5.5 Dextran sulfate sodium-induced colitis in mice

Animals like mouse, hamster, and rat can be used and are given dextran sulfate sodium (DSS) to cause colitis in this model. The animals are maintained in a regular laboratory setting with free access to animal food. DSS in the drinking water can be used to cause colon inflammation. DSS with a molecular weight of 40–44kDa and sulfur content of 15.4%–17.0% is dissolved in ultra-pure water at 2.5% and 5.0% levels, respectively, at a pII of 8.5. DSS' properties and its stability are examined in solution form [72]. The animals are allowed unlimited access to DSS solutions. The sulfation and molecular weight of the DSS, as well as the dosage and duration of DSS treatment, all influence the appearance of DSS-induced animal colitis [4].

5.6 Skin inflammation

Many skin conditions, like psoriasis, atopic dermatitis, contact sensitivity, acne, are marked by inflammation [73]. These illnesses impact more than 20% of the population, and dermatologists have devised a variety of therapeutic options. Since its debut in 1952, topical corticosteroids have been standard treatments [74]. While these potent antiinflammatory medicines effectively cure both acute and chronic skin inflammation, they are not suitable for continued use in chronic illnesses like psoriasis due to adverse effects. Topically applied steroids cause skin shrinkage, shortening the therapy period [75]. Furthermore, topical steroid administration to large areas of body surface causes hypothalamic-pituitary-adrenal suppression due to absorption in the systemic circulation, necessitating therapy discontinuation. In some situations, the illness resurfaces, often in a more severe form than before therapy. New nonsteroidal antiinflammatory medicines with effectiveness comparable to topical steroids but devoid of steroid-related adverse effects are urgently needed. Various molecular targets have been the subject of study at many pharmaceutical research facilities, and they continue to be. There are a plethora of potential targets implicated in inflammatory cascades, and biochemical screens can be used to find inhibitors and antagonists. Molecular targets are frequently chosen based on increased target expression or activity in illnesses of human beings. Cytokines, lipid mediators, protein kinases, adhesion molecules, and growth factors have been recognized as potential sources of cancer. Potential possibilities include cytokines, lipid mediators, protein kinases, adhesion molecules, and growth factors. To evaluate proof-of-principle, inhibitors or antagonists are discovered and checked for efficacy in cell-based and animal models. Antiinflammatory actions will be found if the target has a major role in inflammation. One type of inflammagens that have been investigated in this way are lipid mediators of inflammation, which are collectively known as eicosanoids. Since 1975, eicosanoids are found to be increased in psoriatic skin [24]. Many of these substances have pro-inflammatory properties, and their synthesis has been thoroughly studied [76]. Because arachidonic acid is a precursor of leukotrienes and prostaglandins, inhibiting phospholipase A2 activity that releases arachidonate from membrane phospholipids, may block the entire family of the mediator [77]. Inhibitors that prevent arachidonic acid release in cells have been discovered using enzyme screens. This in vitro proof-of-concept implies that such chemicals might be beneficial in disorders of skin like psoriasis, which have high levels of leukotrienes and prostaglandins. However, psoriasis does not seem to occur naturally in animals, and there is no consensus on whether generated models adequately resemble human illness. Researchers have built models that simulate certain features of the pathophysiology that happens in the human state to overcome this shortcoming. The results of such models have been used to make decisions on which drugs to test in clinical trials. Of course, human disease activity is the final check for determining the therapeutic effectiveness of new antiinflammatory medicines for the treatment of skin inflammation. Clinical evaluations, on the other hand, are expensive and have a lot of possible factors that need to be controlled,; therefore, they should only be used to evaluate candidates which demonstrate potential in the most rigorous models available [78]. Some of the models used have been discussed below.

5.6.1 TPA-induced skin inflammation

The most frequent test for both steroidal and nonsteroidal antiinflammatory drugs is croton oil or 12-O-tetradecanoyl-phorbol-13-acetate or a TPA-induced skin irritation model. Croton oil has been phased out in favor of the active ingredient TPA [79]. In the instance of TPA, just one topical dosage applied to the ears of mice causes an edematous reaction that lasts for 6 h. The phorbol ester also causes neutrophil infiltration, with peak levels 20–24 h later [80]. As the acute injury heals, these reactions fade away. The exact method through which phorbol ester induces inflammation

is unknown, although it seems to be related to the release of eicosanoid mediators in part. TPA causes a brief rise in prostaglandin levels in the skin. Alterations in the permeability of the vasculature and cell infiltration cause LTB4 levels to rise [76]. The effects of antiinflammatory medications given orally and topically on phorbol ester-induced mouse ear inflammation have been studied. Carlson et al. investigated the effects of several different pharmacological drugs in this animal model [81]. Betamethasone and other topical steroids effectively prevent phorbol ester-induced edema. Traditional NSAIDs, such as indomethacin, diclofenac, and piroxicam, are also highly effective when applied topically. Substances that prevent leukotriene production, like prednisone, BW755c, and zileuton, are also effective. It has also been demonstrated that LTB4 antagonists are effective. Phospholipase A2 inhibitors have been found to prevent edema induced by phorbol ester and cell infiltration. In general, cyclooxygenase and/or lipoxygenase or phospholipase A2 inhibitors, which regulate eicosanoid production, exhibit topical action in this animal model. This paradigm seems to be a viable screen for the in vivo assessment of leukotriene/cyclooxygenase inhibitors that have been chosen based on enzyme and cell-based tests, based on these results. Given the fact that antihistamines and serotonin antagonists are topically active, it is clear that additional mediators, apart from eicosanoids, are involved in this kind of inflammation. Mast cells are a requirement for the full manifestation of the increase in permeability of the vasculature and cell infiltration caused by TPA, as demonstrated by the use of mast cell defective animals. The fact that antihistamines can stop the inflammatory reaction from fully developing indicates that mast cells participate significantly in the development of acute inflammation. Hydrochlorothiazide, chlorpromazine, haloperidol, and nifedipine are examples of nontraditional antiinflammatory medicines that have demonstrated activity. The efficacy of this model to forecast new, antiinflammatory drugs for human skin inflammation has been called into doubt because of the activity of these latter molecules. The traditional NSAID action can potentially be problematic. Indomethacin is ineffective in the treatment of psoriasis, whether it is used orally or topically. In fact, according to one study, indomethacin worsens the illness. Before evaluating active substances as clinical trial candidates, supplementary models should be examined to eliminate these false positives [82].

5.6.2 Immune-driven models of skin inflammation

Psoriasis and atopic dermatitis are genetically manifested immunologic disorders in which T cells and cytokines play a key role, according to mounting data. Immunosuppressive drugs, for example, methotrexate, cyclosporine A, FK-506, and interleukin-2-diphtheria toxin fusion protein have recently been discovered. The effectiveness of these medicines in clinical trials has prompted researchers to look for immunosuppressive compounds that can block initial T cell activation and serve as local immune suppressants following topical administration. Most often employed in in vivo assays for evaluation of drug-induced immunosuppression, apart from transplantation models, evaluate changes in inflammatory skin reactions in delayed-type hypersensitivity (DTH) models. These models represent normal cellular immune responses. Humans get classic DTH after contracting Mycobacterium tuberculosis. Antigen sensitivity may be induced in mice, guinea pigs, and pigs. The infiltration of lymphocytes, occurring 4–6 h after antigen challenge in all of these animals, is the most important histological characteristic. Extravasated plasma is present in the inflammatory cell infiltrate, which explains the swelling and induration seen in most DTH reactions. Inflammatory and immune-modulating drugs have been assessed using a variety of common methods and species [83].

5.6.3 Oxazalone-induced delayed-type hypersensitivity in mice

The mouse has long been used to test the effects of new anti-inflammatory drugs on DTH reactions. DTH reactions in sensitized animals can be easily evaluated by measuring ear thickness by a micrometer or weight increases in ears or paws following the sacrifice. Histological assessment of tissue samples or the use of a neutrophil marker like myeloperoxidase can also be used to determine cell infiltration. Animals are made sensitive to the antigen oxazolone, in general, by applying a solution (1%–3% in acetone) to the shaved belly. A modest dosage of oxazolone (0.5%–1%) is given to the mice 4 or 5 days later to elicit a DTH response. It's important to choose the challenge dose carefully so that an irritating reaction is not generated. In the mouse, the DTH reaction, the pattern of cell infiltration has been extensively described. Edema is significant and the cell infiltration is mild 24 h after the challenge. Mononuclear cells and PMNs are almost similar in number (31:27). The preponderance of mononuclear cells over PMNs is apparent after 48 and 72 h (40:12 and 26:7, respectively). The mouse DTH is distinguished from other animal species and humans by its early and substantial PMN cell infiltration. The diapedesis of lymphocytes, with varying involvement of monocytes and macrophages, is an important microscopic characteristic of typical human DTH. The most common infiltrating cell is lymphocytes. Furthermore, investigations have revealed that the bulk of these lymphocytes are of the helper/inducer phenotype, while there are a few killer/suppressor cells as well. In DTH procedures, mutant mice missing the CD4 gene exhibit significant hyporesponsiveness. DTH responses in mice have been reported to be inhibited by immune modifying medications. Methotrexate, azathioprine, and thioquanine are all active drugs that alter T cell activity. All of these substances have an inhibiting impact on growing cells and are commonly used in cancer treatment. Noncytotoxic immunosuppressive medications such as cyclosporin A and FK-506 are effective in inhibiting mouse DTH. In the management of psoriasis, therapy has been discovered to be effective. Topical FK-506 has also exhibited effectiveness in psoriasis and atopic dermatitis [84].

References

[1] R.K. Sindhu, N. Sood, V. Puri, S. Arora, Various animal models for preclinical testing of anti-inflammatory agents, Int. J. Pharmaceut. Sci. Res. 8 (4) (2017) 1550.

[2] J.Y. Kim, J.M. Baek, S.J. Ahn, Y.H. Cheon, S.H. Park, M. Yang, M.K. Choi, J. Oh, Ethanolic extract of Schizonepeta tenuifolia attenuates osteoclast formation and activation in vitro and protects against lipopolysaccharide-induced bone loss in vivo, BMC Complement. Altern. Med. 16 (1) (2016) 1–9.

[3] J.E. Graham, T.F. Robles, J.K. Kiecolt-Glaser, W.B. Malarkey, M.G. Bissell, R. Glaser, Hostility and pain are related to inflammation in older adults, Brain Behav. Immun. 20 (4) (2006) 389–400.

[4] M.I. Umara, R. Altafa, M.A. Iqbalb, M.B. Sadiqc, In vivo experimental models to investigate the anti-inflammatory activity of herbal extracts, Sci Int. 22 (3) (2010) 199–203.

[5] I. Negut, V. Grumezescu, A.M. Grumezescu, Treatment strategies for infected wounds, Molecules 23 (9) (2018) 2392.

[6] S. Dewanjee, T.K. Dua, R. Sahu, Potential anti-inflammatory effect of Leea macrophylla Roxb. leaves: a wild edible plant, Food Chem. Toxicol. 59 (2013) 514–520.

[7] R.K. Sindhu, S. Arora, Anti-inflammatory potential of different extracts isolated from the roots of Ficus lacor Buch. Hum and Murraya koenigii L. Spreng, Arch. Biol. Sci. 66 (3) (2014) 1261–1270.

[8] R.K. Sindhu, S. Arora, Therapeutic effect of Ficus lacor aerial roots of various fractions on adjuvant-induced arthritic rats, Int. Schol. Res. Not. 09 (2013) 1261–1270, https://doi.org/10.1155/2013/634106.

[9] S. Verma, Medicinal plants with anti-inflammatory activity, J. Phytopharmacol. 5 (4) (2016) 157–159.

[10] H.J. Chung, H.S. Lee, J.S. Shin, S.H. Lee, B.M. Park, Y.S. Youn, S.K. Lee, Modulation of acute and chronic inflammatory processes by a traditional medicine preparation GCSB-5 both in vitro and in vivo animal models, J. Ethnopharmacol. 130 (3) (2010) 450–459.

[11] S. Debnath, S. Ghosh, B. Hazra, Inhibitory effect of Nymphaea pubescens Willd. flower extract on carrageenan-induced inflammation and CCl4-induced hepatotoxicity in rats, Food Chem. Toxicol. 59 (2013) 485–491.

[12] N. Singh, D. Baby, J.P. Rajguru, P.B. Patil, S.S. Thakkannavar, V.B. Pujari, Inflammation and cancer, Ann. Afr. Med. 18 (3) (2019) 121.

[13] K.R. Patil, U.B. Mahajan, B.S. Unger, S.N. Goyal, S. Belemkar, S.J. Surana, S. Ojha, C.R. Patil, Animal models of inflammation for screening of anti-inflammatory drugs: Implications for the discovery and development of phytopharmaceuticals, Int. J. Mol. Sci. 20 (18) (2019) 4367.

[14] W.S. Jo, K.M. Yang, Y.J. Choi, C.H. Jeong, K.J. Ahn, B.H. Nam, S.W. Lee, S.Y. Seo, M.H. Jeong, In vitro and in vivo anti-inflammatory effects of pegmatite, Mol. Cellular Toxicol. 6 (2) (2010) 195–202.

[15] M.O. Sofidiya, E. Imeh, C. Ezeani, F.R. Aigbe, A.J. Akindele, Antinociceptive and anti-inflammatory activities of ethanolic extract of Alafia barteri, Rev. Bras. Farm. 24 (2014) 348–354.

[16] R. Gautam, S.M. Jachak, Recent developments in anti-inflammatory natural products, Med. Res. Rev. 29 (5) (2009) 767–820.

[17] S. Gorzalczany, P. López, C. Acevedo, G. Ferraro, Anti-inflammatory effect of Lithrea molleoides extracts and isolated active compounds, J. Ethnopharmacol. 133 (3) (2011) 994–998.

[18] G. Uddin, A. Rauf, B.S. Siddiqui, N. Muhammad, A. Khan, S.U. Shah, Anti-nociceptive, anti-inflammatory and sedative activities of the extracts and chemical constituents of Diospyros lotus L, Phytomedicine 21 (7) (2014) 954–959.

[19] Y. Bellik, L. Boukraâ, H.A. Alzahrani, B.A. Bakhotmah, F. Abdellah, S.M. Hammoudi, M. Iguer-Ouada, Molecular mechanism underlying anti-inflammatory and anti-allergic activities of phytochemicals: an update, Molecules 18 (1) (2013) 322–353.

[20] R.G. de Oliveira, C.P. Mahon, P.G. Ascêncio, S.D. Ascêncio, S.O. Balogun, D.T. de Oliveira Martins, Evaluation of anti-inflammatory activity of hydroethanolic extract of Dilodendron bipinnatum Radlk, J. Ethnopharmacol. 155 (1) (2014) 387–395.

[21] M. Eddouks, D. Chattopadhyay, N.A. Zeggwagh, Animal models as tools to investigate antidiabetic and anti-inflammatory plants, Evid. Based Complement. Alternat. Med. 2012 (2012), https://doi.org/10.1155/2012/142087. Article No.: 142087.

[22] C. Dubois, F.V. Abeele, V.Y. Lehen'kyi, D. Gkika, B. Guarmit, G. Lepage, C. Slomianny, A.S. Borowiec, G. Bidaux, M. Benahmed, Y. Shuba, Remodeling of channel-forming ORAI proteins determines an oncogenic switch in prostate cancer, Cancer Cell 26 (1) (2014) 19–32.

[23] M.J. Stables, D.W. Gilroy, Old and new generation lipid mediators in acute inflammation and resolution, Prog. Lipid Res. 50 (1) (2011) 35–51.

[24] E.A. Dennis, P.C. Norris, Eicosanoid storm in infection and inflammation, Nat. Rev. Immunol. 15 (8) (2015) 511–523.

[25] C. Franceschi, J. Campisi, Chronic inflammation (inflammaging) and its potential contribution to age-associated diseases, J. Gerontol. Ser. A: Biomed. Sci. Med. Sci. 69 (Suppl_1) (2014) S4-9.

[26] S.K. Biswas, Does the interdependence between oxidative stress and inflammation explain the antioxidant paradox? Oxid. Med. Cell. Longev. (2016).

[27] B. Heras, S. Hortelano, Molecular basis of the anti-inflammatory effects of terpenoids, Inflam. Allergy-Drug Targets 8 (1) (2009) 28–39, https://doi.org/10.2174/187152809787582534.

[28] Y. Yadav, P.K. Mohanty, S.B. Kasture, Anti-inflammatory activity of hydroalcoholic extract of Quisqualis indica Linn. flower in rats, Int. J. Pharm. Life Sci. 2 (8) (2011) 977–981.

[29] A.F. Pires, N.V. Rodrigues, P.M. Soares, R.R. de Albuquerque, K.S. Aragao, M.M. Marinho, M.T. da Silva, B.S. Cavada, A.M. Assreuy, A novel N-acetyl-glucosamine lectin of Lonchocarpus araripensis attenuates acute cellular inflammation in mice, Inflamm. Res. 65 (1) (2016) 43–52.

[30] M. Patel, G. Murugananthan, K.P. Gowda, In vivo animal models in preclinical evaluation of anti-inflammatory activity—a review, Int. J. Pharm. Res. Allied Sci. 1 (2) (2012) 1–5.

[31] F. Navid, L. Kolbe, F. Stäb, T. Korff, G. Neufang, UV radiation induces the release of angiopoietin-2 from dermal microvascular endothelial cells, Exp. Dermatol. 21 (2) (2012) 147–153.

[32] R.K. Sindhu, S. Arora, Therapeutic effect of Ficus lacor aerial roots of various fractions on adjuvant-induced arthritic rats, ISRN Pharmacol. 1–8 (2013), https://doi.org/10.1155/2013/634106.

[33] H. Rachmawati, D. Safitri, A.T. Pradana, I.K. Adnyana, TPGS-stabilized curcumin nanoparticles exhibit superior effect on carrageenan-induced inflammation in wistar rat, Pharmaceutics 8 (3) (2016) 24.

[34] E.K. Tamura, R.S. Jimenez, K. Waismam, L. Gobbo-Neto, N.P. Lopes, E.A. Malpezzi-Marinho, E.A. Marinho, S.H. Farsky, Inhibitory effects of Solidago chilensis Meyen hydroalcoholic extract on acute inflammation, J. Ethnopharmacol. 122 (3) (2009) 478–485.

[35] Y. Wu, C. Zhou, L. Song, X. Li, S. Shi, J. Mo, H. Chen, H. Bai, X. Wu, J. Zhao, R. Zhang, Effect of total phenolics from Laggera alata on acute and chronic inflammation models, J. Ethnopharmacol. 108 (2) (2006) 243–250.

[36] K.I. Hulkower, J.S. Pollock, R.E. Walsh, R. Huang, E.R. Otis, C.D. Brooks, R.L. Bell, Leukotrienes do not regulate nitric oxide production in RAW 264.7 macrophages, Prostaglandins Leukot. Essent. Fatty Acids 55 (3) (1996) 145–149.

[37] H. Sadeghi, M. Parishani, M. Akbartabar Touri, M. Ghavamzadeh, M. Jafari Barmak, V. Zarezade, H. Delaviz, H. Sadeghi, Pramipexole reduces inflammation in the experimental animal models of inflammation, Immunopharmacol. Immunotoxicol. 39 (2) (2017) 80–86.

[38] S. Boller, C. Soldi, M.C. Marques, E.P. Santos, D.A. Cabrini, M.G. Pizzolatti, A.R. Zampronio, M.F. Otuki, Anti-inflammatory effect of crude extract and isolated compounds from Baccharis illinita DC in acute skin inflammation, J. Ethnopharmacol. 130 (2) (2010) 262–266.

[39] E. Bas, M.C. Recio, M. Abdallah, S. Máñez, R.M. Giner, M. Cerdá-Nicolás, J.L. Ríos, Inhibition of the pro-inflammatory mediators' production and anti-inflammatory effect of the iridoid scrovalentinoside, J. Ethnopharmacol. 110 (3) (2007) 419–427.

[40] Y. Fujii, H. Takeuchi, K. Tanaka, S. Sakuma, Y. Ohkubo, S. Mutoh, Effects of FK506 (tacrolimus hydrate) on chronic oxazolone-induced dermatitis in rats, Eur. J. Pharmacol. 456 (1–3) (2002) 115–121.

[41] B. Botz, S.M. Brunner, Á. Kemény, E. Pintér, J.J. McDougall, B. Kofler, Z. Helyes, Galanin 3 receptor-deficient mice show no alteration in the oxazolone-induced contact dermatitis phenotype, Exp. Dermatol. 25 (9) (2016) 725–727.

[42] R. Huggenberger, S.S. Siddiqui, D. Brander, S. Ullmann, K. Zimmermann, M. Antsiferova, S. Werner, K. Alitalo, M. Detmar, An important role of lymphatic vessel activation in limiting acute inflammation, Blood, J. Am. Soc. Hematol. 117 (17) (2011) 4667–4678.

[43] H. Bouriche, S. Kada, A.M. Assaf, A. Senator, F. Gül, I. Dimertas, Phytochemical screening and anti-inflammatory properties of Algerian Hertia cheirifolia methanol extract, Pharm. Biol. 54 (11) (2016) 2584–2590.

[44] J.C. Fehrenbacher, M.R. Vasko, D.B. Duarte, Models of inflammation: carrageenan- or complete freund's adjuvant (CFA)–induced edema and hypersensitivity in the rat, Curr. Protocols Pharmacol. 56 (1) (2012) 4–5.

[45] A. Panthong, P. Norkaew, D. Kanjanapothi, T. Taesotikul, N. Anantachoke, V. Reutrakul, Anti-inflammatory, analgesic and antipyretic activities of the extract of gamboge from Garcinia hanburyi Hook f, J. Ethnopharmacol. 111 (2) (2007) 335–340.

[46] S. Sarkhel, Evaluation of the anti-inflammatory activities of Quillaja saponaria Mol. saponin extract in mice, Toxicol. Rep. 3 (2016) 1–3.

[47] M. Duwiejua, E. Woode, D.D. Obiri, Pseudo-akuammigine, an alkaloid from Picralima nitida seeds, has anti-inflammatory and analgesic actions in rats, J. Ethnopharmacol. 81 (1) (2002) 73–79.

[48] K.R. Patil, C.R. Patil, Anti-inflammatory activity of bartogenic acid containing fraction of fruits of Barringtonia racemosa Roxb. in acute and chronic animal models of inflammation, J. Tradit. Complement. Med. 7 (1) (2017) 86–93.

[49] G.R. Battu, R. Parimi, K.B. Chandra Shekar, In vivo and in vitro pharmacological activity of Aristolochia tagala (syn: Aristolochia acuminata) root extracts, Pharm. Biol. 49 (11) (2011) 1210–1214.

[50] G. Garrido, D. González, Y. Lemus, D. Garcia, L. Lodeiro, G. Quintero, C. Delporte, A.J. Núñez-Sellés, R. Delgado, In vivo and in vitro anti-inflammatory activity of Mangifera indica L. extract (VIMANG®), Pharmacol. Res. 50 (2) (2004) 143–149.

[51] O.A. Olajide, S.O. Awe, J.M. Makinde, A.I. Ekhelar, A. Olusola, O. Morebise, D.T. Okpako, Studies on the anti-inflammatory, antipyretic and analgesic properties of Alstonia boonei stem bark, J. Ethnopharmacol. 71 (1–2) (2000) 179–186.

[52] J. Cheng, T. Ma, W. Liu, H. Wang, J. Jiang, Y. Wei, H. Tian, N. Zou, Y. Zhu, H. Shi, X. Cheng, In in vivo evaluation of the anti-inflammatory and analgesic activities of compound Muniziqi granule in experimental animal models, BMC Complement. Altern. Med. 16 (1) (2015) 1.

[53] I.O. Ben, O.E. Etim, N.M. Udo, Anti-inflammatory effects of Napoleona imperialis *P. Beauv.* (Lecythidaceae) on rat model of inflammation, Ind. J. Health Sci. Biomed. Res. (KLEU) 9 (1) (2016) 89.

[54] J. Silva, W. Abebe, S.M. Sousa, V.G. Duarte, M.I. Machado, F.J. Matos, Analgesic and anti-inflammatory effects of essential oils of Eucalyptus, J. Ethnopharmacol. 89 (2–3) (2003) 277–283.

[55] M.S. Vilar, G.L. De Souza, D.D. Vilar, J.A. Leite, F.N. Raffin, J.M. Barbosa-Filho, F.H. Nogueira, S. Rodrigues-Mascarenhas, T.F. Moura, Assessment of phenolic compounds and anti-inflammatory activity of ethyl acetate phase of Anacardium occidentale L. bark, Molecules 21 (8) (2016) 1087.

[56] C.O. Coura, R.B. Souza, J.A. Rodrigues, E.D. Vanderlei, I.W. de Araújo, N.A. Ribeiro, A.F. Frota, K.A. Ribeiro, H.V. Chaves, K.M. Pereira, R.M. da Cunha, Mechanisms involved in the anti-inflammatory action of a polysulfated fraction from Gracilaria cornea in rats, PLoS One 10 (3) (2015), e0119319.

[57] N.P. Babu, P. Pandikumar, S. Ignacimuthu, Anti-inflammatory activity of Albizia lebbeck Benth., an ethnomedicinal plant, in acute and chronic animal models of inflammation, J. Ethnopharmacol. 125 (2) (2009) 356–360.

[58] I.L. Calil, A.C. Zarpelon, A.T. Guerrero, J.C. Alves-Filho, S.H. Ferreira, F.Q. Cunha, T.M. Cunha, W.A. Verri Jr., Lipopolysaccharide induces inflammatory hyperalgesia triggering a TLR4/MyD88-dependent cytokine cascade in the mice paw, PLoS One 9 (3) (2014), e90013.

[59] K. Lalrinzuali, M. Vabeiryureilai, G.C. Jagetia, Investigation of the anti-inflammatory and analgesic activities of ethanol extract of stem bark of Sonapatha Oroxylum indicum in vivo, Int. J. Inflamm. 2016 (2016).

[60] A.J. Vargas, D.S. Geremias, G. Provensi, P.E. Fornari, F.H. Reginatto, G. Gosmann, E.P. Schenkel, T.S. Fröde, Passiflora alata and Passiflora edulis spray-dried aqueous extracts inhibit inflammation in mouse model of pleurisy, Fitoterapia 78 (2) (2007) 112–119.

[61] G.G. Meshram, A. Kumar, W. Rizvi, C.D. Tripathi, R.A. Khan, Evaluation of the anti-inflammatory activity of the aqueous and ethanolic extracts of the leaves of Albizzia lebbeck in rats, J. Tradit. Complement. Med. 6 (2) (2016) 172–175.

[62] G. Amresh, G.D. Reddy, C.V. Rao, P.N. Singh, Evaluation of the anti-inflammatory activity of *Cissampelos pareira* root in rats, J. Ethnopharmacol. 110 (3) (2007) 526–531.

[63] Z. Ghlissi, N. Sayari, R. Kallel, A. Bougatef, Z. Sahnoun, Antioxidant, antibacterial, anti-inflammatory and wound healing effects of Artemisia campestris aqueous extract in rat, Biomed. Pharmacother. (84) (2016) 115–122.

[64] P.H. Wooley, H.S. Luthra, J.M. Stuart, C.S. David, Type II collagen-induced arthritis in mice. I. Major histocompatibility complex (I region) linkage and antibody correlates, J. Exp. Med. 154 (3) (1981) 688–700.

[65] X. Han, D. Su, X. Xian, M. Zhou, X. Li, J. Huang, J. Wang, H. Gao, Inhibitory effects of Saussurea involucrata (Kar. et Kir.) Sch.-Bip. on adjuvant arthritis in rats, J. Ethnopharmacol. 194 (2016) 228–235.

[66] R. Kumar, Y.K. Gupta, S. Singh, A. Patil, Glorisa superba hydroalcoholic extract from tubers attenuates experimental arthritis by downregulating inflammatory mediators, and phosphorylation of ERK/JNK/p-38, Immunol. Invest. 45 (7) (2016) 603–618.

[67] O.P. Gupta, S. Sing, S. Bani, N. Sharma, S. Malhotra, B.D. Gupta, S.K. Banerjee, S.S. Handa, Anti-inflammatory and anti-arthritic activities of silymarin acting through inhibition of 5-lipoxygenase, Phytomedicine 7 (1) (2000) 21–24.

[68] J.B. Warren, R.K. Loi, M.L. Coughlan, Involvement of nitric oxide synthase in the delayed vasodilator response to ultraviolet light irradiation of rat skin in vivo, Br. J. Pharmacol. 109 (3) (1993) 802.

[69] Á. Montilla-García, M.Á. Tejada, G. Perazzoli, J.M. Entrena, E.-Portillo-Salido, E. Fernández-Segura, F.J. Canizares, E.J. Cobos, Grip strength in mice with joint inflammation: a rheumatology function test sensitive to pain and analgesia, Neuropharmacology 125 (2017) 231–242.

[70] M. Mbiantcha, J. Almas, S.U. Shabana, D. Nida, F. Aisha, Anti-arthritic property of crude extracts of Piptadeniastrum africanum (Mimosaceae) in complete Freund's adjuvant-induced arthritis in rats, BMC Complement. Altern. Med. 17 (1) (2017) 1–6.

[71] Kshirsagar A.D., Panchal P.V., Harle U.N., Nanda R.K., Shaikh H.M. Anti-inflammatory and antiarthritic activity of anthraquinone derivatives in rodents. Int. J. Inflamm. 2014; 2014.

[72] D.W. Kim, K.H. Son, H.W. Chang, K. Bae, S.S. Kang, H.P. Kim, Anti-inflammatory activity of Elsholtzia splendens, Arch. Pharm. Res. 26 (3) (2003) 232–236.

[73] J. Schwingen, M. Kaplan, F.C. Kurschus, current concepts in inflammatory skin diseases evolved by transcriptome analysis: in-depth analysis of atopic dermatitis and psoriasis, Int. J. Mol. Sci. 21 (3) (2020) 699.

[74] L.A. Bernard, L.F. Eichenfield, Eczematous and papulosquamous disorders, Neonatal Dermatol. E-Book 20 (2007) 229–244.

[75] A. Coondoo, M. Phiske, S. Verma, K. Lahiri, Side-effects of topical steroids: a long overdue revisit, Indian Dermatol. Online J. 5 (4) (2014) 416.

[76] E. Ricciotti, G.A. FitzGerald, Prostaglandins and inflammation, Arterioscler. Thromb. Vasc. Biol. 31 (5) (2011) 986–1000.

[77] A.M. Johnson, E.K. Kleczko, R.A. Nemenoff, Eicosanoids in cancer: new roles in immunoregulation, Front. Pharmacol. 11 (2020), https://doi.org/10.3389/fphar.2020.595498.

[78] K.M. Tramposch, Skin inflammation, in: In Vivo Models of Inflammation, Birkhäuser, Basel, 1999, pp. 179–204.

[79] A. Pagani, S. Gaeta, A.I. Savchenko, C.M. Williams, G. Appendino, An improved preparation of phorbol from croton oil, Beilstein J. Org. Chem. 13 (1) (2017) 1361–1367.

[80] E.E. Bralley, P. Greenspan, J.L. Hargrove, L. Wicker, D.K. Hartle, Topical anti-inflammatory activity of Polygonum cuspidatum extract in the TPA model of mouse ear inflammation, J. Inflamm. 5 (1) (2008) 1–7.

[81] S.H. Lee, D.W. Kim, S. Eom, S.Y. Jun, M.Y. Park, D.S. Kim, H.J. Kwon, H.Y. Kwon, K.H. Han, J.S. Park, H.S. Hwang, Suppression of 12-O-tetradecanoylphorbol-13-acetate (TPA)-induced skin inflammation in mice by transduced Tat-Annexin protein, BMB Rep. 45 (6) (2012) 354–359.

[82] C.S. Stevenson, L.A. Marshall, D.W. Morgan (Eds.), In Vivo Models of Inflammation, vol. 2, Springer Science & Business Media, 2006.

[83] C. Jardet, A. David, E. Braun, P. Descargues, J.L. Grolleau, J. Hebsgaard, H. Norsgaard, P. Lovato, Development and characterization of a human Th17-driven ex vivo skin inflammation model, Exp. Dermatol. 29 (10) (2020) 993–1003.

[84] D. Aebischer, A.H. Willrodt, C. Halin, Oxazolone-induced contact hypersensitivity reduces lymphatic drainage but enhances the induction of adaptive immunity, PLoS One 9 (6) (2014), e99297.

Further reading

J.M. da Silva, J.L. Conegundes, R.D. Mendes, N.D. Pinto, A.C. Gualberto, A. Ribeiro, J. Gameiro, J.A. de Aguiar, M.C. Castañon, E. Scio, Topical application of the hexane fraction of Lacistema pubescens reduces skin inflammation and cytokine production in animal model, J. Pharm. Pharmacol. 67 (11) (2015) 1613–1622.

S.K. Gupta, Analgesic Agents. Drug Screening Methods, second ed., Jaypee Brothers, New Delhi, India, 2009, pp. 461–479.

S. Hortelano, Molecular basis of the anti-inflammatory effects of terpenoids, Inflamm. Allergy Drug Targets 8 (1) (2009) 28–39.

R.G. Kulkarni, G. Achaiah, S.G. Narahari, Novel targets for antiinflammatory and antiarthritic agents, Curr. Pharm. Des. 12 (19) (2006) 2437–2454.

A. Lama, L. Ferreiro, M.E. Toubes, A. Golpe, F. Gude, J.M. Álvarez-Dobaño, F.J. González-Barcala, E. San Jose, N. Rodríguez-Núñez, C. Rabade, C. Rodríguez-García, Characteristics of patients with pseudochylothorax—a systematic review, J. Thorac. Dis. 8 (8) (2016) 2093.

S.W. Martin, A.J. Stevens, B.S. Brennan, D. Davies, M. Rowland, J.B. Houston, The six-day-old rat air pouch model of inflammation: characterization of the inflammatory response to carrageenan, J. Pharmacol. Toxicol. Methods 32 (3) (1994) 139–147.

F.R. Nonato, T.M. Nogueira, T.A. de Almeida Barros, A.M. Lucchese, C.E. Oliveira, R.R. dos Santos, M.B. Soares, C.F. Villarreal, Antinociceptive and antiinflammatory activities of Adiantum latifolium Lam.: Evidence for a role of IL-1β inhibition, J. Ethnopharmacol. 136 (3) (2011) 518–524.

A.M. Pedernera, T. Guardia, C.E. Calderón, A.E. Rotelli, N.E. de la Rocha, J.R. Saad, M.A. Verrilli, S.G. Aseff, L.E. Pelzer, Anti-inflammatory effect of Acacia visco extracts in animal models, Inflammopharmacology 18 (5) (2010) 253–260.

O.S. Qureshi, A. Zeb, M. Akram, M.S. Kim, J.H. Kang, H.S. Kim, A. Majid, I. Han, S.Y. Chang, O.N. Bae, J.K. Kim, Enhanced acute anti-inflammatory effects of CORM-2-loaded nanoparticles via sustained carbon monoxide delivery, Eur. J. Pharm. Biopharm. 108 (2016) 187–195.

S.M. Satyam, K.L. Bairy, S. Musharraf, D.L. Fernandes, Inhibition of croton oil-induced oedema in rat ear skin by topical nicotinamide gel, Pharmacology 3 (2014) 22–25.

D.P. Silva, I.F. Florentino, L.P. Oliveira, R.C. Lino, P.M. Galdino, R. Menegatti, E.A. Costa, Anti-nociceptive and anti-inflammatory activities of 4-[(1-phenyl-1H-pyrazol-4-yl) methyl] 1-piperazine carboxylic acid ethyl ester: a new piperazine derivative, Pharmacol. Biochem. Behav. 137 (2015) 86–92.

J.Y. Sun, C.Y. You, K. Dong, H.S. You, J.F. Xing, Anti-inflammatory, analgesic and antioxidant activities of 3, 4-oxo-isopropylidene-shikimic acid, Pharm. Biol. 54 (10) (2016) 2282–2287.

T. Tamura, T. Amano, K. Ohmori, H. Manabe, The effects of olopatadine hydrochloride on the number of scratching induced by repeated application of oxazolone in mice, Eur. J. Pharmacol. 524 (1–3) (2005) 149–154.

B. Weinkauf, M. Main, M. Schmelz, R. Rukwied, Modality-specific nociceptor sensitization following UV-B irradiation of human skin, J. Pain 14 (7) (2013) 739–746.

B. Weinkauf, R. Rukwied, H. Quiding, L. Dahllund, P. Johansson, M. Schmelz, Local gene expression changes after UV-irradiation of human skin, PLoS One 7 (6) (2012), e39411.

I. Wilches, V. Tobar, E. Peñaherrera, N. Cuzco, L. Jerves, Y. Vander Heyden, F. León-Tamariz, E. Vila, Evaluation of anti-inflammatory activity of the methanolic extract from Jungia rugosa leaves in rodents, J. Ethnopharmacol. 173 (2015) 166–171.

Chapter 21

Clinical trials and future perspectives of antiinflammatory agents

Kamini[a], Anoop Kumar[a,b], Pooja A. Chawla[c], and Bhupinder Kapoor[d]

[a]Department of Pharmacology, Delhi Institute of Pharmaceutical Sciences and Research, New Delhi, India, [b]School of Pharmaceutical Sciences, Delhi Pharmaceutical Sciences and Research University, New Delhi, India, [c]Department of Pharmaceutical Chemistry and Analysis, ISF College of Pharmacy, Moga, Punjab, India, [d]School of Pharmaceutical Sciences, Lovely Professional University, Phagwara, Punjab, India

1 Introduction

Inflammation is a protective response to eliminate the initial cause of cell injury. The physiological inflammation is required for diluting, destroying, and neutralizing the harmful agents. It removes the damaged tissue and generates new tissues. It is a defensive process that a living body initiates against local tissue damage. It takes the form of a complex reaction of blood vessels, certain plasma components, and blood cells, and cellular and structural components of connective tissue [1]. The signs of inflammation are redness (rubor), swelling (tumor), heat (calor), pain or discomfort (dollar), and loss of function. These signs may not appear always, sometimes inflammation is also silent without any symptom. Fever and tiredness can also be observed. The symptoms of acute inflammation last a few days whereas chronic inflammation may last for months or years. The etiology of inflammation are physical agents such as extreme temperature (heat or cold), electric shock, radiation, mechanical injures, etc.; chemical agents such as products of metabolism, acids, alkalis, drugs, tissue necrosis, etc.; biological agents such as microorganisms (bacteria, viruses, fungi), parasites (helminths, insects), immune cells and complexes, etc.; endogenous such as circulatory disorder, hypoxia, endogenous protease release, immune complex formation, etc. [2].

Inflammation is broadly classified into two types, i.e., acute and chronic inflammation as presented in Fig. 1. Acute inflammation is of short duration and represents early body reaction and is usually followed by repair. It lasts from several days up to several months; in the focus of inflammation are neutrophils and intravascular platelet activation. The chronic inflammation lasts from a few months up to tens of years.

The controlled inflammatory response is beneficial such as providing protection to the body against infection, however, it become harmful in uncontrolled conditions.

The undesired inflammation is associated with various diseases, such as diabetes [3], cardiovascular disease (CVD) [4], arthritis [5] and other joint diseases, allergies [6], chronic obstructive pulmonary disease (COPD) [7], psoriasis [8], etc.

2 Mediators of inflammation

Various chemicals play a role as a mediator in the process of inflammation. Broadly, these are categorized as cell-derived and plasma protein-derived mediators. The cell-derived mediators such as histamine are produced from mast cells and basophils; serotonin from platelets; leukotrienes from leukocytes and mast cells; platelet-activating factor (PAF) from leukocytes; reactive oxygen species (ROS) from leukocytes; and prostaglandins (PGs) from leukocytes and mast cells. The plasma protein-derived mediators such as complement achration and factor XII achration (bradykinin coagulation) are produced from liver. The various mediators are presented in Fig. 2.

3 Mechanism of inflammation in physiological and pathological process

Irrespective of the type of injury, immediate vascular response is of transient vasoconstriction of arterioles followed by persistent progressive vasodilation which results in increased blood volume in microvascular bed of the area, which is responsible for redness and warmth at site of acute inflammation. Endothelial activation result in the release of histamine; thrombin; TNF immediate vascular changes, vasodilatation of the arterioles, capillaries, and postcapillary venules; erythema, swelling, and pain in the inflamed area. Vasodilatation and fluid exudation are accompanied by leukocyte margination, adhesion, and migration. Neutrophils are the first and most abundant

Recent Developments in Anti-Inflammatory Therapy. https://doi.org/10.1016/B978-0-323-99988-5.00012-7

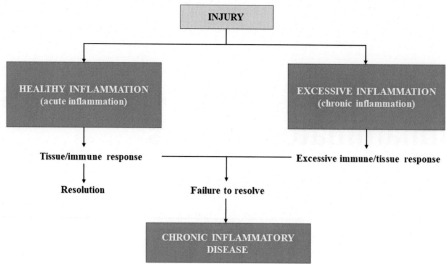

FIG. 1 Different types of inflammation.

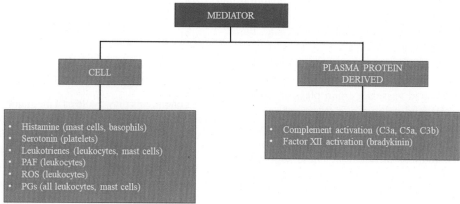

FIG. 2 Mediators of inflammation.

leukocytes to be delivered to the site of infection or inflammation. The transmigration phenomenon is divided into several distinct steps: margination, rolling, adhesion, diapedesis, and chemotaxis (Fig. 3). Margination is the process of neutrophil movement from the central bloodstream to the periphery of the vessel. This phenomenon is facilitated by stasis following fluid exudation at the site of inflammation and physical interactions between erythrocytes and neutrophils. After margination, a weak adhesive interaction develops between neutrophils and vascular endothelial cells, causing neutrophils to remain in close proximity to the vascular endothelium. Neutrophil rolling is facilitated by the shear stress of passing erythrocytes. The neutrophils move across the endothelial cells, i.e., transendothelial migration, and enter into the extravascular space followed by chemotaxis. Finally, various cytokines are released which kill the microbes as shown in Fig. 3.

The mediators derived from lipids also play a significant role in inflammation. These mediators are generally produced from action of phospholipase which degrades phospholipids of membranes resulting in the production of arachidonic acid. The 5-LOX and COX enzymes convert the arachidonic acid into leukotrienes (LTs) and prostaglandins (PGs), respectively (Fig. 4). The excess production of these mediators results in various pathological conditions.

In pathological conditions, excessive inflammatory mediators are released which destroy body cells. In sepsis (a severe systemic inflammation), vasodilation process could result in systemic hypotension and shock. The undesired inflammation could also result in the formation of edema due to transvascular flux of protein-rich fluid from the intravascular compartment into the interstitium as a result of the actions of histamine, bradykinin, leukotrienes, complement components, substance P, and platelet-activating factor (PAF). These factors markedly alter the barrier functions of small blood vessels and increase the permeability of capillaries and venules for both water and protein. At the same time, capillary hydrostatic pressure increases at the site of injury early during inflammation

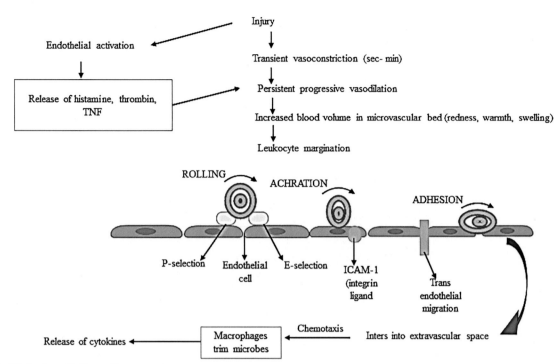

FIG. 3 Mechanism of inflammation.

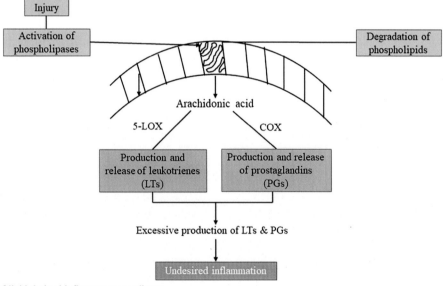

FIG. 4 Production of lipid-derived inflammatory mediators.

or injury as a result of local vasodilatation. The outpouring of protein-rich fluid causes a concentration of erythrocytes in small vessels and increases viscosity of the blood. This transvascular fluid flux eventually returns intravascular pressures at the site of inflammation to normal. At the same time, the loss of plasma proteins decreases the intravascular oncotic pressure. Together, the increase in vascular permeability, transient augmentation of capillary hydrostatic pressure, and fall in plasma oncotic pressure act to induce a

transvascular flux of fluid and protein into the inflamed interstitium. The function of these alterations is to allow the delivery of soluble factors such as antibodies and acute-phase proteins to the site of injury. Severe systemic inflammation can, however, cause inappropriate increase in vascular permeability that can result in edema formation in the lungs and extremities. The accumulation of fluid in the lungs causes the acute respiratory distress syndrome, a major source of morbidity and mortality in critically ill patients.

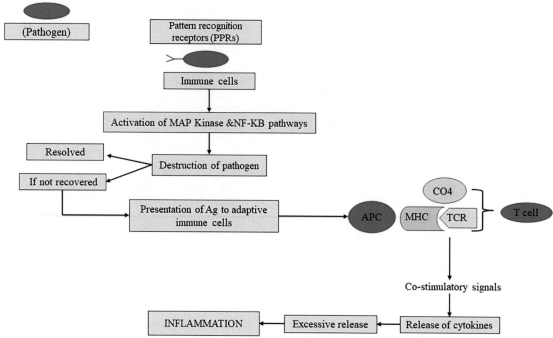

FIG. 5 Immune system and inflammation.

Edema accumulation in the extremities may lead to compartment syndrome and the loss of vital perfusion in the distal extremities.

4 Inflammation and immune system

Inflammation consists of a tightly regulated cascade of immunological, physiological, and behavioral processes that are orchestrated by soluble immune signaling molecules called cytokines. The first step of the inflammatory cascade involves recognition of infection or damage. The pathogens possess specific structures outside the surface called pathogen-associated molecular patterns (PAMPs) which are sensed by innate immune cells through pattern recognition receptors (PRRs). The well-known PRRs are Toll-like receptors (TLRs), NOD-like receptors, etc. The innate immune system contains first line of defense, i.e., skin and mucous membrane and second line of defense, i.e., white blood cells (WBCs). The skin contains a keratin protein that protects us from pathogens whereas mucous membrane contains various enzymes that destroy pathogens. If pathogens enter into the systemic circulation, WBCs sense the pathogen and activate innate immune signaling pathways (NF-κB and MAP kinase) followed by translocation to the nucleus and production of cytokines such as interleukin-1-beta (IL-1β), IL-6, tumor necrosis factor-alpha (TNF-α), etc., which destroy pathogens. Other toxic chemicals such as ROS, RNS, and various proteinases also released, which destroy pathogens. Overall, this process eliminates the pathogen with

cardinal signs of inflammation, i.e., heat, swelling, redness, pain, and loss of function.

However, adaptive immune system is activated if innate immune system is not able to handle the pathogen. The antigenic peptide is presented by antigen-presenting cells (APCs) to the T cells (adaptive immune system). The major histocompatibility complex proteins (MHC-1 and 2), costimulatory signals, T-cell receptors (TCRs), CD4 (helper T cells), CD8 (cytotoxic T cells), etc., play a significant role in presenting antigenic peptides to adaptive immune cells (Fig. 5). It results in the activation and proliferation of T cells. The activated T cells (helper T cells, cytotoxic T cells, regulated T cells) release various that destroy pathogens. Also, these released cytokines activate B cells to produce antibodies. However, the overactivation of adaptive immune system results in various pathological conditions.

5 Clinical trials of antiinflammatory drugs

Various clinical trials have been conducted to find the efficacy and safety of antiinflammatory drugs against various inflammatory diseases. The information is compiled below.

5.1 Back pain

Various classes of antiinflammatory drugs have been tested for the treatment of various types of back pains.

Marcu et al. [9] have tested etoricoxib in a randomized, longitudinal, controlled trial, and concluded that etoricoxib facilitates the application of individualized exercise programs in patients with ankylosing spondylitis. Various clinical trials of antiinflammatory drugs in the treatment of various types of back pains are compiled in Table 1.

5.2 Osteoarthritis

Osteoarthritis is one the major inflammatory disorder affecting millions of peoples. Various clinical trials of antiinflammatory molecules in the treatment of osteoarthritis are being conducted. Recently, Nuelle et al. [16] have tested ibuprofen in a prospective, randomized, parallel, single-blind study in the treatment of osteoarthritis. The clinical trials conducted so far with antiinflammatory drugs in osteoarthritis are compiled in Table 2.

5.3 Migraine and headache

Inflammation is also involved in migraine and headache. The antiinflammatory molecules have been tested in different phases of clinical trials and mixed results were observed. Gertsch et al. [63] have tested acetazolamide in a prospective, double-blind, randomized, placebo-controlled trial and found that acetazolamide or ibuprofen has similar efficacy in moderate or severe headache. However, both these drugs have been found to be more effective than placebo. Various clinical trials of antiinflammatory drugs in the treatment of migraine and headache are compiled in Table 3.

5.4 Rheumatoid arthritis

Rheumatoid arthritis is one of the autoimmune diseases which mainly affects the joints. Inflammation plays a significant role in rheumatoid arthritis. Thus, various classes of antiinflammatory drugs have been tested in clinical trials in the treatment of rheumatoid arthritis. Bakhtiari et al. [69] have tested guluronic acid in phase I/II clinical trial and found immunological mechanism of G2013 as a novel antiinflammatory that could reduce pro-inflammatory cytokine and its transcription factors. Vanags et al. [70] have tested chaperonin 10 in randomized, double-blind, multicentric study, and found that it is well tolerated and efficacious in the treatment of the symptoms of rheumatoid arthritis. The clinical trials of antiinflammatory drugs tested for rheumatoid arthritis are compiled in Table 4.

5.5 Conjunctivitis and cataract surgery

Various classes of antiinflammatory drugs have been tested for the treatment of conjunctivitis and cataract surgery. Kontadakis et al. [82] conducted a prospective, comparative, contralateral randomized study, and concluded that nepafenac 0.3% ophthalmic suspension in a daily regimen after PRK seems to be an effective treatment for pain and ocular discomfort with effects similar to the 0.1% suspension. Donnenfeld and Holland [83] have tested dexamethasone in a prospective, randomized, double-masked, multicentric trial, and the concluded that the IBI-10090 dexamethasone drug delivery suspension placed in the anterior chamber after cataract surgery at concentrations of 342 and 517 μg was safe and effective in treating inflammation occurring after cataract surgery. Various clinical trials of antiinflammatory drugs tested for conjunctivitis and cataract surgery are compiled in Table 5.

5.6 Throat infections

Antiinflammatory drugs have been tested for the treatment of throat infections. Agarwal et al. [114] have tested a benzydamine hydrochloride in a prospective, randomized, placebo-controlled single-blind study and found significant reduction in the incidence and severity of postoperative of sore throat. Kiderman et al. [115] have tested prednisone in randomized, placebo-controlled trial and experienced more rapid throat pain resolution than those in the placebo group. Watson et al. [116] have found flurbiprofen as effective and well-tolerated treatment for sore throat in a randomized, double-blind, placebo-controlled study (Table 6).

5.7 Asthma

Asthma is hyperresponsiveness of bronchial smooth muscle which is considered not only an airway disease but also an inflammatory disorder. Thus, various powerful antiinflammatory drugs are already being used for its management and many are under clinical trials. Malizia et al. [117] have tested beclomethasone dipropionate in an open label, randomized controlled study and found it to be more effective than CTZ in improving nasal patency, nasal cytology, sleep quality, and quality of life. Asai et al. [118] have tested a combination of salmeterol and fluticasone (SFC 250) in a randomized, double-blind, parallel group, placebo-controlled trial and found that SFC 250 did not produce significant changes from baseline in sputum neutrophil levels or other sputum or serum inflammatory markers compared with placebo. The clinical trials of antiinflammatory drugs tested for the management of asthma are compiled in Table 7.

5.8 Acne

Various antiinflammatory drugs have been tested for the treatment of acne. Kircik [154] have tested doxycycline in a single-center, open label pilot study and concluded that

TABLE 1 Clinical trials related to antiinflammatory drugs in treatment of back pain.

Sr no.	Name of drug	Type of study	Dose	Route of administration	Duration	Effects	References
1.	Etoricoxib	Randomized, longitudinal, controlled trial	90 mg/day	Oral	52 weeks	Etoricoxib, facilitate the application of individualized exercise programs in patients with ankylosing spondylitis.	[9]
2.	Ketorolac	Randomized, double-blind trial	10, 15, and 30 mg	i.v.	120 min	Ketorolac has similar analgesic efficacy at intravenous doses of 10, 15, and 30 mg, showing that intravenous ketorolac administered at the analgesic ceiling dose (10 mg) provided effective pain relief to ED patients with moderate-to-severe pain without increased adverse effects.	[10]
3.	Diclofenac	Randomized, double-blind, active comparator- and placebo-controlled, parallel-group phase III multicenter study	25, 50, or 75 mg	s.c.	8 h	Single SC doses of diclofenac HPbCD of 25 and 50 mg are effective and well tolerated for relieving pain compared with placebo.	[11]
4.	Tizanidine	Double-blind, double-dummy, randomized, comparative, multicentric, parallel group study	100 mg	Oral	7 days	Aceclofenac-tizanidine combination was more effective than aceclofenac alone and had a favorable safety profile in the treatment of acute low back pain.	[12]
5.	Cyclobenzaprine	Prospective, randomized, open-label, multicenter, community-based study	5 mg t.i.d.	Oral	7 days	Combination therapy with cyclobenzaprine 5 mg t. i.d. plus ibuprofen was not superior to cyclobenzaprine 5 mg t.i.d. alone in adult patients with acute neck and back pain with muscle spasm. All treatments were well tolerated.	[13]
6.	Piroxicam-beta-cyclodextrin	An open-label noncomparative study	20 mg	Oral	6 months	Newly developed dosage form of piroxicam is effective and well tolerated in the treatment of patients with chronic BP.	[14]
7	Nimesulide	A prospective, randomized double-blind comparative trial	10 mg	Oral	10 days	Nimesulide is an effective and well-tolerated agent for use in general practices to treat acute low back pain. The incidence of gastrointestinal side effects seems to be lower with nimesulide than with ibuprofen.	[15]
8.	Nimesulide	Randomized, double-blind comparative trial	100–300 mg	Oral	10 days	Nimesulide was found to be more effective than ibuprofen in improved lateral bending measurements.	[15]

BP, blood pressure; *ED*, emergency department; *HPbCD*, hydroxypropyl b-cyclodextrin; *t.i.d.*, three times in a day.

TABLE 2 Clinical trials related to antiinflammatory drugs in treatment of osteoarthritis.

Sr no.	Name of drug	Design	Dose	Route of administration	Duration	Effects	References
1.	Ibuprofen	A prospective, randomized, parallel, single-blind study	4–10 mg/kg/dose	Oral	10–12 weeks	Ibuprofen is an effective medication for fracture pain in children and its use does not impair clinical or radiographic long bone fracture healing in skeletally immature patients.	[16]
2.	ONO-4474	Multicenter, placebo-controlled, randomized, double-blind, parallel-group comparative study	100 mg	Oral	28 days	ONO-4474 was well tolerated overall and may offer an improved safety profile compared with NSAIDs or weak opioids for the treatment of moderate-to-severe knee pain in OA patients.	[17]
3.	Loxoprofen	A phase III, parallel, randomized, double-blind, double-dummy, noninferiority comparative trial	100 mg	Topical	8 days	LX-P has a comparable efficacy to LX-T, but with a better safety profile, being a therapeutic option for the treatment of posttraumatic injury pain.	[18]
4.	Ustekinumab	Phase III, randomized, placebo-controlled PSUMMIT 1 and PSUMMIT 2 studies	45 and 90 mg	s.c.	24 weeks	Ustekinumab demonstrated greater clinical response at week 24 compared with placebo.	[19]
5.	Zaltoprofen	An assessor-blinded, randomized controlled trial with three parallel arms	80 mg t.i.d.	Oral	7 weeks	–	[20]
6.	Resveratrol	A prospective, parallel-group, double-blind, randomized controlled multicenter study	40 mg	Oral	6 months	–	[21]
7.	Pelubiprofen	A randomized, open-label, crossover study	45 mg	Oral	4 months	No clinically significant pharmacokinetic interactions between pelubiprofen and eperisone hydrochloride exist after the administration of 75-mg sustained-release eperisone hydrochloride and 45-mg sustained-release pelubiprofen.	[22]

Continued

TABLE 2 Clinical trials related to antiinflammatory drugs in treatment of osteoarthritis—cont'd

Sr no.	Name of drug	Design	Dose	Route of administration	Duration	Effects	References
8.	Tramadol hydrochloride/acetaminophen combination (TRAM/APAP)	A prospective, randomized, open-label clinical trial	75/650 mg	Oral	14 days	TKA of TRAM/APAP was shown to be superior to that of NSAID in the treatment of perioperative pain management.	[23]
9.	Diclofenac patch	A randomized, double-blind, placebo-controlled trial	140 mg		7 days	The diclofenac patch could be a safe and effective alternative to the oral administration of nonsteroidal antiinflammatory drugs in the treatment of minor sport injuries.	[24]
10.	Diclofenac sodium	A phase II, 4-week, randomized, double-blind, parallel-group, two-arm, vehicle-controlled study	2%	Topical	4 weeks	Significantly greater improvement in pain reduction in patients with OA of the knee vs vehicle control and was well tolerated.	[25]
11.	Hydroxychloroquine	Multicenter, randomized, double-blind, placebo-controlled trial	200/400 mg	Oral	12 months	–	[26]
12.	Naproxen sodium-codeine phosphate	A prospective, randomized, double-blind study	550 mg + 30 mg	Oral	6 months	Provided more effective analgesia than naproxen sodium and did not increase side effects.	[27]
13.	Betamethasone	An open-label parallel-group randomized trial.	7 mg	Oral	7 days	Betamethasone 7 mg i.m. once for all was more effective and had quicker effects than diclofenac sodium 75 mg oral administration b.i.d. for 7 days for acute attack of gout within 24 h.	[28]
14.	Traumeel ointment	Prospective, multicenter, randomized, blinded, active-controlled and noninferiority study	2 g	Topical	12 weeks	Traumeel ointment decreased pain and improved joint function to the same extent as diclofenac gel in acute ankle sprain, and was well tolerated.	[29]
15.	Celecoxib	Randomized, double-blind, parallel-group study	200 mg	Oral	6 weeks	Celecoxib was as effective as naproxen in reducing OA pain. Celecoxib was well tolerated and demonstrated favorable upper gastro-intestinal tolerability.	[30]

16.	OMS103HP	Prospective, double-blind, randomized, vehicle-controlled, parallel-group study	30mL	Intraarticular injection	90days	The use of OMS103HP resulted in reduced acute postoperative pain, reduced pain during recovery, improved postoperative knee motion, and improved functional outcomes as assessed with the KOOS Knee Survey.	[31]
17.	Ibuprofen	a multicenter, randomized, double-blind placebo-controlled trial	800mg	i.v.	7 days	Pre- and postoperative administration of i.v.-ibuprofen significantly reduced both pain and morphine use in orthopedic surgery patients.	[32]
18.	Flavocoxid	Randomized, double-blind study	500mg b.i.d.	Oral	12 weeks	Flavocoxid was as effective as naproxen in managing the signs and symptoms of OA of the knee.	[33]
19.	Morphine sulfate and naltrexone hydrochloride (MS-sNT)	Phase III, randomized-withdrawal, double-blind, multicenter design	20–160mg/day	Oral	9 months	MS-sNT provided effective analgesia in patients with chronic, moderate-to-severe osteoarthritis pain, with a safety profile typical of morphine-containing products. Naltrexone sequestered in MS-sNT had no clinically relevant effect when MS-sNT was taken as directed.	[34]
20.	Venlafaxine	Single-blind placebo run-in trial	150–225mg	Oral	12 weeks	Venlafaxine significantly reduced pain intensity on the BPI and marginally improved self-reported function.	[35]
21.	Golimumab	A randomized, double-blind, placebo-controlled phase III study	50 or 100mg	Subcutaneous	4 weeks	Antibody-to-golimumab status, baseline C-reactive protein level, and smoking status were identified as significant covariates on apparent clearance.	[36]
22.	Acetaminophen extended-release (APAP ER)	A randomized, controlled study	1300mg.t.i.d.	Oral	4 weeks	APAP ER 3900mg daily was noninferior to rofecoxib 12.5 mg daily, but noninferiority was not established to rofecoxib 25 mg daily. APAP ER was well tolerated and no safety issues were identified.	[37]
23.	Combination of nimesulide and racemethionine	Open, randomized, comparative clinical trial	100mg+50mg	Oral	3 months	Combination of nimesulide and racemethionine is found to be better for the long-term treatment of osteoarthritis in patients.	[38]

Continued

TABLE 2 Clinical trials related to antiinflammatory drugs in treatment of osteoarthritis—cont'd

Sr no.	Name of drug	Design	Dose	Route of administration	Duration	Effects	References
24.	Aceclofenac	A double-blind, parallel-group, multicenter clinical trial.	200 mg/day	Oral	6 weeks	Patients with symptomatic OA of the knee showed a greater improvement in pain and functional capacity with aceclofenac than paracetamol with no difference in tolerability.	[39]
25.	Sodium hyaluronate	Controlled, randomized, an intention-to-treat, masked-observer study		Intraarticular	24 weeks	A single course of three SH injections is effective in relieving pain and improving joint function in patients with OA of the CMC joint of the thumb. Although in comparison with triamcinolone its effects are achieved more slowly, the results indicate a superior long-lasting effect of hyaluronan at 6 months after end of treatment period.	[40]
26.	Lumiracoxib	Randomized, double-blind multicenter study	400 mg once daily	Oral	96 h	Lumiracoxib is an effective alternative to traditional nonselective nonsteroidal antiinflammatory drugs (NSAIDs) for the treatment of postoperative pain.	[41]
27.	Etoricoxib	A randomized, double-blind, placebo-controlled trial	30 mg once daily	Oral	12 weeks	Primary end points (WOMAC) ranged from −16.53 to −13.55 mm, −27.89 to −23.68 mm, and −26.53 to −22.97 mm in the placebo, etoricoxib, and ibuprofen groups, respectively. For patients with OA, treatment with etoricoxib, 30 mg/day is well tolerated and provides sustained clinical effectiveness that is superior to placebo and comparable to ibuprofen, 2400 mg/day.	[42]
28.	Rofecoxib	Prospective, randomized, double-blinded study	50 mg	Oral	12–24 h	Preoperative rofecoxib is as effective as ketorolac for the treatment of pain after knee arthroscopy. Higher frequency of pain reporting at 24 h by patients in ketorolac group is explained by the longer analgesic effect of rofecoxib.	[43]

No.	Drug	Study design	Dose	Route	Duration	Outcome	Reference
29.	Bupivacaine	A prospective, randomized, controlled trial	0.5%	Epidural	1 year	There was a significant reduction in pain early on in those having an epidural steroid injection but no difference in the long term between the two groups.	[44]
30.	Lumiracoxib	Randomized, double-blind multicenter study	400 mg	Oral	96 h	Lumiracoxib and naproxen were comparable and both treatments were superior to placebo for the treatment of postoperative pain.	[41]
31.	Tramadol	Multicenter, randomized, double-blind, placebo-controlled trial	37.5 mg	Oral	91 days	Tramadol 37.5 mg/APAP 325 mg combination tablets were effective and safe as add-on therapy with COX-2 NSAID for treatment of OA pain.	[45]
32.	Oxaprozin	Open, multicenter, randomized, controlled study	1200 mg/day	Oral	15 days	Once-daily oxaprozin proved to be as effective as diclofenac t.i.d. in reducing the primary efficacy variable of patient-assessed shoulder pain score in patients with periarthritis of the shoulder refractory to previous treatments with other NSAIDs. Oxaprozin was shown to be superior to diclofenac in improving shoulder function.	[46]
33.	Lumiracoxib	Multicenter, randomized, double-blind study	400 mg OD	Oral	13 weeks	Lumiracoxib demonstrated significant improvement in OA pain intensity, patient's global assessment of disease activity, and the WOMAC pain subscale and total scores compared with celecoxib.	[47]
34.	5% Ibuprofen cream	Double-blind, randomized, placebo-controlled, parallel-group study with an adaptive sequential design	Each strip contains 200 mg		7 days	Effective against pain at rest, overall pain, Lequesne index, no adverse event was recorded.	[48]
35.	Etoricoxib	Double-blind, active comparator controlled, parallel-group study	60 mg	Oral	6 weeks	Etoricoxib is clinically effective in the therapy of osteoarthritis providing a magnitude of effect comparable to that of the maximum recommended daily dose of diclofenac.	[49]

Continued

TABLE 2 Clinical trials related to antiinflammatory drugs in treatment of osteoarthritis—cont'd

Sr no.	Name of drug	Design	Dose	Route of administration	Duration	Effects	References
36.	Acetaminophen	A randomized, double-blind, placebo-controlled trial	1000 mg	Oral	2 weeks	Diclofenac is effective in the symptomatic treatment of OA of the knee, but acetaminophen is not.	[50]
37.	Nimesulide vs rofecoxib	A prospective, randomized, double-blind, double-dummy, parallel group study	300 mg (nimesulide) 25 mg (rofecoxib)	Oral	30 days	Both drugs were equally effective in terms of overall improvement of pain and the quality of life; they were equally well tolerated.	[51]
38.	Dexibuprofen (S(+)-ibuprofen)	Randomized, parallel-group, double-blind, active-controlled clinical trial	400 mg b.i.d.	Oral	15 days	Dexibuprofen has at least equal efficacy and a comparable safety/tolerability profile as celecoxib in adult patients suffering from osteoarthritis of the hip.	[52]
39.	Pamidronate	Randomized, double-blind, controlled trial	60 mg vs 10 mg	i.v.	6 months	Pamidronate has dose-dependent therapeutic properties in AS.	[53]
40.	Acemetacin	Double-blind, randomized, controlled parallel group	60 mg t.i.d.	Oral	28 days	Acemetacin is effective as indomethacin for the treatment of OA and incidence of gastrointestinal side effects was significantly lower for acemetacin than for indomethacin.	[54]
41.	Ibuprofen syrup	Randomized in a double-blind, placebo-controlled trial	10 mg/kg	Oral	5 days	Ibuprofen shortened the duration of symptoms in children with a clinical diagnosis of transient synovitis of the hip.	[55]
42.	Valdecoxib	A randomized, double-blind, placebo-controlled comparison	5 and 10 mg b.i.d.	Oral	12 weeks	Single daily doses of valdecoxib 5 and 10 mg were similar to naproxen and superior to placebo, in treating symptomatic OA of the hip. Both doses of valdecoxib were well tolerated and demonstrated improved GI tolerability compared to naproxen.	[56]

		Dose	Route	Duration	Outcome	Ref
43.	Acemetacine	Prospective, unblinded, randomized clinical trial with an 8-week follow-up	120 mg/kg	Oral	8 weeks	Significant improvement in carpal tunnel syndrome.	[57]
44.	Celecoxib	A multicenter, parallel group, double-blind, double-dummy, randomized, controlled trial	200 mg	Oral	6 weeks	Patients receiving celecoxib experienced less edema and less destabilization of blood pressure control compared with those receiving rofecoxib.	[58]
45.	Rofecoxib	A multicenter, randomized, controlled trial	12.5 and 25 mg once daily	Oral	6 weeks	In patients 80 years and older, rofecoxib, 12.5 and 25 mg once daily demonstrated clinical efficacy for the treatment for OA as did 1500 mg of nabumetone. Rofecoxib and nabumetone were generally well tolerated in this elderly population.	[59]
46.	Tiaprofenic acid	A randomized placebo-controlled trial	300 mg (b.i.d.)	Oral	5 years	NSAIDs significantly reduce overall pain over 4 weeks.	[60]
47.	Piroxicam	Randomized, parallel study	1 mg/kg/day	Oral		Oral piroxicam is an effective and safe treatment in the management of the osteoarticular painful crisis in sickle cell anemia.	[61]
48.	Diacerein	Randomized, double-blind, placebo-controlled, parallel study	50, 100, and 150 mg/day (b.i.d.)	Oral	16 weeks	Diacerein have been shown to be an effective treatment for patients with knee OA.	[62]

AS, ankylosing spondylitis; *BP*—blood pressure; *OA*, osteoarthritis; *SH*, sodium hyaluronate.

TABLE 3 Clinical trials related to antiinflammatory drugs in the treatment of migraine and headache.

Sr no.	Name of drug	Design	Dose	Route	Duration	Effect	References
1.	DFN-15	Single-dose randomized crossover study	120, 180, and 240 mg	Oral	26 days	DFN-15 oral solution peak plasma concentration were found to be higher than capsule oral formulation. DFN-15 oral solution peak plasma concentration was found to be higher than capsule oral formulation. DFN-15 was more rapidly absorbed and eliminated than 400 mg celecoxib oral capsules.	[64]
2.	Acetazolamide	A prospective, double-blind, randomized, placebo-controlled trial	85 mg	Oral		Moderate or severe headache incidence was similar when treated with acetazolamide or ibuprofen and both agents were significantly more effective than placebo.	[63]
3.	Dexketoprofen	Prospective randomized, double-blind, placebo-controlled trial	50 mg	i.v.	3 months	Intravenous dexketoprofen is superior to placebo in relieving migraine headaches in the ED.	[65]
4.	Diclofenac-K	A single-dose multicenter, randomized, double-blind, double-dummy, clinical trial	12.5 and 25 mg	Oral	3–6 h evaluation time	Relieves ETH and is comparable to ibuprofen 400 mg.	[66]
5.	Ketoprofen	Double-blind, placebo-controlled, randomized crossover trial	75/150 mg	Oral	2 h short-term study	Effective and well-tolerated drug in the acute treatment of migraine attacks.	[67]
6.	Rofecoxib	Randomized, open-label study	10 mg	Oral		Combining a fast acting triptan such as rizatriptan with rofecoxib reduced headache recurrence rates, was well tolerated.	[68]
7.	Ketoprofen	A double-blind, placebo-controlled, randomized crossover trial of a dual-release formulation	75 or 150 mg	Oral		Effective and well-tolerated drug in the treatment of acute migraine attacks.	[67]

ETH, episodic tension-type headache.

TABLE 4 Clinical trials related to antiinflammatory drugs in the treatment of rheumatoid arthritis.

Sr no.	Name of drug	Type of study	Dose	Route	Duration	Effects	References
1.	Guluronic acid	Phase I/II clinical trial	500 mg	Oral	12 weeks	Immunological mechanism of G2013 as a novel antiinflammatory that could reduce pro-inflammatory cytokine and their transcription factors.	[69]
2.	Chaperonin 10	Randomized, double-blind, multicenter study	5 mg	i.v.	12 weeks	Well tolerated and efficacious in the treatment of the symptoms of rheumatoid arthritis.	[70]
3.	Indomethacin, diclofenac, and ibuprofen	Single-dose, randomized, crossover trial with a 1-week washout period	25, 5 0 mg 50, 100, 400, 600 mg	Oral		The NSAIDs indomethacin, ibuprofen, and diclofenac produced concentration-related suppression of prostaglandin synthesis.	[71]
4.	Artrofoon	A randomized, open-label, comparative trial	8 tablets daily	Oral	6 months	A half-dose treatment with artrofoon (4 tablets daily) was able to sustain clinical improvements over a 6-month follow-up period.	[72]
5.	Adalimumab	A double-blind, randomized, placebo-controlled study	40 mg	Oral	24 weeks	Adalimumab significantly improved joint and skin manifestations, inhibited structural changes on radiographs, lessened disability due to joint damage, and improved quality of life in patients with moderate to severe active PsA.	[73]
6.	Amtolmetin guacyl (AMG)	Randomized, parallel group, double-blind, double-dummy, multicenter trial	600 mg	Oral	24 weeks	AMG and celecoxib proved to be equivalent, showing comparable gastrointestinal safety and therapeutic efficacy in the treatment of rheumatoid arthritis.	[74]
7.	Etanercept	An open-label trial	20 mg	Oral	12 months	Useful adjunct to glucocorticoids in the treatment of TA.	[75]
8.	Tacrolimus (FK506)	Double-blind, multicenter, randomized, placebo-controlled study	1.5 mg/day	Oral	16 weeks		[76]
9.	Nabumetone	An open label, multicenter study	30 mg/kg/day	Oral	12 weeks	Nabumetone 30 mg/kg/day (up to 2000 mg/day) demonstrated a safe profile with no loss of efficacy compared to previous treatment in children with JRA.	[77]
10.	Meloxicam	Phase I/II study	0.25 mg/kg	Oral	52 weeks	Meloxicam suspension once daily seems to be effective and safe for treating active JRA over a period of 52 weeks.	[78]
11.	Pirfenidone	Open-label study			3–24 months	Pirfenidone appeared to be safe and reduced the incidence of clinical relapses over the 24 months of the study. No new nonenhancing or enhancing MRI lesions were detected over the 24 months of treatment in patients on pirfenidone.	[79]
12.	Celecoxib	Randomized, double-blind, placebo-controlled trial with three treatment arms: placebo,	Ketoprofen 100 mg b.i.d., and celecoxib 100 mg b.i.d.	Oral	6 weeks	Confirm the clinically relevant antiinflammatory effect of celecoxib at a 200-mg daily dosage, with significant improvement in both pain and function in patients with AS.	[80]
13.	1	Randomized, double-blind, multicenter, parallel-group study	2000 mg/day	Oral	12 weeks	Effective as naproxen 1000 mg/day in relieving the signs and symptoms of RA. No serious GI adverse events were observed with either NSAID, but nabumetone was associated with a higher incidence of diarrhea.	[81]

AS, ankylosing spondylitis.

TABLE 5 Clinical trials related to antiinflammatory drugs in the treatment of conjunctivitis and cataract surgery.

Sr no.	Name of drug	Type of study	Dose	Route	Duration	Effects	References
1.	Nepafenac	A prospective, comparative, contralateral randomized study	0.3%	Topical	2 weeks	Nepafenac 0.3% ophthalmic suspension in a daily regimen after PRK seems to be an effective treatment for pain and ocular discomfort with effects similar to the 0.1% suspension.	[82]
2.	Dexamethasone	Prospective, randomized, double-masked, multicenter trial	5 μL	Intracameral injection	21 days	The IBI-10090 dexamethasone drug-delivery suspension placed in the anterior chamber after cataract surgery at concentrations of 342 and 517 μg was safe and effective in treating inflammation occurring after cataract surgery.	[83]
3.	Indomethacin 0.1%	Prospective randomized clinical trial		Topical	6 months	SLT induces little inflammation: antiinflammatory drops do not make a significant difference in pain, redness, cells in anterior chamber, or peak IOP following SLT. The IOP-lowering effect of the SLT is not influenced by the use of indomethacin or dexamethasone.	[84]
4.	PEA (defluxa)	A pilot clinical trial		Topical	30 days	Topical PEA (defluxa) is a safe, effective, and generally well-tolerated treatment to prevent or suppress ocular surface inflammation attributable to chronic glaucoma treatment.	[85]
5.	Clacier	Multicenter (six-study centers) double-masked study	0.05%	Topical	12 weeks	Treatment with clacier alleviated clinical signs and symptoms of DES comparably to the commercially available restasis, resulting in improved quality of life for patients. Clacier is an effective and safe therapeutic agent for DES.	[86]
6.	Nepafenac	Randomized double-masked clinical trial	0.1%	Topical	6 weeks	The combination of topical nepafenac and steroid treatment reduced subclinical macular swelling and inflammation as well as subjective complaints, indicating that it is an efficient antiinflammatory regimen after cataract surgery.	[87]
7.	Prednisolone acetate	Single-center, masked, randomized clinical study	1%	Topical	1 year	Preoperative use of ketorolac, prednisolone, and nepafenac was effective in maintaining intraoperative mydriasis when compared with placebo.	[88]

No.	Drug	Study type	Concentration	Route	Duration	Description	Ref.
8.	Triamcinolone acetonide	Randomized controlled study		Intracameral injections	1 month	Intracameral injections of triamcinolone acetonide and gentamicin appear to be a promising treatment option for the control of postoperative inflammation following cataract surgery.	[89]
9.	Bromfenac ophthalmic solution	Randomized, double-masked, vehicle-controlled or active-controlled, multicenter, clinical trials.	0.09%	Topical	22 days	Bromfenac 0.09% once daily was clinically safe and effective for reducing and treating ocular inflammation and pain associated with cataract surgery.	[90]
10.	Nepafenac 0.1%	Randomized double-masked single-center clinical trial		Topical	5 weeks	Nepafenac was more effective than fluorometholone in preventing angiographic CME and BAB disruption, and results indicate that nepafenac leads to more rapid visual recovery.	[91]
11.	5% Povidone-iodine drop	Prospective randomized study		Subconjunctival injection	6 months	Antiinflammatory, antiinfective effects and visual outcome are similar in both groups, 5% povidone iodine drop and dexamethasone and gentamicin combination group.	[92]
12.	Durezol	Difluprednate given two or four times a day cleared postoperative inflammation and reduced pain rapidly and effectively	0.05%	Ocular	15 days	Difluprednate given two or four times a day cleared postoperative inflammation and reduced pain rapidly and effectively. Fewer adverse events were reported in the difluprednate-treated groups than in the placebo group.	[93]
13.	Bepotastine besilate	Phase III, single-center, prospective, randomized, double-masked, placebo-controlled, CAC clinical trial	1.0% and 1.5%	Topical		CAC model of allergic conjunctivitis in adults and children, bepotastine besilate ophthalmic solutions 1.0% and 1.5% were associated with clinically and statistically significant reductions in ocular itching, but not conjunctival hyperemia, within 15 min that were maintained for at least 8 h after administration.	[94]
14	Ketorolac tromethamine	Open-label nonmasked randomized (random number assignment) study	0.5%	Topical	31 days	Ketorolac 0.5% was efficacious in decreasing postoperative macular edema.	[95]
15	Azithromycin ophthalmic solution	Randomized in an open-label study	1%	Topical	14 days	Azithromycin ophthalmic solution in combination with warm compresses provided a significantly greater clinical benefit than warm compresses alone in treating the signs and symptoms of posterior blepharitis.	[96]

Continued

TABLE 5 Clinical trials related to antiinflammatory drugs in the treatment of conjunctivitis and cataract surgery—cont'd

Sr no.	Name of drug	Type of study	Dose	Route	Duration	Effects	References
16.	Triamcinolone acetonide	Eyes were randomized	40 mg in mL	Subcutaneous	4 weeks	A single posterior subtenon injection of TA can be as effective and safe as a 4-week regimen of prednisolone acetate 1% eye drops in controlling intraocular inflammation after PPV.	[97]
17.	Bromfenac ophthalmic solution	Two phase III, multicenter, randomized, double-masked, parallel, placebo-controlled, clinical trials	0.09%	Topical	14 days	Bromfenac ophthalmic solution 0.09% demonstrated neither treatment-related systemic adverse events nor evidence of hepatic toxicity.	[98]
18.	0.1% prednisolone	Prospective, double-masked, randomized, comparative clinical trial		Topical	14–28 days	Keratoconjunctivitis sicca patients showed elevated levels of tear NGF, which were decreased by treatment with 0.1% prednisolone.	[99]
19.	Dexamethasone-	A randomized clinical trial	0.7%	Topical	3 weeks	Use of 0.7% dexamethasone-cyclodextrin eye drops may be useful especially in elderly people who cannot apply themselves the eye drops onto the eye.	[100]
20.	Ketotifen fumarate	Randomized, double-masked, artificial tear substitute (ATS)-controlled clinical trial	0.025% ophthalmic solution	Topical	30 days	Ketotifen and olopatadine diminished the expression of CAMs and inflammatory markers on the conjunctival surface cells effectively. Both active treatments were more efficacious compared with ATS and were well tolerated.	[101]
21.	Epinastine hydrochloride	Randomized (age-stratified), double-masked, parallel-group, active- and vehicle-controlled, environmental, phase III clinical trial	0.05% ophthalmic solution	Topical	8 weeks	Ophthalmic epinastine instilled twice daily was more effective than vehicle for the control of ocular itching and was similar in efficacy to levocabastine for the control of ocular itching and hyperemia. Epinastine was well tolerated.	[102]
22.	Rimexolone	One eye was randomized to receive topical 1% rimexolone while the contralateral eye received topical 0.1% fluorometholone	1% four times daily	topical	8 weeks	Rimexolone seems to be a more effective antiinflammatory agent than fluorometholone.	[103]
23.	Bromfenac sodium hydrate	A prospective, crossover and observer masked clinical trial		Topical	2 weeks	Results indicate that bromfenac sodium interferes with IOP reduction by latanoprost ophthalmic solution in normal volunteers and that we should take this into account when treating patients with glaucoma using latanoprost ophthalmic solution.	[104]
24.	Nedocromil sodium	A multicenter, open-label evaluation	2% twice	Topical	1 month	Effective and safe for the treatment of symptoms of allergic conjunctivitis, significantly improving quality of life and producing high rates of user and physician satisfaction.	[105]

#	Drug	Study type	Dose	Route	Duration	Findings	Ref.
25.	Ketorolac tromethamine	Prospectively and randomly assigned double masked study	5% solution	Topical		Effective as loteprednol etabonate ophthalmic suspension 0.5% in reducing inflammation after routine phacoemulsification and IOL implantation.	[106]
26.	Indomethacin	A randomized, multicenter study comparing two parallel groups	0.1%	Topical	30 days	Both antiinflammatory eye drops were effective in reducing subclinical conjunctival inflammation before filtering surgery. Regarding superficial punctate keratitis, the corneal tolerance of preservative-free indomethacin 0.1% eye drops seemed to be better than that of preserved fluorometholone eye drops.	[107]
27.	Indomethacin/gentamicin eye drops	A multicenter, randomized, double-masked study comparing two parallel treatment groups	0.1%	Topical	7 days	Combined indomethacin/gentamicin eye drops were effective and well tolerated in reducing the pain and discomfort associated with traumatic corneal abrasion.	[108]
28.	Dexamethasone phosphate eye gel	A prospective, multicenter, clinical parallel group study	0.1%	Topical		Effective and safe steroidal antiinflammatory agent for topical use following cataract surgery and intraocular lens implantation.	[109]
29.	Surodex	Randomized, masked, controlled trial		Intraocular	4 weeks to 1 year	Safe and effective treatment method to reduce intraocular inflammation after cataract surgery and clearly is superior to eye drops in reducing inflammatory symptoms and aqueous flare.	[110]
30.	Fluorometholone	Prospective clinical trial with randomization of fellow eyes to different postoperative treatment. Thirty-one consecutive children undergoing bilateral symmetrical strabismus operation.	6 drops and 1 drop	Ocular	4 weeks	No significant difference in antiinflammatory response between the two groups.	[111]
31.	Diclofenac	Prospective randomized double-masked double-dummy study	0.1% solution drops t.i.d.	Topical	28 days	The diclofenac-gentamicin combination followed by diclofenac alone was significantly better at suppressing flare and cells but showed a slightly higher incidence of punctate keratitis and eye discomfort.	[112]
32.	Ketorolac	A randomized, double-masked trial	0.5% four times daily	Topical	3–4 days follow-up visit	Topical ketorolac 0.5% used four times daily is no better than artificial tears at relieving the symptoms or signs of viral conjunctivitis and produces more stinging than artificial tears.	[113]

BAB, blood-aqueous barrier; *CME*, cystoid macular edema; *IOL*, intraocular lens; *NGF*, nerve growth factor; *PPV*, pars plana vitrectomy; *SLT*, selective laser trabeculoplasty.

TABLE 6 Clinical trials related to antiinflammatory drugs in the treatment of throat infections.

Sr no.	Name of drug	Type of study	Dose	Route	Duration	Effect	References
1.	Benzydamine hydrochloride	Prospective, randomized, placebo-controlled, single-blind study	0.15% gargle	Oral	24h	Significantly reduced the incidence and severity of postoperative sore throat.	[114]
2	Prednisone	Randomized placebo-controlled trial	60mg	Orally	2 weeks	Experienced more rapid throat pain resolution than those in the placebo group	[115]
3.	Flurbiprofen	A randomized, double-blind, placebo-controlled study	8.75mg	Oral	4 days	Provide an effective and well-tolerated treatment for sore throat.	[116]

combination treatment, i.e., doxycycline combined with adapalene 0.3% and benzoyl peroxide 2.5% gel is safe and effective for the management of severe acne. Dréno et al. [155] have tested A0.3/BPO2.5 gel in a randomized, investigator-blinded, split-face design and found additional improvement in atrophic scar count with 48 weeks' treatment. Various clinical trials of antiinflammatory drugs tested for acne treatment are compiled in Table 8.

5.9 Psoriasis

Various antiinflammatory drugs have also been tested for the treatment of psoriasis. Reich et al. [163] have reported the efficacy of mirikizumab at 300mg in a randomized phase II study. Bhatia et al. [164] have tested halobetasol propionate in two randomized, double-blind, vehicle-controlled clinical studies and results confirm the safety and effectiveness of HBP foam in the treatment of plaque psoriasis. Various clinical trials of antiinflammatory drug tested for the treatment of psoriasis are compiled in Table 9.

5.10 Other associated inflammation

Nguyen et al. [178] have tested ibuprofen in a study and demonstrated that the preoperative ibuprofen significantly decreased the levels of most pro-inflammatory cytokines in the dental pulp, which could possibly help with the anesthesia in IRREVERSIBLE cases. Kumar et al. [179] have tested tramadol in a randomized parallel, double-blind active-controlled pilot study and found that both tramadol and diclofenac are equally effective in controlling pain in AP with similar safety profile. The clinical trials are compiled in Table 10.

5.11 COVID-19

As we know that SARS-COv-2 infection results in undesired inflammation in the body. Therefore, existing antiinflammatory drugs such as indomethacin, mefenamic acid, etc., are being used for its management. Various clinical trials are also ongoing to test antiinflammatory molecules for its management. Saeedi-Boroujeni et al. [274] have tested tranilast and found its efficacy in the improvement of severe COVID-19 cases by preventing key inflammatory transcription factors such as NF-κB and inhibiting NLRP-3 inflammasome. Lopes et al. [275] have tested colchicine in a randomized, double-blind, placebo-controlled trial, and concluded that colchicine reduced the length of both supplemental oxygen therapy and hospitalization due to its antiinflammatory mechanism. Various clinical trials of antiinflammatory drugs tested for the treatment of COVID-19 are compiled in Table 11.

6 Conclusions

Many antiinflammatory drugs are under experimental investigation and some of them are in different phases of clinical trials in the management of various diseases associated with inflammation. We hope that many safe and effective antiinflammatory drugs for various conditions will reach in market soon.

Acknowledgments

The authors are thankful to Vice-Chancellor Professor (Dr.) R.K. Goyal, Delhi Pharmaceutical Sciences & Research University (DPSRU), New Delhi, 110017, India and Mr. Parvin Garg (Chairman) and Dr. G.D. Gupta (Director) of ISF College of Pharmacy, Moga, Punjab, 142001, India for continuous support and motivation.

TABLE 7 Clinical trials related to antiinflammatory drugs in the treatment of asthma.

Sr no.	Name of drug	Type of study	Dose	Route	Duration	Effects	References
1.	Prednisone	An open-label, proof of concept study	0.5 mg/kg		12 months	The addition of pirfenidone to the antiinflammatory treatment in patients with chronic HP may improve the outcome with acceptable safety profile.	[119]
2.	Beclomethasone dipropionate (nBDP)	Open-label, randomized controlled study	100 μg	Nasal	21 days	nBDP is more effective than CTZ in improving nasal patency, nasal cytology, sleep quality, and quality of life.	[117]
3.	Salmeterol + fluticasone propionate (SFC 250)	A randomized, double-blind, parallel group, placebo-controlled trial	50 + 25 μg	Inhalation	12 weeks	SFC 250 did not produce significant changes from baseline in sputum neutrophil levels or other sputum or serum inflammatory markers compared with placebo.	[118]
4.	Salmeterol/fluticasone propionate (SFC)	A randomized, controlled, parallel-group multicenter trial	50/100 μg	Inhalation	24 weeks	Maintenance therapy with SFC provides further improvements in cough symptoms, pulmonary function and airway inflammation, and discontinuation of the therapy causes worsening of the disease.	[120]
5.	Zileuton ER	A randomized controlled study	2400 mg/day	Oral	12 weeks	Zileuton ER seems to be more efficacious than Montelukast and well tolerated for the treatment of mild-to moderate chronic persistent asthma in adult patient population.	[121]
6.	Mometasone furoate/ formoterol (MF/F)	Open-label run-in, randomized controlled study	100/10, 200/ 10, or 400/ 10 μg	Inhalation	2 weeks	All three MF/F doses demonstrated pronounced, clinically meaningful, dose-dependent reductions in FENO, with reduced sputum eosinophil levels for MF/F 200/10 μg and MF/F 400/10 μg.	[122]
7.	Budesonide + formoterol	Placebo-controlled crossover design, including healthy males	400 mg + 12 mg	Inhalation	240 min	Combined budesonide and formoterol may reduce airway inflammation and immune reactivity of circulating lymphocytes through its local and systemic effects.	[123]
8.	Amoxicillin-clavulanic acid	Multicenter, parallel, single-blinded placebo-controlled, randomized clinical trial	500 mg/125	Oral	10 days	No significant differences were observed in the number of days with cough between patients with uncomplicated acute bronchitis and discolored sputum treated with ibuprofen, amoxicillin–clavulanic acid, or placebo.	[124]
9.	Levocetirizine	Randomized, parallel-group study	5 mg	Oral	4–8 weeks	Levocetirizine bases on its rate of response and relapse was superior to budesonide in the treatment of the high symptom group and is comparable in the low symptom group.	[125]

Continued

TABLE 7 Clinical trials related to antiinflammatory drugs in the treatment of asthma—cont'd

Sr no.	Name of drug	Type of study	Dose	Route	Duration	Effects	References
10.	Inhaled budesonide	The study was a prospective, double-blind, placebo-controlled, randomized, three-period crossover design	200 μg	Inhalation	33 days	This study demonstrated that 11 days of treatment with the combination of budesonide/formoterol significantly attenuated allergen-induced early and late asthmatic airway responses compared with placebo and significantly attenuated early asthmatic airway responses compared with budesonide alone.	[126]
11.	UK-500,001	Multicentered, 6-week, randomized, double-blind, placebo-controlled, parallel group study	0.1, 0.4, and 1.0 mg b.i.d.	Inhalation	6 weeks	The inhaled isotype-nonspecific, selective phosphodiesterase type-4 inhibitor UK-500,001 did not demonstrate efficacy at any dose, up to and including the maximum tolerated dose, in patients with moderate-to-severe chronic obstructive pulmonary disease.	[127]
12.	HFA beclomethasonediproprionate	Randomized, double-blind study	400 and 200 μg b.i.d.	Inhalation	14 days	Extra-fine HFA-BDP leads to a more rapid reduction of cough frequency at the beginning of treatment.	[128]
13.	Budesonide	A randomized, controlled-open study	250 μg (b.i.d.)	Inhalation	7–10 days	Short-term treatment with budesonide inhalation suspension, used for an indication out of label, may significantly reduce local neutrophilic inflammation, and nasal obstruction in children with recurrent upper airway infections.	[129]
14.	Hydrofluoroalkane formulation of beclomethasone dipropionate (HFA-BDP)	A randomized, placebo-controlled trial		Inhalation	10 weeks	HFA-BDP reduced eosinophilic inflammation and T helper 2-type cytokine expression in both early- and late-induced sputa, whereas the effect of DPI-BUD on inflammation was predominantly demonstrated in early-induced sputum.	[130]
15.	Rofecoxib Valdecoxib	Patients with challenge-proven NSAID cutaneous sensitivity were submitted to single-blinded controlled oral challenge	50 mg 40 mg	Oral		Rofecoxib and valdecoxib can be safely used by most NSAID-sensitive patients with cutaneous reactions.	[131]
16.	Fluticasone propionate	Randomized, controlled trial	125 μg b.i.d.	Inhalation	>3 weeks	Fluticasone propionate reduces neither supplemental O_2 use nor the need for ventilatory support in this patient population.	[132]
17.	Etoricoxib		90 mg	Oral		Low rate of adverse reactions to etoricoxib, tested by oral challenge, suggests that patients with previous cutaneous hypersensitivity reactions to NSAIDs (primarily urticaria and angioedema) may tolerate this drug.	[133]

No.	Drug	Study design	Dose	Route	Duration	Outcome	Ref.
18.	Ciclesonide	Phase III, randomized, double-dummy, open-label study	160 µg q.d.	Inhalation	12 weeks	Ciclesonide was as effective as budesonide in adults with persistent asthma. Both treatments were well tolerated.	[134]
19.	Nasal budesonide	Double-blind two-way crossover design	100 µg	Nasal		Single dose of nasal steroid has the capacity to selectively abolish IL-5 and IL-13 responses following NAC.	[135]
20.	Nebulized budesonide	Double-blind, placebo-controlled study	1 mg/dose	Inhalat on		Statistically significant difference between the two groups with respect to the increase in PEFR.	[136]
21.	Salmeterol/fluticasone propionate	A double-blind, randomized placebo-controlled trial	50/250 µg b.i.d.	Inhaler	3 months	Reduced airway hyperresponsiveness, FENO and tryptase density in the airway mucosa as markers of airway inflammation.	[137]
22.	Pirfenidone	A double-blind, placebo-controlled, randomized, multicenter, prospective clinical trial	200,400, and 80mg	Oral	9months	Treatment with pirfenidone improved VC and prevented acute exacerbation of IPF during the 9 months of follow-up.	[138]
23.	Fluticasone propionate (FP)	A randomized, double-blind, placebo-controlled trial	500mg (b.i.d.)	Inhalation	2 weeks	Antiinflammatory treatment with the inhaled steroid fluticasone propionate reduces cough in otherwise healthy adults who do not smoke.	[139]
24.	Etoricoxib	A double-masked, placebo-controlled design	120mg	Oral		Most NSAID-sensitive individuals with cutaneous reactions to classic NSAIDs will tolerate specific COX-2 inhibitors.	[140]
25.	Clarithromycin (CAM)		400mg/day	Oral	21 days	CAM may suppress the postoperative systemic inflammatory response syndrome in lung cancer patients.	[141]
26.	Montelukast		10mg	Oral	4 weeks	Improves nasal function and nasal response to aspirin substantially in ASA-sensitive asthmatics.	[142]
27.	Budesonide/ formoterol	Double-blind, randomized, parallel-group study conducted at 246 centers in 22 countries	80/4.5 µg b.i.d.	Oral	12months	Reduces the risk and rate of severe asthma exacerbations and the need for systemic steroids and improves asthma symptoms, nocturnal awakenings, and lung function compared with traditional fixed dosing regimens, thereby reducing the morbidity and potentially the mortality from asthma.	[126]
28.	Fluticasone propionate/ salmeterol	Randomized, double-blind, parallel group, placebo-controlled study	88/42 mg daily	Inhalation	12 weeks	Fluticasone propionate/salmeterol HFA MDI given as two inhalations, resulted in significantly greater improvements in overall asthma control than treatment with FP or S alone in patients previously uncontrolled on a short-acting or long-acting b2-agonist or inhaled corticosteroid alone.	[143]
29.	Albuterol	A randomized, double-blind trial	(0.1mg/kg/dose) three times per day	Oral	7 days	No significant group differences in any secondary outcome. Health care revisit and admission rates were similar between groups.	[144]

Continued

TABLE 7 Clinical trials related to antiinflammatory drugs in the treatment of asthma—cont'd

Sr no.	Name of drug	Type of study	Dose	Route	Duration	Effects	References
30.	Budesonide	Randomized, double-blind, double-dummy, parallel group, multicenter, dose-reduction trial	800 μg/day	Dry powder inhaler	4–6 weeks	The budesonide-to-fluticasone ratio for the geometric mean MED was 123% (95% CI, 99–153 [not significant]).	[145]
31.	Azelastine eye drops	A randomized, placebo-controlled, double-blind, parallel-group study			30 min to 6 h	Azelastine, in comparison to placebo, significantly reduced symptom scores, number of inflammatory cells, and intercellular adhesion molecule-1 expression during the early- and late-phase reaction.	[146]
32.	Budesonide	Prospective, double-blind, double-dummy, placebo-controlled, randomized, four-period crossover design	400 μg/day	Inhalation	12 months	Attenuated allergen-induced sputum eosinophilia	[147]
33.	Azelastine hydrochloride	Two multicenter, randomized, double-blind, placebo-controlled, parallel-group clinical trials	Two sprays per nostril b.i.d., 1.1 mg/day	Nasal	1 year	Azelastine nasal spray significantly reduced the TVRSS from baseline when compared with placebo.	[148]
34.	Fluticasone propionate	A double-blind placebo-controlled trial	1 mg/day	Inhalation		In COPD, the capability of inflammatory cells to produce certain AA metabolites was decreased after inhaled FP treatment.	[149]
35.	Salmeterol xinafoate	Randomized, controlled, blinded, double-dummy, parallel-group trial	42 μg b.i.d.	Inhalation	24 weeks	In patients with persistent asthma suboptimally controlled by triamcinolone. Total elimination of triamcinolone therapy results in a significant deterioration in asthma control.	[150]
36	Budesonide	A double-blind, placebo-controlled, crossover study	400 mg	Inhalation	4 weeks	Long-term treatment with inhaled budesonide reduces airway cell generation of cytokines, specifically IL-5, which then decreases circulating eosinophils and their availability for recruitment to the airway after allergen exposure.	[151]
37.	Triamcinolone acetonide	A randomized, three-way placebo-controlled, crossover design	225 μg	Inhalation	35 days	Both products were generally well tolerated	[152]
38.	Clarithromycin	A prospective, double-blind, controlled trial	500 mg	Oral	8 days	Little or no effect on the severity of cold symptoms or the intensity of neutrophilic nasal inflammation in experimental rhinovirus-16 cold.	[153]

AA, arachidonic acid; ASA, acetylsalicylic acid; CTZ—chemoreceptor trigger zone; FENO, fraction of exhaled nitric oxide; FP, fluticasone propionate; NAC, nasal allergen challenge; PEFR, peak expiratory flow rate; TVRSS, total vasomotor rhinitis symptom score; VC, vital capacity.

TABLE 8 Clinical trials related to antiinflammatory drugs in the treatment of acne.

Sr no.	Name of drug	Type of study	Dose	Route	Duration	Effects	References
1.	Doxycycline	Single-center, open-label pilot study	40 mg	Oral	12 weeks	Combination treatment with antiinflammatory dose doxycycline plus combination adapalene 0.3% and benzoyl peroxide 2.5% gel is safe and effective for management of severe acne.	[154]
2.	A0.3/BPO2.5 gel	A randomized, investigator-blinded, split-face design		Topical	48 weeks	The additional improvement in atrophic scar count with 48 weeks was observed.	[155]
3.	Afamelanotide	Phase II open-label pilot study	16 mg	s.c.	56 days	Afamelanotide appears to have antiinflammatory effects in patients with mild-to-moderate acne vulgaris.	[156]
4.	0.1% adapalene gel	A multicenter, open-label, randomized parallel-group controlled trial		Topical	2 weeks	Combination therapy with oral antibiotics and adapalene results in earlier improvement in patients with moderate-to-severe inflammatory acne compared to the application of adapalene alone, and 4 weeks of the combination therapy is preferable to 2 weeks of treatment.	[157]
5	Dapsone + tazarotene	Randomized study.	5% + 0.1%	Topical	12 weeks	Combination therapy with dapsone gel 5% plus tazarotene cream 0.1% was more effective than tazarotene monotherapy for the treatment of comedonal acne.	[158]
6.	Clindamycin phosphate 1% with benzoyl peroxide 5% (CDP/BPO)	Prospective, randomized, open-label comparative study		Topical	12 weeks	Combination formulation of CDP/BPO and ADA were shown to be both effective in decreasing total, inflammatory, and noninflammatory lesion counts along with well tolerability in Asian patients with mild-to-moderate acne vulgaris.	[159]
7.	Clindamycin phosphate 1.2%-tretinoin 0.025% gel (CLIN/RA)	Three multicenter, double-blind, randomized, phase III trials		Topical	2 weeks	Participants with moderate-to-severe acne showed no signs of RA-induced flaring. In each comparison, the CLIN/RA combination showed the lowest percentage of increased inflammatory lesions.	[160]
8.	Taurine bromamine	A randomized, double-blind, placebo-controlled study		Topical	4 weeks	Comparable reductions of acne lesions were observed in the TauBr and clindamycin groups	[161]
9.	Azithromycin	An open, multicentric, noncomparative study	500 mg	Oral	3 months	Three monthly pulses of azithromycin 500 mg for three consecutive days are safe, well tolerated, effective, and promote increased patient adhesion to the treatment.	[162]

TABLE 9 Clinical trials related to antiinflammatory drugs in the treatment of psoriasis.

Sr no.	Name of drug	Type of study	Dose	Route	Duration	Effects	References
1.	Mirikizumab	Randomized, phase II study	30 mg/10 mg/100 mg	s.c.	16 weeks	At week 16, 67% of patients treated with mirikizumab 300 mg at 8-week intervals achieved PASI 90. The percentage of patients reporting at least one treatment-emergent adverse event was similar among patients treated with placebo or mirikizumab.	[163]
2.	Halobetasol propionate	Two randomized, double-blind, vehicle-controlled clinical studies	0.05%	Topical	14 days	Confirms the safety and effectiveness of HBP-foam in the treatment of plaque psoriasis.	[164]
3.	ZPL-3893787	A randomized, double-blind, placebo-controlled, parallel-group study	30 mg	Oral	8 weeks	ZPL-3893787 improved inflammatory skin lesions in patients with AD, confirming H_4 receptor antagonism as a novel therapeutic option.	[165]
4.	UR-1505	Unicenter randomized, double-blind, within-patient, controlled phase II exploratory trial	0.5%, 1%, or 2%	Topical	28 days	UR-1505 may not be a suitable option for the treatment of atopic dermatitis due to its lack of clinically relevant effect compared with its vehicle and 0.1% tacrolimus ointment.	[166]
5.	Lipoxins cream	Two-center, double-blind, placebo-controlled, randomized, parallel-group comparative study		Topical	10 days	A skin inflammation disease in humans, i.e., eczema can be effectively and safely treated with 15(R/S)-methyl-LXA4, and provides a second human disease that can be temporarily controlled with LXA4 analog.	[6]
6.	WBI-1001	Multicenter, randomized, placebo-controlled double-blind trial	0.5%	Topical	12 weeks	WBI-1001 is an efficacious novel topical antiinflammatory molecule for the treatment of AD.	[167]
7.	CF101	A phase II, multicenter, randomized, double-blind, dose-ranging, placebo-controlled study	1, 2, and 4 mg	Oral	12 weeks	CF101 was well tolerated and demonstrated clear evidence of efficacy in patients with moderate-to-severe plaque psoriasis.	[168]
8.	Ciclopirox	Open-label study	0.77 mg	Topical	14 days	Treatment provided statistically significant improvement in both the rate of mycological cure and reduction in severity score at each time point compared with baseline.	[169]
9.	Tacrolimus	Randomized double-blind controlled trial	0.03%	Topical	3 weeks	0.03% tacrolimus ointment applied once or twice daily is significantly more efficacious than 1% HA in treating moderate-to-severe AD in children. Twice daily application of 0.03% tacrolimus ointment results in the greatest improvement in mEASI, and is especially effective in patients with severe baseline disease.	[170]

#	Drug	Study design	Concentration	Route	Duration	Findings	Ref
10.	Diclofenac-Na	A randomized, double-blind, single-center, vehicle-controlled clinical trial	0.1% gel		30h	Pain relief was rapid with a reduction in erythema, which was apparent within the first few hours after the first application of the trial medication with a maximum effect observed up to 30h after sun exposure.	[171]
11.	Betamethasone valerate (BVM)	An open-label, prospective, multicenter trial study	0.1%	Topical	8 weeks	85% of patients considered BVM foam to be a better topical formulation both in terms of both efficacy and acceptability compared with previous treatments used. BVM is an effective and well-tolerated topical treatment of scalp SD. Its clinical effect is also maintained after a 2-month wash-out period.	[172]
12.	Tazarotene	Multicenter, investigator-masked, randomized, parallel-group study	0.1% gel	Topical	12 weeks	This study indicates that tazarotene plus a topical corticosteroid offers superior clinical improvement to tazarotene monotherapy with a reduced incidence of adverse effects. Maximum improvements were achieved within 8 weeks. The best-tolerated regimen was tazarotene plus mometasone furoate 0.1% ointment and the optimal balance between efficacy and tolerability was achieved with this regimen.	[173]
13.	Fluticasone propionate		0.005%	Topical	10 weeks	Limited application of fluticasone propionate ointment over a period of 10 weeks is effective and delays lesion recurrence without causing skin atrophy in patients with moderate-to-severe psoriasis in areas at risk for corticosteroid application	[174]
14.	Clobetasone butyrate (CB)	A single-center, double-blind, intra-individual, comparative study	0.05%	Topical	7 days	CB 0.05% (as Eumovate 0.05% cream) has both more effective antiinflammatory activity and better moisturizing properties than hydrocortisone 1% cream	[175]
15.	SDZ ASM 981	A randomized, double-blind controlled study	1% cream	Topical	4 weeks	The lack of atrophogenic properties of SDZ ASM demonstrates its potential as long-term treatment for inflammatory skin diseases.	[176]
16.	Hydrocortisone-17-butyrate cream	Multicenter, double-blind, randomized, active-controlled study		Topical	4 weeks	Cleared, excellent, or good end-of-treatment response rates for fluticasone propionate compared with hydrocortisone-17-butyrate. Adverse events were limited to mild-to-moderate pruritus with fluticasone propionate and hydrocortisone-17-butyrate and mild skin warmth with hydrocortisone-17-butyrate.	[177]

TABLE 10 Clinical trials of antiinflammatory drugs in the treatment of various disorders.

Sr no.	Drug	Type of study	Dosage	Route of administration	Duration	Condition and effect	References
1.	Ibuprofen plus acetaminophen	A randomized, double-blind study	600 mg + 500 mg	Oral	1 week	Among ED patients with acute, nontraumatic, nonradicular LBP, adding acetaminophen to ibuprofen does not improve outcomes within 1 week.	[180]
2.	Ibuprofen		600 mg	Oral		The data demonstrated that the preoperative ibuprofen significantly decreased the levels of most pro-inflammatory cytokines in the dental pulp, which could possibly help with anesthesia in irreversible cases.	Nguyen et al. (2020)
3.	Tramadol	A randomized parallel group double-blind active-controlled pilot study	1 mg/kg	i.v.	7 days	Both diclofenac and tramadol are equally effective in controlling pain in AP with similar safety profile.	Kumar et al. (2020)
4.	Hydroxychloroquine	A randomized pilot, open-label study	200 mg	Oral	12 weeks	Low-dose HCQ and ASA was associated with a significant decrease in the proportion of HIV target cells in the blood and genital tract, respectively.	[181]
5.	Vamorolone (VBP15)	Phase I clinical trials	20 mg/kg/day		14 days	Vamorolone is a dissociative steroid that retains high affinity binding and nuclear translocation of both glucocorticoid (agonist) and mineralocorticoid (antagonist) receptors, but does not show pharmacodynamic safety concerns of existing glucocorticoid drugs at up to 20 mg/kg/day.	[75]
6.	Diclofenac	Randomized, double-blind, noninferiority trial	75 mg	Oral	1 month	Diclofenac is inferior to norfloxacin for symptom relief of UTI and is likely to be associated with an increased risk of pyelonephritis, even though it reduces antibiotic use in women with uncomplicated lower UTI.	[182]

No.	Compound	Study type	Dose	Route	Duration	Findings	Ref.
7.	Oral budesonide suspension (MB-9)	A phase II, randomized, double-blind, placebo-controlled study with an open-label extension	10 mL	Oral	16 weeks	Treatment with BOS was well tolerated in adolescent and young adult patients with EoE and resulted in improvement in symptomatic, endoscopic, and histologic parameters using validated outcome instruments.	[183]
8.	Paracetamol	Multisite, randomized comparative effectiveness trial		Oral	6 months	Use of NSAIDs and paracetamol, alone or in combination, does not affect lithium- or quetiapine-based bipolar disorder mood-stabilizing treatment outcomes. Results support findings indicating no detrimental effects of NSAIDs or paracetamol on affective disorder treatment.	[184]
9.	Acetaminophen		1000 mg	i.v.	1 month	Acetaminophen produces an equivalent analgesic effect to flurbiprofen in postpartial mastectomy patients.	[185]
10.	Mefenamic acid	Randomized clinical trial	250 mg	Oral	2 months	Mefenamic acid effective as ginger on pain relief in primary dysmenorrhea.	[186]
11.	Diclofenac	A prospective, double-blinded, placebo-controlled, two-period, crossover study		Oral	2 weeks	Diclofenac attenuated acid-induced heartburn by inhibiting PGE2 overproduction in the esophagus. Esophageal PGE2 might be involved in producing heartburn symptoms.	[187]
12.	Resveratrol	Randomized, double-blinded, controlled clinical trial	50 mg	Oral	12 weeks	Resveratrol supplementation was associated with a significant reduction in liver enzyme alanine aminotransferase, inflammatory cytokines, nuclear factor κB activity, serum cytokeratin-18, and hepatic steatosis grade, as compared with placebo supplementation.	[188]

Continued

TABLE 10 Clinical trials of antiinflammatory drugs in the treatment of various disorders—cont'd

Sr no.	Drug	Type of study	Dosage	Route of administration	Duration	Condition and effect	References
13.	Piroxicam	A single-center, randomized, single-dose, laboratory-blinded, two-period, two-sequence, crossover study	20 mg	Oral	3 weeks	From PK perspectives, the two piroxicam formulations were considered bioequivalent, based on the rate and extent of absorption.	[189]
14.	Aosuvastatin	A randomized, double-blind, placebo-controlled study	10 mg		24 weeks	Rosuvastatin treatment effectively lowered markers of monocyte activation in HIV-infected subjects on antiretroviral therapy.	[190]
15.	Flurbiprofen	Phase I clinical trial	8.75 mg	Oral	15 days	The average ODT was about 7.5 min in both groups, and there was no significant difference between the ODTs associated with each compound	[191]
16.	Omega-3 fatty acids	A randomized, placebo-controlled trial	180 mg eicosapentaenoic acid and 120 mg docosahexaenoic acid	Oral	4 months	Supplemental use of omega-3 fatty acids decreases depressive symptoms in hemodialysis patients apart from their antiinflammatory effects.	[192]
17.	Linagliptin	Open label study	5 mg	Oral	6 months	The antiinflammatory effects of linagliptin monotherapy indicate that it may serve as a useful glucose control strategy for HD patients with diabetes.	[193]
18.	LY2189102	Double-blind, randomized study	0.6, 18, and 180 mg	s.c.	12 weeks	Weekly subcutaneous LY2189102 for 12 weeks was well tolerated, modestly reduced HbA1c and fasting glucose, and demonstrated significant antiinflammatory effects in T2DM patients.	[194]
19.	Pravastatin	A randomized, double-blind, controlled, and crossover clinical trial	20 mg	Oral	2 months	Pravastatin significantly reduced serum levels of CRP and total and LDL cholesterol compared to placebo. This treatment may be of great help to decrease the inflammatory status and probably the cardiovascular disease of CAPD patients.	[195]

No.	Drug	Study type	Dose	Route	Duration	Comments	Ref.
20.	ʟ-Carnitine+celecoxib	A phase III, randomized noninferiority study	4 g/day+ 300 mg/day		4 months	The results of the present study showed a noninferiority of arm 1 (two-drug combination) vs arm 2	[196]
21.	Ezetimibe	A prospective, randomized, placebo-controlled study	10 mg	Oral	90 days	The results of this study indicate that simvastatin is superior to ezetimibe in producing lymphocyte-suppressing, systemic antiinflammatory and endothelial protective effects in patients with elevated cholesterol levels.	[197]
22.	Diclofenac	Prospective randomized, double-blind	150 mg	Oral	18 months	Baseline BP, but not change in BP, was significantly associated with risk of thrombotic CVEs through 18 months.	[198]
23.	Exenatide	Prospectively randomized study	10 µg	s.c	12 weeks	Exenatide exerts a rapid antiinflammatory effect at the cellular and molecular level. This may contribute to a potentially beneficial antiatherogenic effect. This effect was independent of weight loss.	[199]
24.	Astaxanthin	Randomized, double-blind, placebo-controlled study	12 mg	Oral	4 weeks	Administration of AXT over a 4-week period can elevate the choroidal blood flow velocity without any adverse effects.	[200]
25.	CG100649	A controlled, double-blind randomized trial	8 mg	Oral	240 h	CG100649 and celecoxib are both relatively selective inhibitors of COX-2, but they differ in duration of action. Whether they have similar impact on cardiovascular events remains to be determined.	[201]
26.	HZT-501 (800 mg ibuprofen and 26.6 mg famotidine)	Double-blind randomized trials		Oral	24 weeks	Combined results of the REDUCE studies indicate that double-dose famotidine plus ibuprofen, given as a combination tablet, decreases endoscopic upper GI ulcers as compared with ibuprofen alone.	[202]

Continued

TABLE 10 Clinical trials of antiinflammatory drugs in the treatment of various disorders—cont'd

Sr no.	Drug	Type of study	Dosage	Route of administration	Duration	Condition and effect	References
27.	Tenoxicam	A prospective double-blind randomized trial	20 mg in 10 mL saline	i.v.	120 min	Intravenous tenoxicam, lornoxicam, and dexketoprofen are all effective in the treatment of renal colic, although lornoxicam appears to reduce VAS pain scores with the fastest rate in this comparison.	[203]
28.	Dalteparin	A randomized, controlled, double-blind, double-dummy trial	200 units kg^{-1}	s.c.	14 days	Dalteparin is superior to the NSAID ibuprofen in preventing extension of superficial thrombophlebitis during the 14-day treatment period with similar relief of pain and no increase in bleeding.	[204]
29.	Prednisolone	Single-center, double-blind, randomized, placebo-controlled study	5 mg	Oral	2 weeks	The identified genes may be useful as biomarkers for GC-induced side effects or provide a starting point for the development of improved GCs, which demonstrate the same antiinflammatory effects, but have a better safety profile.	[205]
30.	Mesalamine	A multicenter, double-blind, randomized study	2.4, 2.25, and 3.6 g/day		3–8 weeks	Higher dose of the pH-dependent release formulation was more effective for the induction of remission in patients with mild-to-moderate active UC.	[206]
31.	Budesonide-MMX	Randomized, placebo-controlled study	9 mg	Oral	4–8 weeks	Budesonide-MMX 9 mg tablets induced a fast and significant clinical improvement in active left-sided UC without suppression of adrenocortical functions and without important toxicity.	[207]
32.	Desmopressin	A double-blind controlled clinical trial study	40 μg	Intranasally	30 min	Intranasal desmopressin plus diclofenac sodium suppository caused prompt pain relief with significant decreases in pain scores after 15 and 30 min.	[208]

No.	Drug	Study type	Dose	Route	Duration	Outcome	Ref.
33.	Aceclofenac-drotaverine combination	Double-blind, double-dummy, randomized, comparative, multicentric study	100 mg + 80 mg	Oral	4–8 h	The fixed-dose combination of aceclofenac and drotaverine should therefore be considered as a suitable, effective, and well-tolerated treatment option for primary dysmenorrhoea.	[209]
34.	Doxycycline	A community-based assessment (ORCA) trial, a phase IV trial	40 mg	Oral	>12 weeks	The results of the ORCA trial support the effectiveness and safety of the 40-mg formulation of doxycycline in patients with papulopustular rosacea.	[210]
35.	Mesalamine	Randomized, multicenter, parallel-group, noninferiority study	1 g	Topical	6 weeks	Mesalamine 500-mg BID and 1-g QHS suppositories are safe and effective for patients with UP. Most patients reported significant improvement within 3 weeks and UP remission and reduced disease extension after 6 weeks of treatment. Validity of QHS administration was confirmed.	[211]
36.	Sulindac	Phase Ib trial	50 mg		6 weeks	Results are the first to show partitioning of sulindac and metabolites to human breast tissue and the first evidence for a potential dose-dependent effect of sulindac on growth differentiation factor 15 levels in NAF.	[212]
37.	Melatonin	A randomized, double-blind, placebo-controlled study	5 mg	Oral	24 h	The preoperative anxiolysis with melatonin or clonidine reduced postoperative pain and morphine consumption in patients undergoing abdominal hysterectomy. The effects these two drugs were equivalent and greater than with placebo.	[213]
38.	Ketoprofen 100 mg + acetaminophen 1000 mg	Single-dose randomized, double-blind, active- and placebo-controlled study		Oral	1.5 h	Combination of ketoprofen 100 mg + acetaminophen 1000 mg provided a significantly more rapid onset of analgesia than either drug given alone in the management of pain after oral surgery in this patient population.	[214]

Continued

TABLE 10 Clinical trials of antiinflammatory drugs in the treatment of various disorders—cont'd

Sr no.	Drug	Type of study	Dosage	Route of administration	Duration	Condition and effect	References
39.	Ibuprofen	A prospective double-blind controlled study	400 mg	Oral	10–14 days	Ibuprofen was found to be statistically significantly more effective for pain relief after medical abortion compared with paracetamol.	[215]
40.	Flurbiprofen axetil	Prospective, randomized, double-blind, placebo-controlled study	50 mg	i.v.	24 h	Pretreatment with flurbiprofen axetil 50 mg preceded by venous occlusion was found to be more effective in reducing pain on injection of propofol.	[216]
41.	Pimecrolimus	A randomized, placebo-controlled, observer-blinded study		Topical		Pimecrolimus cream and 1% hydrocortisone cream significantly reduced the SLS-induced erythema.	[217]
42.	Triflusal	A randomized, double-blind, placebo-controlled trial	900 mg	Oral	18 months	Significant difference in the probability of progression to dementia of Alzheimer's type with a lower risk in the Triflusal compared with the placebo group (hazard ratio, 2.10).	[218]
43.	Fluocinolone acetonide	Retrospective, single-center case series		Intraocular	27 months	A fluocinolone acetonide implant insertion can be combined safely with phacoemulsification plus IOL implantation during the same surgical session in eyes with uveitis. VA generally was improved, uveitis recurrences decreased, and the need for immunosuppression decreased.	[219]
44.	Flurbiprofen axetil (FA)	A prospective, randomized, double-blind, placebo-controlled study	1 mg/kg	i.v.	4 days	Flurbiprofen axetil may have an antiinflammatory effect in major abdominal surgery. The combination of perioperative intravenous FA, intraoperative thoracic epidural anesthesia, and postoperative PCEA facilitated recovery of bowel function, enhanced analgesia, and attenuated the cytokine response.	[220]

No.	Drug	Study type	Dose	Route	Duration	Outcome	Ref.
45.	Ropivacaine	A randomized, single-blinded, study	2 mL	Intravesical	8 h	Intravesical injection of ropivacaine before ureteroscopic surgery demonstrated trends toward decreased pain and voiding symptoms in this small-sample study. Inclusion of a larger sample should definitively address the effectiveness of intravesical ropivacaine and its impact on stent-related symptoms.	[221]
46.	Celecoxib	Randomized, double-blind, placebo-controlled, parallel group trial	200 or 400 mg	Oral	18 months	Celecoxib use may improve cognitive performance and increase regional brain metabolism in people with age-associated memory decline.	[222]
47.	Diflunisal	A prospective, randomized, single-blind, crossover study	1000 mg	Oral	24 h	Preemptive administration of both NSAIDs proved to be effective in the management of pain following the surgical removal of impacted third molar teeth.	[223]
48.	Simvastatin	A randomized, placebo-controlled trial	20 mg/day	Oral	1 month	Simvastatin decreased the serum TNF-alpha level in PD patients with a noninflammatory status. A decrease in the TNF-alpha level could be one of the possible mechanisms of the antiatherogenic effect of simvastatin.	[224]
49.	40% DMSO	A prospective randomized study	10 g	Topical		Pain scores were significantly lower for the DMSO group than for the EMLA group.	[225]
50.	Short-acting insulin	Prospective, randomized and unblinded clinical study	1 IU/kg/h	i.v.	24 h	High-dose insulin treatment has potential antiinflammatory properties independent of its ability to lower blood glucose levels. Even profound suppression of free fatty acid levels, the attenuation of myocardial ischemia–reperfusion injury was not detected.	[226]

Continued

TABLE 10 Clinical trials of antiinflammatory drugs in the treatment of various disorders—cont'd

Sr no.	Drug	Type of study	Dosage	Route of administration	Duration	Condition and effect	References
51.	Piroxicam	Randomized, double-blind study	40mg	Sublingual	24h	Preoperative s.l. piroxicam is more effective than the postoperative administration.	[227]
52.	Aceclofenac	The trial was controlled, comparative, randomized, and double-blind	10mg	Oral	2–8weeks	Aceclofenac was found to be statistically superior to diclofenac in terms of epigastric discomfort, dyspepsia and abdominal pain. Compliance was also better with aceclofenac.	[228]
53.	Hydrocortisone	Prospective, randomized, double-blind clinical study of cardiac surgical patients. Sixty elective cardiac surgical patients scheduled for coronary artery bypass graft, cardiac valve replacement, or both.	0, 0.4, 4, and 8μg/mg/min for 6h	i.v.		At the doses studied, cortisol-induced suppression of plasma interleukin-6 during and after cardiac surgery appears to be a saturable phenomenon at the concentration of plasma cortisol that is normally achieved after surgery in untreated patients.	[229]
54.	Candesartan	Randomized, double-blind, placebo-controlled, crossover in design	16mg		2 months	Candesartan therapy significantly reduced inflammation and increased adiponectin levels and improved insulin sensitivity in hypertensive patients.	[230]
55.	Budesonide	Double-blind, placebo-controlled, multicenter trial	6mg	Oral	52weeks	Patients treated with budesonide 6mg once daily had a trend toward a prolonged time to relapse and lower CDAI scores compared with patients treated with placebo, but relapse rates were not significantly different at the 1-year end point.	[231]
56.	Valdecoxib	Single-center, double-blind study with a four-period, four-sequence crossover design	20 or 40mg	Oral	≤3 days	Valdecoxib provided a fast onset of analgesic action, a level of efficacy similar to naproxen sodium, and a high level of patient satisfaction in the relief of menstrual pain due to primary dysmenorrhea.	[232]

57.	Alendronate	A randomized placebo-controlled study	70 mg	Oral	3 months	Once weekly mg used concomitantly with nonsteroidal antiinflammatory drugs did not increase upper gastrointestinal adverse events relative to placebo over 3 months.	[233]
58.	Aceclofenac	A prospective randomized double-blind clinical trial	100 mg	Oral	3 days	Efficacy of pain control over baseline data documented in both the treatment groups was statistically significant. There was no significant difference between the two drugs.	[234]
59.	Diclofenac hydroxyethyl pyrrolidine	A randomized double-blind controlled trial	100 mg	Oral	48 h	Diclofenac hydroxyethyl pyrrolidine and ketoprofen had similar analgesic properties. Diclofenac hydroxyethyl pyrrolidine may be the preferred choice because it is associated with less adverse reactions, together with a faster action in the relief of pain.	[235]
60.	Simvastatin	A randomized, double-blind study	40 mg/day		4–12 weeks	Statins and fibrates can exert antithrombotic and antiinflammatory effects as early as after 3 days of therapy.	[236]
61.	Oxycodone 5 mg/ibuprofen 400 mg	A multicenter, randomized, double-blind, placebo- and active-controlled, parallel-group, single-dose study				In patients with moderate-to-severe pain after surgery to remove impacted third molars, oxycodone 5 mg/ibuprofen 400 mg provided significantly better analgesia throughout the 6-h study compared with the other opioid/nonopioid combinations tested, and was associated with fewer adverse events.	[237]

Continued

TABLE 10 Clinical trials of antinflammatory drugs in the treatment of various disorders—cont'd

Sr no.	Drug	Type of study	Dosage	Route of administration	Duration	Condition and effect	References
62.	Piroxicam-FDDF	Randomly assigned comparative study	20 mg/day	Sublingual	3 days	Results indicate that when given alone in the preoperative period, piroxicam-FDDF effectively counteracts postsurgical pain and inflammatory reactions in oral tissues. Upon combined treatment with piroxicam-FDDF and azithromycin, the macrolide antibiotic may reduce the influence of piroxicam on postoperative inflammation, without affecting its beneficial effect on surgical pain.	[238]
63.	Licofelone	Randomized, parallel-group trial	400 mg b.i.d.	Oral	4 weeks	Licofelone has a potential gastrointestinal safety advantage over conventional NSAID therapy, as licofelone was associated with significantly superior gastric tolerability and a lower incidence of ulcers compared with naproxen in healthy volunteers.	[239]
64.	Acetaminophen	A randomized, double-blind, placebo-controlled crossover trial		Oral	48 h	Acetaminophen improved pain and well-being without major side effects in patients with cancer and persistent pain despite a strong opioid regimen.	[240]
65.	Infliximab	Patients were randomly assigned	5 mg/kg	i.v.	3–13 weeks	The median baseline activity scores were 13.5 (12–18) in group A (infliximab) and 14.0 (11–18) in group B (prednisolone). Infliximab could be effective in the treatment of acute, moderate, or severe ulcerative colitis.	[241]

#	Drug	Study design	Dose	Route	Duration	Outcome	Ref.
66.	Nitroflurbiprofen	A crossover study	100 mg	Oral		Nitroflurbiprofen was undetectable in the systemic circulation, suggesting metabolism to 15N nitrate/nitrite and flurbiprofen in the presystemic circulation. Levels of gastric NO were significantly higher after the ingestion of nitroflurbiprofen than flurbiprofen.	[242]
67.	Infliximab	A randomized, open-label, methylprednisolone-controlled trial	5 mg/kg	i.v.	6–8 months	The potential efficacy of repeated treatment with infliximab for short-term maintenance of remission and steroid withdrawal in glucocorticoid-dependent ulcerative colitis.	[243]
68.	Rofecoxib	A randomized, comparative study	50 mg	Oral	6 days	The effectiveness of rofecoxib in this study, plus considerations of the toxicity profile of nimesulide, support the conclusion that rofecoxib is preferable to nimesulide for relief of postoperative pain in patients undergoing surgical extraction of molars.	[244]
69.	Loxoprofen	A prospective nonrandomized study	60 mg	Oral	14 days	The effects were better in patients whose baseline nocturia was more than two times than in those with a lesser frequency at enrollment. Loxoprofen can be an effective and useful treatment option for patients with BPH complaining of refractory nocturia.	[245]
70.	Lenercept	A multicenter phase III, prospective, double-blind, placebo-controlled, randomized study	0.125 mg/kg	i.v.	28 days	Lenercept-treated patients experienced a protracted TNF-alpha half-life, leading to higher total TNF-alpha levels throughout the study. However, the treatment had no effects on antiinflammatory mediators.	[246]

Continued

TABLE 10 Clinical trials of antiinflammatory drugs in the treatment of various disorders—cont'd

Sr no.	Drug	Type of study	Dosage	Route of administration	Duration	Condition and effect	References
71.	NSAIDs	A prospective, randomized, blinded, placebo-corflormed study was performed to evaluate the effects of topical NSAIDs on cyclic and noncyclic mastalgia. A total of 108 patients, 60 with cyclic (group I) and 48 with noncyclic (group II) breast pain were enrolled		Topical	6 months	The pain score decreased significantly when the mean initial breast pain score was compared with the sixth-month breast pain score of the treatment or the placebo group of cyclic or noncyclic mastalgia.	[247]
72.	Pimecrolimus	A single-dose, randomized, double-blind, placebo-controlled, dose-rising, parallel-group study in healthy male volunteers, and a multiple dose, randomized, double-blind, placebo-controlled, dose-rising study in patients with psoriasis	5–60 mg	Oral	28 days	Oral administration of pimecrolimus was well tolerated up to the highest dose (60 mg). Pimecrolimus was rapidly absorbed (time to maximum blood concentration 0.7–2 h). A high-fat meal before drug administration delayed the time to peak concentration.	[248]
73.	Valdecoxib,	This is a multicenter, double-blind, randomized, study	500 mg (b.i.d.)	Oral	7 days	Valdecoxib, even at supratherapeutic doses, was associated with an ulcer rate significantly lower than naproxen but similar to placebo in healthy elderly subjects, despite the short duration of therapy (6.5 days). Naproxen and valdecoxib were as well tolerated as placebo.	[249]
74.	AZD3582	Randomized, double-blind three-period crossover volunteer study	750 mg b.i.d.	Oral	12 days	The potential combination of effective pain relief and gastrointestinal protection offered by AZD3582	[250]
75.	Nitroglycerin	A randomized, double-blind, placebo-controlled pilot study	15 mg/24 h	Transdermal	6 weeks	Nitroglycerin has an antiinflammatory action in patients with peripheral vascular disease.	[251]

No.	Drug	Study type	Dose	Route	Duration	Outcome	Ref.
76.	Predocol	Open label study	47.1 mg b.i.d.	Topical	8–14 days	Total scintigraphic score improved by a mean of 2.5. Mean individual scores improved in the rectum by 0.7 and in the descending colon by 0.8. Predocol is an oral preparation of a poorly absorbed salt of prednisolone that is effective in reducing inflammation over short treatment periods in patients with active ulcerative colitis.	[252]
77.	Naproxen	A randomized controlled trial	500 mg		3 days	Adding regular doses of naproxen to conventional "on request" acetaminophen and codeine therapy provides small reductions in pain on the second day after cesarean delivery. The greatest effects occur at 36h, when pain peaks.	[253]
78.	Benzydamine	Single-blind, placebo-controlled				Benzydamine is a well-tolerated drug in patients with nimesulide-induced urticaria, and it may represent a valid alternative NSAID in nimesulide-sensitive patients.	[254]
79.	Ketorolac	Two prospective, randomized, controlled, double-blind, parallel group–design studies were performed sequentially	30 mg	i.v. i.m.	2 h	Administration of 30mg ketorolac tromethamine produced parallel decreases in pain, PGE2 levels, and TxB2 levels at the surgical site. Administration of 1mg ketorolac tromethamine intramuscularly or directly at the surgical site was analgesic but without measurable effects on PGE2 levels.	[255]
80.	Nimesulide	Randomized, controlled, parallel-group trial, double-blind phase	100 mg b.i.d.	Oral	12 weeks to 2 years	Findings support the feasibility of nimesulide therapy in AD; assessment of efficacy will require a larger, long-term treatment study.	[256]

Continued

TABLE 10 Clinical trials of antiinflammatory drugs in the treatment of various disorders—cont'd

Sr no.	Drug	Type of study	Dosage	Route of administration	Duration	Condition and effect	References
81.	Nabumetone	Open, randomized, crossover trial	1000 mg b.i.d.	Oral	4 weeks	In the maximum registered dosage, nabumetone inhibits thromboxane production much more than meloxicam, signifying less COX-2 nabumetone and meloxicam cause only minor impairment in platelet function in selectivity of the former. However, both comparison with indomethacin and the difference between them is not significant.	[257]
82.	Tenoxicam	Randomized into two groups	40 mg	i.v.	>24 h	The tenoxicam group had significant lower uterine contraction pain scores and required less supplemental meperidine medication than did the placebo group.	[258]
83.	Dexamethasone	A prospective placebo-controlled double-blind study	0.6 mg/kg/day		14 days	Neurological complications and hearing loss were more common and severe in placebo group as compared to the dexamethasone group. Dexamethasone may be beneficial in some aspects of bacterial meningitis, in adults.	[259]
84.	Glyceryl trinitrate	An open, randomized, crossover trial	2.5 mg/24 h	Transdermal		Headache was significantly increased by GTN but not by DCF.	[260]
85.	0.3% triclosan/0.3% flurbiprofen gels	A comparative clinical study		Intracrevicularly	10 days	Local delivery of 0.3% triclosan/0.3% flurbiprofen gel can be used as an antiinflammatory agent either alone or as an adjunct to scaling in periodontal therapy.	[261]
86.	Tamoxifen	P-1 trial was a multicenter randomized, double-blind, placebo-controlled clinical trial	20 mg/day	Oral	6 months	Tamoxifen demonstrated effects on inflammatory markers such as CRP that were consistent with reduced cardiovascular risk.	[262]

No.	Drug	Study type	Dose	Route	Duration	Description	Ref.
87.	Hydroxychloroquine	Pilot study	200 mg	Oral	12 weeks	Regimens of antiinflammatory therapy are well tolerated in subjects with AD, indicating the feasibility of large-scale therapeutic trials of these agents.	[263]
88.	Pravastatin	Community-based, prospective, randomized, double-blind trial	40 mg/day	Oral	24 weeks	Pravastatin reduced CRP levels at both 12 and 24 weeks in a largely LDL-C-independent manner.	[264]
89.	Methylprednisolone	Randomized, controlled study	60 mg	Intrathecal	2 years	In the patients who received methylprednisolone, interleukin-8 concentrations decreased by 50%, and this decrease correlated with the duration of neuralgia and with the extent of global pain relief.	[265]
90.	Methylprednisolone	This is a randomized 'prospective' double-blind, placebo-controlled trial	125 mg	i.v.	48 h	A 48 h course of antiinflammatory therapy with methylprednisolone given at the doses of this study did not improve the short-term outcome of patients with unstable angina.	[266]
91.	Dexamethasone	A randomized, prospective, double-blind study	1 mg/kg	i.v.		Dexamethasone administration prior to CPB in children leads to a reduction in the postbypass inflammatory response as assessed by cytokine levels and clinical course.	[267]
92.	Rofecoxib	Randomized, double-blind group study	25 or 50 mg once daily	Oral	5 weeks	In healthy subjects, treatment with rofecoxib, at two to four times the doses that are currently recommended for the treatment of patients with osteoarthritis, produced significantly less fecal blood loss than a therapeutic dose of ibuprofen and was equivalent to placebo.	[268]

Continued

TABLE 10 Clinical trials of antiinflammatory drugs in the treatment of various disorders—cont'd

Sr no.	Drug	Type of study	Dosage	Route of administration	Duration	Condition and effect	References
93.	Mesalazine	Multicenter, randomized, double-blind, parallel-group study	2 g/day	Rectal	6 weeks	Mesalazine foam enema was well tolerated and was more effective than placebo in the treatment of patients with distal ulcerative colitis.	[269]
94.	Dextromethorphan	This was a double-blind, randomized (computer-generated random numbers) and placebo-controlled study.	120 mg	Oral		No analgesic effects of oral dextromethorphan 120 mg on pain after surgical termination of labor, and no additive analgesic effects when combined with ibuprofen 400 mg, were observed. Ibuprofen reduced both VAS pain scores and analgesic consumption compared with placebo.	[270]
95.	Misoprostol	A double-blind placebo-controlled parallel group	100 mg daily		28 days	Misoprostol 100 µg daily can prevent low-dose aspirin-induced gastric mucosal injury without causing identifiable adverse effects.	[271]
96.	LY293558	A randomized, double-blind, parallel-group study	0.4 or 1.2 mg/kg	i.v.	240 min	LY293558 was well tolerated, with dose-dependent and reversible side effects including hazy vision.	[272]
97.	Tenoxicam	A double-blinded, randomized, patient-controlled study	20 mg, 40 mg	i.v.	24 h	The preoperative administration of 20 or 40 mg i.v. tenoxicam does not reduce fentanyl consumption via patient-controlled analgesia, compared with placebo, after total abdominal hysterectomy. Additionally, tenoxicam may increase intraoperative bleeding and gastrointestinal side effects.	[273]

CPB, cardiopulmonary bypass; *DCF*, diclofenac; *IOL*, intraocular lens.

TABLE 11 Clinical trials of antiinflammatory drugs in COVID-19.

Sr no.	Drug	Type of study	Dosage	Route of administration	Time frame	Effects	References
1.	Tranilast		300 mg/day		3 months	Controlling inflammation, which even act as an effective antichemotactic factor, thereby resulting in an improvement in severe COVID-19 by preventing key inflammatory transcription factors like NF-κB and inhibiting NLRP-3 inflammasome.	[274]
2.	Mometasone furoate	A prospective, randomized, controlled trial	100 μg	Inhalation	3 weeks	Mometasone furoate nasal spray as a topical corticosteroid in the treatment of post-COVID-19 anosmia offers no superiority benefits over the olfactory training, regarding smell scores, duration of anosmia, and recovery rates.	[276]
3.	Colchicine	A randomized, double-blinded, placebo-controlled clinical trial	0.5 mg		>3 months	Colchicine reduced the length of both, supplemental oxygen therapy and hospitalization. The drug was safe and well tolerated.	Lopes et al. (2021)
4.	Hydroxychloroquine	An open label, randomized, parallel assignment group phase I and II study	200 mg	Oral	1–6 months	Adding HCQ to standard care did not add an extra benefit for the patients. Hydroxychloroquine arm was similar in all outcomes.	[277]
5.	Methylprednisolone	A single-blind, randomized controlled clinical trial	250 mg	i.v.	2 months	Methylprednisolone pulse could be an efficient therapeutic agent for hospitalized severe COVID-19 patients at the pulmonary phase.	[278]
6.	Colchicine	Prospective, open-label, randomized clinical trial	0.5 mg		24 days	Colchicine had statistically significant improved time to clinical deterioration compared with a control group that did not receive colchicine.	[279]
7.	Dexamethasone	Controlled, open-label trial	6 mg	i.v. or oral	28 days	Dexamethasone resulted in lower 28-day mortality among those who were receiving either invasive mechanical ventilation or oxygen alone at randomization but not among those receiving no respiratory support.	[280]
8.	Azithromycin	ATOMIC2 is a phase II/III, multicenter, prospective, open-label, two-arm randomized superiority clinical trial	500 mg	Oral	14–28 days	Clinical utility of azithromycin in patients with moderately severe, clinically diagnosed COVID-19 and could be rapidly applied worldwide.	[281]

References

[1] A.U. Ahmed, An overview of inflammation: mechanism and consequences, Front. Biol. 6 (4) (2011) 274.

[2] R. Medzhitov, Origin and physiological roles of inflammation, Nature 454 (7203) (2008) 428–435.

[3] N.G. Cruz, L.P. Sousa, M.O. Sousa, N.T. Pietrani, A.P. Fernandes, K.B. Gomes, The linkage between inflammation and Type 2 diabetes mellitus, Diabetes Res. Clin. Pract. 99 (2) (2013) 85–92.

[4] A. Lopez-Candales, P.M.H. Burgos, D.F. Hernandez-Suarez, D. Harris, Linking chronic inflammation with cardiovascular disease: from normal aging to the metabolic syndrome, J. Nat. Sci. 3 (4) (2017).

[5] R.E. Simmonds, B.M. Foxwell, Signalling, inflammation and arthritis: NF-κ B and its relevance to arthritis and inflammation, Rheumatology 47 (5) (2008) 584–590.

[6] S.H. He, H.Y. Zhang, X.N. Zeng, D. Chen, P.C. Yang, Mast cells and basophils are essential for allergies: mechanisms of allergic inflammation and a proposed procedure for diagnosis, Acta Pharmacol. Sin. 34 (10) (2013) 1270–1283.

[7] S. Sethi, D.A. Mahler, P. Marcus, C.A. Owen, B. Yawn, S. Rennard, Inflammation in COPD: implications for management, Am. J. Med. 125 (12) (2012) 1162–1170.

[8] E.A. Dowlatshahi, E.A.M. Van Der Voort, L.R. Arends, T. Nijsten, Markers of systemic inflammation in psoriasis: a systematic review and meta-analysis, Br. J. Dermatol. 169 (2) (2013) 266–282.

[9] I.R. Marcu, D. Dop, V. Padureanu, S.A. Niculescu, R. Padureanu, C.E. Niculescu, O.C. Rogoveanu, Non-steroidal anti-inflammatory drug etoricoxib facilitates the application of individualized exercise programs in patients with ankylosing spondylitis, Medicina (Kaunas) 56 (6) (2020) 270.

[10] S. Motov, M. Yasavolian, A. Likourezos, I. Pushkar, R. Hossain, J. Drapkin, V. Cohen, N. Filk, A. Smith, F. Huang, B. Rockoff, P. Homel, C. Fromm, Comparison of intravenous ketorolac at three single-dose regimens for treating acute pain in the emergency department: a randomized controlled trial, Ann. Emerg. Med. 70 (2) (2017) 177–184.

[11] T. Dietrich, R. Leeson, B. Gugliotta, B. Petersen, Efficacy and safety of low dose subcutaneous diclofenac in the management of acute pain: a randomized double-blind trial, Pain Pract. 14 (4) (2014) 315–323.

[12] A. Pareek, N. Chandurkar, A.S. Chandanwale, R. Ambade, A. Gupta, G. Bartakke, Aceclofenac-tizanidine in the treatment of acute low back pain: a double-blind, double-dummy, randomized, multicentric, comparative study against aceclofenac alone, Eur. Spine J. 18 (12) (2009) 1836–1842.

[13] M.K. Childers, D. Borenstein, R.L. Brown, S. Gershon, M.E. Hale, M. Petri, G.J. Wan, C. Laudadio, D.D. Harrison, Low-dose cyclobenzaprine versus combination therapy with ibuprofen for acute neck or back pain with muscle spasm: a randomized trial, Curr. Med. Res. Opin. 21 (9) (2005) 1485–1493.

[14] M.R. Pijak, P. Turcani, Z. Turcaniova, I. Buran, I. Gogolak, A. Mihal, F. Gazdik, Efficacy and tolerability of piroxicam-beta-cyclodextrin in the outpatient management of chronic back pain, Bratisl. Lek. Listy 103 (12) (2002) 467–472.

[15] T. Pohjolainen, A. Jekunen, L. Autio, H. Vuorela, Treatment of acute low back pain with the COX-2-selective anti-inflammatory drug nimesulide: results of a randomized, double-blind comparative trial versus ibuprofen, Spine (Phila Pa 1976) 25 (12) (2000) 1579–1585.

[16] J.A.V. Nuelle, K.M. Coe, H.A. Oliver, J.L. Cook, D.G. Hoernschemeyer, S.K. Gupta, Effect of NSAID use on bone healing in pediatric fractures: a preliminary, prospective, randomized, blinded study, J. Pediatr. Orthop. 40 (8) (2020) e683–e689.

[17] N. Ishiguro, S. Oyama, R. Higashi, K. Yanagida, Efficacy, safety, and tolerability of ONO-4474, an orally available pan-tropomyosin receptor kinase inhibitor, in Japanese patients with moderate to severe osteoarthritis of the knee: a randomized, placebo-controlled, double-blind, parallel-group comparative study, J. Clin. Pharmacol. 60 (1) (2020) 28–36.

[18] E.N. Fujiki, N.A. Netto, D.C. Kraychete, M.T. Daher, R. Tardini, A. Nakamoto, D.G. Lopes, Efficacy and safety of loxoprofen sodium topical patch for the treatment of pain in patients with minor acute traumatic limb injuries in Brazil: a randomized, double-blind, non-inferiority trial, Pain 160 (7) (2019) 1606–1613.

[19] I.B. McInnes, S.D. Chakravarty, I. Apaolaza, S. Kafka, E.C. Hsia, Y. You, A. Kavanaugh, Efficacy of ustekinumab in biologic-naïve patients with psoriatic arthritis by prior treatment exposure and disease duration: data from PSUMMIT 1 and PSUMMIT 2, RMD Open 5 (2) (2019) e000990.

[20] S. Jun, J.H. Lee, H.M. Gong, Y.J. Chung, J.R. Kim, C.A. Park, S.H. Choi, G.M. Lee, H.J. Lee, J.S. Kim, Efficacy and safety of combined treatment of miniscalpel acupuncture and non-steroidal anti-inflammatory drugs: an assessor-blinded randomized controlled pilot study, Trials 19 (1) (2018) 36.

[21] C. Nguyen, I. Boutron, G. Baron, E. Coudeyre, F. Berenbaum, S. Poiraudeau, F. Rannou, Evolution of pain at 3 months by oral resveratrol in knee osteoarthritis(ARTHROL): protocol for a multicentre randomised double-blind placebo-controlled trial, BMJ Open 7 (9) (2017) e017652.

[22] J.H. Ryu, J.I. Kim, H.S. Kim, G.J. Noh, K.T. Lee, E.K. Chung, Pharmacokinetic interactions between pelubiprofen and eperisone hydrochloride: a randomized, open-label, crossover study of healthy Korean men, Clin. Ther. 39 (1) (2017) 138–149.

[23] T. Mochizuki, K. Yano, K. Ikari, R. Hiroshima, H. Takaoka, K. Kawakami, N. Koenuma, M. Ishibashi, T. Shirahata, S. Momohara, Tramadol hydrochloride/acetaminophen combination versus non-steroidal anti-inflammatory drug for the treatment of perioperative pain after total knee arthroplasty: a prospective, randomized, open-label clinical trial, J. Orthop. Sci. 21 (5) (2016) 625–629.

[24] H.G. Predel, H. Pabst, A. Schäfer, D. Voss, N. Giordan, Diclofenac patch for the treatment of acute pain caused by soft tissue injuries of limbs: a randomized, placebo-controlled clinical trial, J. Sports Med. Phys. Fitness 56 (1–2) (2015) 92–99.

[25] L.T. Wadsworth, J.D. Kent, R.J. Holt, Efficacy and safety of diclofenac sodium 2% topical solution for osteoarthritis of the knee: a randomized, double-blind, vehicle-controlled, 4 week study, Curr. Med. Res. Opin. 32 (2) (2016) 241–250.

[26] J. Detert, P. Klaus, J. Listing, V. Höhne-Zimmer, T. Braun, S. Wassenberg, R. Rau, F. Buttgereit, G.R. Burmester, Hydroxychloroquine in patients with inflammatory and erosive osteoarthritis of the hands (OA TREAT): study protocol for a randomized controlled trial, Trials 15 (2014) 412.

[27] C. Bali, P. Ergenoglu, O. Ozmete, S. Akin, N.B. Ozyilkan, O.Y. Cok, A. Aribogan, Comparison of the postoperative analgesic effects of naproxen sodium and naproxen sodium-codeine phosphate for arthroscopic meniscus surgery, Braz. J. Anesthesiol. 66 (2) (2016) 151–156.

[28] Y.K. Zhang, H. Yang, J.Y. Zhang, L.J. Song, Y.C. Fan, Comparison of intramuscular compound betamethasone and oral diclofenac sodium in the treatment of acute attacks of gout, Int. J. Clin. Pract. 68 (5) (2014) 633–638.

[29] C. González de Vega, C. Speed, B. Wolfarth, J. González, Traumeel vs. diclofenac for reducing pain and improving ankle mobility after acute ankle sprain: a multicentre, randomised, blinded, controlled and non-inferiority trial, Int. J. Clin. Pract. 67 (10) (2013) 979–989.

[30] M.N. Essex, M. O'Connell, P. Bhadra Brown, Response to nonsteroidal anti-inflammatory drugs in African Americans with osteoarthritis of the knee, J. Int. Med. Res. 40 (6) (2012) 2251–2266.

[31] W.E. Garrett, C.C. Kaeding, N.S. ElAttrache, J.W. Xerogeanes, M.S. Hewitt, N.V. Skrepnik, J.D. Papilion, J.B. O'Donnell, D.L. Fox, F. Ruvuna, J.S. Whitaker, G.A. Demopulos, Novel drug OMS103HP reduces pain and improves joint motion and function for 90 days after arthroscopic meniscectomy, Arthroscopy 27 (8) (2011) 1060–1070.

[32] N. Singla, A. Rock, L. Pavliv, A multi-center, randomized, double-blind placebo-controlled trial of intravenous-ibuprofen (IV-ibuprofen) for treatment of pain in post-operative orthopedic adult patients, Pain Med. 11 (8) (2010) 1284–1293.

[33] R. Levy, A. Khokhlov, S. Kopenkin, B. Bart, T. Ermolova, R. Kantemirova, V. Mazurov, M. Bell, P. Caldron, L. Pillai, B. Burnett, Efficacy and safety of flavocoxid compared with naproxen in subjects with osteoarthritis of the knee—a subset analysis, Adv. Ther. 27 (12) (2010) 953–962.

[34] N. Katz, M. Hale, D. Morris, J. Stauffer, Morphine sulfate and naltrexone hydrochloride extended release capsules in patients with chronic osteoarthritis pain, Postgrad. Med. 122 (4) (2010) 112–128.

[35] M. Sullivan, S. Bentley, M.Y. Fan, G. Gardner, A single-blind placebo run-in study of venlafaxine XR for activity-limiting osteoarthritis pain, Pain Med. 10 (5) (2009) 806–812.

[36] Z. Xu, T. Vu, H. Lee, C. Hu, J. Ling, H. Yan, D. Baker, A. Beutler, C. Pendley, C. Wagner, H.M. Davis, H. Zhou, Population pharmacokinetics of golimumab, an anti-tumor necrosis factor-alpha human monoclonal antibody, in patients with psoriatic arthritis, J. Clin. Pharmacol. 49 (9) (2009) 1056–1070.

[37] T.J. Schnitzer, J.R. Tesser, K.M. Cooper, R.D. Altman, A 4-week randomized study of acetaminophen extended-release vs rofecoxib in knee osteoarthritis, Osteoarthr. Cartil. 17 (1) (2008) 1–7.

[38] V.V. Prabhu, A comparative clinical trial evaluating efficacy and safety of fixed dose combination of nimesulide (100 mg) and racemethionine (50 mg)(namsafe) versus reference drug (nimesulide) and other NSAIDs in the treatment of osteoarthritis, J. Indian Med. Assoc. 106 (6) (2008) 402–404.

[39] E. Batlle-Gualda, J. Román Ivorra, E. Martín-Mola, J. CarbonellAbelló, L.F. Linares Ferrando, Tornero, J. Molina, A. RaberBéjar, J. Fortea Busquets, Aceclofenac vs paracetamol in the management of symptomatic osteoarthritis of the knee: a double-blind 6-week randomized controlled trial, Osteoarthr. Cartil. 15 (8) (2007) 900–908.

[40] S. Fuchs, R. Mönikes, A. Wohlmeiner, T. Heyse, Intra-articular hyaluronic acid compared with corticoid injections for the treatment of rhizarthrosis, Osteoarthr. Cartil. 14 (1) (2006) 82–88.

[41] V.W. Chan, A.J. Clark, J.C. Davis, R.S. Wolf, D. Kellstein, S. Jayawardene, The post-operative analgesic efficacy and tolerability of lumiracoxib compared with placebo and naproxen after total knee or hip arthroplasty, Acta Anaesthesiol. Scand. 49 (10) (2005) 1491–1500.

[42] C.W. Wiesenhutter, J.A. Boice, A. Ko, E.A. Sheldon, F.T. Murphy, B.A. Wittmer, M.L. Aversano, A.S. Reicin, Protocol 071 Study Group, Evaluation of the comparative efficacy of etoricoxib and ibuprofen for treatment of patients with osteoarthritis: a randomized, double-blind, placebo-controlled trial, Mayo Clin. Proc. 80 (4) (2005) 470–479.

[43] J.T. Kim, O. Sherman, G. Cuff, A. Leibovits, M. Wajda, A.Y. Bekker, A double-blind prospective comparison of rofecoxib vs ketorolac in reducing postoperative pain after arthroscopic knee surgery, J. Clin. Anesth. 17 (6) (2005) 439–443.

[44] J. Wilson-MacDonald, G. Burt, D. Griffin, C. Glynn, Epidural steroid injection for nerve root compression. A randomised, controlled trial, J. Bone Joint Surg. Br. Vol. 87 (3) (2005) 352–355.

[45] R. Emkey, N. Rosenthal, S.C. Wu, D. Jordan, M. Kamin, CAPSS-114 Study Group, Efficacy and safety of tramadol/acetaminophen tablets (Ultracet) as add-on therapy for osteoarthritis pain in subjects receiving a COX-2 nonsteroidal antiinflammatory drug: a multicenter, randomized, double-blind, placebo-controlled trial, J. Rheumatol. 31 (1) (2004) 150–156.

[46] B. Heller, R. Tarricone, Oxaprozin versus diclofenac in NSAID-refractory periarthritis pain of the shoulder, Curr. Med. Res. Opin. 20 (8) (2004) 1279–1290.

[47] H. Tannenbaum, F. Berenbaum, J.Y. Reginster, J. Zacher, J. Robinson, G. Poor, H. Bliddal, S. Uebelhart, S. Adami, F. Navarro, A. Lee, A. Moore, A. Gimona, Lumiracoxib is effective in the treatment of osteoarthritis of the knee: a 13 week, randomised, double blind study versus placebo and celecoxib, Ann. Rheum. Dis. 63 (11) (2004) 1419–1426.

[48] K. Trnavský, M. Fischer, U. Vögtle-Junkert, F. Schreyger, Efficacy and safety of 5% ibuprofen cream treatment in knee osteoarthritis. Results of a randomized, double-blind, placebo-controlled study, J. Rheumatol. 31 (3) (2004) 565–572.

[49] J. Zacher, D. Feldman, R. Gerli, D. Scott, S.M. Hou, D. Uebelhart, I. W. Rodger, Z.E. Ozturk, etoricoxib OA study group, A comparison of the therapeutic efficacy and tolerability of etoricoxib and diclofenac in patients with osteoarthritis, Curr. Med. Res. Opin. 19 (8) (2003) 725–736.

[50] J.P. Case, A.J. Baliunas, J.A. Block, Lack of efficacy of acetaminophen in treating symptomatic knee osteoarthritis: a randomized, double-blind, placebo-controlled comparison trial with diclofenac sodium, Arch. Intern. Med. 163 (2) (2003) 169–178.

[51] J.A. Herrera, M. González, Comparative evaluation of the effectiveness and tolerability of nimesulide versus rofecoxib taken once a day in the treatment of patients with knee osteoarthritis, Am. J. Ther. 10 (6) (2003) 468–472.

[52] R. Hawel, G. Klein, F. Singer, F. Mayrhofer, S.T. Kähler, Comparison of the efficacy and tolerability of dexibuprofen and celecoxib in the treatment of osteoarthritis of the hip, Int. J. Clin. Pharmacol. Ther. 41 (4) (2003) 153–164.

[53] W.P. Maksymowych, G.S. Jhangri, A.A. Fitzgerald, S. LeClercq, P. Chiu, A. Yan, K.J. Skeith, S.L. Aaron, J. Homik, P. Davis, D. Sholter, A.S. Russell, A six-month randomized, controlled, double-blind, dose-response comparison of intravenous pamidronate(60 mg versus 10 mg) in the treatment of nonsteroidal antiinflammatory drug-refractory ankylosing spondylitis, Arthritis Rheum. 46 (3) (2002) 766–773.

[54] C.T. Hou, Y.Y. Tsai, A double-blind, randomized, controlled parallel group study evaluating the efficacy and safety of acemetacin for the management of osteoarthritis, Int. J. Clin. Pharmacol. Res. 22 (1) (2002) 1–6.

[55] S. Kermond, M. Fink, K. Graham, J.B. Carlin, P. Barnett, A randomized clinical trial: should the child with transient synovitis of the hip be treated with nonsteroidal anti-inflammatory drugs? Ann. Emerg. Med. 40 (3) (2002) 294–299.

[56] W. Makarowski, W.W. Zhao, T. Bevirt, D.P. Recker, Efficacy and safety of theCOX-2 specific inhibitor valdecoxib in the management of osteoarthritis of the hip: a randomized, double-blind, placebo-controlled comparison with naproxen, Osteoarthr. Cartil. 10 (4) (2002) 290–296.

[57] R. Çeliker, Ş. Arslan, F. İnanc, Corticosteroid injection vs. nonsteroidal antiinflammatory drug and splinting in carpal tunnel syndrome, Am. J. Phys. Med. Rehabil. 81 (3) (2002) 182–186.

[58] A. Whelton, J.G. Fort, J.A. Puma, D. Normandin, A.E. Bello, K.M. Verburg, SUCCESS VI Study Group, Cyclooxygenase-2–specific inhibitors and cardiorenal function: a randomized, controlled trial of celecoxib and rofecoxib in older hypertensive osteoarthritis patients, Am. J. Ther. 8 (2) (2001) 85–95.

[59] K.E. Truitt, R.S. Sperling, W.H. Ettinger Jr., M. Greenwald, L. DeTora, Q. Zeng, J. Bolognese, E. Ehrich, Phase III Rofecoxib Geriatric Study Group, A multicenter, randomized, controlled trial to evaluate the safety profile, tolerability, and efficacy of rofecoxib in advanced elderly patients with osteoarthritis, Aging (Milano) 13 (2) (2001) 112–121.

[60] D.L. Scott, H. Berry, H. Capell, J. Coppock, T. Daymond, D.V. Doyle, L. Fernandes, B. Hazleman, J. Hunter, E.C. Huskisson, A. Jawad, R. Jubb, T. Kennedy, P. McGill, F. Nichol, J. Palit, M. Webley, A. Woolf, J. Wotjulewski, The long-term effects of non-steroidal anti-inflammatory drugs in osteoarthritis of the knee: a randomized placebo-controlled trial, Rheumatology (Oxford) 39 (10) (2000) 1095–1101.

[61] F.U. Eke, A. Obamyonyi, N.N. Eke, E.A. Oyewo, An open comparative study of dispersible piroxicam versus soluble acetylsalicylic acid for the treatment of osteoarticular painful attack during sickle cell crisis, Tropical Med. Int. Health 5 (2) (2000) 81–84.

[62] J.P. Pelletier, M. Yaron, B. Haraoui, P. Cohen, M.A. Nahir, D. Choquette, I. Wigler, I.A. Rosner, A.D. Beaulieu, Efficacy and safety of diacerein in osteoarthritis of the knee: a double-blind, placebo-controlled trial. The Diacerein Study Group, Arthritis Rheum. 43 (10) (2000) 2339–2348.

[63] J.H. Gertsch, G.S. Lipman, P.S. Holck, A. Merritt, A. Mulcahy, R.S. Fisher, B. Basnyat, E. Allison, K. Hanzelka, A. Hazan, Z. Meyers, J. Odegaard, B. Pook, M. Thompson, B. Slomovic, H. Wahlberg, V. Wilshaw, E.A. Weiss, K. Zafren, Prospective, double-blind, randomized, placebo-controlled comparison of acetazolamide versus ibuprofen for prophylaxis against high altitude headache: the Headache Evaluation at Altitude Trial (HEAT), Wilderness Environ. Med. 21 (3) (2010) 236–243.

[64] A. Pal, S. Shenoy, A. Gautam, S. Munjal, J. Niu, M. Gopalakrishnan, J. Gobburru, Pharmacokinetics of DFN-15, a novel Oral solution of celecoxib, versus celecoxib 400-mg capsules: a randomized crossover study in fasting healthy volunteers, Clin. Drug Investig. 37 (10) (2017) 937–946.

[65] F. Gungor, K.C. Akyol, M. Kesapli, A. Celik, A. Karaca, M.N. Bozdemir, C. Eken, Intravenous dexketoprofen vs placebo for migraine attack in the emergency department: a randomized, placebo-controlled trial, Cephalalgia 36 (2) (2016) 179–184.

[66] F. Kubitzek, G. Ziegler, M.S. Gold, J.M. Liu, E. Ionescu, Low-dose diclofenac potassium in the treatment of episodic tension-type headache, Eur. J. Pain 7 (2) (2003) 155–162.

[67] M. Dib, H. Massiou, M. Weber, P. Henry, S. Garcia-Acosta, M.G. Bousser, Bi-Profenid Migraine Study Group, Efficacy of oral ketoprofen in acute migraine: a double-blind randomized clinical trial, Neurology 58 (11) (2002) 1660–1665.

[68] A.V. Krymchantowski, J.S. Barbosa, Rizatriptan combined with rofecoxib vs. rizatriptan for the acute treatment of migraine: an open label pilot study, Cephalalgia 22 (4) (2002) 309–312.

[69] T. Bakhtiari, S. Azarian, A. Ghaderi, A. Ahmadzadeh, A. Mirshafiey, Effect of guluronic acid (G2013), as a new anti-inflammatory drug on gene expression of pro-inflammatory and anti-inflammatory cytokines and their transcription factors in rheumatoid arthritis patients, Iran. J. Allergy Asthma Immunol. 18 (6) (2019) 639–648.

[70] D. Vanags, B. Williams, B. Johnson, S. Hall, P. Nash, A. Taylor, J. Weiss, D. Feeney, Therapeutic efficacy and safety of chaperonin 10 in patients with rheumatoid arthritis: a double-blind randomised trial, Lancet 368 (9538) (2006) 855–863.

[71] G. Giagoudakis, S.L. Markantonis, Relationships between the concentrations of prostaglandins and the nonsteroidal antiinflammatory drugs indomethacin, diclofenac, and ibuprofen, Pharmacotherapy 25 (1) (2005) 18–25.

[72] J.L. Dugina, V.I. Petrov, A.R. Babayeva, A.V. Martyushev-Poklad, E.V. Tcherevkova, O.I. Epstein, S.A. Sergeeva, A randomized, open-label, comparative, 6-month trial of oral ultra-low doses of antibodies to tumor necrosis factor-alpha and diclofenac in rheumatoid arthritis, Int. J. Tissue React. 27 (1) (2005) 15–21.

[73] P.J. Mease, D.D. Gladman, C.T. Ritchlin, E.M. Ruderman, S.D. Steinfeld, E.H. Choy, J.T. Sharp, P.A. Ory, R.J. Perdok, M.A. Weinberg, Adalimumab Effectiveness in Psoriatic Arthritis Trial Study Group, Adalimumab for the treatment of patients with moderately to severely active psoriatic arthritis: results of a double-blind, randomized, placebo-controlled trial, Arthritis Rheum. 52 (10) (2005) 3279–3289.

[74] Z. Jajić, M. Malaise, K. Nekam, E. Koó, K. Dankó, M. Kovacs, C. Scarpignato, Gastrointestinal safety of amtolmetin guacyl in comparison with celecoxib in patients with rheumatoid arthritis, Clin. Exp. Rheumatol. 23 (6) (2005) 809–818.

[75] G.S. Hoffman, P.A. Merkel, R.D. Brasington, D.J. Lenschow, P. Liang, Anti-tumornecrosis factor therapy in patients with difficult to treat Takayasu arteritis, Arthritis Rheum. 50 (7) (2004) 2296–2304.

[76] H. Kondo, T. Abe, H. Hashimoto, S. Uchida, S. Irimajiri, M. Hara, S. Sugawara, Efficacy and safety of tacrolimus (FK506) in treatment of rheumatoid arthritis: a randomized, double blind, placebo controlled dose-finding study, J. Rheumatol. 31 (2) (2004) 243–251.

[77] S. Goodman, P. Howard, A. Haig, S. Flavin, B. Macdonald, An open label study to establish dosing recommendations for nabumetone in juvenile rheumatoid arthritis, J. Rheumatol. 30 (4) (2003) 829–831.

[78] I. Foeldvari, R. Burgos-Vargas, A. Thon, D. Tuerck, High response rate in the phase I/II study of meloxicam in juvenile rheumatoid arthritis, J. Rheumatol. 29 (5) (2002) 1079–1083.

[79] J.E. Walker, S.B. Margolin, Pirfenidone for chronic progressive multiplesclerosis, Mult. Scler. J. 7 (5) (2001) 305–312.

[80] M. Dougados, J.M. Béhier, I. Jolchine, A. Calin, D. van der Heijde, I. Olivieri, H. Zeidler, H. Herman, Efficacy of celecoxib, a cyclooxygenase 2-specificinhibitor, in the treatment of ankylosing spondylitis: a six-week controlled study with comparison against placebo and against a conventional nonsteroidal antiinflammatory drug, Arthritis Rheum. 44 (1) (2001) 180–185.

[81] H. Krug, L.K. Broadwell, M. Berry, R. DeLapp, R.H. Palmer, M. Mahowald, Tolerability and efficacy of nabumetone and naproxen in the treatment of rheumatoid arthritis, Clin. Ther. 22 (1) (2000) 40–52.

[82] G.A. Kontadakis, K.G. Chronopoulou, R. Tsopouridou, D. Tabibian, G.D. Kymionis, Nepafenac ophthalmic suspension 0.3% for the management of ocular pain after photorefractive keratectomy, J. Refract. Surg. 34 (3) (2018) 171–176.

[83] E. Donnenfeld, E. Holland, Dexamethasone intracameral drug-delivery suspension for inflammation associated with cataract surgery: a randomized, placebo-controlled, phase III trial, Ophthalmology 125 (6) (2018) 799–806.

[84] M. De Keyser, M. De Belder, V. De Groot, Randomized prospective study of the use of anti-inflammatory drops after selective laser trabeculoplasty, J. Glaucoma 26 (2) (2017) e22–e29.

[85] A. Di Zazzo, G. Roberti, A. Mashaghi, T.B. Abud, D. Pavese, S. Bonini, Use of topical cannabinomimetic palmitoylethanolamide in ocular surface disease associated with antiglaucoma medications, J. Ocul. Pharmacol. Ther. 33 (9) (2017) 670–677.

[86] H.S. Kim, T.I. Kim, J.H. Kim, K.C. Yoon, J.Y. Hyon, K.U. Shin, C.Y. Choi, Evaluation of clinical efficacy and safety of a novel cyclosporin A nanoemulsion in the treatment of dry eye syndrome, J. Ocul. Pharmacol. Ther. 33 (7) (2017) 530–538.

[87] A. Zaczek, D. Artzen, C.G. Laurell, U. Stenevi, P. Montan, Nepafenac 0.1% plus dexamethasone 0.1% versus dexamethasone alone: effect on macular swelling aftercataract surgery, J Cataract Refract Surg 40 (9) (2014) 1498–1505.

[88] F.R. Zanetti, E.A. Fulco, F.R. Chaves, A.P. da Costa Pinto, C.E. Arieta, R.P. Lira, Effect of preoperative use of topical prednisolone acetate, ketorolac tromethamine, nepafenac and placebo, on the maintenance of intraoperative mydriasis during cataract surgery: a randomized trial, Indian J. Ophthalmol. 60 (4) (2012) 277–281.

[89] P. Simaroj, P. Sinsawad, K. Lekhanont, Effects of intracameral triamcinoloneand gentamicin injections following cataract surgery, J. Med. Assoc. Thail. 94 (7) (2011) 819–825.

[90] B.A. Henderson, J.L. Gayton, S.P. Chandler, J.A. Gow, S.M. Klier, T.R. McNamara, Bromfenac Ophthalmic Solution (Bromday) Once Daily Study Group, Safety and efficacy of bromfenac ophthalmic solution (Bromday) dosed once daily for postoperative ocular inflammation and pain, Ophthalmology 118 (11) (2011) 2120–2127.

[91] K. Miyake, I. Ota, G. Miyake, J. Numaga, Nepafenac 0.1% versus fluorometholone 0.1% for preventing cystoid macular edema after cataract surgery, J Cataract Refract Surg 37 (9) (2011) 1581–1588.

[92] M.S. Ahmed, K.N. Moly, M.A. Aziz, Use of povidone-iodine drop instead of sub-conjunctival injection of dexamethasone and gentamicin combination at the end of phacoemulsification cataract surgery, Mymensingh Med. J. 19 (2) (2010) 232–235.

[93] M.S. Korenfeld, S.M. Silverstein, D.L. Cooke, R. Vogel, R.S. Crockett, Difluprednate Ophthalmic Emulsion 0.05% (Durezol) Study Group, Difluprednate ophthalmic emulsion 0.05% for postoperative inflammation and pain, J Cataract Refract Surg 35 (1) (2009) 26–34.

[94] M.B. Abelson, G.L. Torkildsen, J.I. Williams, J.A. Gow, P.J. Gomes, T.R. McNamara, Bepotastine Besilate Ophthalmic Solutions Clinical Study Group, Time to onset and duration of action of the antihistamine bepotastine besilate ophthalmic solutions 1.0% and 1.5% in allergic conjunctivitis: a phase III, single-center, prospective, randomized, double-masked, placebo-controlled, conjunctival allergen challenge assessment in adults and children, Clin. Ther. 31 (9) (2009) 1908–1921.

[95] D.R. Almeida, D. Johnson, H. Hollands, D. Smallman, S. Baxter, K.T. Eng, V. Kratky, M.W. ten Hove, S. Sharma, S. El-Defrawy, Effect of prophylactic nonsteroidal antiinflammatory drugs on cystoid macular edema assessed using optical coherence tomography quantification of total macular volume after cataract surgery, J. Cataract Refract. Surg. 34 (1) (2008) 64–69.

[96] J. Luchs, Efficacy of topical azithromycin ophthalmic solution 1% in the treatment of posterior blepharitis, Adv. Ther. 25 (9) (2008) 858–870.

[97] L. Paccola, R. Jorge, J.C. Barbosa, R.A. Costa, I.U. Scott, Anti-inflammatory efficacy of a single posterior subtenon injection of triamcinolone acetonide versus prednisolone acetate 1% eyedrops after pars plana vitrectomy, Acta Ophthalmol. Scand. 85 (6) (2007) 603–608.

[98] R.H. Stewart, L.R. Grillone, M.L. Shiffman, E.D. Donnenfeld, J.A. Gow, Bromfenac Ophthalmic Solution 0.09% Study Group, The systemic safety of bromfenac ophthalmic solution 0.09%, J. Ocul. Pharmacol. Ther. 23 (6) (2007) 601–612.

[99] H.K. Lee, I.H. Ryu, K.Y. Seo, S. Hong, H.C. Kim, E.K. Kim, Topical 0.1% prednisolone lowers nerve growth factor expression in kerato conjunctivitis sicca patients, Ophthalmology 113 (2) (2006) 198–205.

[100] K.M. Saari, L. Nelimarkka, V. Ahola, T. Loftsson, E. Stefánsson, Comparison of topical 0.7% dexamethasone-cyclodextrin with 0.1% dexamethasone sodium phosphate for postcataract inflammation, Graefes Arch. Clin. Exp. Ophthalmol. 244 (5) (2006) 620–626.

[101] A.M. Avunduk, Y. Tekelioglu, A. Turk, N. Akyol, Comparison of the effects of ketotifen fumarate 0.025% and olopatadine HCl 0.1% ophthalmic solutions in seasonal allergic conjunctivities: a 30-day, randomized, double-masked, artificial tear substitute-controlled trial, Clin. Ther. 27 (9) (2005) 1392–1402.

[102] S.M. Whitcup, R. Bradford, J. Lue, R.M. Schiffman, M.B. Abelson, Efficacy and tolerability of ophthalmic epinastine: a randomized, double-masked, parallel-group, active- and vehicle-controlled environmental trial in patients with seasonal allergic conjunctivitis, Clin. Ther. 26 (1) (2004) 29–34.

[103] D.S. Fan, C.B. Yu, T.Y. Chiu, C.Y. Wong, J.S. Ng, C.P. Pang, D.S. Lam, Ocular-hypertensive and anti-inflammatory response to rimexolone therapy in children, Arch. Ophthalmol. 121 (12) (2003) 1716–1721.

[104] K. Kashiwagi, S. Tsukahara, Effect of non-steroidal anti-inflammatory ophthalmic solution on intraocular pressure reduction by latanoprost, Br. J. Ophthalmol. 87 (3) (2003) 297–301.

[105] J. Tauber, Alocril Community Allergy Trial Study Group, Nedocromil sodium ophthalmic solution 2% twice daily in patients with allergic conjunctivitis, Adv. Ther. 19 (2) (2002) 73–84.

[106] M.P. Holzer, K.D. Solomon, H.P. Sandoval, D.T. Vroman, Comparison of ketorolac tromethamine 0.5% and loteprednol etabonate 0.5% for inflammation after phacoemulsification: prospective randomized double-masked study, J Cataract Refract Surg 28 (1) (2002) 93–99.

[107] C. Baudouin, J.P. Nordmann, P. Denis, C. Creuzot-Garcher, C. Allaire, C. Trinquand, Efficacy of indomethacin 0.1% and fluorometholone 0.1% on conjunctival inflammation following chronic application of antiglaucomatous drugs, Graefes Arch. Clin. Exp. Ophthalmol. 240 (11) (2002) 929–935.

[108] M.M. Alberti, C.G. Bouat, C.M. Allaire, C.J. Trinquand, Combined indomethacin/gentamicin eyedrops to reduce pain after traumatic corneal abrasion, Eur. J. Ophthalmol. 11 (3) (2001) 233–239.

[109] H.G. Struck, A. Bariszlovich, Comparison of 0.1% dexamethasone phosphate eye gel (Dexagel) and 1% prednisolone acetate eye suspension in the treatment of post-operative inflammation after cataract surgery, Graefes Arch. Clin. Exp. Ophthalmol. 239 (10) (2001) 737–742.

[110] D.T. Tan, S.P. Chee, L. Lim, J. Theng, M. Van Ede, Randomized clinical trial of Surodex steroid drug delivery system for cataract surgery: anterior versus posterior placement of two Surodex in the eye, Ophthalmology 108 (12) (2001) 2172–2181.

[111] D.S. Fan, J.S. Ng, D.S. Lam, A prospective study on ocular hypertensive and antiinflammatory response to different dosages of fluorometholone in children, Ophthalmology 108 (11) (2001) 1973–1977.

[112] C.P. Herbort, A. Jauch, P. Othenin-Girard, J.J. Tritten, M. Fsadni, Diclofenacdrops to treat inflammation after cataract surgery, Acta Ophthalmol. Scand. 78 (4) (2000) 421–424.

[113] Y. Shiuey, B.K. Ambati, A.P. Adamis, A randomized, double-masked trial of topical ketorolac versus artificial tears for treatment of viral conjunctivitis, Ophthalmology 107 (8) (2000) 1512–1517.

[114] A. Agarwal, S.S. Nath, D. Goswami, D. Gupta, S. Dhiraaj, P.K. Singh, An evaluation of the efficacy of aspirin and benzydamine hydrochloride gargle for attenuating postoperative sore throat: a prospective, randomized, single-blind study, Anesth. Analg. 103 (4) (2006) 1001–1003.

[115] A. Kiderman, J. Yaphe, J. Bregman, T. Zemel, A.L. Furst, Adjuvant prednisone therapy in pharyngitis: a randomised controlled trial from general practice, Br. J. Gen. Pract. 55 (512) (2005) 218–221.

[116] N. Watson, W.S. Nimmo, J. Christian, A. Charlesworth, J. Speight, K. Miller, Relief of sore throat with the anti-inflammatory throat lozenge flurbiprofen 8.75 mg: a randomised, double-blind, placebo-controlled study of efficacy and safety, Int. J. Clin. Pract. 54 (8) (2000) 490–496.

[117] V. Malizia, S. Fasola, G. Ferrante, G. Cilluffo, R. Gagliardo, M. Landi, L. Montalbano, D. Marchese, S. La Grutta, Comparative effect of beclomethasone dipropionate and cetirizine on acoustic rhinometry parameters in children with perennial allergic rhinitis: a randomized controlled trial, J. Investig. Allergol. Clin. Immunol. 28 (6) (2018) 392–400.

[118] K. Asai, A. Kobayashi, Y. Makihara, M. Johnson, Anti-inflammatory effects of salmeterol/fluticasone propionate 50/250 mcg combination therapy in Japanese patients with chronic obstructive pulmonary disease, Int. J. Chron. Obstruct. Pulmon. Dis. 10 (2015) 803–811.

[119] H. Mateos-Toledo, M. Mejía-Ávila, Ó. Rodríguez-Barreto, J.G. Mejía-Hurtado, J. Rojas-Serrano, A. Estrada, J. Castillo-Pedroza, K.- Castillo-Castillo, M. Gaxiola, I. Buendía-Roldan, M. Selman, An open-label study with pirfenidone on chronic hypersensitivity pneumonitis, Arch. Bronconeumol. (Engl. Ed.) 56 (3) (2020) 163–169.

[120] E. Tagaya, M. Kondo, S. Kirishi, M. Kawagoe, N. Kubota, J. Tamaoki, Effects of regular treatment with combination of salmeterol/fluticasone propionate and salmeterol alone in cough variant asthma, J. Asthma 52 (5) (2015) 512–518.

[121] A.H. Kubavat, N. Khippal, S. Tak, P. Rijhwani, S. Bhargava, T. Patel, N. Shah, R.R. Kshatriya, R. Mittal, A randomized, comparative, multicentric clinical trial to assess the efficacy and safety of zileuton extended-release tablets with montelukast sodium tablets in patients suffering from chronic persistent asthma, Am. J. Ther. 20 (2) (2013) 154–162.

[122] H. Nolte, I. Pavord, V. Backer, S. Spector, T. Shekar, D. Gates, P. Nair, F. Hargreave, Dose-dependent anti-inflammatory effect of inhaled mometasone furoate/formoterol in subjects with asthma, Respir. Med. 107 (5) (2013) 656–664.

[123] J.J. Rüdiger, M. Gencay, J.Q. Yang, M. Bihl, M. Tamm, M. Roth, Fast beneficial systemic anti-inflammatory effects of inhaled budesonide and formoterol on circulating lymphocytes in asthma, Respirology 18 (5) (2013) 840–847.

[124] C. Llor, A. Moragas, C. Bayona, R. Morros, H. Pera, O. Plana-Ripoll, J.M. Cots, M. Miravitlles, Efficacy of anti-inflammatory or antibiotic treatment in patients with non-complicated acute bronchitis and discoloured sputum: randomised placebo controlled trial, BMJ 347 (2013) f5762.

[125] B. Kulapaditharom, K. Pornprasertsuk, V. Boonkitticharoen, Clinical assessment of levocetirizine and budesonide in treatment of persistent allergic rhinitis regarding to symptom severity, J. Med. Assoc. Thail. 93 (2) (2010) 215–223.

[126] M.M. Kelly, T.M. O'Connor, R. Leigh, J. Otis, C. Gwozd, G.M. Gauvreau, J. Gauldie, P.M. O'Byrne, Effects of budesonide and formoterol on allergen-induced airway responses, inflammation, and airway remodeling in asthma, J. Allergy Clin. Immunol. 125 (2) (2010) 349–356.e13.

[127] J. Vestbo, L. Tan, G. Atkinson, J. Ward, UK-500,001 Global Study Team, A controlled trial of 6-weeks' treatment with a novel inhaled phosphodiesterasetype-4 inhibitor in COPD, Eur. Respir. J. 33 (5) (2009) 1039–1044.

[128] A. Gillissen, A. Richter, H. Oster, Clinical efficacy of short-term treatment with extra-fine HFA beclomethasone dipropionate in patients with post-infectious persistent cough, J. Physiol. Pharmacol. 58 (Suppl. 5(Pt 1)) (2007) 223–232.

[129] S. Bellodi, M.A. Tosca, G. Pulvirenti, L. Petecchia, L. Serpero, M. Silvestri, F. Sabatini, E. Battistini, G.A. Rossi, Activity of budesonide on nasal neutrophilic inflammation and obstruction in children with recurrent upper airway infections. A preliminary investigation, Int. J. Pediatr. Otorhinolaryngol. 70 (3) (2006) 445–452.

[130] H. Hauber, R. Taha, C. Bergeron, V. Migounov, Q. Hamid, R. Olivenstein, Effects of hydrofluoroalkane and dry powder-formulated corticosteroids on sputum inflammatory markers in asthmatic patients, Can. Respir. J. 13 (2) (2006) 73–78.

[131] M. Sánchez-Borges, F. Caballero-Fonseca, A. Capriles-Hulett, Tolerance of nonsteroidal anti-inflammatory drug-sensitive patients to the highly specific cyclooxygenase 2 inhibitors rofecoxib and valdecoxib, Ann. Allergy Asthma Immunol. 94 (1) (2005) 34–38.

[132] M.A. Dugas, D. Nguyen, L. Frenette, C. Lachance, O. St-Onge, A. Fougères, S. Bélanger, G. Caouette, E. Proulx, M.C. Racine, B. Piedboeuf, Fluticasone inhalation in moderate cases of bronchopulmonary dysplasia, Pediatrics 115 (5) (2005) e566–e572.

[133] E. Nettis, M.C. Colanardi, A. Ferrannini, A. Vacca, A. Tursi, Short-term tolerability of etoricoxib in patients with cutaneous hypersensitivity reactions to nonsteroidal anti-inflammatory drugs, Ann. Allergy Asthma Immunol. 95 (5) (2005) 438–442.

[134] P. Niphadkar, K. Jagannath, J.M. Joshi, N. Awad, H. Boss, S. Hellbardt, D.A. Gadgil, Comparison of the efficacy of ciclesonide 160 microg QD and budesonide 200 microg BID in adults with persistent asthma: a phase III, randomized, double-dummy, open-label study, Clin. Ther. 27 (11) (2005) 1752–1763.

[135] E.M. Erin, B.R. Leaker, A.S. Zacharasiewicz, L.A. Higgins, T.J. Williams, M.J. Boyce, P. de Boer, S.R. Durham, P.J. Barnes, T.T. Hansel, Single dose topical corticosteroid inhibits IL-5 and IL-13 in nasal lavage following grass pollen challenge, Allergy 60 (12) (2005) 1524–1529.

[136] Y. Nuhoglu, E. Atas, C. Nuhoglu, M. Iscan, S. Ozcay, Acute effect of nebulized budesonide in asthmatic children, J. Investig. Allergol. Clin. Immunol. 15 (3) (2005) 197–200.

[137] L.M. van den Toorn, J.B. Prins, J.C. de Jongste, K. Leman, P.G. Mulder, H.C. Hoogsteden, S.E. Overbeek, Benefit from anti-inflammatory treatment during clinical remission of atopic asthma, Respir. Med. 99 (6) (2005) 779–787.

[138] A. Azuma, T. Nukiwa, E. Tsuboi, M. Suga, S. Abe, K. Nakata, Y. Taguchi, S. Nagai, H. Itoh, M. Ohi, A. Sato, S. Kudoh, Double-blind, placebo-controlled trial of pirfenidone in patients with idiopathic pulmonary fibrosis, Am. J. Respir. Crit. Care Med. 171 (9) (2005) 1040–1047.

[139] B.P. Ponsioen, W.C. Hop, N.A. Vermue, P.N. Dekhuijzen, A.M. Bohnen, Efficacy of fluticasone on cough: a randomised controlled trial, Eur. Respir. J. 25 (1) (2005) 147–152.

[140] M. Sánchez-Borges, F. Caballero-Fonseca, A. Capriles-Hulett, Safety of etoricoxib, a new cyclooxygenase 2 inhibitor, in patients with nonsteroidal anti-inflammatory drug-induced urticaria and angioedema, Ann. Allergy Asthma Immunol. 95 (2) (2005) 154–158.

[141] T. Hirata, E. Ogawa, K. Takenaka, F. Kawashita, Suppression of postoperative systemic inflammatory response syndrome with clarithromycin following lung cancer surgery, Eur. Surg. Res. 36 (1) (2004) 13–19.

[142] C. Micheletto, S. Tognella, M. Visconti, C. Pomari, F. Trevisan, R.W. Dal Negro, Montelukast 10 mg improves nasal function and nasal response to aspirin in ASA-sensitive asthmatics: a controlled study vs placebo, Allergy 59 (3) (2004) 289–294.

[143] D.S. Pearlman, D. Peden, J.J. Condemi, S. Weinstein, M. White, L. Baitinger, C. Scott, S.Y. Ho, K. House, P. Dorinsky, Efficacy and safety of fluticasone propionate/salmeterol HFA 134A MDI in patients with mild-to-moderate persistent asthma, J. Asthma 41 (8) (2004) 797–806.

[144] H. Patel, S. Gouin, R.W. Platt, Randomized, double-blind, placebo-controlled trial of oral albuterol in infants with mild-to-moderate acute viral bronchiolitis, J. Pediatr. 142 (5) (2003) 509–514.

[145] P. Kuna, J.R. Joubert, L.A. Greefhorst, H. Magnussen, A randomized, double-blind, double-dummy, parallel-group, multicenter, dose-reduction trial of the minimal effective doses of budesonide and fluticasone dry-powder inhalers in adults with mild to moderate asthma, Clin. Ther. 25 (8) (2003) 2182–2197.

[146] G. Ciprandi, C. Cosentino, M. Milanese, M.A. Tosca, Rapid anti-inflammatory action of azelastine eyedrops for ongoing allergic reactions, Ann. Allergy Asthma Immunol. 90 (4) (2003) 434–438.

[147] R. Leigh, D. Vethanayagam, M. Yoshida, R.M. Watson, T. Rerecich, M.D. Inman, P.M. O'Byrne, Effects of montelukast and budesonide on airway responses and airway inflammation in asthma, Am. J. Respir. Crit. Care Med. 166 (9) (2002) 1212–1217.

[148] C.H. Banov, P. Lieberman, Vasomotor Rhinitis Study Groups, Efficacy of azelastine nasal spray in the treatment of vasomotor (perennial nonallergic) rhinitis, Ann. Allergy Asthma Immunol. 86 (1) (2001) 28–35.

[149] G.T. Verhoeven, I.M. Garrelds, H.C. Hoogsteden, F.J. Zijlstra, Effects of fluticasone propionate inhalation on levels of arachidonic acid metabolites in patients with chronic obstructive pulmonary disease, Mediat. Inflamm. 10 (1) (2001) 21–26.

[150] R.F. Lemanske Jr., C.A. Sorkness, E.A. Mauger, S.C. Lazarus, H.A. Boushey, J.V. Fahy, J.M. Drazen, V.M. Chinchilli, T. Craig, J.E. Fish, J.G. Ford, E. Israel, M. Kraft, R.J. Martin, S.A. Nachman, S.P. Peters, J.D. Spahn, S.J. Szefler, Asthma Clinical Research Network for the National Heart, Lung, and Blood Institute, Inhaled corticosteroid reduction and elimination in patients with persistent asthma receiving salmeterol: a randomized controlled trial, JAMA 285 (20) (2001) 2594–2603.

[151] E.A. Kelly, W.W. Busse, N.N. Jarjour, Inhaled budesonide decreases airway inflammatory response to allergen, Am. J. Respir. Crit. Care Med. 162 (3 Pt 1) (2000) 883–890.

[152] D. Argenti, B. Shah, D. Heald, A study comparing the clinical pharmacokinetics, pharmacodynamics, and tolerability of triamcinolone acetonide HFA-134a metered-dose inhaler and budesonide dry-powder inhaler following inhalation administration, J. Clin. Pharmacol. 40 (5) (2000) 516–526.

[153] J.A. Abisheganaden, P.C. Avila, J.L. Kishiyama, J. Liu, S. Yagi, D. Schnurr, H.A. Boushey, Effect of clarithromycin on experimental rhinovirus-16 colds: a randomized, double-blind, controlled trial, Am. J. Med. 108 (6) (2000) 453–459.

[154] L.H. Kircik, Anti-inflammatory dose doxycycline plus adapalene 0.3% and benzoyl peroxide 2.5% gel for severe acne, J. Drugs Dermatol. 18 (9) (2019) 924–927.

[155] B. Dréno, R. Bissonnette, A. Gagné-Henley, B. Barankin, C. Lynde, R. Chavda, N. Kerrouche, J. Tan, Long-term effectiveness and safety of up to 48 weeks' treatment with topical adapalene 0.3%/benzoyl peroxide 2.5% gel in the prevention and reduction of atrophic acne scars in moderate and severe facial acne, Am. J. Clin. Dermatol. 20 (5) (2019) 725–732.

[156] M. Böhm, J. Ehrchen, T.A. Luger, Beneficial effects of the melanocortin analogue Nle4-D-Phe7-α-MSH in acne vulgaris, J. Eur. Acad. Dermatol. Venereol. 28 (1) (2014) 108–111.

[157] N. Hayashi, M. Kawashima, Multicenter randomized controlled trial on combination therapy with 0.1% adapalene gel and oral antibiotics for acne vulgaris: comparison of the efficacy of adapalene gel alone and in combination with oral faropenem, J. Dermatol. 39 (6) (2012) 511–515.

[158] E. Tanghetti, S. Dhawan, L. Green, M. Ling, J. Downie, M.A. Germain, J.S. Kasteler, L. Kircik, M.G. Oefelein, Z. Draelos, Clinical evidence for the role of a topical anti-inflammatory agent in comedonal acne: findings from a randomized study of dapsone gel 5% in combination with tazarotene cream 0.1% in patients with acne vulgaris, J. Drugs Dermatol. 10 (7) (2011) 783–792.

[159] H.C. Ko, M. Song, S.H. Seo, C.K. Oh, K.S. Kwon, M.B. Kim, Prospective, open-label, comparative study of clindamycin 1%/benzoyl peroxide 5% gel with adapalene 0.1% gel in Asian acne patients: efficacy and tolerability, J. Eur. Acad. Dermatol. Venereol. 23 (3) (2009) 245–250.

[160] J.J. Leyden, M. Wortzman, A novel gel formulation of clindamycin phosphate-tretinoin is not associated with acne flaring, Cutis 82 (2) (2008) 151–156.

[161] J. Marcinkiewicz, A. Wojas-Pelc, M. Walczewska, S. Lipko-Godlewska, R. Jachowicz, A. Maciejewska, A. Białecka, A. Kasprowicz, Topical taurine bromamine, a new candidate in the treatment of moderate inflammatory acne vulgaris: a pilot study, Eur. J. Dermatol. 18 (4) (2008) 433–439.

[162] J.R. Antonio, J.R. Pegas, T.F. Cestari, L.V. Do Nascimento, Azithromycin pulses in the treatment of inflammatory and pustular acne: efficacy, tolerability and safety, J. Dermatol. Treat. 19 (4) (2008) 210–215.

[163] K. Reich, P. Rich, C. Maari, R. Bissonnette, C. Leonardi, A. Menter, A. Igarashi, P. Klekotka, D. Patel, J. Li, J. Tuttle, M. Morgan-Cox, E. Edson-Heredia, S. Friedrich, K. Papp, AMAF Investigators, Efficacy and safety of mirikizumab (LY3074828) in the treatment of moderate-to-severe plaque psoriasis: results from a randomized phase II study, Br. J. Dermatol. 181 (1) (2019) 88–95.

[164] N. Bhatia, L. Stein Gold, L.H. Kircik, R. Schreiber, Two multicenter, randomized, double-blind, parallel group comparison studies of a novel foam formulation of halobetasol propionate, 0.05% vs its vehicle in adult subjects with plaque psoriasis, J. Drugs Dermatol. 18 (8) (2019) 790–796.

[165] T. Werfel, G. Layton, M. Yeadon, L. Whitlock, I. Osterloh, P. Jimenez, W. Liu, V. Lynch, A. Asher, A. Tsianakas, L. Purkins, Efficacy and safety of the histamine H_4 receptor antagonist ZPL-3893787 in patients with atopic dermatitis, J. Allergy Clin. Immunol. 143 (5) (2019) 1830–1837.e4.

[166] R. Vives, C. Pontes, M. Sarasa, A. Millier, Safety and activity of UR-1505 in atopic dermatitis: a randomized, double-blind phase II exploratory trial, Clin. Ther. 37 (9) (2015) 1955–1965.

[167] R. Bissonnette, Y. Poulin, Y. Zhou, J. Tan, H.C. Hong, J. Webster, W. Ip, L. Tang, M. Lyle, Efficacy and safety of topical WBI-1001 in patients with mild to severe atopic dermatitis: results from a 12-week, multicentre, randomized, placebo-controlled double-blind trial, Br. J. Dermatol. 166 (4) (2012) 853–860.

[168] M. David, L. Akerman, M. Ziv, M. Kadurina, D. Gospodinov, F. Pavlotsky, R. Yankova, V. Kouzeva, M. Ramon, M.H. Silverman, P. Fishman, Treatment of plaque-type psoriasis with oral CF101: data from an exploratory randomized phase 2 clinical trial, J. Eur. Acad. Dermatol. Venereol. 26 (3) (2012) 361–367.

[169] E. Gallup, T. Plott, Ciclopirox TS Investigators, A multicenter, open-label study to assess the safety and efficacy of ciclopirox topical suspension 0.77% in the treatment of diaper dermatitis due to *Candida albicans*, J. Drugs Dermatol. 4 (1) (2005) 29–34.

[170] S. Reitamo, J. Harper, J.D. Bos, F. Cambazard, C. Bruijnzeel-Koomen, P. Valk, C. Smith, C. Moss, A. Dobozy, R. Palatsi, European Tacrolimus Ointment Group, 0.03% Tacrolimus ointment applied once or twice daily is more efficacious than 1%hydrocortisone acetate in children with moderate to severe atopic dermatitis: results of a randomized double-blind controlled trial, Br. J. Dermatol. 150 (3) (2004) 554–562.

[171] J. Magnette, J.L. Kienzler, I. Alekxandrova, E. Savaluny, A. Khemis, S. Amal, M. Trabelsi, J.P. Césarini, The efficacy and safety of low-dose diclofenac sodium 0.1% gel for the symptomatic relief of pain and erythema associated with superficial natural sunburn, Eur. J. Dermatol. 14 (4) (2004) 238–246.

[172] M. Milani, S.A. Di Molfetta, R. Gramazio, C. Fiorella, C. Frisario, E. Fuzio, V. Marzocca, M. Zurilli, G. Di Turi, G. Felice, Efficacy of betamethasone valerate 0.1% thermophobic foam in seborrhoeic dermatitis of the scalp: an open-label, multicentre, prospective trial on 180 patients, Curr. Med. Res. Opin. 19 (4) (2003) 342–345.

[173] L. Green, W. Sadoff, A clinical evaluation of tazarotene 0.1% gel, with and without a high- or mid-high-potency corticosteroid, in patients with stable plaque psoriasis, J. Cutan. Med. Surg. 6 (2) (2002) 95–102.

[174] M.G. Lebwohl, M.H. Tan, S.L. Meador, G. Singer, Limited application of fluticasone propionate ointment, 0.005% in patients with psoriasis of the face and intertriginous areas, J. Am. Acad. Dermatol. 44 (1) (2001) 77–82.

[175] A. Parneix-Spake, P. Goustas, R. Green, Eumovate (clobetasone butyrate) 0.05% cream with its moisturizing emollient base has better healing properties than hydrocortisone 1% cream: a study in nickel-induced contact dermatitis, J. Dermatol. Treat. 12 (4) (2001) 191–197.

[176] C. Queille-Roussel, C. Paul, L. Duteil, M.C. Lefebvre, G. Rapatz, M. Zagula, J.P. Ortonne, The new topical ascomycin derivative SDZ ASM 981 does not induce skin atrophy when applied to normal skin for 4 weeks: a randomized, double-blind controlled study, Br. J. Dermatol. 144 (3) (2001) 507–513.

[177] M. James, A randomized, double-blind, multicenter trial comparing fluticasone propionate cream, 0.05%, and hydrocortisone-17-butyrate cream, 0.1%, applied twice daily for 4 weeks in the treatment of psoriasis, Cutis 67 (4 Suppl) (2001) 2–9.

[178] V. Nguyen, Y.W. Chen, J.D. Johnson, A. Paranjpe, In vivo evaluation of effect of preoperative ibuprofen on proinflammatory mediators in irreversible pulpitis cases, J. Endodont. 46 (9) (2020) 1210–1216.

[179] N.S. Kumar, G. Muktesh, T. Samra, P. Sarma, J. Samanta, S.K. Sinha, N. Dhaka, T.D. Yadav, V. Gupta, R. Kochhar, Comparison of efficacy of diclofenac and tramadol in relieving pain in patients of acute pancreatitis: a randomized parallel group double blind active controlled pilot study, Eur. J. Pain 24 (3) (2020) 639–648.

[180] B.W. Friedman, E. Irizarry, A. Chertoff, C. Feliciano, C. Solorzano, E. Zias, E.J. Gallagher, Ibuprofen plus acetaminophen versus ibuprofen alone for acute low Back pain: an emergency department–based randomized study, Acad. Emerg. Med. 27 (3) (2020) 229–235.

[181] J. Lajoie, L. Mwangi, K.R. Fowke, Preventing HIV infection without targeting the virus: how reducing HIV target cells at the genital tract is a new approach to HIV prevention, AIDS Res. Ther. 14 (1) (2017) 1–5.

[182] A. Kronenberg, L. Bütikofer, A. Odutayo, K. Mühlemann, B.R. da Costa, M. Battaglia, D.N. Meli, P. Frey, A. Limacher, S. Reichenbach, P. Jüni, Symptomatic treatment of uncomplicated lower urinary tract infections in the ambulatory setting: randomised, double blind trial, Br. Med. J. 359 (2017).

[183] E.S. Dellon, D.A. Katzka, M.H. Collins, M. Hamdani, S.K. Gupta, I. Hirano, A. Kagalwalla, J. Lewis, J. Markowitz, S. Nurko, J. Wo, Budesonide oral suspension improves symptomatic, endoscopic, and histologic parameters compared with placebo in patients with eosinophilic esophagitis, Gastroenterology 152 (4) (2017) 776–786.

[184] O. Köhler-Forsberg, L. Sylvia, M. Thase, J.R. Calabrese, T. Deckersbach, M. Tohen, C.L. Bowden, M. McInnis, J.H. Kocsis, E.S. Friedman, T.A. Ketter, Nonsteroidal anti-inflammatory drugs (NSAIDs) and paracetamol do not affect 6-month mood-stabilizing treatment outcome among 482 patients with bipolar disorder, Depress. Anxiety 34 (3) (2017) 281–290.

[185] T. Nonaka, M. Hara, C. Miyamoto, M. Sugita, T. Yamamoto, Comparison of the analgesic effect of intravenous acetaminophen with that of flurbiprofen axetil on post-breast surgery pain: a randomized controlled trial, J. Anesth. 30 (3) (2016) 405–409.

[186] M.A. Shirvani, N. Motahari-Tabari, A. Alipour, The effect of mefenamic acid and ginger on pain relief in primary dysmenorrhea: a randomized clinical trial, Arch. Gynecol. Obstet. 291 (6) (2015) 1277–1281.

[187] T. Kondo, T. Oshima, T. Tomita, H. Fukui, H. Okada, J. Watari, H. Miwa, The nonsteroidal anti-inflammatory drug diclofenac reduces acid-induced heartburn symptoms in healthy volunteers, Clin. Gastroenterol. Hepatol. 13 (7) (2015) 1249–1255.

[188] F. Faghihzadeh, P. Adibi, R. Rafiei, A. Hekmatdoost, Resveratrol supplementation improves inflammatory biomarkers in patients with nonalcoholic fatty liver disease, Nutr. Res. 34 (10) (2014) 837–843.

[189] S.A. Helmy, H.M. El-Bedaiwy, Piroxicam immediate release formulations: a fasting randomized open-label crossover bioequivalence study in healthy volunteers, Clin. Pharmacol. Drug Dev. 3 (6) (2014) 466–471.

[190] N.T. Funderburg, Y. Jiang, S.M. Debanne, N. Storer, D. Labbato, B. Clagett, J. Robinson, M.M. Lederman, G.A. McComsey, Rosuvastatin treatment reduces markers of monocyte activation in HIV-infected subjects on antiretroviral therapy, Clin. Infect. Dis. 58 (4) (2014) 588–595.

[191] R. Imberti, S. De Gregori, L. Lisi, P. Navarra, Influence of the oral dissolution time on the absorption rate of locally administered solid formulations for oromucosal use: the flurbiprofen lozenges paradigm, Pharmacology 94 (3–4) (2014) 143–147.

[192] A. Gharekhani, M.R. Khatami, S. Dashti-Khavidaki, E. Razeghi, A. A. Noorbala, S.S. Hashemi-Nazari, M.A. Mansournia, The effect of omega-3 fatty acids on depressive symptoms and inflammatory markers in maintenance hemodialysis patients: a randomized, placebo-controlled clinical trial, Eur. J. Clin. Pharmacol. 70 (6) (2014) 655–665.

[193] Y. Nakamura, M. Tsuji, H. Hasegawa, K. Kimura, K. Fujita, M. Inoue, T. Shimizu, H. Gotoh, Y. Goto, M. Inagaki, K. Oguchi, Anti-inflammatory effects of linagliptin in hemodialysis patients with diabetes, Hemodial. Int. 18 (2) (2014) 433–442.

[194] J. Sloan-Lancaster, E. Abu-Raddad, J. Polzer, J.W. Miller, J.C. Scherer, A. De Gaetano, J.K. Berg, W.H. Landschulz, Double-blind, randomized study evaluating the glycemic and anti-inflammatory effects of subcutaneous LY2189102, a neutralizing IL-1β antibody, in patients with type 2 diabetes, Diabetes Care 36 (8) (2013) 2239–2246.

[195] A.M. Cueto-Manzano, J.R. Ángel-Zúñiga, G. Ornelas-Carrillo, E. - Rojas-Campos, H.R. Martínez-Ramírez, L. Cortés-Sanabria, Anti-inflammatory interventions in end-stage kidney disease: a randomized, double-blinded, controlled and crossover clinical trial on the use of pravastatin in continuous ambulatory peritoneal dialysis, Arch. Med. Res. 44 (8) (2013) 633–637.

[196] C. Madeddu, M. Dessì, F. Panzone, R. Serpe, G. Antoni, M.C. Cau, L. Montaldo, Q. Mela, M. Mura, G. Astara, F.M. Tanca, Randomized phase III clinical trial of a combined treatment with carnitine+ celecoxib±megestrol acetate for patients with cancer-related anorexia/cachexia syndrome, Clin. Nutr. 31 (2) (2012) 176–182.

[197] R. Krysiak, W. Zmuda, B. Okopien, The effect of ezetimibe, administered alone or in combination with simvastatin, on lymphocyte cytokine release in patients with elevated cholesterol levels, J. Intern. Med. 271 (1) (2012) 32–42.

[198] H. Krum, G. Swergold, A. Gammaitoni, P.M. Peloso, S.S. Smugar, S.P. Curtis, D.C. Brater, H. Wang, A. Kaur, L. Laine, M.R. Weir, Blood pressure and cardiovascular outcomes in patients taking nonsteroidal antiinflammatory drugs, Cardiovasc. Ther. 30 (6) (2012) 342–350.

[199] A. Chaudhuri, H. Ghanim, M. Vora, C.L. Sia, K. Korzeniewski, S. Dhindsa, A. Makdissi, P. Dandona, Exenatide exerts a potent antiinflammatory effect, J. Clin. Endocrinol. Metab. 97 (1) (2012) 198–207.

[200] M. Saito, K. Yoshida, W. Saito, A. Fujiya, K. Ohgami, N. Kitaichi, H. Tsukahara, Ishida, S. Ohno, Astaxanthin increases choroidal blood flow velocity, Graefes Arch. Clin. Exp. Ophthalmol. 250 (2) (2012) 239–245.

[201] C. Skarke, N. Alamuddin, J.A. Lawson, L. Cen, K.J. Propert, G.A. Fitzgerald, Comparative impact on prostanoid biosynthesis of celecoxib and the novel nonsteroidal anti-inflammatory drug CG100649, Clin. Pharmacol. Ther. 91 (6) (2012) 986–993.

[202] L. Laine, A.J. Kivitz, A.E. Bello, A.Y. Grahn, M.H. Schiff, A.S. Taha, Double-blind randomized trials of single-tablet ibuprofen/high-dose famotidine vs. ibuprofen alone for reduction of gastric and duodenal ulcers, Am. J. Gastroenterol. 107 (3) (2012) 379.

[203] E. Cevik, O. Cinar, N. Salman, A. Bayir, I. Arziman, S. Ardic, S.T. Youngquist, Comparing the efficacy of intravenous tenoxicam, lornoxicam, and dexketoprofen trometamol for the treatment of renal colic, Am. J. Emerg. Med. 30 (8) (2012) 1486–1490.

[204] S.W. Rathbun, C.E. Aston, T.L. Whitsett, A randomized trial of dalteparin compared with ibuprofen for the treatment of superficial thrombophlebitis, J. Thromb. Haemost. 10 (5) (2012) 833–839.

[205] E.J. Toonen, W.W. Fleuren, U. Nässander, M.J.C. Van Lierop, S. Bauerschmidt, W.H. Dokter, W. Alkema, Prednisolone-induced changes in gene-expression profiles in healthy volunteers, Pharmacogenomics 12 (7) (2011) 985–998.

[206] H. Ito, M. Iida, T. Matsumoto, Y. Suzuki, H. Sasaki, T. Yoshida, Y. Takano, T. Hibi, Direct comparison of two different mesalamine formulations for the induction of remission in patients with ulcerative colitis: a double-blind, randomized study, Inflamm. Bowel Dis. 16 (9) (2010) 1567–1574.

[207] G.R. D'Haens, A. Kovacs, P. Vergauwe, F. Nagy, T. Molnar, Y. Bouhnik, W. Weiss, H. Brunner, A. Lavergne-Slove, D. Binelli, A.F.D. Di Stefano, Clinical trial: Preliminary efficacy and safety study of a new Budesonide-MMX® 9 mg extended-release tablets in patients with active left-sided ulcerative colitis, J. Crohn's Colitis 4 (2) (2010) 153–160.

[208] A. Roshani, S. Falahatkar, I. Khosropanah, Z.A. Roshan, T. Zarkami, M. Palizkar, S.A. Emadi, M. Akbarpour, N. Khaki, Assessment of clinical efficacy of intranasal desmopressin spray and diclofenac sodium suppository in treatment of renal colic versus diclofenac sodium alone, Urology 75 (3) (2010) 540–542.

[209] A. Pareek, N.B. Chandurkar, R.T. Patil, S.N. Agrawal, R.B. Uday, S.G. Tambe, Efficacy and safety of aceclofenac and drotaverine fixed-dose combination in the treatment of primary dysmenorrhoea: a double-blind, double-dummy, randomized comparative study with aceclofenac, Eur. J. Obstet. Gynecol. Reprod. Biol. 152 (1) (2010) 86–90.

[210] G.F. Webster, An open-label, community-based, 12-week assessment of the effectiveness and safety of monotherapy with doxycycline 40 mg (30-mg immediate-release and 10-mg delayed-release beads), Cutis 86 (5 Suppl) (2010) 7–15.

[211] M. Lamet, A multicenter, randomized study to evaluate the efficacy and safety of mesalamine suppositories 1 g at bedtime and 500 mg twice daily in patients with active mild-to-moderate ulcerative proctitis, Digest. Dis. Sci. 56 (2) (2011) 513–522.

[212] P.A. Thompson, C.H. Hsu, S. Green, A.T. Stopeck, K. Johnson, D.S. Alberts, H.S. Chow, Sulindac and sulindac metabolites in nipple aspirate fluid and effect on drug targets in a phase I trial, Cancer Prev. Res. 3 (1) (2010) 101–107.

[213] W. Caumo, R. Levandovski, M.P.L. Hidalgo, Preoperative anxiolytic effect of melatonin and clonidine on postoperative pain and morphine consumption in patients undergoing abdominal hysterectomy: a double-blind, randomized, placebo-controlled study, J. Pain 10 (1) (2009) 100–108.

[214] E.I. Akural, V. Järvimäki, A. Länsineva, A. Niinimaa, S. Alahuhta, Effects of combination treatment with ketoprofen 100 mg+ acetaminophen 1000 mg on postoperative dental pain: a single-dose, 10-hour, randomized, double-blind, active-and placebo-controlled clinical trial, Clin. Ther. 31 (3) (2009) 560–568.

[215] A. Livshits, R. Machtinger, L.B. David, M. Spira, A. Moshe-Zahav, D.S. Seidman, Ibuprofen and paracetamol for pain relief during medical abortion: a double-blind randomized controlled study, Fertil. Steril. 91 (5) (2009) 1877–1880.

[216] Y. Fujii, M. Itakura, Pretreatment with flurbiprofen axetil, flurbiprofen axetil preceded by venous occlusion, and a mixture of flurbiprofen axetil and propofol in reducing pain on injection of propofol in adult Japanese surgical patients: a prospective, randomized, double-blind, placebo-controlled study, Clin. Ther. 31 (4) (2009) 721–727.

[217] K. Engel, J. Reuter, C. Seiler, J.S. Mönting, T. Jakob, C.M. Schempp, Anti-inflammatory effect of pimecrolimus in the sodium lauryl sulphate test, J. Eur. Acad. Dermatol. Venereol. 22 (4) (2008) 447–450.

[218] T. Gómez-Isla, R. Blesa, M. Boada, J. Clarimón, T. Del Ser, G. Domenech, J.M. Ferro, B. Gómez-Ansón, J.M. Manubens, J. M. Martínez-Lage, D. Muñoz, A randomized, double-blind, placebo controlled-trial of triflusal in mild cognitive impairment: the TRIMCI study, Alzheimer Dis. Assoc. Disord. 22 (1) (2008) 21–29.

[219] J.J. Chieh, A.N. Carlson, G.J. Jaffe, Combined fluocinolone acetonide intraocular delivery system insertion, phacoemulsification, and intraocular lens implantation for severe uveitis, Am. J. Ophthalmol. 146 (4) (2008) 589–594.

[220] Y. Xu, Z. Tan, J. Chen, F. Lou, W. Chen, Intravenous flurbiprofen axetil accelerates restoration of bowel function after colorectal surgery, Can. J. Anesth. 55 (7) (2008) 414–422.

[221] R.L. Sur, G.E. Haleblian, D.A. Cantor, W.P. Springhart, D.M. Albala, G.M. Preminger, Efficacy of intravesical ropivacaine injection on urinary symptoms following ureteral stenting: a randomized, controlled study, J. Endourol. 22 (3) (2008) 473–478.

[222] G.W. Small, P. Siddarth, D.H. Silverman, L.M. Ercoli, K.J. Miller, H. Lavretsky, S.Y. Bookheimer, S.C. Huang, J.R. Barrio, M.E. Phelps, Cognitive and cerebral metabolic effects of celecoxib versus placebo in people with age-related memory loss: randomized controlled study, Am. J. Geriatr. Psychiatry. 16 (12) (2008) 999–1009.

[223] Z.O. Pektas, M. Sener, B. Bayram, T. Eroglu, N. Bozdogan, A. Donmez, G. Arslan, S. Uckan, A comparison of pre-emptive analgesic efficacy of diflunisal and lornoxicam for postoperative pain management: a prospective, randomized, single-blind, crossover study, Int. J. Oral. Maxillofac. Surg. 36 (2) (2007) 123–127.

[224] M. Tugrul Sezer, S. Katirci, M. Demir, J. Erturk, S. Adana, S. Kaya, Short-term effect of simvastatin treatment on inflammatory parameters in peritoneal dialysis patients, Scand. J. Urol. Nephrol. 41 (5) (2007) 436–441.

[225] E. Demir, M. Kilciler, S. Bedir, K. Erten, Y. Ozgok, Comparing two local anesthesia techniques for extracorporeal shock wave lithotripsy, Urology 69 (4) (2007) 625–628.

[226] J.K. Koskenkari, P.K. Kaukoranta, J. Rimpiläinen, V. Vainionpää, P. P. Ohtonen, H.M. Surcel, T. Juvonen, T.I. Ala-Kokko, Anti-inflammatory effect of high-dose insulin treatment after urgent coronary revascularization surgery, Acta Anaesthesiol. Scand. 50 (8) (2006) 962–969.

[227] H.F. Gramke, J.J. Petry, M.E. Durieux, J.P. Mustaki, M. Vercauteren, G. Verheecke, M.A. Marcus, Sublingual piroxicam for postoperative analgesia: preoperative versus postoperative administration: a randomized, double-blind study, Anesth. Analg. 102 (3) (2006) 755–758.

[228] A. Pareek, A.S. Chandanwale, J. Oak, U.K. Jain, S. Kapoor, Efficacy and safety of aceclofenac in the treatment of osteoarthritis: a randomized double-blind comparative clinical trial versus diclofenac–an Indian experience, Curr. Med. Res. Opin. 22 (5) (2006) 977–988.

[229] M.P. Yeager, A.J. Rassias, M.P. Fillinger, A.W. DiScipio, K.E. Gloor, J.A. Gregory, P.M. Guyre, Cortisol antiinflammatory effects are maximal at postoperative plasma concentrations, Crit. Care Med. 33 (7) (2005) 1507–1512.

[230] K.K. Koh, M.J. Quon, S.H. Han, W.J. Chung, Y. Lee, E.K. Shin, Anti-inflammatory and metabolic effects of candesartan in hypertensive patients, Int. J. Cardiol. 108 (1) (2006) 96–100.

[231] S. Hanauer, W.J. Sandborn, A. Persson, T. Persson, Budesonide as maintenance treatment in Crohn's disease: a placebo-controlled trial, Aliment. Pharmacol. Ther. 21 (4) (2005) 363–371.

[232] S.E. Daniels, S. Torri, P.J. Desjardins, Valdecoxib for treatment of primary dysmenorrhea, J. Gen. Intern. Med. 20 (1) (2005) 62–67.

[233] B. Cryer, P. Miller, R.A. Petruschke, E. Chen, G.P. Geba, A.E. De Papp, Upper gastrointestinal tolerability of once weekly alendronate 70 mg with concomitant non-steroidal anti-inflammatory drug use, Aliment. Pharmacol. Ther. 21 (5) (2005) 599–607.

[234] S. Chalini, U. Raman, Comparative efficacy of aceclofenac and etoricoxib in post extraction pain control: randomized control trial, Indian J. Dent. Res. 16 (2) (2005) 47–50.

[235] F. Facchinetti, M.L. Casini, L. Costabile, B. Malavasi, V. Unfer, Diclofenac pyrrolidine versus Ketoprofen for the relief of pain from episiotomy: a randomized controlled trial, Acta Obstet. Gynecol. Scand. 84 (10) (2005) 951–955.

[236] A. Undas, M. Celinska-Löwenhoff, T.B. Domagala, T. Iwaniec, J. Dropinski, T. Löwenhoff, A. Szczeklik, Early antithrombotic and anti-inflammatory effects of simvastatin versus fenofibrate in patients with hypercholesterolemia, Thromb. Haemost. 94 (07) (2005) 193–199.

[237] L.J. Litkowski, S.E. Christensen, D.N. Adamson, T. Van Dyke, S.H. Han, K.B. Newman, Analgesic efficacy and tolerability of oxycodone 5 mg/ibuprofen400 mg compared with those of oxycodone 5 mg/acetaminophen 325 mg and hydrocodone 7.5 mg/acetaminophen 500 mg in patients with moderate to severe postoperative pain: a randomized, double-blind, placebo-controlled, single-dose, parallel-group study in a dental pain model, Clin. Ther. 27 (4) (2005) 418–429.

[238] F. Graziani, L. Corsi, M. Fornai, L. Antonioli, M. Tonelli, S. Cei, R. Colucci, C. Blandizzi, M. Gabriele, M. Del Tacca, Clinical evaluation of piroxicam-FDDF and azithromycin in the prevention of complications associated with impacted lower third molar extraction, Pharmacol. Res. 52 (6) (2005) 485–490.

[239] P. Bias, A. Buchner, B. Klesser, S. Laufer, The gastrointestinal tolerability of the LOX/COX inhibitor, licofelone, is similar to placebo

and superior to naproxen therapy in healthy volunteers: results from a randomized, controlled trial, Am. J. Gastroenterol. 99 (4) (2004) 611–618.

[240] M. Stockler, J. Vardy, A. Pillai, D. Warr, Acetaminophen (paracetamol) improves pain and well-being in people with advanced cancer already receiving a strong opioid regimen: a randomized, double-blind, placebo-controlled cross-over trial, J. Clin. Oncol. 22 (16) (2004) 3389–3394.

[241] T. Ochsenkühn, M. Sackmann, B. Göke, Infliximab for acute, not steroid-refractory ulcerative colitis: a randomized pilot study, Eur. J. Gastroenterol. Hepatol. 16 (11) (2004) 1167–1171.

[242] P. Zacharowski, K. Zacharowski, C. Donnellan, A. Johnston, I. Vojnovic, P. Forte, P. Del Soldato, N. Benjamin, S. O'Byrne, The effects and metabolic fate of nitroflurbiprofen in healthy volunteers, Clin. Pharmacol. Ther. 76 (4) (2004) 350–358.

[243] A. Armuzzi, B. De Pascalis, A. Lupascu, P. Fedeli, D. Leo, M.C. Mentella, F. Vincenti, D. Melina, G. Gasbarrini, P. Pola, A. Gasbarrini, Infliximab in the treatment of steroid-dependent ulcerative colitis, Eur. Rev. Med. Pharmacol. Sci. 8 (5) (2004) 231–233.

[244] P. Bracco, C. Debernardi, D. Coscia, D. Pasqualini, F. Pasqualicchio, N. Calabrese, Efficacy of rofecoxib and nimesulide in controlling post-extraction pain in oral surgery: a randomised comparative study, Curr. Med. Res. Opin. 20 (1) (2004) 107–112.

[245] T. Araki, T. Yokoyama, H. Kumon, Effectiveness of a nonsteroidal anti-inflammatory drug for nocturia on patients with benign prostatic hyperplasia: a prospective non-randomized study of loxoprofen sodium 60 mg once daily before sleeping, Acta Med. Okayama 58 (1) (2004) 45–49.

[246] V.L. Butty, P. Roux-Lombard, J. Garbino, J.M. Dayer, B. Ricou, Geneva Sepsis Network, Anti-inflammatory response after infusion of p55 soluble tumor necrosis factor receptor fusion protein for severe sepsis, Eur. Cytokine Netw. 14 (1) (2003) 15–19.

[247] T. Colak, T. Ipek, A. Kanik, Z. Ogetman, S. Aydin, Efficacy of topical nonsteroidal antiinflammatory drugs in mastalgia treatment, J. Am. Coll. Surg. 196 (4) (2003) 525–530.

[248] G. Scott, S.A. Osborne, G. Greig, S. Hartmann, M.E. Ebelin, P. Burtin, K. Rappersberger, M. Komar, K. Wolff, Pharmacokinetics of pimecrolimus, a novel nonsteroid anti-inflammatory drug, after single and multiple oral administration, Clin. Pharmacokinet. 42 (14) (2003) 1305–1314.

[249] J.L. Goldstein, A.J. Kivitz, K.M. Verburg, D.P. Recker, R.C. Palmer, J.D. Kent, A comparison of the upper gastrointestinal mucosal effects of valdecoxib, naproxen and placebo in healthy elderly subjects, Aliment. Pharmacol. Ther. 18 (1) (2003) 125–132.

[250] C.J. Hawkey, J.I. Jones, C.T. Atherton, M.M. Skelly, J.R. Bebb, U. Fagerholm, B. Jonzon, P. Karlsson, I.T. Bjarnason, Gastrointestinal safety of AZD3582, a cyclooxygenase inhibiting nitric oxide donor: proof of concept study in humans, Gut 52 (11) (2003) 1537–1542.

[251] J.R. de Berrazueta, I. Sampedro, M.T. Garcia-Unzueta, J. Llorca, M. Bustamante, J.A. Amado, Effect of transdermal nitroglycerin on inflammatory mediators in patients with peripheral atherosclerotic vascular disease, Am. Heart J. 146 (4) (2003) 746.

[252] E.A.B. Cameron, J.A.H. Binnie, K. Balan, S.A. Skerratt, A. Swift, C. Solanki, S.J. Middleton, Oral prednisolone metasulphobenzoate in the treatment of active ulcerative colitis, Scand. J. Gastroenterol. 38 (5) (2003) 535–537.

[253] P.J. Angle, S.H. Halpern, B.L. Leighton, J.P. Szalai, K. Gnanendran, J.E. Kronberg, A randomized controlled trial examining the effect of naproxen on analgesia during the second day after cesarean delivery, Anesth. Analg. 95 (3) (2002) 741–745.

[254] E. Nettis, R. Di Paola, G. Napoli, A. Ferrannini, A. Tursi, Benzydamine: an alternative nonsteroidal anti-inflammatory drug in patients with nimesulide-induced urticaria, Allergy 57 (5) (2002) 442–445.

[255] S.M. Gordon, J.S. Brahim, J. Rowan, A. Kent, R.A. Dionne, Peripheral prostanoid levels and nonsteroidal anti-inflammatory drug analgesia: replicate clinical trials in a tissue injury model, Clin. Pharmacol. Ther. 72 (2) (2002) 175–183.

[256] P.S. Aisen, J. Schmeidler, G.M. Pasinetti, Randomized pilot study of nimesulide treatment in Alzheimer's disease, Neurology 58 (7) (2002) 1050–1054.

[257] D.J.W. Van Kraaij, A.H.I. Hovestad-Witterland, De Metz, E.J. Vollaard, A comparison of the effects of nabumetone vs meloxicam on serum thromboxane B2 and platelet function in healthy volunteers, Br. J. Clin. Pharmacol. 53 (6) (2002) 644–647.

[258] Y.C. Huang, S.K. Tsai, C.H. Huang, M.H. Wang, P.L. Lin, L.K. Chen, C.J. Lin, W.Z. Sun, Intravenous tenoxicam reduces uterine cramps after Cesarean delivery, Can. J. Anesth. 49 (4) (2002) 384–387.

[259] D. Gijwani, M.R. Kumhar, V.B. Singh, V.S. Chadda, P.K. Soni, K.C. Nayak, B.K. Gupta, Dexamethasone therapy for bacterial meningitis in adults: a double blind placebo control study, Neurol. India 50 (1) (2002) 63.

[260] F. Facchinetti, L. Sgarbi, F. Piccinini, A. Volpe, A comparison of glyceryl trinitrate with diclofenac for the treatment of primary dysmenorrhea: an open, randomized, cross-over trial, Gynecol. Endocrinol. 16 (1) (2002) 39–43.

[261] D.K. Suresh, K.L. Vandana, D.S. Mehta, Intracrevicular application of 0.3% Flurbiprofen gel and 0.3% Triclosan gel as anti inflammatory agent. A comparative clinical study, Indian J. Dent. Res 12 (2) (2001) 105–112.

[262] M. Cushman, J.P. Costantino, R.P. Tracy, K. Song, L. Buckley, J.D. Roberts, D.N. Krag, Tamoxifen and cardiac risk factors in healthy women: suggestion of an anti-inflammatory effect, Arterioscler. Thromb. Vasc. Biol. 21 (2) (2001) 255–261.

[263] P.S. Aisen, D.B. Marin, A.M. Brickman, J. Santoro, M. Fusco, Pilot tolerability studies of hydroxychloroquine and colchicine in Alzheimer disease, Alzheimer Dis. Assoc. Disord. 15 (2) (2001) 96–101.

[264] M.A. Albert, E. Danielson, N. Rifai, P.M. Ridker, Prince Investigators, PRINCE Investigators, Effect of statin therapy on C-reactive protein levels: the pravastatin inflammation/CRP evaluation (PRINCE): a randomized trial and cohort study, JAMA 286 (1) (2001) 64–70.

[265] N. Kotani, T. Kushikata, H. Hashimoto, F. Kimura, M. Muraoka, M. Yodono, M. Asai, A. Matsuki, Intrathecal methylprednisolone for intractable postherpetic neuralgia, New Engl. J. Med. 343 (21) (2000) 1514–1519.

[266] R.R. Azar, S. Rinfret, P. Theroux, P.H. Stone, R. Dakshinamurthy, Y.J. Feng, A.H.B. Wu, G. Rangé, D.D. Waters, A randomized placebo-controlled trial to assess the efficacy of antiinflammatory therapy with methylprednisolone in unstable angina (MUNA trial), Eur. Heart J. 21 (24) (2000) 2026–2032.

[267] R.A. Bronicki, C.L. Backer, H.P. Baden, C. Mavroudis, S.E. Crawford, T.P. Green, Dexamethasone reduces the inflammatory

response to cardiopulmonary bypass in children, Ann. Thoracic Surg. 69 (5) (2000) 1490–1495.

[268] R.H. Hunt, B. Bowen, E.R. Mortensen, T.J. Simon, C. James, A. Cagliola, H. Quan, J.A. Bolognese, A randomized trial measuring fecal blood loss after treatment with rofecoxib, ibuprofen, or placebo in healthy subjects, Am. J. Med. 109 (3) (2000) 201–206.

[269] J. Pokrotnieks, K. Marlicz, L. Paradowski, B. Margus, P. Zaborowski, R. Greinwald, Efficacy and tolerability of mesalazine foam enema (Salofalk foam) for distal ulcerative colitis: a double-blind, randomized, placebo-controlled study, Aliment. Pharmacol. Ther. 14 (9) (2000) 1191–1198.

[270] S. Ilkjaer, P.A. Nielsen, L.F. Bach, M. Wernberg, J.B. Dahl, The effect of dextromethorphan, alone or in combination with ibuprofen, on postoperative pain after minor gynaecological surgery, Acta Anaesthesiol. Scand. 44 (7) (2000) 873–877.

[271] M.T. Donnelly, A.F. Goddard, B. Filipowicz, S.V. Morant, M.J. Shield, C.J. Hawkey, Low-dose misoprostol for the prevention of low-dose aspirin-induced gastroduodenal injury, Aliment. Pharmacol. Ther. 14 (5) (2000) 529–534.

[272] I. Gilron, M.B. Max, G. Lee, S.L. Booher, C.N. Sang, A.S. Chappell, R.A. Dionne, Effects of the 2-amino-3-hydroxy-5-methyl-4-isoxazole-proprionic acid/kainate antagonist LY293558 on spontaneous and evoked postoperative pain, Clin. Pharmacol. Ther. 68 (3) (2000) 320–327.

[273] F. Danou, A. Paraskeva, T. Vassilakopoulos, A. Fassoulaki, The analgesic efficacy of intravenous tenoxicam as an adjunct to patient-controlled analgesia in total abdominal hysterectomy, Anesth. Analg. 90 (3) (2000) 672–676.

[274] A. Saeedi-Boroujeni, M.R. Mahmoudian-Sani, R. Nashibi, S. Houshmandfar, S. TahmasebyGandomkari, A. Khodadadi, Tranilast: a potential anti-inflammatory and NLRP3inflammasome inhibitor drug for COVID-19, Immunopharmacol. Immunotoxicol. 43 (3) (2021) 247–258.

[275] M.I. Lopes, L.P. Bonjorno, M.C. Giannini, N.B. Amaral, P.I. Menezes, S.M. Dib, S.L. Gigante, M.N. Benatti, U.C. Rezek, L.L. Emrich-Filho, B.A. Sousa, Beneficial effects of colchicine for moderate to severe COVID-19: a randomised, double-blinded, placebo-controlled clinical trial, RMD Open 7 (1) (2021) e001455.

[276] A.A. Abdelalim, A.A. Mohamady, R.A. Elsayed, M.A. Elawady, A.F. Ghallab, Corticosteroid nasal spray for recovery of smell sensation in COVID-19 patients: a randomized controlled trial, Am. J. Otolaryngol. 42 (2) (2021) 102884.

[277] S. Abd-Elsalam, E.S. Esmail, M. Khalaf, E.F. Abdo, M.A. Medhat, M.S. Abd El Ghafar, O.A. Ahmed, S. Soliman, G.N. Serangawy, M. Alboraie, Hydroxychloroquine in the treatment of COVID-19: a multicenter randomized controlled study, Am. J. Trop. Med. Hyg. 103 (4) (2020) 1635–1639.

[278] M. Edalatifard, M. Akhtari, M. Salehi, Z. Naderi, A. Jamshidi, S. Mostafaei, S.R. Najafizadeh, E. Farhadi, N. Jalili, M. Esfahani, B. Rahimi, H. Kazemzadeh, M. MahmoodiAliabadi, T. Ghazanfari, M. Sattarian, H. Ebrahimi Louyeh, S.R. Raeeskarami, S. Jamalimoghadamsiahkali, N. Khajavirad, M. Mahmoudi, A. Rostamian, Intravenous methylprednisolone pulse as a treatment for hospitalised severe COVID-19 patients: results from a randomised controlled clinical trial, Eur. Respir. J. 56 (6) (2020) 2002808.

[279] S.G. Deftereos, G. Giannopoulos, D.A. Vrachatis, G.D. Siasos, S.G. Giotaki, P. Gargalianos, S. Metallidis, G. Sianos, S. Baltagiannis, P. Panagopoulos, K. Dolianitis, Effect of colchicine vs standard care on cardiac and inflammatory biomarkers and clinical outcomes in patients hospitalized with coronavirus disease 2019: the GRECCO-19 randomized clinical trial, JAMA Netw. Open 3 (6) (2020). e2013136–e2013136.

[280] RECOVERY Collaborative Group, Dexamethasone in hospitalized patients with Covid-19, New Engl. J. Med. 384 (8) (2021) 693–704.

[281] T.S. Hinks, V.S. Barber, J. Black, S.J. Dutton, M. Jabeen, J. Melhorn, N.M. Rahman, D. Richards, D. Lasserson, I.D. Pavord, M. Bafadhel, A multi-centre open-label two-arm randomised superiority clinical trial of azithromycin versus usual care in ambulatory COVID-19: study protocol for the ATOMIC2 trial, Trials 21 (1) (2020) 1–8.

Index

Note: Page numbers followed by *f* indicate figures and *t* indicate tables.